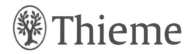

Handbook of Pediatric Neurosurgery

George I. Jallo, MD
Professor of Neurosurgery, Pediatrics and Oncology
Institute for Brain Protection Sciences
Johns Hopkins All Children's Hospital
St. Petersburg, Florida

Karl F. Kothbauer, MD
Associate Professor of Neurosurgery
University of Basel
Basel, Switzerland
Chief of Neurosurgery
Lucerne Cantonal Hospital
Lucerne, Switzerland

Violette M.R. Recinos, MD
Assistant Professor
Department of Neurosurgery
Cleveland Clinic Lerner College of Medicine of Case Western Reserve University
Division of Pediatric Neurosurgery, Cleveland Clinic
Cleveland, Ohio

275 illustrations

Thieme
New York • Stuttgart • Delhi • Rio de Janeiro

Acquisitions Editor: Timothy Hiscock
Managing Editor: Prakash Naorem
Director, Editorial Services: Mary Jo Casey
Production Editor: Shivika
International Production Director: Andreas Schabert
Editorial Director: Sue Hodgson
International Marketing Director: Fiona Henderson
International Sales Director: Louisa Turrell
Senior Vice President and Chief Operating
    Officer: Sarah Vanderbilt
President: Brian D. Scanlan

Library of Congress Cataloging-in-Publication Data

Names: Jallo, George I., editor. | Kothbauer, Karl F., editor. |
    Recinos, Violette M. R., editor.
Title: Handbook of pediatric neurosurgery / [edited by]
    George I. Jallo, Karl F. Kothbauer, Violette M.R. Recinos.
Description: New York : Thieme, [2018] | Includes
    bibliographical references and index.
| Identifiers: LCCN 2018008565 (print) | LCCN 2018009192
    (ebook) | ISBN 9781604068801 | ISBN 9781604068795
    (softcover) | ISBN 9781604068801 (e-book)
Subjects: | MESH: Nervous System Diseases–surgery | Child |
    Infant | Neurosurgical Procedures | Nervous System
    Diseases–diagnostic imaging
Classification: LCC RD593 (ebook) | LCC RD593 (print) | NLM
    WS 340 | DDC 617.4/8–dc23
LC record available at https://lccn.loc.gov/2018008565

© 2018 Thieme Medical Publishers, Inc.
Thieme Publishers New York
333 Seventh Avenue, New York, NY 10001 USA
+1 800 782 3488, customerservice@thieme.com

Thieme Publishers Stuttgart
Rüdigerstrasse 14, 70469 Stuttgart, Germany
+49 [0]711 8931 421, customerservice@thieme.de

Thieme Publishers Delhi
A-12, Second Floor, Sector-2, Noida-201301
Uttar Pradesh, India
+91 120 45 566 00, customerservice@thieme.in

Thieme Publishers Rio de Janeiro
Thieme Publicações Ltda.
Edifício Rodolpho de Paoli, 25º andar
Av. Nilo Peçanha, 50 – Sala 2508
Rio de Janeiro 20020-906 Brasil
+55 21 3172-2297

Cover design: Thieme Publishing Group
Typesetting by Thomson Digital, India

Printed in Germany by CPI books, Leck   5 4 3 2

ISBN 978-1-60406-879-5

Also available as an e-book:
eISBN 978-1-60406-880-1

Important note: Medicine is an ever-changing science undergoing continual development. Research and clinical experience are continually expanding our knowledge, in particular our knowledge of proper treatment and drug therapy. Insofar as this book mentions any dosage or application, readers may rest assured that the authors, editors, and publishers have made every effort to ensure that such references are in accordance with **the state of knowledge at the time of production of the book.**

Nevertheless, this does not involve, imply, or express any guarantee or responsibility on the part of the publishers in respect to any dosage instructions and forms of applications stated in the book. **Every user is requested to examine carefully** the manufacturers' leaflets accompanying each drug and to check, if necessary in consultation with a physician or specialist, whether the dosage schedules mentioned therein or the contraindications stated by the manufacturers differ from the statements made in the present book. Such examination is particularly important with drugs that are either rarely used or have been newly released on the market. Every dosage schedule or every form of application used is entirely at the user's own risk and responsibility. The authors and publishers request every user to report to the publishers any discrepancies or inaccuracies noticed. If errors in this work are found after publication, errata will be posted at www.thieme.com on the product description page.

Some of the product names, patents, and registered designs referred to in this book are in fact registered trademarks or proprietary names even though specific reference to this fact is not always made in the text. Therefore, the appearance of a name without designation as proprietary is not to be construed as a representation by the publisher that it is in the public domain.

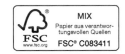

To my children, Maxwell, Nicholas, and Alexis, who have helped shape my career
and interests in pediatric neurosurgery.

George I. Jallo

To my son, Florian, whose talents and dedication fascinate and continue to inspire me.

Karl F. Kothbauer

For Pablo, Elisa, Sebastian, and Nicolas, who are my daily reminders that life is beautiful.

Violette M.R. Recinos

Contents

4 Ultrasonography 28

Thierry A.G.M. Huisman

5 Computed Tomography 32

Thierry A.G.M. Huisman

6 Conventional Magnetic Resonance Imaging. 35

Thierry A.G.M. Huisman

Section V   Cerebrovascular Disorders

Section VI   Developmental and Congenital Cranial Disorders

Section VIII Functional Disorders

51   Management of Pediatric Head Trauma 409
Linda W. Xu, Gerald A. Grant

52   Abusive Head Trauma.. 423
Mark S. Dias

Section X   Infections

53   Evaluation and Management of Pediatric Intracranial Infections 430
Jonathan R. Ellenbogen, Richard P.D. Cooke, Conor L. Mallucci

Foreword

George I. Jallo and his distinguished collaborators have assembled a succinct and practical guide for the field of pediatric neurosurgery, and yet have managed to beautifully cover the depth and breadth of the discipline.

The organization, evenness of coverage, and the consistency bespeak a strong editorial hand.

This book is destined to become a classic reference for those involved in the care of pediatric neurosurgery patients at every level. The greatest beneficiaries of this wonderful text will undoubtedly be the patients for whom we care.

Mark S. Greenberg, MD, FAANS
Associate Professor of Neurosurgery
University of South Florida
Morsani College of Medicine, Tampa, Florida
Author of "Handbook of Neurosurgery"

Foreword

Residents, fellows, and neurosurgeons have for long needed a crisp, condensed, and authoritative book in pediatric neurosurgery. Residents starting in pediatric neurosurgery firms have needed a book to rapidly get an overview of this very broad specialty. The pediatric neurosurgery fellows have required a book to help them master the core knowledge required of them and in revising for board exams. Consultants have required a quick reference to refresh their knowledge, where parents of their patients come to see them having done varying levels of reading off the web. At last, such a book is now available in the form of Dr George I. Jallo's *Handbook of Pediatric Neurosurgery*!

The *Sine qua non* of any handbook is to identify the "trees" and direct the readers for further study. Dr Jallo has assembled international experts to contribute to such an excellent multiauthored manual. Each chapter is a compendium of distilled key concepts, facts, and nuances; the remarkable achievement of this book is that in each chapter, these have been incorporated into a cohesive narrative, aided and abetted by exquisite diagrams and illustrative images, in an immensely appealing way. The book can be read from cover to cover or be dipped into and out of, as desired. At the end of each chapter, the authors have listed relevant references.

Besides his mastery over operative pediatric neurosurgery and prodigious research, Dr Jallo has been at the forefront of pediatric neurosurgical education through training residents and fellows at Johns Hopkins, lectures at courses, invited webinars, internet-based academic conferences, his other previously published highly regarded books, and through co-organizing the International Neurosurgery Resident Course (INRC). This *Handbook of Pediatric Neurosurgery* adds to his already impressive holistic contribution to world-wide pediatric neurosurgical education.

I am confident that like Youman's and Greenberg's, this "Jallo's" will become a neurosurgery classic in its own right. The relevance, lucidity, and beauty of this book, which makes it such a joy to study from, will no doubt garner converts to pediatric neurosurgery—a book that pediatric neurosurgery can be very proud of. More importantly, the *Handbook of Pediatric Neurosurgery* would constantly help all neurosurgeons who care for children to provide better care!

G. 'Naren' Narenthiran, BSc (MedSci) (Hons), MB, ChB, MRCSE, FEBNS, FRCS (SN)
Charing Cross Hospital, London, UK
Penn State University, Hershey, Pennsylvania
Neurosurgery Research Listserv, Southampton, UK

Foreword

"The most valuable of all talents is that of never using two words when one will do."

Thomas Jefferson

This is a no-nonsense, concise, thoughtfully compiled handbook that will serve as an invaluable reference for those interested in pediatric neurosurgery. There is no fluff here, just the facts. And there are lots of facts indeed, ranging from the fundamentals of intracranial pressure monitoring to advanced neuroimaging and state-of-the-art adjuvant therapy for complex brain tumors.

What makes the work unique is its ease of use as a pocket reference about pediatric neurosurgery. It provides the busy reader with on-the-fly rapid access to nuts-and-bolts essentials along with focused details and handy clinical pearls. We owe a debt of gratitude to George I. Jallo and the international group of authors he has assembled for putting together this indispensable resource.

Alan R. Cohen, MD, FACS, FAAP, FAANS
Chief of Pediatric Neurosurgery
Professor of Neurosurgery, Oncology and Pediatrics
Carson-Spiro Professor of Pediatric Neurosurgery
The Johns Hopkins University School of Medicine, Baltimore, Maryland

Preface

Many textbooks have been published focusing on pediatric neurosurgery, and while these texts are available in print or online, they remain inaccessible for the neurosurgery resident or midlevel provider who is on call to manage these children. We have developed this first edition of the handbook to provide a concise and practical text that covers the important aspects of caring for these children. It is comprehensive, readable, and distilled for the pertinent pearls that are important in managing the neurosurgical disease processes that may arise in the hospital, emergency room, or outpatient setting.

This text was not meant to be a comprehensive reference book on pediatric neurosurgery, as many such texts already exist. The strength and benefits of this handbook lie in its portability and its practical approach to the most common disease processes. There is a list of references at the end of each chapter to provide more comprehensive understanding for all the topics.

George I. Jallo, MD
Karl F. Kothbauer, MD
Violette M.R. Recinos, MD

Acknowledgments

We are grateful to all our contributors for the quality of their submission. We also thank the staff at Thieme, Timothy Hiscock and Prakash Naorem, without whom this text would not have been possible. We also cannot forget all the midlevel providers, students, residents, and fellows who have contributed to the shaping of this handbook. In particular, we are grateful to Nir Shimony, Rajiv Iyer, Meleine Sosa-Martinez, and Brooks Osburn who were the real force behind the topics and chapters.

George I. Jallo, MD
Karl F. Kothbauer, MD
Violette M.R. Recinos, MD

About the Editors

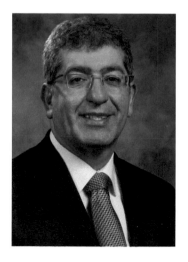

George Jallo, MD, Professor of Neurosurgery, Pediatrics and Oncology at the Johns Hopkins University School of Medicine, joined the faculty in 2003 after training under Dr. Fred Epstein. He was the Chief of Pediatric Neurosurgery at Johns Hopkins Hospital before relocating to Johns Hopkins All Children's Hospital (St. Petersburg, Florida) in September 2015 as Director of the Institute for Brain Protection Sciences (IBPS). He leads a team of neurosurgeons, neurologists, psychiatrists, psychologists, developmental pediatricians, sports medicine physicians, and physiatrists, who all care for pediatric neurological disorders and conditions. As an internationally respected pediatric neurosurgeon, with expertise in epilepsy, tumors of the brain and spinal cord, intraoperative neurophysiological monitoring for eloquent tumors, and use of minimally invasive technologies such as endoscopy and keyhole surgery, he felt the need for a handbook in pediatric neurosurgery for the neurosurgery trainee and midlevel provider.

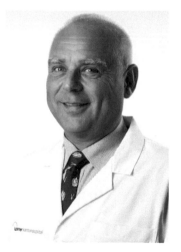

Karl F. Kothbauer, MD, Associate Professor of Neurosurgery at the University of Basel, Switzerland, and Chief of Neurosurgery at the Lucerne Cantonal Hospital, Lucerne, Switzerland, completed fellowship training in pediatric neurosurgery under Fred J. Epstein in New York. In 2004, he founded and since then developed the Division of Neurosurgery in Lucerne. As a neurosurgeon and pediatric neurosurgeon, his broad experience and expertise centers on brain tumor surgery, endoscopic neurosurgery, surgery for dysraphic conditions, and, in particular, surgery for intramedullary spinal cord tumors in children and adults.

He is an internationally recognized expert and researcher in the field of application of intraoperative neurophysiology in neurosurgery, particularly the development of neuromonitoring of the motor pathways. From 2009 to 2011, he served as president of the International Society for Intraoperative Neurophysiology (ISIN).

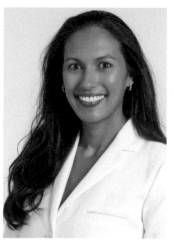

Violette M.R. Recinos, MD, Assistant Professor of Neurosurgery at the Cleveland Clinic Lerner College of Medicine, is an ABNS- and ABPNS-certified pediatric neurosurgeon who is the Section Head of Pediatric Neurosurgery at the Cleveland Clinic. She graduated with a major in Neuroscience from the Johns Hopkins University, and stayed on to complete her medical school, neurosurgical residency, and pediatric neurosurgery fellowship at the Johns Hopkins School of Medicine. In residency, she also completed a 2-year NIH fellowship in Neuro-Oncology, investigating local delivery of chemotherapeutic agents in the treatment of brain tumors. She maintains an active research laboratory focused on the investigation of CNS tumors.

Contributors

Richard C.E. Anderson, MD, FACS, FAAP
Associate Professor of Neurological Surgery
Division of Pediatric Neurosurgery
Columbia University
Morgan Stanley Children's Hospital of New York
    Presbyterian
New York, New York

Luis A. Arredondo, MD
Head
Pediatric Neurosurgery Department
Hospital Civil Fray Antonio Alcalde
Jalisco, Mexico

Micol Babini, MD
Neurosurgeon
Pediatric Neurosurgery
Institute of Neurosurgery
University Hospital of Verona
Verona, Italy

Liat Ben-Sira, MD
Director
Pediatric Imaging, "Dana" Children's Hospital
Gilbert Israeli Neurofibromatosis Center (GINFC),
    Tel-Aviv Medical Center
Tel-Aviv University
Tel-Aviv, Israel

Felix Bokstein, MD
Co-director, Adult Neuro-oncology Program and
    Adult NF1 Clinic
Department of Oncology
    Gilbert Israeli Neurofibromatosis Center (GINFC)
Tel Aviv Sourasky Medical Center
Tel Aviv, Israel

Douglas Brockmeyer, MD
Professor of Neurosurgery
Marion L Walker Endowed Chair
Division Chief
Pediatric Neurosurgery
University of Utah
Salt Lake City, Utah

Rafael U. Cardenas, MD, MHS
Fellow
Division of Pediatric Neurosurgery
Department of Neurosurgery
Weill Cornell Medicine
New York, New York

Oguz Cataltepe, MD
Professor of Neurosurgery and Pediatrics
Director, Pediatric Neurosurgery and Epilepsy
    Surgery
Department of Neurosurgery UMass-Memorial
    Medical Center
University of Massachusetts Medical School
Worcester, Massachusetts

Vikram B. Chakravarthy, MD
Resident Physician
Department of Neurosurgery
Cleveland Clinic Lerner College of Medicine
Cleveland Clinic
Cleveland, Ohio

Peter A. Christiansen, MD
Resident Physician
Department of Neurosurgery
University of Virginia Health System
Charlottesville, Virginia

Alan R. Cohen, MD, FACS, FAAP
Professor of Neurosurgery, Oncology and Pediatrics
Chief, Division of Pediatric Neurosurgery
The Johns Hopkins University School of Medicine
Baltimore, Maryland

Shlomi Constantini, MD, MSc
Professor and Chair
Department of Pediatric Neurosurgery, "Dana"
    Children's Hospital;
Gilbert Israeli Neurofibromatosis Center (GINFC),
    Tel-Aviv Medical Center,
Tel-Aviv University
Tel-Aviv, Israel

Richard P.D. Cooke, MD
Consultant Microbiologist
Department of Microbiology
Alder Hey Children's Hospital
Liverpool, UK

Moise Danielpour, MD, FACS
Vera and Paul Guerin Family Chair in Pediatric
    Neurosurgery
Associate Professor, Neurosurgery
Director, Pediatric Neurosurgery and Center for
    Pediatric Neurosciences
Cedars Sinai Medical Center
Advanced Health Sciences Pavilion
Los Angeles, California

Chandrashekhar Deopujari, MCh, MSc
Professor and Head
Department of Neurosurgery
Bombay Hospital Institute of Medical Sciences
Mumbai, India

Mark S. Dias, MD, FAANS, FAAP
Professor of Neurosurgery and Pediatrics
Vice Chair for Neurosurgical Education
Director of Pediatric Neurosurgery
Penn State Health, Penn State College of Medicine
Hershey, Pennsylvania

Amir H. Dorafshar, MBChB, FACS, FAAP
Associate Professor
Department of Plastic Surgery
Johns Hopkins Medical Institute
Baltimore, Maryland

**Jonathan R. Ellenbogen, BMedSc (Hons),
    MBChB (Hons), FRCS (Neurosurgery)**
Paediatric Neurosurgery Fellow
Department of Neurosurgery
Alder Hey Children's Hospital
Liverpool, UK

Anthony A. Figaji, MD, PhD
Professor and Head of Pediatric Neurosurgery
Pediatric Neurosurgery
Institute for Child Health, Red Cross Children's
    Hospital
Cape Town, South Africa

Jared S. Fridley, MD
Neurosurgery Resident
Department of Neurosurgery
Baylor College of Medicine
Houston, Texas

Neil R. Friedman, MB, ChB
Director
Center for Pediatric Neurosciences
Cleveland Clinic's Neurological Institute
Cleveland Clinic
Cleveland, Ohio

Gerald A. Grant, MD, FACS
Arline and Pete Harman Endowed Faculty Scholar
Stanford Child Health Research Institute
Division Chief, Pediatric Neurosurgery
Vice Chair for Pediatric Neurosurgery and Associate
    Program Director of Neurosurgery
Associate Professor, Department of Neurosurgery
Stanford University/Lucile Packard Children's
    Hospital
Stanford, California

Mari L. Groves, MD
Assistant Professor of Neurosurgery
Department of Neurosurgery
Johns Hopkins Hospital
Baltimore, Maryland

Lorelay Gutierrez, MD
Consultant
Pediatric Neurosurgery Department
Hospital Civil Fray Antonio Alcalde
Jalisco, Mexico

Raphael Guzman, MD
Professor of Neurosurgery and Neurosciences
Vice Chair Department of Neurosurgery
Chief Pediatric Neurosurgery
Department of Neurosurgery
University Hospital Basel
University Children's Hospital Basel (UKBB)
Basel, Switzerland

Adam L. Hartman, MD, FAAP, FANA
Associate Professor of Neurology & Pediatrics
Department of Neurology
Johns Hopkins Hospital
Baltimore, Maryland

Andrew T. Healy, MD
Neurosurgeon
Carolina Neurosurgery and Spine Associate
Concord, North Carolina

David S. Hersh, MD
Resident
Department of Neurosurgery
University of Maryland
Baltimore, Maryland

Anthony J. Herzog, MD
Orthopedic Resident
Department of Orthopedic Surgery
Johns Hopkins University
Baltimore, Maryland

Eveline T. Hidalgo, MD
Clinical Instructor
Division of Pediatric Neurosurgery
Department of Neurosurgery
NYU Langone Health
New York, New York

Eelco W. Hoving, MD, PhD
Professor
Department of Neurosurgery
University Hospital Utrecht
Utrecht, The Netherlands

Gary Hsich, MD
Staff Pediatric Neurologist
Center for Pediatric Neurosciences
Cleveland Clinic
Cleveland, Ohio

Thierry A.G.M. Huisman, MD, EQNR, EDiPNR
Professor of Radiology, Pediatrics, Neurology, and
    Neurosurgery
Chairman, Department of Imaging and Imaging
    Science, JHBMC
Director, Division Pediatric Radiology and Pediatric
    Neuroradiology, JHH
Johns Hopkins Medicine
Baltimore, Maryland

Lee S. Hwang, MD
Resident Physician
Department of Neurosurgery
Cleveland Clinic Lerner College of Medicine
Cleveland Clinic
Cleveland, Ohio

Rajiv R. Iyer, MD
Resident
Department of Neurosurgery
Johns Hopkins Hospital
Baltimore, Maryland

Sonal Jain, MCH
Superspecialty Medical Officer
Department of Neurosurgery
King Edward Memorial Hospital and Seth G.S.
    Medical College
Mumbai, India

George I. Jallo, MD
Professor of Neurosurgery, Pediatrics and Oncology
Institute for Brain Protection Sciences
Johns Hopkins All Children's Hospital
St. Petersburg, Florida

John A. Jane, Jr., MD
Professor of Neurosurgery and Pediatrics
Neurosurgery Residency Program Director
Department of Neurosurgery
University of Virginia Health System
Charlottesville, Virginia

Andrew Jea, MD, MHA
Professor and Chief
Department of Pediatric Neurosurgery
Riley Hospital for Children
Department of Neurological Surgery
Indiana University School of Medicine
Indianapolis, Indiana

Kambiz Kamian, MD, FRCS(C), FAANS
Amber Rollins Endowed Chair in Pediatrics
    Neurosurgery Chair
Department of Pediatrics Neurosurgery
Boonshoft School of Medicine
Wright State University
Dayton Children's Hospital
Dayton, Ohio

Sarah A. Kelley, MD
Assistant Professor, Neurology and Pediatrics
Director, Pediatric Epilepsy Monitoring Unit
Johns Hopkins Hospital
Baltimore, Maryland

Christopher D. Kelly, MD
Attending Neurosurgeon
Kantonsspital Aarau
Aarau, Switzerland

Karl F. Kothbauer, MD
Associate Professor of Neurosurgery
University of Basel
Basel, Switzerland
Chief of Neurosurgery
Lucerne Cantonal Hospital
Lucerne, Switzerland

Elizabeth J. Le, MD
Resident
Department of Neurosurgery
University of Maryland
Baltimore, Maryland

Bryan S. Lee, MD
Resident Physician
Department of Neurosurgery
Cleveland Clinic Lerner College of Medicine
Cleveland Clinic
Cleveland, Ohio

Lydia J. Liang, BS
Student
Johns Hopkins University School of Medicine
Baltimore, Maryland

Tina Lovén, DO
Pediatric Neurosurgeon
Division of Neurosurgery
Mercy Hospital
Springfield, Minnesota

Conor L. Mallucci, MD
Consultant Paediatric Neurosurgeon
Department of Neurosurgery
Alder Hey Children's Hospital
Liverpool, UK

Michael M. McDowell, MD
Resident
Department of Neurological Surgery
University of Pittsburgh
Pittsburgh, Pennsylvania

Miguel A. Medina III, MD
Assistant Professor
Director of Microsurgery
Miami Cancer Institute
Plastic and Reconstructive Surgery
Miami, Florida

Rodrigo Mercado, MD
Head
Functional Neurosurgery Clinic
Hospital Civil de Guadalajara
Functional Neurosurgery
Unit of Movement Disorders and Neurodegenerative
    Diseases
Hospital San Javier
Jalisco, Mexico

Martina Messing-Jünger, MD
Associate Professor of Neurosurgery
Heinrich-Heine-University, Düsseldorf, Germany
Head of Department
Pediatric Neurosurgery
Asklepios Klinik-Sankt Augustin, Germany

Mark A. Mittler, MD
Co-Chief, Division of Pediatric Neurosurgery
Steven and Alexandra Cohen Children's Medical
    Center of New York
Director of Quality Assurance, Department of
    Neurosurgery
Northwell Health
Clinical Associate Professor of Neurosurgery and
    Pediatrics
Hofstra-Northwell School of Medicine
New York, New York

Tiago Morgado, MD
Resident in Neurosurgery
Division of Neurosurgery
Groote Schuur Hospital
Cape Town, South Africa

Debraj Mukherjee, MD, MPH
Chief Neurosurgery Resident
Robert Wood Johnson Foundation Scholar
Congress of Neurological Surgeons Leadership Fellow
Council of State Neurosurgical Societies Washington
    Fellow
American Association of Neurological Surgeons
    Young Neurosurgeons Committee Representative
Department of Neurosurgery
Cedars-Sinai Medical Center
Los Angeles, California

Jeffrey P. Mullin, MD, MBA
Assistant Professor
Department of Neurosurgery
University of Buffalo
Buffalo, New York

Gerhard S. Mundinger, MD
Assistant Professor Craniofacial, Plastic, and
    Reconstructive Surgery
Louisiana State University Health Sciences Center;
Department of Cell Biology and Anatomy
Louisiana State University Health Sciences Center;
Director of Plastic Surgery
Children's Hospital of New Orleans
New Orleans, Louisiana

Dattatraya Muzumdar, MCh, FRCSI, FACS (USA)
Professor
Department of Neurosurgery
King Edward Memorial Hospital and Seth G.S.
    Medical College
Mumbai, India

Greg Olavarria, MD
Faculty, University of Central Florida College of
    Medicine
Co-Director, Craniofacial Program; Co-Director,
    Epilepsy Surgery Program; Trauma Quality Liaison
Department of Neurosurgery
Arnold Palmer Hospital for Children
Orlando, Florida

Aurelia Peraud, MD
Professor of Pediatric Neurosurgery
Department of Neurosurgery
University Hospital Ulm
Ulm, Germany

Michelle Q. Phan, MD
Resident
Department of Neurosurgery
Cincinnati Children's Hospital
Cincinnati, Ohio

Jonathan Pindrik, MD
Assistant Professor
Division of Pediatric Neurosurgery
Department of Neurological Surgery
Nationwide Children's Hospital and The Ohio State
    University College of Medicine
Columbus, Ohio

Violette M.R. Recinos, MD
Assistant Professor
Department of Neurosurgery
Cleveland Clinic Lerner College of Medicine of Case
    Western Reserve University
Division of Pediatric Neurosurgery
Cleveland Clinic
Cleveland, Ohio

Lindsey Ross, MD
Resident Physician
Department of Neurosurgery
Cedars-Sinai Medical Center
West Hollywood, California

Martin H. Sailer, MD, PhD
Attending Neurosurgeon
Department of Neurosurgery
University Hospital Basel
Basel, Switzerland

Francesco Sala, MD
Professor of Neurosurgery
Department of Neurosciences, Biomedicine and
    Movement Sciences
University Hospital Verona
Verona, Italy

Christina Sayama, MD, MPH
Pediatric Neurosurgery Fellow
Department of Neurosurgery
Texas Children's Hospital
Houston, Texas

Christian A. Schneider, MD
Pediatric Neurosurgeon
Department of Neurosurgery
Universitäts-Kinderspital beider Basel
Basel, Switzerland

Joanne E. Shay, MD, MBA
Assistant Professor
Director of Pediatric Remote Anesthesia Services
Pediatric Anesthesiology and Critical Care Medicine
Johns Hopkins University School of Medicine
Baltimore, Maryland

Nir Shimony, MD
Pediatric Neurosurgery Fellow
Department of Neurosurgery
Johns Hopkins University
Institute for Brain Protection Sciences
Johns Hopkins All Children's Hospital
St. Petersburg, Florida

Ben Shofty, MD, PhD
Resident Physician
Department of Neurosurgery
Gilbert Israeli Neurofibromatosis Center (GINFC)
Tel-Aviv Medical Center
Tel-Aviv University
Tel-Aviv, Israel

Edward R. Smith, MD
R. Michael Scott Chair in Neurosurgery
Associate Professor, Harvard Medical School
Department of Neurosurgery
Boston Children's Hospital
Boston, Massachusetts

Paul D. Sponseller, MD, MBA
Professor and Chief of Pediatric Orthopaedics Surgery
Johns Hopkins Children's Center
Baltimore, Maryland

Stacie Stapleton, MD
Director of Pediatric Neuro-Oncology Program
Assistant Professor of Pediatrics
Johns Hopkins Medicine
Cancer and Blood Disorders Institute
Johns Hopkins All Children's Hospital
St. Petersburg, Florida

Scellig S.D. Stone, MD, PhD, FRCSC
Assistant Professor
Department of Neurosurgery
Boston Children's Hospital
Harvard Medical School
Boston, Massachusetts

Gianpiero Tamburrini, MD
Professor
Department of Pediatric Neurosurgery
Institute of Neurosurgery
Catholic University Medical School
Rome, Italy

Ulrich-Wilhelm N. Thomale, MD
Head
Department of Pediatric Neurosurgery
Charité Universitätsmedizin Berlin
Berlin, Germany

Dominic N.P. Thompson, MBBS BSc FRCS (SN)
Paediatric Neurosurgeon
Department of Paediatric Neurosurgery
Great Ormond Street Hospital for Children NHS
    Foundation Trust
London, UK

Hagit Toledano-Alhadef, MD
Clinical Director
The Gilbert Israeli Neurofibromatosis Center (GINFC)
"Dana" Children's Hospital, Tel-Aviv Medical Center
Tel-Aviv University
Tel-Aviv, Israel

Gerald F. Tuite, MD
Pediatric Neurosurgeon
Institute for Brain Protection Sciences
Johns Hopkins All Children's Hospital
St. Petersburg, Florida

Jesus A. Villagómez, MD
Consultant
Centro de Neuro-Radiocirugia San Javier
    Gamma Knife
Hospital San Javier
Jalisco, Mexico

Linda W. Xu, MD
Neurosurgery Resident
Department of Neurosurgery
Stanford University Hospital and Clinics
Stanford, California

Section I

General and Critical Care

I

1 ICP Management

Tiago Morgado, Anthony A. Figaji

1.1 Introduction

Management of raised intracranial pressure (ICP) occupies a central role in neurocritical care, but exact recommendations on how to monitor ICP and how to best respond to elevations in ICP remain somewhat contentious. Moreover, although ICP monitoring and management is usually considered in the context of traumatic brain injury (TBI), several other acute comatose conditions are also subject to the problems of raised ICP and brain ischemia and may benefit from ICP management.[1] This chapter will discuss the management of raised ICP in the setting of TBI in children, but these principles may well apply to other conditions.

Numerous strategies exist for reducing ICP. The control of ICP without a good understanding of cerebral hemodynamics and homeostasis, however, may well cause more harm than good. It is essential that ICP-directed therapies are tailored to individual cases, and that a thought process appraising the potential adverse effects of each treatment modality is applied. Ideally, ICP monitoring should be employed as part of a multimodal neuromonitoring setup, as correlation of ICP and the therapies directed at it with other neurophysiological parameters provides a more complete assessment of the dynamic cerebral pathological state. This ultimately leads to more well-informed, controlled, and safer therapeutic interventions.

Although "normal" ICP is difficult to define, it is generally accepted that in nonpathological states ICP in children is usually less than 10 to 15 mm Hg. The association of raised ICP with poor neurological outcome is widely reported. It is also known that there is an association between increased ICP and pediatric TBI outcomes, as well as between protocol-driven ICP-lowering strategies and improved outcomes. However, recent data have highlighted the potential for getting this wrong. ICP monitoring allows for objective assessment of ICP, but does not necessarily reveal the cause of increased ICP and how the brain responds to various treatments. Studies directly assessing the effect of ICP monitoring on outcome have produced conflicting results. Although some authors go as far as suggesting that ICP monitoring itself is associated with worsening of survival,[2] recent research has found an association between ICP monitoring and reduced mortality in both the adult and pediatric age groups.[3] A randomized controlled trial performed at hospitals in Bolivia and Ecuador that had previously not used ICP monitoring failed to show the expected benefit of ICP monitoring on outcome.[4,5] However, the study has several limitations, and whether these findings can be extrapolated to more organized centers is controversial. Still, it raises the question of whether blindly controlling ICP at a threshold of 20 mm Hg in all patients makes physiological sense. A study looking at the effect of adherence to specific ICP and cerebral perfusion pressure (CPP) targets found that despite acceptable ICP control, many patients still suffered episodes of compromised brain oxygenation.[6]

There are several potential adverse effects of ICP-lowering treatments. For example, injudicious hyperventilation may result in cerebral vasoconstriction and ischemia, overzealous use of diuretics may result in adverse hemodynamic changes and electrolyte abnormalities, and decompressive craniectomy (DC) may directly harm the brain. It is important therefore that ICP management is an individualized process, tailored to each patient, preferably with more information than just the ICP number. Where possible, the etiology of ICP increases should be determined and there should be a feedback loop to determine the effects of the ICP treatment.

1.2 Pathophysiology

1.2.1 Anatomy and Physiology of ICP and Cerebral Perfusion

Changes in ICP

The cranium is a rigid structure with little (in infants) or no ability to increase in volume. Its contents, made up of brain, blood, and cerebrospinal fluid (CSF), are incompressible. As the *Monro–Kellie doctrine* states, an increase in the volume of one intracranial component (brain, blood, or CSF) results in an equal compensatory decrease of another, the total intracranial volume being fixed. CSF egress from the cranial compartment to the spinal cisterns is usually one the first compensatory mechanisms to occur in this scenario, followed by decreased intracranial venous blood volume. As these "buffering" processes become

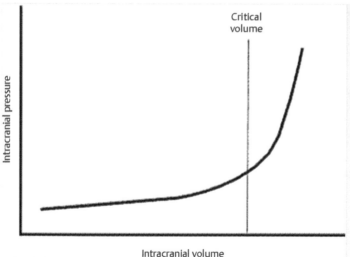

Fig. 1.1 Monro–Kellie doctrine and cerebral compliance curve.

exhausted, ICP begins to rise at an exponential rate. As cerebral compliance (defined as the change in intracranial volume divided by the change in ICP) decreases, even a minimal increase in intracranial volume may result in a rapid rise in ICP (► Fig. 1.1). Infants are more protected from this phenomenon as a result of open fontanels and sutures, but even their reserves of compliance may become quickly exhausted and ICP can rise to very high levels. As this pathological state progresses, cerebral blood flow (CBF) decreases if CPP is significantly compromised. When CBF falls below critical thresholds (approximately 18–20 mL/100 g/min in stroke studies), potentially irreversible hypoxic-ischemic damage to neurons and glia may occur.

ICP and Cerebral Perfusion

CPP is the difference between mean arterial pressure (MAP) and ICP: CPP = MAP – ICP. Calculation of this is affected by where the MAP is zeroed: at the level of the heart or the head. Treatment threshold values for the above parameters remain controversial in adults and even more so in children, who have changing normative blood pressure (BP) and ICP values across the age range. There are no widely accepted data on normal ICP values in infants and children. Although 20 mm Hg is recommended as the ICP cutoff above which intervention is required, it is likely that this value is well above the normal ICP in small children and infants, and that secondary brain injury may occur below this value. At the same time, the cause of the ICP increase should also be considered. For example, hyperemia is likely more common in

children and presumably has different consequences at a given ICP number. The target for CPP is even less clear, as it depends not only on ICP but also on the changing normative values for BP across a wide physiological age range. All of these increase the heterogeneity of TBI and so interaction between ICP and other neurophysiological parameters is complex.[7]

Failure of Cerebral Autoregulation

In adult physiology, autoregulation fails below a CPP of 40 to 50 mm Hg or above a CPP of 150 mm Hg; therefore, CBF decreases, potentially resulting in tissue ischemia and neuronal injury (► Fig. 1.2). Furthermore, increased metabolic demand and the disruption of homeostatic mechanisms (such as pressure autoregulation and flow-metabolism coupling) may result in tissue ischemia despite a CPP range that would be adequate in the uninjured brain.[8] Pediatric guidelines published in 2012 suggested an age-related CPP threshold of 40 to 50 mm Hg below which neurological outcome is significantly worsened; however, the evidence on which this is based is weak.[9]

Herniation

Brain shift occurs when there is compartmentalization of pressure within the cranium. The classic herniation syndromes are subfalcine, transtentorial, and "coning" (across the foramen magnum) (► Fig. 1.3). Brainstem distortion results in cranial nerve palsies (most commonly oculomotor and abducens nerve palsies), hemiparesis, Cushing's

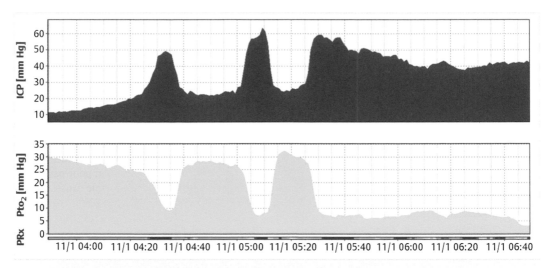

Fig. 1.2 Reduced brain tissue oxygen tension (Pto$_2$) as a result of increase in ICP.

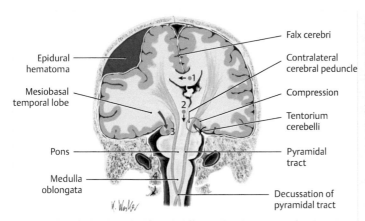

Fig. 1.3 Cerebral herniation syndromes in TBI. 1, subfalcine herniation; 2, central herniation; 3, uncal transtentorial herniation; 4, tonsillar herniation. (Reproduced from Schuenke, Schulte, and Schumacher, Atlas of Anatomy, 2nd edition, ©2016, Thieme Publishers, New York. Illustration by Karl Wesker.)

response, and respiratory arrest. The occurrence of these syndromes depends on the rapidity of the rise in ICP, the cause and location of the increased volume, the tentorial configuration, and the size and shape of the posterior fossa.

1.2.2 Causes of Raised ICP in TBI

▶ Table 1.1 lists several mechanisms that may contribute to a raised ICP in TBI.[10]

Mass Lesions

- In trauma, intracranial mass lesions such as subdural, epidural, and intracerebral hematomas and contusions may contribute to both focal and global increases in ICP.

Table 1.1 Causes of raised ICP in TBI

Expansive	Hematoma (EDH/SDH/ICH)
Parenchymal	Cerebral edema
	Contusion
Vascular	Arterial vasodilation
	Venous congestion
	Loss of cerebral autoregulation
Hydrocephalus	
Seizure	

Abbreviations: EDH, extradural hemorrhage; ICH, intracerebral hemorrhage; SDH, subdural hemorrhage.

Cerebral Edema

- Both diffuse and/or perilesional edema often contributes to raised ICP. This usually involves a combination of both vasogenic and cytotoxic edema as a result of blood–brain barrier dysfunction and cellular energy failure.

- Sodium and water imbalance due to central nervous system and hypothalamic–pituitary axis dysfunction may aggravate this, as may overzealous fluid resuscitation.

Vascular

Loss of Autoregulation, Abnormal Vascular Reactivity, and Hyperemia

- Disrupted vascular reactivity of the injured brain plays a significant role in pathologically raised ICP. Several intrinsic systems regulate perfusion to neuronal tissue and ensure cerebral tissue homeostasis.
- Pressure autoregulation, metabolism-perfusion coupling, and vascular carbon dioxide tension (Pco_2) reactivity are important mechanisms in this regulation.
- Pressure autoregulation, which maintains a constant CBF within a CPP range of approximately 50 to 150 mm Hg (but which may be different in children), may be disrupted to varying degrees, causing BP and CBF (and volume) to assume a passive relationship because of a lack of vasoreactivity. The brain is therefore at greater risk of increased ICP when BP is raised and of ischemia when BP is lowered.
- Similarly, flow-metabolism uncoupling may result in hyperemia and increased ICP.

Changes in Pco_2

- Carbon dioxide is known to have a potent vasoactive effect.
- Head-injured patients with a depressed level of consciousness, diminished respiratory drive and lower cranial nerve dysfunction are prone to hypoventilation and CO_2 retention, potentially resulting in cerebral arterial vasodilation and increased intracranial blood content and ICP.
- Conversely, intentional or accidental iatrogenic hyperventilation is common—especially because the respiratory tidal volume is so small—and may cause profound decreases in CBF. The pediatric brain is very sensitive to changes in arterial Pco_2, which has significant consequences for ICP and CBF.

Intracranial Venous Congestion

- Several factors may contribute to increased venous pressure, which in turn results in decreased venous return from the head and neck, and increased ICP.
- High airway pressures result from several causes, including ventilator settings and patient agitation, and should be avoided whenever possible.
- Other causes for decreased venous return from the head, such as constrictive endotracheal tube fixation tape, cervical collars, and poor patient positioning, are common avoidable causes for potentially harmful increases in ICP.

Hydrocephalus

- Hydrocephalus is not uncommon in TBI, although less so in children than in adults.
- Communicating hydrocephalus may be due to traumatic subarachnoid hemorrhage; noncommunicating hydrocephalus may be due to hematomas or infarcts with mass effect, especially in the posterior fossa.

Seizure

- Epileptic activity (both convulsive and nonconvulsive) may increase both ICP and cerebral metabolic demand in patients with TBI. Sometimes the only evidence of subclinical seizures may be rapid and repeated changes in ICP and BP. Where possible, continuous electroencephalogram (EEG) monitoring should be used.

1.3 ICP Monitoring

1.3.1 Indications

Despite only level III evidence supporting the use of ICP monitoring in infants and children with severe TBI, a significant body of evidence suggests that monitoring ICP may be of benefit in this patient group.[9] There is little evidence to support routine ICP monitoring in moderate TBI, although this may be indicated in specific cases. ICP monitoring in other conditions remains to be defined, but it is likely that an ICP-targeted approach may also benefit these patients.[1]

1.3.2 Methods

► Table 1.2 summarizes the various methods of ICP measurement. Both external ventricular drain (EVD) and dedicated ICP monitoring devices are

Table 1.2 Methods of measuring ICP

External ventricular drain	
ICP monitoring devices	Intraparenchymal Subdural/subarachnoid Epidural
Noninvasive methods	Transcranial Doppler ultrasound Optic nerve sheath diameter measurement Cochlear fluid pressure measurement

Abbreviation: ICP, intracranial pressure.

used to measure ICP. EVD provides the most accurate measurement of ICP and can be used as a therapy for raised ICP, allowing for drainage of CSF. However, there is a higher risk of malposition, infection, and hematoma on insertion. Furthermore, EVD is limited by not being able to measure ICP and drain CSF simultaneously; therefore, episodes of increased ICP may be missed.[11] When manually evaluating the level at which an EVD drains as an indication of ICP, it should be remembered that this pressure measurement is in centimeters of water (cm H_2O), and not millimeters of mercury (mm Hg). Conversion of ICP to mm Hg is achieved by multiplying the value by a factor of 0.74 (e.g., 20 cm $H_2O \times 0.74 = 15$ mm Hg).

Several different ICP monitors are available for invasive monitoring. These devices may function on a fiberoptic, strain gauge, or pneumatic mechanism. The usual accepted pressure range for these monitors is 0 to 100 mm Hg, with an error of no more than 2 mm Hg between 0 and 20 mm Hg (as advised by the Association for the Advancement of Medical Instrumentation). Placement of the pressure monitor probe varies. Intraparenchymal monitors, although perhaps more invasive than extra-axially sited devices, provide the most accurate, reliable pressure measurements in this group, and are the most commonly used type of monitor in the setting of TBI.[9,11] When placed by experienced personnel, the risk of infection or hemorrhage is very low. EVD and ICP monitors are sometimes used in conjunction.[11] The most widely used probes include Camino fiberoptic ICP monitoring device (Integra Neuroscience, Plainsboro, NJ) and the Codman Microsensor ICP transducer (Johnson & Johnson, New Brunswick, NJ). Recently, a combined ICP and brain tissue oxygen probe was introduced (Raumedic AG, Helmbrechts, Germany); however, this still requires wider validation. Noninvasive methods of ICP measurement have attracted interest since the 1960s. Various strategies of indirectly assessing ICP have been developed, including measuring changes in blood flow velocity with transcranial Doppler, measurement of optic nerve sheath diameter, and even measuring cochlear fluid pressure via tympanic membrane displacement, all of which have demonstrated potential in determining ICP, usually as a spot measurement. However, none of these modalities have reached a standard of accuracy and reliability for continuous measurement of ICP to replace invasive monitoring. Although head computed tomography (CT) scanning plays a role in estimating ICP in pediatric TBI, it remains an unreliable method of detecting raised ICP because of its poor sensitivity.[12]

Recording and graphical display of ICP (and other neurophysiological parameters) augments the clinical value of ICP monitoring. Systems such as Intensive Care Monitoring Plus (ICM +, Cambridge University, UK[13]) allow for real-time display of ICP (and calculated variables such as CPP) trends at the bedside. This system not only assists with patient treatment and decision-making in the ICU, but also records a multitude of parameters, forming a database that may later be analyzed and used for research purposes. Continuous recording identifies more episodes of adverse changes in the monitored variables and allows for appreciation of the dynamic interplay, for example, the relationship between BP and ICP.

1.3.3 Raised ICP—When to Treat?

Numerous studies have shown sustained elevation in ICP to be associated with death or poor outcome in severe pediatric TBI. There are, however, little data on normal values for pediatric ICP. Although level II evidence exists that treatment should be initiated at an ICP threshold of 20 mm Hg in adult patients with severe TBI, no such studies exist for the pediatric population. This cutoff is extrapolated to children, but it is highly likely that this value might not be appropriate for smaller children and infants, whose lower MAP and CPP (and less robust autoregulatory capacity) probably necessitate a lower ICP target. The duration of ICP elevation is also significant and should be included in the decision of whether or not ICP should be treated.

A number of ICP waveforms may be observed with continuous visual charting of ICP. *Pulse waves* reflect small changes in ICP related to arterial pulsation within the intracranial compartment. *Breathing waves* represent a second-class wave

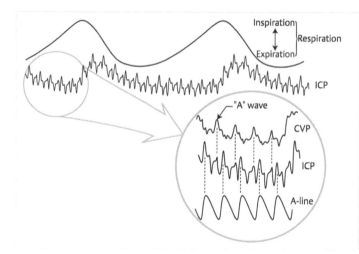

Fig. 1.4 Pathological ICP waveforms. (Reproduced with permission from Greenberg MS. Handbook of Neurosurgery. 8th ed. New York, NY: Thieme; 2016.)

reflecting the varying intracranial blood volume related to the different stages of the respiratory cycle. Both of these represent physiological waveforms, although changes in amplitude may reflect pathology related to ICP.

The well-described pathological ICP waveforms include A- (plateau), B-, and C-waves.[14,15] Plateauwaves are sustained (5–30 minutes) elevations of ICP well above the mean pressure, representing an increase in blood volume within the intracranial compartment. ICP drops quickly to the mean ICP after the wave. B-waves occur as a rise of ICP up to 20 mm Hg and occur with a frequency of 0.5 to 3 per minute. C-waves represent transmission of Herring–Traube waves to the intracranial compartment, and herald terminal vasoparalysis (▶ Fig. 1.4).

1.4 Treatment of Raised ICP

Management of raised ICP should employ a stepwise approach to exclude simple, easily treatable causes first. Numerous simple, risk-free measures can be carried out to ensure that ICP control is maximized before progressing to medical and surgical interventions. ▶ Table 1.3 provides a simple checklist of potential causes of raised ICP and their treatments that should be carried out for patients in the neurocritical care setting with raised ICP prior to considering therapeutic options such as DC or barbiturate coma.

1.4.1 Simple Measures

A number of simple measures can be instituted to minimize the risk of secondary injury related to raised ICP.

Venous drainage may be optimized by ensuring neutral cervical alignment and by loosening cervical collars and endotracheal tube fixation tape that may restrict venous flow from the head and neck. The head of the bed should be raised by 15 to 30 degrees. Adequate patient sedation and analgesia is an essential adjunct in controlling ICP. Agitation and forceful exhalation against a ventilator increase venous pressure in the head and neck veins. Attention must be paid to airway pressures, as these may also compromise venous return. Peak end-expiratory pressure (PEEP) should be kept in the normal to low range. With regard to sedation, both etomidate and thiopental (as a single dose) have been shown to be safe and effective in reducing ICP. Continuous propofol infusion is not recommended in pediatric patients, and there have been no studies aimed at addressing the role of muscular blockade in the setting of severe TBI in pediatric patients.

Hypercarbia must be avoided, as even small changes may cause dramatic changes in vascular tone. Conversely, a drop in Pco_2 causes vessels to constrict, and may result in cerebral ischemia. Targets of ventilation and oxygenation should be Pco_2 of 30 to 37.5 mm Hg and Po_2 of > 80 mm Hg, respectively, but ideally should be adjusted based on monitoring the adequacy of perfusion to the brain (e.g., with brain tissue oxygen monitoring).

Hypovolemia should be avoided at all times. Blood rheology and hydrostatic and oncotic pressure are affected by changes in serum osmolality, and it is essential that these are optimized. To make matters worse, brain-injured patients often have disturbances of sodium and water balance, and may also have hemodynamic abnormalities

Table 1.3 Checklist of causes of raised ICP and suggested action

Potential cause of raised ICP	Action
Cerebral venous congestion	Head of bed up at 30 degrees Head position neutral Cervical collar and head and neck strapping loosened Adequate patient sedation and analgesia Ensure ventilatory pressures not raised Sedate for procedures/maneuvers associated with increases in ICP (suctioning, patient manipulation)
Hypercarbia and hypoxia	Ventilate to Pco_2 of 30 to 37.5 mm Hg. If possible, titrate against some measure of brain oxygenation change Prevent systemic hypoxia. Keep Pao_2 preferably above 80 to 100 mm Hg
Hyponatremia	Maintain serum Na^+ 140 to 150 mmol/L
Cerebral swelling and edema	Osmotherapy with hypertonic saline (monitor serum Na^+) or mannitol
Seizure	Continuous EEG monitoring Administer antiepileptic medication if unable to monitor for seizures or if clinical suspicion of seizure
Pyrexia	Keep normothermic using antipyretics and active cooling
Expanding intracranial hematoma/hydrocephalus	Urgent CT scan and surgery as indicated

Abbreviations: CT, computed tomography; EEG, electroencephalogram; ICP, intracranial pressure.
Note: Prior to initiating any intervention to decrease ICP, confirm that the ICP monitoring device is calibrated and functioning correctly.

related to systemic injury (such as hypovolemia, dehydration, and renal dysfunction), which may compound the situation.

Serum Na fluid balance should be monitored judiciously in these patients, and attention must be paid to hydration status and central venous pressure. Hyponatremia must be avoided. Although there is little evidence to support this, we prefer to maintain serum sodium in the higher range of normal if ICP is a problem.

1.4.2 Medical Therapies

Osmotherapy

Intravenous hyperosmolar agents to reduce ICP have been in use for quite some time. The agents most commonly used are mannitol and hypertonic saline (HTS). Mannitol works by two mechanisms: it decreases the viscosity of blood, inducing a reflex arteriolar vasoconstriction, which results in decreased cerebral blood volume and ICP, while an osmotic mechanism draws fluid from the interstitial space into the cerebral vasculature. Mannitol requires an intact blood–brain barrier to function adequately. HTS exerts an effect on ICP and improves CPP through a number of mechanisms, including improved blood rheology, creating an osmotic gradient, stimulating vascular release of natriuretic peptide, improving cardiac output, and reducing inflammation. Overzealous use of HTS or mannitol is not without its adverse effects, and this should be borne in mind whenever using either of these two agents. Although level II and III evidence exists for the use of HTS in pediatric TBI with intracranial hypertension, the recently published pediatric guidelines for management of severe TBI failed to find any studies supporting the use of mannitol in this setting.[9,16,17] Recent trends have favored HTS above mannitol.

Sedation and Muscle Paralysis

Little evidence exists for the use of muscle paralysis in the treatment of intracranial hypertension. Previous research has shown a benefit from the use of thiopental and etomidate in treating raised ICP, although the risks inherent in the use of these medications should be considered. Both thiopentone and etomidate have been shown to reduce ICP, although correlation with outcome remains unclear.[18,19] Thiopentone is generally used as a second tier therapy, along with craniectomy or hypothermia, to control refractory increased ICP.

Antiepileptic Medication

Subclinical seizures may occur in over 50% of critically ill children and are known to lead to increased ICP and potential secondary injury.[20,21,22] Where resources for continuous electroencephalogram (cEEG) monitoring are not available in the critical care setting, it may be reasonable to treat children with antiepileptic medication empirically.

Hypothermia

Although previous studies had shown promise for moderate hypothermia as a neuroprotective intervention, enthusiasm for this modality has waned in recent years in light of new research showing no significant impact on outcome.[23] At our center, hypothermia is not part of the management protocol for severe TBI in children.

Corticosteroids

Previous studies have failed to show any benefit of steroids in TBI, with the largest trial to date finding an increased risk of mortality in the treatment group.[24] The study did, however, have very broad selection criteria across a wide range of severity and heterogeneity in pathology. It is possible that there are some subgroups of TBI patients that may benefit from corticosteroid therapy.

Barbiturate-induced Coma

Barbiturate-induced coma using thiopentone or pentobarbital is sometimes used as a treatment of intracranial hypertension refractory to both medical and surgical treatments. This modality is limited by its negative cardiorespiratory effects, which necessitate close cardiovascular monitoring and support. No correlation with outcome has been proven.[9]

1.4.3 Surgical Options

Mass Lesion Evacuation

Surgical removal of any significant space-occupying lesion such as traumatic extradural, subdural, and intracerebral hematoma is the first-line surgical treatment of raised ICP. Quite often, ICP and other neurophysiological monitors are placed at this time.

CSF Drainage

CSF drainage via EVD is a relatively simple strategy in trauma to reduce ICP. As previously mentioned, this intervention also allows for monitoring of ICP via EVD transduction. However, EVD placement in this setting is often difficult because of cerebral swelling and small ventricular size, often requiring image-guidance and potentially increasing risks related to drain malposition and multiple attempts at placement. The collapse of ventricles with CSF drainage also limits this intervention. The clinician should keep in mind the risks of increased hematoma on insertion, CSF infection, and failure to diagnose ICP spikes when the EVD is on drainage as opposed to monitoring.

1.4.4 Decompressive Craniectomy

DC for the treatment of raised ICP continues to divide opinion on the management of raised ICP in severe TBI. Although there is a clear potential benefit in reducing ICP via craniectomy in cases where both simple and medical measures have been exhausted, evidence for overall benefit is conflicting. This procedure carries a significant risk of neurological morbidity, and commits the patient to having a second operation at some point to undergo a cranioplasty. Various surgical options have been described, the most common being bifrontal and a large hemicraniectomy on the side of the more injured hemisphere. The bone is placed either in a bone fridge (preferably minus 70 °C) or in an abdominal pocket.

The only randomized trial of DC on outcome in children was a small pilot study by Taylor et al in 2001.[25] They found a significant improvement in outcome in patients managed with DC and conventional medical management as opposed to standard medical management alone; however, the procedure was atypical in comparison to more widespread use—a bilateral small temporal decompression without dural opening—and the ICP reduction was modest.

The DECRA trial, a randomized multicenter trial assessing the impact of early DC in severe TBI in adult patients, showed a decrease in ICP with DC but significantly worse outcome.[26] The study was, however, criticized for having a very low threshold for instituting this surgical option (medically refractory ICP of more than 20 mm Hg for 15 minutes in a 1-hour period) and so most patients who had surgery had modestly elevated ICP Also, ICP was well controlled in the medical arm, the patients of which still had the option of DC if ICP was refractory. The RESCUEicp trial showed reduced mortality but increased disability, so the decision comes down to what disability is acceptable.[27] If a DC is to be performed, it should be done in a controlled manner; loss of control of brain swelling after the dura is opened can lead to disastrous acute herniation through the defect. Brain swelling must be maximally controlled, even if temporarily, before the dura is opened, by using a combination of elevation of the head, good anesthesia, mannitol/HTS, avoidance of hypertension, and temporary hyperventilation. Thereafter, the dura should be grafted with pericranium or a dural substitute. The bone removal should be as large as possible to maximize ICP reduction and minimize fungation of brain across a narrow defect and consequent compression of cortical veins. Postoperative hypertension should be avoided as this may increase edema in the decompressed hemisphere. It is our practice to replace the bone flap as soon as brain swelling has subsided, preferably within 4 to 6 weeks, to minimize delayed injury to the underlying brain and hydrocephalus.

1.5 Summary

Management of ICP in the traumatic setting requires a logical, stepwise approach, employing simple strategies first and moving on to more complex medical and surgical treatment modalities as needed. A good understanding of the cause of the raised ICP as well as the physiological effects and potential risks of the treatment modalities employed leads to safe decision-making and effective treatment in these patients.

1.6 Questions

1. Name the main volume-occupying constituents of the intracranial compartment, and list some of the pathological processes that may increase the ICP in the injured brain.
2. Describe nonoperative methods of reducing pathologically elevated ICP.
3. What are the implications of altered regulatory mechanisms such as pressure autoregulation and flow-metabolism coupling?
4. What are the physiological and clinical consequences of increased ICP?
5. Discuss the surgical options to decrease ICP in terms of indications and complications.

References

[1] Glimåker M, Johansson B, Halldorsdottir H, et al. Neurointensive treatment targeting intracranial hypertension improves outcome in severe bacterial meningitis: an intervention-control study. PLoS One. 2014; 9(3):e91976

[2] Shafi S, Diaz-Arrastia R, Madden C, Gentilello L. Intracranial pressure monitoring in brain-injured patients is associated with worsening of survival. J Trauma. 2008; 64(2):335–340

[3] Farahvar A, Gerber LM, Chiu YL, Carney N, Härtl R, Ghajar J. Increased mortality in patients with severe traumatic brain injury treated without intracranial pressure monitoring. J Neurosurg. 2012; 117(4):729–734

[4] Chesnut RM, Temkin N, Carney N, et al. Global Neurotrauma Research Group. A trial of intracranial-pressure monitoring in traumatic brain injury. N Engl J Med. 2012; 367(26):2471–2481

[5] Chesnut RM. Intracranial pressure monitoring: headstone or a new head start. The BEST TRIP trial in perspective. Intensive Care Med. 2013; 39(4):771–774

[6] Figaji AA, Fieggen AG, Argent AC, Leroux PD, Peter JC. Does adherence to treatment targets in children with severe traumatic brain injury avoid brain hypoxia? A brain tissue oxygenation study. Neurosurgery. 2008; 63(1):83–91, discussion 91–92

[7] Rohlwink UK, Zwane E, Fieggen AG, Argent AC, le Roux PD, Figaji AA. The relationship between intracranial pressure and brain oxygenation in children with severe traumatic brain injury. Neurosurgery. 2012; 70(5):1220–1230, discussion 1231

[8] Figaji AA, Zwane E, Fieggen AG, et al. Pressure autoregulation, intracranial pressure, and brain tissue oxygenation in children with severe traumatic brain injury. J Neurosurg Pediatr. 2009; 4(5):420–428

[9] Kochanek PM, Carney N, Adelson PD, et al. Guidelines for the acute medical management of severe traumatic brain injury in infants, children, and adolescents–second edition. Pediatr Crit Care Med. 2012; 13 Suppl 1:S1–S82

[10] Padayachy LC, Figaji AA, Bullock MR. Intracranial pressure monitoring for traumatic brain injury in the modern era. Childs Nerv Syst. 2010; 26(4):441–452

[11] Exo J, Kochanek PM, Adelson PD, et al. Intracranial pressure-monitoring systems in children with traumatic brain injury: combining therapeutic and diagnostic tools. Pediatr Crit Care Med. 2011; 12(5):560–565

[12] Kouvarellis AJ, Rohlwink UK, Sood V, Van Breda D, Gowen MJ, Figaji AA. The relationship between basal cisterns on CT and time-linked intracranial pressure in paediatric head injury. Childs Nerv Syst. 2011; 27(7):1139–1144

[13] Smielewski P, Czosnyka M, Steiner L, Belestri M, Piechnik S, Pickard JD. ICM+: software for on-line analysis of bedside monitoring data after severe head trauma. Acta Neurochir Suppl (Wien). 2005; 95:43–49

[14] Lundberg N, Troupp H, Lorin H. Continuous recording of the ventricular-fluid pressure in patients with severe acute traumatic brain injury. A preliminary report. J Neurosurg. 1965; 22(6):581–590

[15] Lundberg N. Continuous recording and control of ventricular fluid pressure in neurosurgical practice. Acta Psychiatr Scand Suppl. 1960; 36(149):1–193

[16] Peterson B, Khanna S, Fisher B, Marshall L. Prolonged hypernatremia controls elevated intracranial pressure in head-injured pediatric patients. Crit Care Med. 2000; 28(4):1136–1143

[17] Fisher B, Thomas D, Peterson B. Hypertonic saline lowers raised intracranial pressure in children after head trauma. J Neurosurg Anesthesiol. 1992; 4(1):4–10

[18] Bramwell KJ, Haizlip J, Pribble C, VanDerHeyden TC, Witte M. The effect of etomidate on intracranial pressure and systemic blood pressure in pediatric patients with severe traumatic brain injury. Pediatr Emerg Care. 2006; 22(2):90–93

[19] de Bray JM, Granry JC, Monrigal JP, Leftheriotis G, Saumet JL. Effects of thiopental on middle cerebral artery blood velocities: a transcranial Doppler study in children. Childs Nerv Syst. 1993; 9(4):220–223

[20] Abend NS, Gutierrez-Colina AM, Topjian AA, et al. Nonconvulsive seizures are common in critically ill children. Neurology. 2011; 76(12):1071–1077

[21] Vespa PM, Miller C, McArthur D, et al. Nonconvulsive electrographic seizures after traumatic brain injury result in a delayed, prolonged increase in intracranial pressure and metabolic crisis. Crit Care Med. 2007; 35(12):2830–2836

[22] Vespa PM, Nuwer MR, Nenov V, et al. Increased incidence and impact of nonconvulsive and convulsive seizures after traumatic brain injury as detected by continuous electroencephalographic monitoring. J Neurosurg. 1999; 91(5):750–760

[23] Adelson PD, Wisniewski SR, Beca J, et al. Paediatric Traumatic Brain Injury Consortium. Comparison of hypothermia and normothermia after severe traumatic brain injury in children (Cool Kids): a phase 3, randomised controlled trial. Lancet Neurol. 2013; 12(6):546–553

[24] Roberts I, Yates D, Sandercock P, et al. CRASH trial colla-borators. Effect of intravenous corticosteroids on death within 14 days in 10008 adults with clinically significant head injury (MRC CRASH trial): randomised placebo-controlled trial. Lancet. 2004; 364(9442):1321–1328

[25] Taylor A, Butt W, Rosenfeld J, et al. A randomized trial of very early decompressive craniectomy in children with traumatic brain injury and sustained intracranial hypertension. Childs Nerv Syst. 2001; 17(3):154–162

[26] Chi JH. Craniectomy for traumatic brain injury: results from the DECRA trial. Neurosurgery. 2011; 68(6):N19–N20

[27] Hutchinson PJ, Kolias AG, Timofeev IS, et al. RESCUEicp Trial Collaborators. Trial of decompressive craniectomy for trau-matic intracranial hypertension. N Engl J Med 2016; 375(12): 1119–1130

2 Pain Management for Pediatric Neurosurgical Patients

Joanne E. Shay

2.1 Introduction

Pain management in pediatric neurosurgical patients transcends the usual boundaries for pediatric pain management imposed by developmental pharmacokinetics, pharmacodynamics, and pharmacogenomics. Because of the additional concern for assessing neurological function, especially a potentially deteriorating mental status examination, caution is the keyword. The goal is to provide balanced analgesia that facilitates neurological assessment without clouding neurologic evaluation by providing symptom targeted therapy. There is also evidence that inadequate analgesia may impact future pain responses in children with evidence of hyperalgesia and concerns for ineffective coping behavior.[1]

Pediatric neurosurgical patients must be considered among the most vulnerable patient groups requiring post-operative analgesia owing to their surgical condition that required treatment and their comorbidities often including neurologic dysfunction that produced or resulted from that condition, such as spasticity and hypotonia. Pediatric neurosurgical patients are also at risk for the general comorbidities that affect the population. In light of these considerations, pediatric neurosurgical patients must be considered to be at greater risk of complications from analgesic therapy. This risk can be reduced by caring for patients in a monitored setting with caregivers who are experienced in assessing and treating pediatric pain and the side effects of that therapy. Once the patient is transitioned from parenteral to enteral pain medications and is at baseline neurologic status, the need for cardiorespiratory monitoring can be re-evaluated and eliminated as indicated by the overall medical condition. A multimodal approach to pharmacotherapy that includes narcotic and non-narcotic drugs with a goal of creating synergy is preferable. This strategy can reduce the side effects from larger doses seen with monomodal drug therapy. Nonpharmacologic interventions such as massage, guided imagery, hypnosis, relaxation therapy, and acupressure can be useful as an adjuvant to medical therapy in some pediatric patients.

The general approach to analgesic therapy is to employ intravenous (IV) agents while the patient is unable to tolerate a regular diet and then to transition to oral analgesics once a regular diet is tolerated, be that solid food or tube feedings. The expectation is that after 5 to 7 days the child will require less frequent dosing of oral narcotics, and usually within 7 to 10 days postoperatively the pain will be successfully managed with nonnarcotic and nonpharmacologic interventions.

Pediatric practice includes five distinct patient age demographics, namely neonates (including premature babies), infants and toddlers, preschoolers, school-aged children, and adolescents. Although each demographic includes special considerations that can impact analgesic therapy from the pain assessment perspective, the lion's share of pharmacologic maturation takes place in the first year of life.

2.2 Pediatric Pain Assessment

Pain was defined by the International Association for the Study of Pain in 1994 as "An unpleasant sensory and emotional experience associated with actual or potential tissue damage, or described in terms of such damage."[2] As with any medical intervention, the efficacy of pain management must be considered and assessed in a systematic construct. The anatomic structures necessary for the pain experience, specifically the cortex with thalamic projections and peripheral nerves with projections to the spinal cord, are present as early as 26 weeks of gestation, although in an immature form.[3]

The routine provokes, quality, radiates, severity, time (PQRST) rubric used to characterize pain in adults is sometimes inadequate in children because of a lack of patient experience with the pain environment or an inability to connect nociception with an experience by the child. Additionally, distress and situational factors may influence the reported pain experience. Physiologic markers alone may also be inadequate to assess the pain experience, especially in the face of dehydration and fever. For these reasons, and usually in the first 3 to 4 years of life, caregiver observational measures for pain assessment are used in addition to self-reporting. Assessment of pain in children requires a multimodal approach, utilizing the patient's narrative, family and caregiver observations, and the historical experience of the nursing and medical staff.

2.2.1 Observational Pain Assessment Tools

The FLACC scale, an observational assessment tool which rates Face, Legs, Activity, Cry, and Consolability on a 0 to 2 (0 = none/normal, 1 = some, 2 = frequent/constant) scale for a maximum score of 10, is simple to use and reliable and is validated for use in children ranging from 4 to 18 years of age for assessing post-operative pain and pain associated with painful procedures.[4] A FLACC score of 4 or more is indicative of pain. The FLACC rating scale has also been validated for use in assessing pain after immunization in 2- through 6-month-old infants,[5] and is commonly used for pain assessment in all children.

2.2.2 Self-reported Pain Assessment Tools

For children capable of self-reporting their pain experience, a variety of evaluation tools to assess the intensity of the pain exist. The Poker Chip Tool Method can be used in children as young as 3 years old and involves showing the child four red poker chips and asking them to show how many pieces of hurt they have. Although toddlers may not have counting skills, they are capable of understanding "more" and "less" and this tool has been validated for this age group.[6] The Wong-Baker Faces scale has been validated to assess pain in school-aged children.[7] The visual analog scale (VAS) is a 100-mm horizontal line anchored at each end by nonstandardized verbal descriptor anchors such as "no pain" and "pain as bad as it could be." The VAS can be used for children as young as 5 years old, and is sensitive to changes in pain associated with analgesic therapy. The Numerical Rating Scale (NRS), which is probably the most widely used in verbal school-aged children, and is simply a query for a score from 1 to 10, is validated in children older than 8 years.[8]

Preverbal, nonverbal, developmentally delayed, cognitively impaired, and demented patients are all at risk for inadequate analgesia.[9] Facial expression, while not a reliable pain assessment tool in verbal patients, is of utility in assessing the pain experience in nonverbal patients. The Non-communicating Children's Pain Checklist–Post-operative Version (NCPC-PV) is a formal pain assessment tool that has been used successfully for nonverbal children in the hospital setting. This tool allowed adult caregivers who were unfamiliar with their pediatric patients to accurately assess signs of postoperative pain.[10] The NCPC-CV can be used to supplement clinical judgment in nonverbal children with special needs.

2.3 Pediatric Pharmacokinetics

2.3.1 General

The main body components that affect drug distribution are muscle mass, total body water content, fat content, and plasma protein content. In the neonatal period, there are less muscle mass, less fat content, and greater total body water content as compared to the adult. The plasma proteins responsible for drug distribution and elimination are diminished as well. All of these differences are exaggerated in preterm infants. Hepatic phase 1 oxidative reactions carried out by the cytochrome P450 enzymes reach adult values generally within the first year of life. Phase 2 conjugation reactions, such as glucuronidation, generally reach adult levels by 6 to 12 months of age. Renal clearance of drugs for drugs predominantly cleared in the kidney is decreased in the first month of life, and reaches adult values after 6 months of age. Lipophilic drugs such as diazepam can be expected to have a smaller volume of distribution, less plasma protein binding, and lower hepatic clearance in neonates. Hydrophilic drugs such as morphine will have a greater volume of distribution; however, clearance and elimination are decreased. Considering these differences and the lack of predictability during illness, it is imperative that infants and toddlers receiving analgesic therapy are in a monitored setting with caregivers who are skilled at assessing and treating pain in children. Furthermore, physicians prescribing analgesics for children must be aware of the complications and side effects of these medications and be prepared to manage them.

2.4 Impact of Preexisting Comorbidities on Analgesic Management

Fortunately, most pediatric patients do not share the acquired health problems of adults; however, as more children survive previously life-threatening conditions, we do see pediatric patients with chronic health problems from varying stages of corrected or palliated congenital heart defects, genetic metabolic errors, and malignancies. In addition, the neurosurgical patient population has a higher incidence of preexisting neurologic deficits from congenital defects such as spina bifida and myopathies. Pediatric patients who have survived traumatic brain and spinal cord injury (SCI) also present challenges for analgesic management.

2.4.1 Childhood Obesity

It is estimated that one out of six children and adolescents in the United States are either overweight or obese.[11] Obesity-related comorbidities that are of particular importance in pain management are obstructive sleep apnea and obesity hypoventilation syndrome, suspicion of which (unless specifically ruled out by polysomnogram) requires cardiorespiratory monitoring in the perioperative period to guide safe administration of opioid analgesics and other sedating adjuvants. In children, tonsillectomy and adenoidectomy (T&A) surgery is assumed to cure most airway obstructive symptoms; however, in obese children who have undergone T&A, there may be persistent respiratory rhythmogenic failure postoperatively.[12]

Nonalcoholic steatohepatitis is also a feature of childhood obesity; however, its implication for pain management other than following weekly liver function enzyme testing in the face of prolonged acetaminophen dosing is unknown.

Therapeutic Modifications

In general, pharmacokinetic considerations for hydrophilic drugs such as morphine and hydromorphone suggest that bolus dosing be based on lean body weight instead of total body weight.[13] For lipophilic drugs such as fentanyl, initial dosing based on lean body mass may undertreat pain; however, subsequent maintenance dosing based on lean body weight is advisable.[13] Strategies for administering analgesics in children with obstructive sleep apnea include consideration of nonopioid analgesics (acetaminophen, nonsteroidal anti-inflammatory drugs [NSAIDs]), initiating opioid therapy with lower than standard dosing and increasing if needed. If using IV patient-controlled analgesia (PCA), the strategy includes starting with lower than standard basal rates and transitioning to oral/enteral medications as quickly as possible. Wound infiltration with local anesthetics during wound closure, if possible, is advisable, as is using preemptive scalp blocks for intracranial procedures.

2.4.2 Seizures

Pediatric neurosurgical patients have an increased risk of seizures because of both preoperative congenital and acquired comorbidities such as neurofibromatosis, cerebral palsy, and brain tumors. Drugs used to treat seizures exhibit varying degrees of protein binding and hepatic enzyme induction that impact the pharmacokinetics of analgesic and sedative drugs by causing a relative resistance to their effects.[14] In addition, antiepileptic drugs exhibit side effects such as sedation, hypotension, encephalopathy, and gastrointestinal (GI) disturbances that may be mistakenly attributed to analgesics or their withdrawal. These considerations highlight the need for conservative dosing, careful patient monitoring, and consideration of subjective and objective pain assessment tools.

2.4.3 Myopathies, Myotonias, and Spinal Muscular Atrophy

Myopathies present a heterogeneous group of disorders sharing a common trait of mitochondrial origin and lactic acidosis from an inefficient metabolism of pyruvate with a resultant shift to anaerobic metabolism. Children with myopathies exhibit generalized weakness and are at risk for respiratory insufficiency.

Myotonic dystrophy is a degenerative disease of the skeletal muscles linked to the myotonin-protein kinase gene and a resulting sodium and chloride channel defect ("channelopathies") producing pathologic muscle membrane depolarization, which results in muscle wasting.

Spinal muscular atrophy, caused by degeneration of spinal motor neurons, is one of the most common inherited lethal diseases in childhood, and results in floppy limbs and swallowing difficulties.[15]

Although these disorders have different etiologies and varying severity of presentation, they share common features of progressive functional deterioration especially with stress. Patients with these conditions are at increased risk for respiratory failure postoperatively, and may require invasive or noninvasive respiratory support. As in the other special needs populations, these considerations highlight the need for conservative dosing, use of nonsedating adjuvants and local anesthetics, careful patient monitoring, and implementation of subjective and objective pain assessment tools.

2.4.4 Chronic Pain and Preexisting Painful Conditions

Postoperative pain management may be confounded by preoperative conditions incidental to the surgical procedure, such as headaches with Chiari I malformation and back pain from scoliosis. Demographic factors such as female gender, adolescence, and surgical approach may predispose patients to more intense postoperative pain.[16] Patients who have been maintained on an analgesic regimen prior to surgical intervention should be expected to require supplemental analgesics in addition to resumption of the preoperative medications. The extent of supplementation is variable, and is related to the dosing and schedule of administration. The additional duration of analgesic therapy in this setting is variable as well, considering that in many cases the impetus for surgery is the elimination of chronic pain. This result may take time to achieve, and may coincide with increased analgesic requirements to treat acute postoperative pain. Children who have been receiving opioid analgesics for more than 2 weeks preoperatively may be at risk for abstinence syndrome and may require gradual medication tapering before complete discontinuation of the opioid. Abstinence syndrome is manifest by symptoms including irritability, diarrhea, fever, tachypnea, anorexia, insomnia, sweating tremors, hyperreflexia, and emesis. In addition, children receiving long-term therapy with benzodiazepines and α-2 adrenergic agonists may require dose tapering before discontinuation of these drugs as well, in consideration of similar physical dependence. Occasionally, patients will have been taking medications preoperatively that are discontinued abruptly postoperatively. This may result in rebound hyperalgesia, and may require reinstating an existing medication or initiating a new drug class to optimize analgesia.

2.5 Analgesic Considerations for Specific Neurosurgical Procedures

2.5.1 Intracranial Tumors

In the pediatric population, brain tumors are the most common type of solid tumors and, along with leukemia, account for more than half of all new cases of cancer.[17] Intracranial tumors in the pediatric population may be broadly classified as either supratentorial or infratentorial, based on the anatomical location, in relation to the tentorium cerebelli. The importance of the site of the craniotomy has been demonstrated in adult studies, where pain in infratentorial region, for example, posterior fossa surgery, is significantly higher in comparison to frontal craniotomy, i.e., supratentorial location.[18] This may be explained by the need for greater muscle and soft-tissue dissection in infratentorial areas, particularly especially in the region of the neck.

The perception that craniotomies are "painless" may have originated from the fact that the brain is considered to be insensate. Yet, pain from other structures cannot be ignored as significant sources of postoperative pain. Postcraniotomy pain is of somatic origin originating from the scalp, pericranial muscles, soft tissue, and dura mater manipulation.[19]

Several studies have shown that contrary to historical perception, the adult population does experience significant pain following craniotomies.[20] Adult studies have reported 10 to 15% of patients experience severe pain in the immediate postoperative period, with 15 to 50% of patients reporting severe chronic postcraniotomy headaches. Postcraniotomy headaches may be debilitating and are often closely correlated to inadequate analgesia in the acute postcraniotomy period.

The literature is limited on postcraniotomy pain specifically in the pediatric population. Yet, there are studies that have demonstrated an inverse relationship between age and incidence of postcraniotomy pain.[21]

The mainstay of postoperative analgesia after craniotomy is intraoperative scalp block combined with NSAIDs and opioids. Preoperative scalp block using local anesthetic can decrease intraoperative anesthetic requirements and can influence intensity and duration of postoperative craniotomy pain.[22] The value of a nerve block performed prior to incision is based on the theory of "preemptive analgesia," which blunts intense nociceptor stimulation and thus prevents central sensitization. Central sensitization is the process of dynamic range adjustment by neurons of the central nervous system so that subsequent noxious stimuli are experienced with even greater intensity.

A scalp block alone will not provide prolonged analgesia in a neurosurgical patient who has undergone an invasive surgery such as craniotomy. Opioids are clearly the most effective analgesic agent, but are often withheld because of the side effects that may impact assessment and management perioperatively. Aggressive pain management may result in an overly sedated patient, which may mask signs of neurological deterioration.

Additionally, the direct respiratory depressant effect of opioids may result in hypoventilation and hypercarbia, which will directly result in increased cerebral blood flow and increased intracranial pressure. On the other hand, pain that is poorly treated may result in hypertension and increased intracranial pressure and cause unwanted neurological effects. Thus, pain management with opioids requires a delicate balance, and may be safely undertaken especially if combined with non-opioid analgesics in order to reduce the total amount of opioid given to the patient.

2.5.2 Intracranial Cerebrovascular Disease

Intracranial cerebrovascular disease, in respect of the pediatric population, includes arteriovenous (AV) malformations and moyamoya disease. Moyamoya is a rare chronic cerebrovascular disease which presents with variable clinical symptoms that are progressive in nature. Clinically, the disease may present with: ischemic stroke, intracranial hemorrhage, seizures, headache, and transient ischemic attack.

Physiologically, it occurs due to progressive stenosis/occlusion of terminal portions of the internal carotid arteries and the proximal portion of the anterior and middle cerebral arteries. The name of the disease originates from Japan, where moyamoya means a "puff of smoke," in reference to the angiographic demonstration of the collaterals that form due to the stenosis, giving it such an appearance.

The most effective treatment for this disease is surgical, and optimal pain management postoperatively is a necessity. Pain in these children must be avoided because of an increase in cerebral metabolism that occurs with pain. Recurrence of symptoms such as headache and transient ischemic attacks may be triggered by pain and straining during crying or coughing. Inadequate analgesia may even cause postoperative cerebral infarction.[23]

Despite the sedation and side effect profile of opioids, they are considered the mainstay of a pain regimen to manage analgesia in a child with moyamoya. Effective analgesia must be achieved while preventing oversedation, since frequent neurological checks will be required in a disease that can cause neurological deterioration unexpectedly and rapidly. Again, adopting the multimodal analgesic approach is most beneficial, with the goal of avoiding the side effects of larger doses of each individual agent.

AV malformations are another cerebrovascular condition which may be seen in children. These occur when there is a connection between an intracranial artery and vein, which bypasses the capillary system. Clinically, these present if the malformation expands or bleeds, causing seizure, focal neurological deficit, or pain.[24] AV malformations present acutely; thus, it is important to once again provide analgesia while avoiding oversedation as frequent neurological checks will be necessary. Since extremes of blood pressure may be detrimental, with hypertension possibly causing bleeding and hypotension preventing adequate brain perfusion, it is essential to maintain analgesia and sedation, while also maintaining hemodynamic stability.

2.5.3 Craniofacial Reconstruction/ Calvarial Bone Tumors

Craniofacial reconstruction for craniosynostosis is a fairly high-risk, invasive surgery. Many children will receive blood transfusions because of blood loss which mainly occurs at the scalp and cranium. Early repair will allow expansion of the intracranial vault and prevent hydrocephalus from a rapidly growing brain within a confined space. The postoperative pain is much less dramatic in comparison to the surgical repair that has been performed. Most of these children will be kept comfortable with opioids usually in the form of intermittent IV dosing or PCA pump. In the pediatric population, this pump is controlled either by parent or nurse, depending on individual institutional guidelines and experience.

Continuous infusion of opioids is sometimes avoided in order to allow for early clinical recognition of neurological deficits.

2.5.4 Spinal Cord Disorders

Scoliosis in the pediatric age group is differentiated by etiology and includes congenital scoliosis, idiopathic adolescent scoliosis, and neuromuscular scoliosis. The complexity of the surgery is usually dictated by the curvature of the spine that is to be corrected. Because of extensive involvement of muscles and bones of the spine, as well as placement of hardware such as screws and rods, the postoperative course may be challenging and often requires trial and error to find a regimen that manages pain while also minimizing side effects.

These patients benefit from a true multimodal regimen, including opioids, initially in the form of an IV PCA. Because of extensive muscle resection, the patients will be at high risk of muscle spasm; thus, diazepam or a similar drug given around the clock can help prevent severe muscle spasm pain. Usually, because of concerns for bone growth healing, NSAIDs such as ibuprofen and ketorolac are avoided. Acetaminophen is also beneficial and may help decrease the opioid requirement. An effective analgesic plan for the postscoliosis repair patient is essential to aid in physical therapy and mobilization. Poor pain control often delays discharge from the hospital, and as one of the most painful procedures that a child may undergo, progress often goes hand in hand with sufficient analgesia.

2.5.5 Chiari Malformation

Chiari malformations are anatomic abnormalities of the posterior fossa causing cephalad displacement of the cerebellar vermis through the foramen magnum. The malformations are categorized by the severity of the disorder and by the parts of the brain that protrude into the spinal canal. Symptoms vary depending on the type of malformation, but may include such complaints as neck pain, imbalance, muscle weakness, and paresthesias.

Treatment of the malformation is often dependent on the symptoms. Extreme cases may require neurosurgical intervention.[25] Chiari type 1 malformation is of a milder variety; these patients are often treated conservatively for chronic headache and neck pain. Pain treatments may include traditional agents such as opioids, NSAIDs, muscle relaxants, and antidepressants drugs. Patients may also benefit from physical therapy.

2.5.6 Traumatic Brain Injury

Patients sustaining traumatic brain injury (TBI) can present with neurological impairment along a spectrum of incapacitation ranging from mild headache and memory loss through coma. In this setting, loss of cognitive and communicative function may necessitate implementation of pain assessment tools used for nonverbal or cognitively impaired children. Parental input is essential when trying to assess pain levels and provide analgesic therapy. A reasonable rule of thumb is to assume that obvious tissue injury is painful (e.g., long bone fracture), and will require analgesia. As in other instances of neurological injury, overmedication resulting in persistent sedation will prevent assessment of the neurological examination and must be avoided. Strategies for pain management in this setting include lowering doses and using nonnarcotic adjuvants to synergize the narcotic effects. In some situations, it may be possible to include local anesthetics in the management of musculoskeletal injuries, in the form of either field blocks or peripheral nerve blocks.

Days or weeks after severe TBI (Glasgow Coma Scale [GCS] < 8) patients may develop sympathetic storming, which manifests as episodic agitation, fever, posturing, and diaphoresis. These episodes place the patient at risk for secondary brain injury, hypertension, and arrhythmias. This storming is often observed concomitantly with weaning of analgesics and sedatives in the intensive care unit (ICU) setting. Therapeutic strategies include prolonging or foregoing the narcotic weaning process, transitioning to longer-acting narcotics to avoid the peak and trough effect, and initiating adjuvant therapies, such as clonidine, an α-2 receptor agonist that reduces circulating levels of norepinephrine and epinephrine.

2.5.7 Spinal Cord Injury

SCI patients may initially exhibit loss of sensation both above and below the level of spinal injury, and it is common to find that patients who have sustained upper body injuries in addition to the spinal injury will report these "new" pain symptoms days after the initial trauma. In this setting, new pain complaints must be evaluated for etiology in addition to treating pain symptoms. In addition, once the initial spinal shock resolves, with spinal injuries above the level of the splanchnic outflow (T6) autonomic dysreflexia (AD) may occur. AD results from the stimulation of intact peripheral sensory nerves below the SCI and the interruption of the course of the ascending sympathetic neurons combined with the interruption of the descending inhibitory pathways which produce hypertension and vasodilation above the SCI results in headache. Vasomotor brainstem reflexes attempt to lower the blood pressure by increasing parasympathetic tone to the heart, producing bradycardia, and parasympathetic signs of sweating and flushing above the level of spinal injury. A balanced analgesic approach may mitigate signs of AD.

2.5.8 Hydrocephalus and Interventricular Shunts

Whether the cause of hydrocephalus is obstruction to cerebrospinal fluid (CSF) outflow or CSF overproduction, hydrocephalus causes headache. The treatment of hydrocephalus is surgical;

indeed, administration of narcotics in the setting of hydrocephalus can result in rapid and potentially lethal decompensation. In addition to post-op pain from the procedure, there may be a component of superimposed chronic headache pain. Furthermore, in the immediate post-operative phase, pain management may be complicated by chronic analgesic use, inappropriate coping skills, and withering family dynamics. The overall analgesic strategies remain the same, and include careful narcotic titration and use of nonnarcotic adjuvants to diminish sedation and unwanted narcotic side effects. In addition, behavioral psychology and liaison psychiatry services may be required to manage the longstanding issues associated with chronic headaches and analgesic dependence.

2.5.9 Peripheral Nerve Injury/Repair

Peripheral nerve injury and pain that arises from repair of such injury usually result in neuropathic pain. In addition to the pain, patients will also have motor and sensory deficits from the nerve injury itself. Mild pain may initially be treated with NSAIDs. More moderate pain may respond to tricyclic antidepressants (TCAs), such as nortriptyline or antiepileptics such as gabapentin. If these more conservative approaches are unsuccessful, opioids may be useful, although opioids have limited success with neuropathic pain and oftentimes lead to escalating doses and dependence. Neuropathic pain may be also be amenable to more aggressive treatment such as spinal cord stimulators.[26]

2.5.10 Implantable Devices

Post-operative analgesia for implantable devices (vagal nerve stimulators, baclofen pumps) in children requires an appreciation for the preoperative status of the patient and any home medications that may impact post-operative analgesic therapy such as antiepileptics that induce hepatic enzymes and may increase clearance of narcotics and sedatives. (See the section Seizures earlier.) In addition, patients may be receiving medications such as valium at home that have sedative effects that may be synergized by residual anesthetic agents and perioperative analgesics. In this setting, it is advisable for patients to be cared for in a monitored setting with caregivers skilled in assessing and treating pain in children. Special monitoring should be maintained until the child resumes their regular diet and is able to tolerate enteral analgesics and is neurologically at baseline.

2.6 Common Analgesics Used in Children

2.6.1 Opioids

Opioids can be used safely in children. ▶ Table 2.1 and ▶ Table 2.2 list the most commonly used enteral and parenteral narcotic medications and their doses.[27] Opioids can be prescribed in an "as needed" schedule for patients with mild pain; however, scheduled dosing is preferable in acute painful conditions, especially the postoperative setting. PCA has been shown to be safe and

Table 2.1 Oral agents

Drug	Parenteral/oral ratio	Starting doses and intervals	
		<50 kg (mg/kg)	>50 kg and adult (mg flat dose)
Oxycodone	N/A	0.1 mg/kg every 3–4 h	5–10 mg every 3–4 h
Morphine			
Immediate release	1:3	0.3 mg/kg every 3–4 h	15–20 mg every 3–4 h
Sustained release	1:5	Flat dose only!! 20–35 kg: 10–15 mg every 8–12 h 35–50 kg: 15–30 mg every 8–12 h	30–45 mg every 8–12 h
Hydromorphone	1:2–1:4	0.03–0.08 mg/kg every 3–4 h	1–2 mg every 3–4 h
Methadone	1:2	0.2 mg/kg every 4–8 h	10 mg every 4–8 h
Codeine	NR[a]		30–60 mg every 3–4 h

[a]Because of the FDA Black Box warning against use of this drug in post-operative pediatric T&A patients, and evidence of pharmacogenetic metabolic variation, the use of this drug is not recommended for pediatric neurosurgical patients.[28]

Table 2.2 Parenteral agents

Drug	Equianalgesic IV dose (mg)	Starting doses and intervals	
		<50 kg (mg/kg)	>50 kg and adult (mg flat dose)
Fentanyl	0.1	0.5–1.0 µg/kg every 1–2 h	25–50 µg/kg every 1–2 h
Morphine	10	Bolus: 0.05–0.1 mg/kg every 1–2 h Infusion: 0.025 mg/kg/h	Bolus: 2.5–5 mg every 0.5–2 h Infusion: 1–2 mg/h
Hydromorphone	1.5–2	Bolus: 0.02 mg/kg every 1–2 h Infusion: 0.03–0.04 mg/kg/h	Bolus: 1 mg every 1–2 h Infusion: 0.2–0.3 mg/h
Methadone	10	0.1 mg/kg every 4–8 h	5–10 mg every 4–8 h
Meperidine	75–100	NR[a]	NR

[a]Meperidine is metabolized to normeperidine, which can cause seizures.

Table 2.3 Common drugs for treatment of narcotic side effects

Side effect	Drug	Starting doses and intervals	
		<50 kg (mg/kg)	>50 kg and adult (mg flat dose)
Constipation	Senna (oral only)	10 mg/kg Bedtime	187–364 mg Bedtime
Constipation	Docusate (oral only)	10 mg/kg Every 4 h	50–500 mg In 1–4 doses Not to exceed 500 mg per day
Nausea	Serotonin receptor antagonists (IV only)	Zofran 0.15 mg/kg every 6 h	4 mg every 6 h
		Dolasetron 0.35 mg/kg every 6 h	12.5 mg every 6 h
Nausea and itching	Diphenhydramine (IV or oral)	0.5–1 mg/kg every 4–6 h Can be sedating	25–50 mg every 4–6 h Can be sedating

Abbreviation: IV, intravenous.

effective in children; however, managing PCA for children should not be undertaken by novices and is outside the scope of this textbook.

Side Effects of Opioids

Common side effects of opioids include sedation, pruritus, and opioid-induced bowel dysfunction, which is manifested by nausea or combined constipation and nausea. ▶ Table 2.3 lists the common drugs for treatment of narcotic side effects most patients receiving narcotics will develop some degree of bowel dysfunction ranging from constipation to nausea and vomiting. Itching is also a common side effect of narcotic therapy, usually worse with parenteral administration of narcotics and narcotic infusions. Low-dose naloxone infusions have been shown to be effective for treating itching related to IV narcotic therapy; however, this should only be undertaken by practitioners who are expert in the management of pain in children. Sedation is an effect of narcotics, although sometimes unwanted. Strategies to avoid sedation include dose reduction and increasing interval of dosing, although this can be difficult if the pain is severe. Another alternative is to switch from one drug to another, in equianalgesic doses.

2.6.2 Nonnarcotic Analgesics
NSAIDs

NSAIDs inhibit the enzymes COX-1 and COX-2, thereby preventing production of central and peripheral prostaglandins. This group of drugs include: acetaminophen, aspirin, ibuprofen, naproxen, and ketorolac. Inhibition of COX-1 is responsible for GI complications such as ulceration and bleeding. Certain NSAIDs (particularly ketorolac) also have other undesirable actions such as reversible antiplatelet adhesion and aggregation effects and negative effect on bone growth and healing.[29] Concerns about bleeding limit the use of NSAIDs in the perioperative setting (▶ Table 2.4).

Despite these side effects, there remains an effective role for NSAIDs within the realm of pain management. NSAIDs are considered "weaker" analgesics and are combined with other pharmacological therapies in order to effectively treat postoperative pain from neurosurgical procedures.

The analgesic properties of NSAIDs make them useful as adjuvant, opioid-sparing agents.

Acetaminophen

Acetaminophen primarily prevents central production of prostaglandin, with minimal anti-inflammatory action. It may also produce analgesia

Table 2.4 Nonopioid analgesics

Drug	Starting doses and intervals	
	<50 kg (mg/kg)	>50 kg and adult (mg flat dose)
Ketorolac	0.5 mg/kg IM/IV every 6 h, up to maximum of 72 h	30 mg every 6 h, not to exceed 120 mg/d
Ibuprofen	5–10 mg/kg orally; not to exceed 40 mg/kg/d	300–800 mg orally every 6 h
Acetaminophen	**Oral** **Neonates** Dose: 10–15 mg/kg orally every 6–8 h. Maximum: 60 mg/kg/d **Infants/children** Dose: 10–15 mg/kg orally every 4–6 h. Maximum: 75 mg/kg/d up to 1 g/4 h and 4 g/d **>12 y** Dose: 325–650 mg orally every 4–6 h. Maximum: 1 g/4 h and 4 g/d	**Oral** 325–650 mg orally every 4 h or 500 mg orally every 8 h
	IV 12.5 mg/kg IV every 4 h or 15 mg/kg IV every 6 h Not to exceed 750 mg/dose or 3.75 g/d	**IV** 650 mg IV every 4 h or 1,000 mg IV every 6 h Not to exceed 4 g/d
	Clonidine	**Oral and transdermal** 1 µg/kg/dose every 4 h orally
Oral and transdermal 1 µg/kg/dose every 4 h orally		
Diazepam	**Oral** 0.12–0.8 mg/kg/d every 6–8 h	**Oral** 2–10 mg/kg/d every 6–8 h
	IV 0.05–0.1 mg/kg every 4–6 h	**IV** 2–10 mg IV/IM every 3–4 h No more than 30 mg/8 h
Gabapentin	**3–12 y** 10–15 mg/kg/d divided every 8 h **>12 y** 300 mg orally every 8 h, may increase up to 600 mg orally every 8 h	300 mg orally at bedtime, then gradually increase as tolerated to 300 mg every 8 h
Amitriptyline	**Load:** 0.1 mg/kg orally at bedtime; increase as tolerated over 2–3 wk	**Load:** 75 mg/d orally
	Maintenance 0.5–2 mg/kg orally at bedtime	**Maintenance** 150–300 mg/d orally in single or divided doses

Abbreviations: IM, intramuscular; IV, intravenous.

by antagonizing substance P and the N-methyl-D-aspartate (NMDA) receptor at the level of spinal cord. It may be administered in a variety of routes: oral, IV, or rectal. It is considered a weaker analgesic and must usually be combined with other analgesics in order to effectively treat postoperative pain.

Acetaminophen has toxic potential, and is one of the main causes of liver failure in the United States; thus, dosages must be kept well within daily limit (less than 4 gm/day, though Food and Drug Administration (FDA) has proposed decreasing this limit to 3.25 gm/day in adults).[30] Acetaminophen has historically been combined with opioids in such formulations as Vicodin, but these formulations are becoming increasingly rare because of the risk of acetaminophen toxicity. In the pediatric age group, this is especially an area of concern and acetaminophen/opioid combination analgesics are not recommended.

Ibuprofen

Ibuprofen has analgesic, anti-inflammatory, and antipyretic properties. It acts by nonselectively inhibiting COX-1 and COX-2. Ibuprofen has a strong association with gastric ulceration and bleeding, and thus must be used with caution.

Ketorolac

Ketorolac acts by nonselectively inhibiting COX-1 and COX-2 and also has analgesic, anti-inflammatory, and antipyretic activity. Ketorolac must be used with caution perioperatively and postoperatively because of inhibition of platelet aggregation. Because of known side effects, its use is limited to 5 days or less, with most practitioners cautiously discontinuing it after 3 days of use. Other adverse effects include gastric ulcers/bleeding and renal dysfunction. It is most commonly administered intravenously or intramuscularly; although oral formulations are manufactured, they are not widely available.

Acetylsalicylic Acid

Salicylate, one of the oldest nonopioid drugs available, suppresses production of prostaglandin and thromboxane by irreversible inactivation of COX-1 and COX-2 enzymes. Aspirin has been widely abandoned as adjuvant in postoperative pain management, secondary to platelet inhibition and its known association with gastric ulcers and bleed-

ing. In the pediatric population, it has also been long abandoned because of its possible implication with Reye's syndrome.[29]

Clonidine

Clonidine is a widely used drug with a variety of indications and routes of administration. Though primarily known as an antihypertensive, it is also an effective analgesic. Clonidine can be administered by a variety of routes: IV, oral, transdermal, epidural, and intrathecal. It provides sedation and analgesia and is very effective in the treatment of withdrawal symptoms from opioids and benzodiazepines.

Clonidine is an α-2 agonist, which works presynaptically and causes a decrease in norepinephrine release, at central as well as peripheral adrenergic receptors. The pain pathway includes inhibition of these signals at the dorsal horn of the spinal cord and then continues to higher CNS centers. Norepinephrine is released in the dorsal horn as an inhibitory pain neurotransmitter, when there is stimulation of the α-2 receptor. The modulation of pain transmission produces analgesia and makes clonidine an effective nonopioid adjuvant. Clonidine also produces analgesia by cholinergic activation in the dorsal horn of the spinal cord by increasing acetylcholine levels in CSF when administered intrathecally.

Clonidine is used as an adjuvant analgesic, primarily as an opioid-sparing agent, for the neurosurgical patient. With judicious use of clonidine, it is possible to reduce the amount of opioid used postoperatively. Clonidine may cause bradycardia, hypotension, and excessive sedation. Dexmedetomidine is another α-2 agonist, which has more selective action in comparison to clonidine and produces potent sedation without respiratory depression, thus explaining its popularity in postoperative ICU sedation as well as for deep procedural sedation.

Antidepressants

This group of medications includes TCAs, such as amitriptyline, and newer drugs, such as duloxetine. Antidepressants produce analgesia by inhibition of re-uptake of 5-HT and norepinephrine, and also have other effects such as NMDA antagonism, decrease in sympathetic α-2 receptor activity and sodium channel blockade.[29]

The older group of antidepressants, the TCAs, has greater analgesic effect compared to newer agents and is beneficial for treating neuropathic. The cleaner pharmacological profile of the newer antidepressants seems to have decreased its utility as an analgesic.

Antiepileptic Analgesics

This group of drugs is most beneficial in the treatment of neuropathic pain. The original drug of this group that was most studied is carbamazepine. Carbamazepine has a long list of drug interactions, which are not seen with the newer drugs, including gabapentin and pregabalin, a group of weak anticonvulsants which bind at voltage-gated calcium channels. Despite their names, these drugs do not have any involvement with gammaaminobutyric acid (GABA) receptors. They produce analgesia by decreasing the presynaptic release of neurotransmitters that are responsible for producing pain, such as glutamate, norepinephrine, and substance P.

NMDA Receptor Antagonists

This group of drugs includes ketamine and methadone, both of which have been proven to be beneficial in the treatment of chronic pain. Ketamine is primarily used as a general anesthetic adjuvant and is helpful in decreasing opioid usage perioperatively. Ketamine also acts by decreasing central hypersensitivity. Its use is limited by its hallucinogenic properties, which may be prevented by co-administering a benzodiazepine, although this side effect limits its use outside of the perioperative arena.

Methadone, another well-established drug for pediatric pain management, has dual mechanism of action, acting at both opioid receptors and NMDA receptors. It is an excellent long-lasting analgesic agent, especially beneficial in weaning protocols for patients who have opioid dependence. Methadone does affect the cardiac QT interval, and electrocardiographic (ECG) monitoring is indicated with initiation and long-term use of the drug.

Muscle Relaxants

Muscle relaxants are divided into two groups: neuromuscular blockers and spasmolytic. In reference to pain management, the focus is on spasmolytic, which is centrally acting and help to relieve spasms and musculoskeletal pain. These medications also confer an element of sedation, which may be beneficial in the immediate postoperative period, but are undesirable once a patient seeks to return to normal daily activities.

The commonly used muscle relaxants include benzodiazepines, such as diazepam, baclofen, and cyclobenzaprine. Muscle relaxants are beneficial in postoperative analgesia and help to alleviate painful muscle spasms that are not relieved with opioids. By adding spasmolytics to a pain regimen, opioid consumption may be drastically reduced.

Local Anesthetics

Local anesthetic wound infiltration can provide sensory analgesia and diminish the need for narcotics in the postoperative setting. Local anesthetics can be used for most incision wounds, including craniotomy and implantable device battery generator pockets. It is not advisable to perform peripheral nerve blocks in patients who have undergone peripheral nerve procedures, since the sensory and motor blockade seen with these blocks will cloud the postoperative neural exam. The most common local anesthetics used for wound infiltration are lidocaine, which should not exceed a dose of 5 mg/kg, and bupivacaine, which should not exceed a dose of 2.5 mg/kg. Epinephrine is often added to these local anesthetics to provide vasoconstriction, and the dose of epinephrine is 0.5 to 1 µg/kg, unless contraindicated by a pre-existing patient condition.

Local Anesthetic Toxicity

Direct intravascular local anesthetic injection must be avoided, and aspiration before injection and slow injection can prevent catastrophe. Local anesthetics have varying degrees of cardiotoxicity, and can cause arrhythmias as well as complete heart block. Local anesthetic overdose can also cause seizures, and the lactic acidosis produced from the seizure combined with the cardiotoxic effects is lethal.

Treatment of Local Anesthetic Toxicity

Supportive therapy of local anesthetic toxicity includes seizure suppression, effective cardiopulmonary resuscitation (CPR) if needed, and airway management. Treatment is with 20% lipid emulsion, 1.5 mL/kg bolus over 1 minute, repeated every 5 minutes for persistent circulatory collapse and an infusion of 0.25 mL/kg/min (can be doubled to 0.5 mL/kg/min if hypotension persists) for a minimum of 30 minutes.

2.6.3 Opioid and Sedative Weaning

General

Weaning of opioid analgesics is necessary in the setting of prolonged opioid therapy. In some children this can be as short as 10 days, and is most likely attributable to some currently unknown pharmacogenomic expression. Certainly after taking narcotics for more than 3 weeks, a weaning plan must be made. In the setting of oral narcotics at usual doses, this weaning may entail nothing more than scheduled spacing of the dose from every 4 to 5 to 6 to 8 to 12 to 24 hours. More frequent dosing, demands for higher doses, and usage beyond the usual postoperative phase should be concerning and the primary care physician or pediatrician should be involved in addressing the problem and may require consultation of an expert in Pediatric Chronic Pain Management.

Calculating the Narcotic Drug Weaning Schedule

Narcotic weaning in the setting of supraphysiologic dosing and multiple drugs can be complicated, and should be guided by experts in pediatric pain medicine. The general approach is to transition the total calculated IV and oral narcotic drug dose to a 24-hour morphine equivalent, taking 60% of that morphine equivalent and converting to a daily methadone dose. The calculated methadone dose (IV or oral) can be given every 6 hours in the first day of transition, and should then be spaced to three times a day (every 8 hours) thereafter. During the transition to methadone, rescue doses of either oral or IV opioid should be available, in a standard dose, such as oxycodone 0.1 mg/kg every 4 hours. During the transition phase and for the duration of weaning, pain scores and withdrawal scores, such as the Neonatal Abstinence Score, must be followed with vigilance for signs and symptoms of withdrawal, which include tachycardia, low-grade fever, diaphoresis, emesis, and diarrhea. Each day the methadone dose should be weaned from 5 to 20% depending on the patient's condition and duration of therapy. Once the methadone is at a normal 0.1 mg/kg or less, the dose interval can be stretched from 8 to 12 hours, and subsequently to a daily dose for a few days and then discontinued. It is suggested that an expert in pediatric pain management be consulted for weaning of narcotics and sedatives in chronically ill children.

Weaning Adjuvant Drugs

Dexmedetomidine and clonidine discontinuation may cause abstinence syndrome and require gradual weaning after as few as 5 days of therapy. The total dose for each drug must be calculated, transitioned to an enteral dose, and weaned systematically, as tolerated. Benzodiazepines may also cause physical dependence, and should be weaned as tolerated in a systematic fashion as well, guided by sedation and abstinence scores. In the setting of multiple drugs requiring weaning, it is recommended that not more than one drug be weaned each day. It is also advisable to have an expert in pediatric pain medicine consult and devise a systematic weaning plan with options for breakthrough medications available. The weaning process may be lengthy, and it may be necessary to slow down or retreat from weaning if signs and symptoms of physical withdrawal develop.

2.7 Review Questions (True or False)

1. Pediatric patients less than 1 year of age do not have the neural mechanisms to feel pain, and so it is not necessary to prescribe pain medications for this age group after surgery.
2. Obese children who have had T&As in the past are at no increased risk of respiratory depression when treated with narcotics for post-operative pain.
3. A 3-year-old child develops a low-grade fever, diaphoresis, tremors, and diarrhea 10 days after a tethered cord repair, and the mother reports that she had given the child the oxycodone that was prescribed every 3 to 4 hours since discharge, but she stopped abruptly 2 days ago when the medication ran out. Is it most likely that this child has a wound infection?
4. The most effective drug to treat local anesthetic toxicity is Dilantin.

References

[1] Taddio A, Katz J, Ilersich AL, Koren G. Effect of neonatal circumcision on pain response during subsequent routine vaccination. Lancet. 1997; 349(9052):599–603
[2] Merskey H, Bogduk N, eds. Part III: Pain terms, a current list with definitions and notes on usage. In: Classification of Chronic Pain. 2nd ed. IASP Task Force on Taxonomy. Seattle, WA: IASP Press; 1994:209–214
[3] Derbyshire SWG. Can fetuses feel pain? BMJ. 2006; 332 (7546):909–912

[4] Merkel SI, Voepel-Lewis T, Shayevitz JR, Malviya S. The FLACC: a behavioral scale for scoring postoperative pain in young children. Pediatr Nurs. 1997; 23(3):293–297

[5] Taddio A, Hogan ME, Moyer P, et al. Evaluation of the reliability, validity and practicality of 3 measures of acute pain in infants undergoing immunization injections. Vaccine. 2011; 29(7):1390–1394

[6] Huguet A, Stinson JN, McGrath PJ. Measurement of self-reported pain intensity in children and adolescents. J Psychosom Res. 2010; 68(4):329–336

[7] Garra G, Singer AJ, Domingo A, Thode HC, Jr. The Wong-Baker pain FACES scale measures pain, not fear. Pediatr Emerg Care. 2013; 29(1):17–20

[8] von Baeyer CL, Spagrud LJ, McCormick JC, Choo E, Neville K, Connelly MA. Three new datasets supporting use of the Numerical Rating Scale (NRS-11) for children's self-reports of pain intensity. Pain. 2009; 143(3):223–227

[9] Herr K, Coyne PJ, Key T, et al. American Society for Pain Management Nursing. Pain assessment in the nonverbal patient: position statement with clinical practice recommendations. Pain Manag Nurs. 2006; 7(2):44–52

[10] Breau LM, Finley GA, McGrath PJ, Camfield CS. Validation of the non-communicating children's pain checklist – postoperative version. Anesthesiology. 2002; 96(3):528–535

[11] Ogden CL, Carroll MD, Kit BK, Flegal KM. Prevalence of obesity and trends in body mass index among US children and adolescents, 1999–2010. JAMA. 2012; 307(5):483–490

[12] O'Brien LM, Sitha S, Baur LA, Waters KA. Obesity increases the risk for persisting obstructive sleep apnea after treatment in children. Int J Pediatr Otorhinolaryngol. 2006; 70(9):1555–1560

[13] Cella M, Knibbe C, Danhof M, Della Pasqua O. What is the right dose for children? Br J Clin Pharmacol. 2010; 70(4):597–603

[14] Kofke WA. Anesthetic management of the patient with epilepsy or prior seizures. Curr Opin Anaesthesiol. 2010; 23 (3):391–399

[15] Sasano N, Fujita Y, So M, Sobue K, Sasano H, Katsuya H. Anesthetic management of a patient with mitochondrial myopathy, encephalopathy, lactic acidosis, and stroke-like episodes (MELAS) during laparotomy. J Anesth. 2007; 21(1):72–75

[16] Vetter TR. A clinical profile of a cohort of patients referred to an anesthesiology-based pediatric chronic pain medicine program. Anesth Analg. 2008; 106(3):786–794

[17] Ward E, DeSantis C, Robbins A, Kohler B, Jemal A. Childhood and adolescent cancer statistics. CA: A Cancer Journal for Clinicians. 2014; 64: 83103. doi:10.3322/caac.21219

[18] National Cancer Institute. Childhood cancers. Available at: http://www.cancer.gov/cancertopics/factsheet/Sites-Types/ childhood. Updated January 10, 2008. Accessed November 1, 2013

[19] Thibault M, Girard F, Moumdjian R, Chouinard P, Boudreault D, Ruel M. Craniotomy site influences postoperative pain following neurosurgical procedures: a retrospective study. Can J Anaesth. 2007; 54(7):544–548

[20] Saha P, Chattopadhyay S, Rudra A, Roy S. Pain after craniotomy: a time for reappraisal? Indian J Pain. 2013; 27(1):7–11

[21] Morad AH, Winters BD, Yaster M, et al. Efficacy of intravenous patient-controlled analgesia after supratentorial intracranial surgery: a prospective randomized controlled trial. Clinical article. J Neurosurg. 2009; 111(2):343–350

[22] Mordhorst C, Latz B, Kerz T, et al. Prospective assessment of postoperative pain after craniotomy. J Neurosurg Anesthesiol. 2010; 22(3):202–206

[23] Nguyen A, Girard F, Boudreault D, et al. Scalp nerve blocks decrease the severity of pain after craniotomy. Anesth Analg. 2001; 93(5):1272–1276

[24] Parray T, Martin TW, Siddiqui S. Moyamoya disease: a review of the disease and anesthetic management. J Neurosurg Anesthesiol. 2011; 23(2):100–109

[25] Pubmed Health. Arteriovenous malformation-cerebral. Available at: http://www.ncbi.nlm.nih.gov/pubmedhealth/ PMH0001783/. Updated November 2, 2012. Accessed November 8, 2013

[26] National Institute of Neurological Disorders and Stroke. Chiari malformation fact sheet. Available at: http://www. ncbi.nlm.nih.gov/pubmedhealth/PMH0001783/. Updated September 30, 2013. Accessed November 5, 2013

[27] Kuehn BM. FDA: No codeine after tonsillectomy for children. JAMA. 2013; 309(11):1100

[28] Bunchorntavakul C, Reddy KR. Acetaminophen-related hepatotoxicity. Clin Liver Dis. 2013; 17(4):587–607, viii

[29] eMedicine. Traumatic peripheral nerve lesions treatment & management. Available at: http://emedicine.medscape.com/ article/1172408-treatment. Updated August 1, 2013. Accessed November 8, 2013

[30] Monitto CL, Kost-Byerly S, Yaster M. Pain management. In: Davis PJ, Cladis FP, Motoyama EK, eds. Smith's Anesthesia for Infants and Children. 8th ed. Philadelphia, PA: Elsevier Mosby; 2011:418–440

Section II

Neuroradiology

II

3 Conventional Radiography

Thierry A.G.M. Huisman

3.1 Introduction

Conventional radiography takes advantage of the differential absorption, penetration, and reflection of roentgen rays (X-rays) by biological tissues. Anatomical structures with a high density such as the calvarial bone appear dense (white), while air-filled paranasal sinuses or soft tissues of the neck appear lucent (dark).

The use of plain radiography should be limited as much as possible in children. Children are more susceptible to the deleterious side effects of ionizing radiation and their life expectancy is significantly longer compared to adults. Each request for a conventional radiography should be carefully evaluated. The benefits should outweigh the possible risks. Alternative nonionizing imaging modalities such as ultrasonography or magnetic resonance imaging (MRI) should be considered. The number of images should be limited as much as possible, and suboptimal images (e.g., due to motion artifacts) should not be repeated if diagnostic. Furthermore, all imaging should follow the as low as reasonably achievable (ALARA) principle taking advantage of newest tube and detector technologies, which allow lowering of the radiation dose.

Conventional radiography remains a valuable, fast, and widely available imaging tool for the workup of many acute (e.g., trauma) and chronic (e.g., remodeling of the skull in neurofibromatosis) neurosurgical pathologies. The two-dimensional, projectional technique allows one to study especially the osseous neuroanatomy in detail. The large field of view may be of advantage to get a quick oversight of, for example, the alignment of the vertebral bodies in kyphoscoliosis. Finally, pathological calcifications (e.g., craniopharyngioma), foreign bodies (penetrating injuries), and the location and integrity of various implant devices (e.g., ventriculoperitoneal shunts, vagus nerve stimulator, position of deep electrodes, baclofen pump, spinal rods) can be evaluated.

3.2 Skull Radiography

Typically, skull radiography is performed in two planes, an anteroposterior (AP) and a lateral projection. Depending on the indication for the study, additional focused views may be completed, including dedicated views of the orbits, sella turcica, paranasal sinuses, and programmable shunt reservoirs.

Nowadays, skull radiography plays only a very limited role in the acute workup of head trauma. Similarly, skull radiography is nowadays rarely used for the preoperative workup of isolated or syndromal craniosynostosis, positional plagiocephaly, or skeletal dysplasias. Computed tomography (CT) allows one to study both the bony calvarium and the brain. In addition, multiplanar two-dimensional as well as three-dimensional image reconstructions render valuable additional diagnostic information, replacing skull radiography in nearly all cases.

Skull and orbital radiography may be performed to rule out ferromagnetic foreign bodies prior to MRI. In addition, skull radiography can be used to follow the position, configuration, and packing of intracranial aneurysm coils and intravascular embolization material.

3.3 Sinus Radiography

Rarely, a preoperative sinus radiography is performed to plan neurosurgical access, in particular for transsphenoidal approaches of sellar pathologies. Similar information can be extracted from a low-dose bone CT study. Acute and chronic sinusitis is nowadays also evaluated by low-dose CT.

3.4 Stenvers and Schüller Radiography

These dedicated focused views of the petrous bone allow evaluation of the inner ear structures and petrous apex in detail. These views have, however, been replaced by low-dose temporal bone CT. On rare occasions, for example, evaluation of the correct positioning of cochlear implants, these views may be considered.

3.5 Shunt Survey

In children with suspected dysfunction of a ventriculoatrial, ventriculopleural, or ventriculoperitoneal shunt, the entire course of the shunt should be evaluated by conventional radiography. The imaging protocol includes radiographies of the skull in two planes (AP and lateral), and single AP views of the neck, chest, and abdomen. Images are evaluated for shunt disconnection, kinking, or fixed positioning of the distal shunt on follow-up imaging possibly within a pseudo-mass lesion, which may indicate that the tip of the shunt is caught within an encapsulated cerebrospinal fluid collection.

3.6 Cervical Spine and Craniocervical Junction

Conventional radiography remains an important tool in the acute workup of craniocervical or cervical spine trauma. Typically, three images are acquired, namely a true AP, lateral, and dedicated transbuccal odontoid view. Imaging can be performed with a neck collar in position. If an instable fracture is ruled out and the child continues to complain about cervical instability and/or pain, functional lateral views in maximal flexion and extension may be added. The cervicothoracic region is frequently obscured by the overlying shoulders. A repeat lateral view with simultaneous downward pulling of the arms may be performed. Alternatively, a "swimmer's view" may offer a better, nonobscured view of the cervicothoracic junction. Oblique lateral views to study the neuroforamina are rarely performed.

Familiarity with the normal developing skeleton is essential to prevent misdiagnosis. Synchondrosis may mimic fractures, the space between the anterior contour of the dens and anterior arch of the first cervical body is wider in children than in adults, and a physiological subluxation between the second and third cervical vertebral body is usually seen. The soft tissues should be scrutinized for soft-tissue swellings. A widening of the prevertebral space may suggest a prevertebral hematoma. Many reference lines have been published in the literature to facilitate diagnosis and quantify pathology. The best known lines include the Swischuk line (spinolaminar line), McRae line, Chamberlain line, Wackenheim line, and many more.

Craniocervical images may also be used to differentiate between a basilar impression, which is often secondary to preexisting conditions, and basilar invagination, which is usually congenital.

Frequently, a CT and/or MRI will follow conventional radiography to rule out, identify, or quantify spinal cord or discoligamentous injury or compression.

3.7 Thoracic and Lumbosacral Radiography

Similar to the cervical spine, AP and lateral views of the thoracic and lumbosacral spinal column may be acquired in trauma, infection, tumor, or malformation. Additional oblique lateral views may be helpful to identify pathologies of the neuroforamina, which may include a widening due to, for example, schwannomas in neurofibromatosis or narrowing related to developmental anomalies such as spondylolysis (dog with neck collar).

3.8 Total Spine Radiography

In the diagnostic workup of multilevel segmentation or formation anomalies (e.g., in Vertebral, anal anomalies, tracheo-esophageal fistula, renal anomalies [VATER] association), in spinal dysraphias, and in cases of idiopathic or acquired scoliosis with or without hyperkyphosis or hyperlordosis, the entire spinal column is examined in an AP and lateral projection. Whenever possible, this should be performed in the upright standing position. The degree of scoliosis is typically quantified by measuring the Cobb angle (named after Dr. John R. Cobb), which refers to the coronal plane deformity seen on an AP view of the spinal column. The Cobb angle is defined as the angle formed between lines perpendicular to a line drawn parallel to the superior end plate and to a line drawn parallel to the inferior end plate of the most tilted superior and inferior vertebral bodies, respectively. The degree of coexistent hyperkyphosis/lordosis is measured on a lateral projection in similar fashion.

Occasionally, an additional AP view of the pelvis will be completed to determine the degree of pelvic tilt.

Whenever possible, the gonads should be shielded for the study.

4 Ultrasonography

Thierry A.G.M. Huisman

4.1 Introduction

Ultrasonography (US) of the central nervous system, orbits, head and neck region, and spine is a safe imaging modality that does not require sedation, can be performed at bedside, is widely available, and is well accepted by patients and their parents.[1] It can be repeated as often as necessary because of the lack of ionizing radiation. Ultrasound can render multiplanar two- and three-dimensional grayscale anatomical images of the central nervous system in high resolution. In addition, color-coded duplex evaluation of the intracranial vasculature with spectral sampling of the arterial pulse waves gives important functional hemodynamic data. US requires a well-trained sonographer or physician familiar with the pediatric pathologies who is able to perform an optimized, personalized study and knows how to take full advantage of technologically advanced, modern US units. Various transducers including vector, curved array, and linear probes capable of scanning at multiple megahertz (MHz) settings should be available and able to attain at least 15 MHz. Moreover, the imaging algorithms within the machine should be optimized for the various age groups (e.g., preterm vs. term neonate). This "tuning" of the machine algorithms in cooperation with the manufacturer's technical representative can dramatically improve resolution, contrast, and conspicuity of pathology.

4.2 Anatomical Ultrasonography of the Brain

Typically, the neonatal brain is sampled in the sagittal and coronal plane through the anterior fontanel. In addition, mastoid fontanel, posterior fontanel, and suboccipital views through the foramen magnum should be included for a better exploration of the contents of the posterior fossa (brain stem and cerebellum). Depending on the probe, three-dimensional data sets may be acquired that allow secondary multiplanar reconstructions, which match the more typical computed tomography (CT) and magnetic resonance imaging (MRI) planes. The used US probe should have a footprint that matches the size of the acoustic window, should be positioned in the center of

the fontanel, and should maintain good contact with the scalp through the use of appropriate amounts of US gel. Depending on the pathology encountered, more detailed assessment of lesions located along the convexity of the cerebral hemispheres may occasionally require additional scanning with higher frequency probes.

Indications for brain US are diverse and depend on the clinical and physical symptoms (e.g., acute onset of seizures, unexplained acute drop in the hematocrit), occurrence of perinatal complications (e.g., perinatal asphyxia or depression), systemic diseases (e.g., coagulation disorders, sepsis), prenatally diagnosed pathologies (e.g., isolated and syndromal ventriculomegaly). In addition, serial brain US studies may be performed as part of routine screening to monitor (e.g., hydrocephalus after intraventricular hemorrhage) or to exclude complications of treatment (e.g., hemorrhage in children on extracorporeal membrane oxygenation). Scanning is also advised before and after major surgery.

With progressing closure of the fontanels, the diagnostic sensitivity of brain ultrasound declines. The time point of fontanel closure varies, but typically highly diagnostic studies are possible until about 4 to 6 months of age. As a rule of thumb, if the fontanel can be palpated, a diagnostic study is possible.

Indications for brain ultrasound:
- Germinal matrix hemorrhage (GMH) grade I, II, and III.
- Periventricular (hemorrhagic) venous infarction, formerly known as grade IV GMH.
- Intraventricular and choroid plexus hemorrhage.
- Parenchymal hemorrhage.
- Extra-axial hemorrhage (epidural, subdural, and subarachnoid hemorrhage).
- Hypoxic ischemic injury (HII).
- Arterial ischemic stroke.
- Brain malformations:
  - Dandy–Walker malformation.
  - Arnold–Chiari II and III malformation.
  - Corpus callosum agenesis/dysgenesis.
  - Septo-optic dysplasia.
  - Holoprosencephaly.
  - Schizencephaly and migrational abnormalities.
  - Vein of Galen aneurysmal malformation.
  - Arachnoid cysts.

- Hydrocephalus:
  - Congenital hydrocephalus (aqueductal stenosis).
  - Acquired (secondary to hemorrhage or infection).
  - Syndromal.
- Infections.
- Trauma.
- Congenital benign and malignant brain tumors (teratoma, lipoma).

Images are evaluated for focal or diffuse imaging findings similar to other cross-sectional imaging modalities.

GMHs are dependent on their age or stage of evolution identified as a focal hyper- or hypoechogenic lesion typically confined to the caudo-thalamic groove (GMH grade I). In grade II GMH, intraventricular extension of the hemorrhage is noted without associated ventriculomegaly, while in GMH grade III intraventricular extension is complicated by ventriculomegaly.

Periventricular venous infarction is believed to be a complication of a GMH at the caudothalamic groove, which compresses the adjacent collector vein that is draining the periventricular white matter into the deep venous system. Consequently, a venous stasis occurs, which may evolve into a venous infarction. The ischemic white matter is typically hyperechogenic in its acute phase and may become progressively hypoechogenic because of progressive tissue resolution. The hyperechogenicity matches the distribution of the venous territory. The periventricular venous ischemia may be complicated by a hemorrhagic transformation resulting in a periventricular hemorrhagic venous infarction. The hemorrhage is typically seen as a focal hyperechogenic mass within the ischemic white matter. These lesions were previously known as grade IV GMH.

Intraventricular hemorrhage is typically recognized by the direct identification of blood products within the ventricles, often with sediment layering in the posterior, dependent parts of the ventricles. In addition, intraventricular blood products may result in a chemical inflammation of the ependymal lining with resultant hyperechogenicity. A focal, hyperechogenic choroid plexus enlargement is strongly suggestive of a choroid plexus hemorrhage.

The imaging characteristics of parenchymal hemorrhages are dependent on their age and are noted as a focal hyperechogenic (acute/subacute) or hypoechogenic (chronic) mass lesion within the brain. Compression of adjacent brain structures may be present dependent on the size of the hemorrhage.

Extra-axial hemorrhages may be challenging because they are frequently obscured secondary to the acoustic shadowing from the osseous boundaries of the fontanels. An asymmetric size of the lateral ventricles or a midline shift is suggestive of an extra-axial hemorrhage. Dedicated imaging that takes advantage of the additional fontanels may enhance detection. Subarachnoid hemorrhages are typically recognized by hyperechogenic material within the hemispheric sulci.

Diffuse HII due to perinatal asphyxia or cardiac arrest with diffuse brain swelling is recognized by a diffuse hyperechogenicity of the hemispheric white matter with resultant increased corticomedullary differentiation, slitlike ventricles, effaced basal cisterns, and a lowered resistive index (RI) value.

Focal arterial ischemic injury may occur secondary to multiple pathologies. In the acute phase, a focal hyperechogenicity is noted, which may affect both the white matter and overlying cortical gray matter typically within the territory of intracranial arteries. On follow-up, the ischemic tissue will progressively resolve and become hypoechogenic, eventually resulting in a porencephalic cyst.

Brain malformations are recognized by identification of the key anatomical features of the malformation. Subtle components may be overlooked by US. Most classic malformations, however, can easily be recognized.

Evaluation of the degree and possible etiology of hydrocephalus typically relies on the subjective analysis of the overall size and configuration of the ventricles on anatomical US images. Recently, more objective quantitative data are collected to detect subtle changes in ventriculomegaly. The ventricular index (VI = total width of the lateral ventricle on coronal view/total biparietal width in the same image) has become a popular, easy-to-measure scalar for monitoring ventricular size.

4.3 Doppler Ultrasonography of the Brain

Doppler sonography allows studying patency of the major intracranial arteries (circle of Willis) and veins (superficial and deep venous system) including evaluation of the flow direction. Moreover, spectral analysis of the arterial pulse waves sampled within major branches of the circle of

Willis allows calculation of the RI values. The RI value is calculated as the ratio between the maximal end-diastolic and end-systolic flow velocities ([peak systolic velocity–minimum diastolic velocity]/peak systolic velocity). The RI value may serve as an objective scalar of the intracranial hemodynamics. For full-term neonates, the normal RI values range between 0.65 and 0.75, while preterm infants have a slightly higher RI value (0.77–0.80).

Measurement of the RI values can give valuable, functional information in addition to the anatomical US images.

Serial evaluation of the RI values is especially helpful in the follow-up of hydrocephalus. An increase in central arterial RI values may occur because of decrease in diastolic flow secondary to elevated intracranial pressure in cases of rapidly progressive ventriculomegaly. In infants and children, RI values exceeding 0.80 and 0.65, respectively, is abnormal. Baseline measurements are useful to distinguish between an overlap in normal and abnormal values. Treated ventriculomegaly may be assessed with serial follow-up of the RI values as needed.

Serial Doppler sonography may be used to evaluate arteriovenous malformations, including the vein of Galen aneurysmal malformation. In particular, Doppler sonography allows evaluation of the effects of endovascular occlusion. In significant arteriovenous shunting, the peak systolic and diastolic flow velocities are elevated. Normalization of these flow scalars indicates successful treatment. In addition, the RI values will normalize.

RI values are lowered in cases of global brain edema, for example, because of hypoxic brain injury or in sepsis. Traumatic brain injury can alter cerebral blood flow dynamics in several ways. First, after subarachnoid hemorrhage, vasospasm may cause elevated cerebral blood flow velocity. Second, if severe injury leads to cerebral edema, elevated RI values reflects increased intracranial pressure. If the intracranial pressure exceeds mean arterial pressure (RI > 1.0), reversed diastolic flow may be identified. Following a traumatic brain injury, Doppler US can be applied to determine the impact of therapy, including hyperventilation. Finally, Doppler US can be used to confirm brain death. Patterns on Doppler US most specific to brain death are near-total absence of antegrade flow or complete absence of flow, timed average mean velocity of less than 10 cm/s over 30 minutes, and prominent bidirectional or "reverberant" flow (high peak systolic velocity and a consistent retrograde diastolic component, away from

the brain). Doppler US for brain death diagnosis should, however, be done cautiously in infants, as reverberant flow may be indicative of circulatory arrest alone.

4.4 Ultrasonography of the Spine

US of the spinal canal and spinal cord can be performed within the first months of life before the progressive ossification of the dorsal elements of the vertebral column obscures the acoustic window. The spinal canal and its contents are typically evaluated in the sagittal and axial plane. The width of the spinal canal, size, configuration and location of the spinal cord, central canal, and cauda equine are evaluated. In addition, cine-loop imaging allows evaluation of the pulsatility and mobility of the spinal cord. Imaging is typically performed with a high-resolution, high-frequency linear transducer. The vertebral bodies are counted either from the cervical spine downward or from the coccyx upward.

Indications for spinal ultrasound:

- Spinal dysraphia:
  - Skin dimple or tag.
  - Cutaneous fistulous tract with or without discharge.
  - Tethered cord.
  - Spectrum of myelomeningoceles and diastematomyelia.
  - Hydromyelia.
- Sacrococcygeal teratoma.
- Spondylitis with or without intraspinal abscess.
- To rule out spinal malformations in genetic disorders.

4.5 Ultrasonography of the Orbits

US of the orbits can give valuable information about the preseptal soft tissues, the eye globe, the optic nerve, and the immediate retrobulbar soft tissues including the central retinal artery and superior ophthalmic vein. Orbital ultrasound is performed with a high-frequency linear transducer through the closed eyelid. Measurement of the optic nerve sheet diameter has been proposed as an additional quantitative marker of increased intracranial pressure, but is rarely used in clinical routine.

Orbital US is depending on the hospital settings performed by ophthalmology or pediatric neuroradiology. Indications include orbital malformations, orbital trauma, intraorbital hemorrhages, tumors (retinoblastoma), retinal detachments, orbital inflammation, and arterial or venous thrombosis.

4.6 Ultrasonography of the Head and Neck

US of the head and neck region are primarily within the field of otorhinolaryngology. The most frequent indications include evaluation of a complicated lymphadenitis or tonsillitis, infected branchial cleft cysts, vascular or lymphatic malformations, and focal mass lesions. Doppler sonography of the major neck vessels may be considered to rule out a spontaneous or posttraumatic arterial dissection or a venous thrombosis (Lemierre's disease).

Reference

[1] Orman G, Benson JE, Kweldam CF, et al. Neonatal head ultrasonography today: a powerful imaging tool! J Neuroimaging. 2015; 25(1):31–55

5 Computed Tomography

Thierry A.G.M. Huisman

5.1 Introduction

Computed tomography (CT) is an imaging technique that uses an X-ray tube that rotates around the object of interest. A simultaneously rotating detector row opposite to the X-ray tube measures the amount of X-rays that have penetrated the body. The simultaneous rotation of X-ray tube and detector row allows us to spatially localize the degree of X-ray attenuation within the body, which gives information about the consistency and quality of examined tissues. The collected raw data are subsequently postprocessed with generation of two-dimensional axial images. Based on the applied reconstruction algorithm, dedicated soft-tissue and bone images are calculated. Nowadays, scanners measure a three-dimensional isotropic volume of data that can be reconstructed in multiple planes (multiplanar reconstructions) typically in the axial, sagittal, and coronal plane. In addition, three-dimensional images in various textures and qualities can be calculated.

5.2 Hounsfield Units

The basic image contrast of CT relies on the differing attenuation of the X-ray beam by the examined tissues. The attenuation level is expressed in Hounsfield units (HU), named after the inventor of the CT, Sir Godfrey N. Hounsfield. By definition, the radiodensity of water is calibrated to zero Hounsfield units. The radiodensity and the number Hounsfield units of other substances and tissues are related to the density of water in a linear fashion (▶ Table 5.1). Typically, the white matter is hypodense compared to the gray matter, resulting in a well-defined corticomedullary differentiation. The density of the white matter is determined by many factors, which include degree of water content, progressing myelination, and packing of white matter tracts. Consequently, the density of the white matter will gradually increase with progressing brain maturation. This variation in density should be carefully considered when studying the brain of very young children. Intracranial hematomas may also show a variation of CT density over time. The imaging appearance of hematomas varies depending on the hematomas' age, size, location, and hematocrit. Hyperacute (< 12 hours) hematomas may be isodense to the brain, rapidly becoming hyperdense in the acute (12 hours to 2 days) and early subacute (2–7 days) phase, and again progressively isodense and later hypodense in the late subacute (8 days to 1 month) and chronic (1 month to years) phase.[1]

5.3 Intravenous Contrast Media

The diagnostic yield of a CT study can be further increased by the simultaneous intravenous injection of iodinated contrast agents. In pathologies where an interrupted blood–brain barrier is expected (e.g., neoplasm, infection), intravenous contrast injection may increase diagnostic sensitivity and specificity. Contrast-enhanced CT is, however, limited in the evaluation of meningitis because the increased enhancement of the meninges may remain undetected because of the obscuring hyperdensity of the adjacent skull.

5.4 CT Angiography, CT Venography, and CT Perfusion

CT angiography (CTA) and CT venography (CTV) take advantage of a rapid intravenous bolus injection of contrast agents, which allows studying the intracranial vasculature in two- and three-dimensional detail. CTA should be considered in the diagnostic workup of acute arterial or venous stroke, congenital or acquired vasculopathies, vascular malformations, aneurysms, and highly vascularized neoplasms. CTV is helpful if a thrombosis of the superficial or deep venous system is suspected. Moreover, perfusion-weighted CT with calculation of multiple hemodynamic maps (e.g., cerebral blood flow and volume, mean transit time, time to peak) may help identify areas of critical perfusion in ischemic stroke.

Table 5.1 Hounsfield units of various tissues

	HU
Air	−1,000
Fat	−100
Water	0
Cerebrospinal fluid	15
White matter	20–30
Gray matter	30–40
Bone	>600

5.5 Limitations of CT Contrast Agents

It should be determined if the patient is allergic to iodinated contrast agents before injection. If there is a previous history of allergic reactions, the patient should receive a prophylactic preparation, which typically includes a combination of prednisone, diphenhydramine, and possibly an additional H_2 antagonist, starting 24 hours prior to the study. In addition, care should be taken to use only non-ionic contrast agents. Finally, the best prevention of contrast reactions is not to give contrast or to choose another imaging modality that does not require the use of iodinated contrast agents.

Furthermore, if there is a history of impaired renal function, the use of intravenous contrast agents should be carefully evaluated. If a contrast-enhanced CT study is considered essential for diagnosis and decisions about treatment, the patients should be well hydrated prior to the study, the amount of contrast agent may be reduced, and hemodialysis should be considered after the study.

5.6 Radiation Exposure

CT studies represent a major source of exposure to ionizing radiation. The use of CT should always be carefully considered in this vulnerably young patient group. If no radiation-free alternative imaging is possible or available, care should be taken to use high-end CT scanners which are equipped with modern dose-reduction techniques. Depending on the clinical question, the imaged region should be limited as much as possible (e.g., avoid unnecessary radiation of the eye lenses), multiphase contrast-enhanced studies should be avoided, and follow-up studies should be tailored to the relevant questions to be answered.[2] The so-called localizer at the beginning of each CT study should also be studied in detail because it may harbor important information (e.g., shunt disconnection), which may be outside of the imaged CT volume.[3]

Finally, when in doubt about the best study to be done, it is worthwhile to seek advice from the radiologist.

5.7 Indications

5.7.1 CT of the Brain

CT of the brain can be diagnostic in a multitude of acute and chronic neurosurgical pathologies. CT should be considered in children with an acute onset of focal or generalized neurological symptoms, unexplained mental deterioration, head trauma, pre- and postoperative workup, follow-up of hydrocephalus, complications of meningitis, stroke, hemorrhage, etc. In most cases, a non-contrast-enhanced CT is diagnostic. If a complex finding is noted, CT will frequently be followed by magnetic resonance imaging (MRI) unless an emergent neurosurgical intervention is necessary, MRI is contraindicated, or the patient cannot be transported to MRI.

In traumatic brain injury, images should be reconstructed using both soft-tissue and bone algorithms. Two- and three-dimensional reconstructions of the skull have proven to be helpful to identify skull fractures that extend along the axial plane. In addition, fracture extension into sutures is easily depicted. Multiplanar coronal and sagittal soft-tissue reconstructions enhance identification of extra-axial hematomas.

Non-contrast-enhanced CT is frequently used for the follow up of children with shunted hydrocephalus in order to rule out shunt malfunction. Various dose-reduced protocols are available. Because many of these children will receive multiple studies over their lifetime, alternative nonionizing imaging techniques should, however, be considered. Nowadays, ultrafast MRI protocols allow imaging the ventricles within minutes. Typically, a single-shot T2-weighted protocol is used in which each slice is measured within 400 to 800 ms, which is in most cases fast enough for even the very young children.

CT is typically limited in the diagnostic workup of children with seizures related to developmental disorders, neurometabolic diseases, or autoimmune inflammatory diseases including Rasmussen's encephalitis. CT may reveal only the tip of the iceberg, while MRI allows studying the malformation in better detail.

Three-dimensional reconstruction of the skull allows preoperative evaluation of skull remodeling in isolated or syndromal craniosynostosis.

Contrast-enhanced CT should be performed if a focal mass lesion is noted, unless an MRI will follow. Similarly, contrast-enhanced CTA or CTV should be considered if a vascular lesion (e.g., aneurysm, arteriovenous malformation) or an arterial or venous thrombosis is suspected.

5.7.2 CT of the Petrous Bone and Skull Base

High-resolution thin-sliced CT of the petrous bone allows us to study the osseous anatomy of the delicate inner ear (cochlea, vestibule, semicircular canals) and middle ear (ossicles) structures. Images are typically reconstructed in multiple planes with separate magnification of both sides. Temporal bone CT is usually performed for otological indications (e.g., cholesteatoma, inner ear deafness). More frequently temporal bone imaging is carried out after traumatic brain injury with fractures involving the skull base. The floor of the middle cranial fossa including clivus, sphenoid body, and sinus should be carefully scrutinized for fractures. Contrast injection is rarely indicated unless a concomitant vascular injury is suspected.

5.7.3 CT of the Orbits

Many pathologies may require a CT of the orbits. In the pediatric age group, one of the most frequent indications is an acutely swollen eye. Contrast-enhanced CT is typically performed to differentiate between a preseptal inflammation and a retrobulbar process. Contrast injection is indicated to rule out abscess formation and/or thrombosis of the superior ophthalmic vein. The adjacent cavernous sinus should also be studied for possible thrombus extension.

The second most frequent indication for orbital CT is a traumatic injury to the orbits. CT images should be reconstructed in both soft-tissue and bone algorithm. Direct injury to the globe, lens, optic nerve, and orbital muscles should be excluded, as well as osseous lesions, which may include orbital wall fractures as well as fractures extending into the optic canal. The adjacent anterior skull base and frontal lobes should also be evaluated for traumatic lesions.

Less frequently, orbital CT is performed because of mass lesions, which may include benign lesions, such as dermoids, venous angiomas, and optic nerve gliomas, malignant lesions, such as rhabdomyosarcomas and retinoblastomas, or metastatic lesions to the orbits such as in systemic neuroblastoma. For these indications, simultaneous contrast injection should be considered if no MRI is scheduled/performed.

In general, CT of the orbits should be done cautiously because of the high sensitivity of the pediatric eye lens for radiation-induced cataract. In addition, in children with retinoblastoma, an increased risk for radiation-induced secondary malignancies, such as osteosarcomas of the orbits, has been reported.

5.7.4 CT of the Paranasal Sinuses

Indications for paranasal sinus CT include sinusitis, trauma, and preoperative workup for transsphenoidal resection of sellar tumors (e.g., pituitary adenoma). CT is typically done in a low-dose approach without the injection of intravenous contrast agents. Mucosal thickening and primary or secondary bony changes are well depicted on bone images. Intrasellar calcifications suggestive of a craniopharyngioma are also easily noted.

5.7.5 CT of the Vertebral Column

Indications for vertebral column CT are multifold and most frequently include trauma, infection, tumor, or malformation. In children, soft-tissue and bone images should be reconstructed in three orthogonal planes and, whenever necessary, additional three-dimensional images may be obtained.

Sagittal soft-tissue reconstructions are especially helpful in children who sustained a traumatic head and neck injury. Because of the unique biomechanical properties of the pediatric craniocervical junction, there is an increased risk for ligamentous injury at this level with possible disruption of the tectal membrane. Retroclival hematomas may result in subsequent compression of the lower brainstem and upper cervical spinal cord. Sagittal soft-tissue images facilitate diagnosis.

Two- and three-dimensional image reconstructions of the spinal column should be considered in complex spinal dysraphia. Preoperative planning may benefit from an exact display of the malformed anatomy.

Occasionally, CT is performed in addition to MRI in children with vertebral infections (e.g., spondylitis, spondylodiscitis) or vertebral tumors (e.g., osteosarcoma, Ewing's sarcoma) to get a better insight into the osseous structure.

Finally, whole-spine CT may serve as baseline study in children with scoliosis.

References

[1] Huisman TA. Intracranial hemorrhage: ultrasound, CT and MRI findings. Eur Radiol. 2005; 15(3):434–440

[2] Pindrik J, Huisman TA, Mahesh M, Tekes A, Ahn ES. Analysis of limited sequence head CT for children with shunted hydrocephalus: potential to reduce diagnostic radiation exposure. J Neurosurg Pediatr. 2013; 12(5):491–500

[3] Orman G, Bosemani T, Aylin T, Poretti A, Huisman TA. Scout view in pediatric CT neuroradiological evaluation: do not underestimate! Childs Nerv Syst. 2014; 30(2):307–311

6 Conventional Magnetic Resonance Imaging

Thierry A.G.M. Huisman

6.1 Introduction

Magnetic resonance imaging (MRI) generates images of the central nervous system based on the distribution and electromagnetic characteristics of protons within the body while exposed to a strong modulated external magnetic field. Depending on the used pulse sequences, various image contrasts can be generated. T1- and T2-weighted sequences serve as the backbone of anatomical MRI. Multiple additional, specialized MR sequences are nowadays available. Many of these sequences represent variations on the T1- and T2-weighted sequences but may offer additional specific contrasts, thereby facilitating diagnosis.

6.2 T1- and T2-weighted Sequences

For anatomical imaging, typically T1- and T2-weighted sequences are being used. On T1-weighted images, fluid (cerebrospinal fluid [CSF]) appears hypointense, and on T2-weighted images, fluid appears hyperintense. The signal intensity of the gray and white matter is highly dependent on the degree of brain maturation. In the first months of life, the gray matter appears T1-hyperintense and T2-hypointense compared to the white matter; around 8 to 10 months of age, the gray and white matter become isointense to each other, before a reversal of contrast occurs in which the gray matter becomes T1-hypointense and T2-hyperintense in relation to the white matter. The time evolution of the changes in signal intensities is somewhat different for the T1- and T2-weighted imaging because the T1 and T2 relaxation phenomena are determined by varying maturational processes. Progressing white matter myelination and increasing fiber packing follow a well-programmed pattern. The first regions to mature include the sensory and motor cortex, including the corticospinal and sensory tracts extending through the corona radiate, internal capsule, and mesencephalon into the brainstem. Almost simultaneously, the visual cortex and optic radiation show an early myelination. These areas appear particularly T1-hyperintense and T2-hypointense. Familiarity with the normal-progressing brain maturation is essential to identify disease processes.

6.3 Contrast-enhanced T1-weighted MRI

Similar to CT, injection of intravenous contrast agents may facilitate diagnosis in pathologies that injure the blood–brain barrier (e.g., neoplasms, infection) or show an intrinsic increased vascularity (e.g., vascular malformations). In MRI, gadolinium-based contrast agents are used. The paramagnetic effects of gadolinium shorten the T1 relaxation times of the examined tissue. Lesions with a leaky blood–brain barrier consequently appear T1-hyperintense. In high concentrations, the paramagnetic properties of gadolinium may result in a focal signal loss or susceptibility artifact. Within the brain, gadolinium does not reach a high enough concentration to induce focal signal loss; this may, however, be observed within the renal pelvis and urinary bladder. Gadolinium-based contrast agents used in diagnostic dosage have no significant impact on the T2 relaxation times; the T2 signal characteristics are not altered. Consequently, T2-weighted sequences may be acquired after gadolinium-based contrast agents have been injected.

Less than 1/1,000 patients may show minor allergic reactions to gadolinium-based contrast agents. Side effects include facial swelling, headache, nausea, and a rash or hives. In patients with an impaired renal function, gadolinium-based contrast agents have been linked to the occurrence of nephrogenic systemic fibrosis and nephrogenic fibrosing dermopathy. To prevent this potentially debilitating or life-threatening complication, the estimated glomerular filtration rate (eGFR) should be calculated prior to the injection of gadolinium-based contrast agents. In children, the eGFR is best calculated using the Schwartz equation, which employs the serum creatinine concentration (mg/dL), the child's height (cm), and an age-dependent constant k: eGFR= $k \times$ height/serum creatinine. In the first year of life, for preterm neonates $k = 0.33$ and for full-term neonates $k = 0.45$. For infants and children age 1 to 12 years, $k = 0.55$. In adolescent males, $k = 0.70$, and in females k remains 0.55 because of the presumed increase in male muscle mass. If the calculated eGFR is below 30 mL/min/1.73 m², no contrast should be given, even when the patient is on dialysis. If the eGFR is between 30 and 60 mL/min/1.73 m^2, the benefits must outweighted the potential risks and an informed consent should be obtained. If the eGFR is above 60 mL/min/1.73 m^2, contrast can be given at a regular dose.

6.4 Fat-saturated T1- and T2-weighted Sequences

The diagnostic sensitivity of T1- and T2-weighted sequences may be further enhanced by the simultaneous use of a fat saturation pulse. The selective suppression of the fat signal can be especially helpful for contrast-enhanced T1-weighted sequences if a focal lesion is embedded within T1-hyperintense fat. Contrast-enhancing metastatic lesions within the diploic space of the skull are typically better appreciated, as well as lesions within the fat-containing epidural space of the vertebral column. Finally, comparing T1-weighted images before and after a fat saturation pulse may prove the presence of fat within a lesion, facilitating diagnosis of, for example, a teratoma.

6.5 Fluid-attenuated Inversion Recovery

In fluid-attenuated inversion recovery (FLAIR) sequences, the signal intensity of free, mobile water is suppressed (e.g., CSF), which facilitates diagnosis of focal or diffuse white matter lesions such as multiple sclerosis plaques along the ventricles, inflammation, trauma, acute or chronic (hemorrhagic) stroke, or white matter gliosis. In addition, FLAIR is beneficial to identify pathology within the subarachnoid space, such as subarachnoid hemorrhage or metastatic seeding of malignancies. Signal suppression of the CSF within the brain sulci may be limited if the study is performed in general anesthesia. The anesthetics and hyperventilation may impair signal suppression. FLAIR imaging is of little value in the neonate because the brain is still very watery.

6.6 T2* - Gradient Echo and Susceptibility-weighted Imaging

T2*-weighted gradient echo (T2*-GRE) and susceptibility-weighted imaging (SWI) are exquisitely sensitive for the magnetic susceptibility effects of blood products and calcifications. These sequences should be added to the standard sequences in children with traumatic brain injury, intracranial hemorrhage, vascular malformations (e.g., cavernomas), TORCH (*t*oxoplasmosis, *o*ther, *r*ubella, *c*ytomegalovirus, *h*erpes) infection, calcifying or hemorrhaging brain tumors (e.g., oligodendroglioma, primitive neuroectodermal tumor, teratoma), and any other pathology that may be complicated by calcifications or hemorrhages. SWI sequences should be preferred above T2*-GRE sequences because of their higher sensitivity. Because the basic design of these sequences is to enhance the magnetic susceptibility effects of substances that interfere with the magnetic field, they are also very susceptible to image distortion related to metallic implants including adjacent dental braces.

6.7 Inversion Recovery Sequences

Inversion recovery (IR) T1-weighted sequences are heavily T1-weighted sequences. Main advantage is that these sequences enhance the contrast between gray and white matter and are consequently frequently used in the diagnostic workup of children with seizures secondary to congenital developmental disorders including cortical dysplasia, polymicrogyria, pachygyria, band heterotopia, or focal nodular heterotopia. In addition, IR T1-weighted sequences enhance detection of gray matter injury secondary to acquired pathologies.

6.8 Heavily T2-weighted MRI

Heavily T2-weighted, thin-sliced, high-resolution three-dimensional MRI (CISS [constructive interference in steady state]) renders images with a high contrast between solid tissues and fluid. This sequence is especially helpful to study detailed anatomical structures containing or outlined by CSF. This sequence is typically used to study the cranial nerves crossing the basal cisterns, the vestibulocochlear nerves within the internal auditory canal, the intraorbital segment of the optic nerve, the spinal cord, and nerve roots of the cauda equine as well as the inner ear structures such as cochlea, vestibule, and semicircular canals. Because this sequence is a three-dimensional acquisition, multiplanar two- and three-dimensional images can be generated. Major limitation is that the sequence does not allow studying subtle differences in T2 relaxation times between structures. Consequently, the sequences cannot be used to study subtle white and gray matter lesions. The gray and white matter appear isointense, for example, the extent of acute stroke may be underestimated.

6.9 Ultrafast MRI

Single-shot, ultrafast half-Fourier acquisition MR sequences is a valuable alternative for imaging children who have difficulty to hold still (young age, anxiety, limited cognitive function). These sequences render images within 400 to 800 ms per slice. Most sequences are T2-weighted. Because this acquisition is a single-shot technique, only those slices will be degraded by motion artifacts that were acquired while the child was moving. The total acquisition time of a triplanar, ultrafast MRI of the brain ranges between 5 and 8 minutes. These sequences are typically used for a rapid evaluation of children with shunted hydrocephalus or to exclude major complications, for example, after surgery.

6.10 Contraindications for MRI

There are various absolute and relative contraindications for MRI. They may vary depending on the magnetic field strength used.

Absolute contraindications:
1. Cardiac pacemaker, implanted neurostimulators, cochlear implants, insulin pumps, baclofen pumps.
2. Ferromagnetic vascular occlusion devices including clips.
3. Ferromagnetic implants or foreign bodies including shrapnel.
4. Metallic fragments within the orbits.

Relative contraindications:
1. Programmable ventricular shunts.
2. Intracranial pressure devices.
3. Claustrophobia.
4. Critically sick, unstable children.
5. Morbid obesity.
6. Ferromagnetic implants within regions adjacent to the field of interest (dental braces).

Care should be taken to inform the MR team members in advance which implants are present, if they are MR compatible, and if they have to be reprogrammed after imaging. Several devices have been FDA-approved for 1.5-tesla MR scanners but may not be imaged at higher field strengths. If there is a clinical concern, the vendor of the device should be contacted prior to imaging. Finally, in rare occasions a conventional radiography may be necessary to rule out, localize, or identify the kind of implanted device or foreign body.

Finally, care should be taken not to have any external electrical wires arranged within a loop close to the patient's skin. These may act as receivers for the used radiofrequency pulses during scanning, and the induced electrical current may heat the wires with possible skin burning. This is of special importance in sedated or intubated children who cannot give a direct feedback. Clothes should always be checked for ferromagnetic objects (e.g., buttons, jewelry).

7 Advanced MRI Techniques

Thierry A.G.M. Huisman

7.1 Introduction

In addition to the anatomical magnetic resonance imaging (MRI) sequences, a multitude of advanced MRI sequences are available that give important additional information about arterial or venous blood flow (magnetic resonance angiography [MRA], magnetic resonance venography [MRV]), cerebrospinal flow dynamics (cerebrospinal fluid [CSF] flow), microstructural neuroarchitecture (diffusion-weighted imaging [DWI]/diffusion tensor imaging [DTI]), brain perfusion (perfusion-weighted imaging [PWI]), biochemical processes (^{1}H magnetic resonance spectroscopy [^{1}H-MRS]), and functional centers (functional MRI [fMRI]).[1] This additional information may help better characterization of the findings or may narrow differential diagnosis. In addition, these functional techniques may show pathology at the microstructural level which remains undetected on anatomical MRI or show pathology before they become apparent on conventional MRI.

7.2 Magnetic Resonance Angiography and Venography

Various two- and three-dimensional MRA and MRV techniques allow study of the vasculature of the central nervous system noninvasively. Depending on the expected hemodynamics, vascular pathology, vasculature of interest, and location of the imaged lesion, time-of-flight (TOF) or phase-contrast (PC) angiographic techniques are applied. In these angiographic techniques, blood flow is translated into an MRI signal. Typically, two-dimensional raw images are generated in which the MRI signal of stationary tissue (gray or white matter) is suppressed, while the signal of moving blood is enhanced. The resultant raw images are subsequently reconstructed as axial, coronal, and sagittal maximum intensity projection (MIP) images or three-dimensional rotational images similar to catheter angiography. Both the raw images and the reconstructed MIP and three-dimensional MRA or MRV images should be studied for pathology.

MRA and MRV suffer from some important limitations. In TOF-MRA/MRV, the short T1 relaxation time of a fresh thrombus may mimic blood flow; slow blood flow, calcifications, or vascular clips may mimic or overestimate a stenosis; small vessels may be overlooked; and finally, blood flow direction and blood flow velocity cannot be determined for certainty. In PC MRA/MRV, inadequate selection of the velocity encoding may result in aliasing artifacts and patency of vessels may be underestimated. In addition, the acquisition time, especially for three-dimensional PC MRA/MRV, is significant.

Dynamic contrast-enhanced MRA/MRV is a valuable alternative angiographic technique in which a bolus of gadolinium-based contrast is injected while images are scanned in a rapid sequence to resolve the various angiographic phases (arterial, parenchymal, venous, and delayed venous). This technique is especially helpful for the hemodynamic analysis of vascular malformations; however, the spatial resolution is somewhat limited.

7.3 Cerebrospinal Fluid Flow Imaging

PC flow–sensitive sequences can also be used to study the CSF flow noninvasively. PC CSF flow techniques are typically used to evaluate flow of CSF at the level of the foramen of magnum (e.g., in Chiari I malformation), sylvian aqueduct (e.g., in aqueductal stenosis), and across the floor of the third ventricle after third ventriculostomy. PC CSF flow imaging gives quantitative information about the CSF flow velocity, direction, and pulsatility.

7.4 Diffusion-weighted Imaging and Diffusion Tensor Imaging

7.4.1 Diffusion-weighted Imaging

In DWI, differences in the diffusion characteristics between various tissues are translated into differences in assigned signal intensity per voxel.[2] Regions with high degree of water mobility or high degree of diffusion such as CSF will be suppressed in their signal, while regions with limited water mobility or low degree of diffusion such as gray and white matter will be less suppressed in their signal. On the resultant trace of diffusion or DWI images, CSF will be hypointense in contrast to the more signal-intense gray and white matter. In addition to the DWI images, an apparent diffusion coefficient (ADC) is being calculated. This quantitative scalar is similarly mapped as a two-dimensional image in which regions with high ADC values or high degree of diffusion are represented bright and regions with low ADC values or low diffusion are displayed dark. Major advantage of this ADC map is that this image is a true image of diffusion and no residual T1 or T2 relaxation phenomena are incorporated. In addition, the ADC values can be extracted by a region of interest approach. These ADC values can be compared between studies and subjects.

The use of DWI and ADC maps has revolutionized early detection of cerebral stroke. In ischemic stroke, cytotoxic edema occurs before vasogenic edema develops. Cytotoxic edema results from a failure of the ischemic membrane pumps with influx of water into the cells; the resultant cell swelling limits diffusion, which can be detected by DWI. The ischemic tissue appears DWI-hyperintense and ADC-dark. The overall amount of water has, however, not changed, explaining why in this early phase conventional T1- and T2-weighted imaging is unremarkable. Within the next phase, efflux of water from the vessels into the extracellular space, known as vasogenic edema, will increase overall diffusion of the ischemic tissue (DWI-hypointense and ADC-bright). Because of the increased overall amount of water, conventional T1- and T2-weighted imaging reveals the ongoing ischemic injury.

DWI has also proven to be helpful in differentiating intracerebral abscesses from necrotic brain tumors. Diffusion within an abscess is typically restricted (DWI-hyperintense, ADC-dark), while diffusion is increased in necrotic tumor (DWI-hypointense, ADC-bright).

7.4.2 Diffusion Tensor Imaging

DTI is a more advanced DWI in which in addition to the magnitude of diffusion (ADC values), the three-dimensional shape and direction of diffusion is also sampled.[1,3] Diffusion within tissues is determined by many factors including the specific microstructural environment. Along white matter tracts, the diffusion of water is predominantly occurring along the main axis of the tract, while the diffusion is limited perpendicular to the main axis of the tract because of the myelin sheet. This directional diffusion is also known as anisotropic diffusion. In CSF, diffusion is equal in all directions,

known as isotropic diffusion. In DTI, the entire tensor of diffusion is sampled by applying diffusion-encoding gradients along at least six directions in space. In DTI, in addition to the DWI and ADC images, maps of anisotropic diffusion are generated. Most frequently, a scalar known as fractional anisotropy (FA) is calculated. The FA scalar varies between 0 and 1. Zero refers to equal diffusion in all direction in space (maximum isotropic diffusion), while an FA value of 1 refers to complete anisotropic diffusion. The magnitude of the FA value can be mapped as a grayscale map similar to the ADC maps. The corpus callosum appears consequently bright on the FA maps matching a high FA value, while CSF appears dark matching a low FA value.

In addition, because not only the three-dimensional shape and magnitude of diffusion, but also the predominant direction of anisotropic diffusion in space is sampled, these FA maps can be color coded. By convention, predominant diffusion from left to right is color coded in red, diffusion from superior to inferior in blue, and anterior to posterior in green.

Finally, powerful postprocessing programs allow reconstruction of fiber tracts from these DTI data. This technique, which is also known as fiber tractography, allows study of the course and integrity of fiber tracts within the brain noninvasively. This technique is helpful in the detailed workup of complex brain malformations but can also be used in the preoperative workup of children who require brain surgery. Displaced, interrupted, or fiber tracts adjacent to a tumor can be studied.

7.5 Perfusion-weighted Imaging

PWI aims to study brain perfusion noninvasively.[4] Various techniques are available. A robust and frequently used approach is the first-pass contrast-enhanced PWI technique. The passage of a compact bolus of gadolinium-based contrast agents through the capillary network of the central nervous system results in a signal loss within the tissue, which gives indirect information about the local hemodynamics. Multiple semi-quantitative maps of cerebral blood flow (CBF), cerebral blood volume, mean transit time, time to peak, and various other hemodynamic parametric maps can be calculated. Alternatively, arterial spin labeling (ASL) labels a volume of blood upstream of the region of interest by a short radiofrequency pulse.

Signal acquisition is carried out after a delay TI (time of inversion of 1–2 seconds). The difference in signal between measurements with and without ASL reflects the amount of labeled blood arriving in the volume of interest during the delay TI, to calculate maps of CBF. Major advantages of this technique are that the patient's blood is used as an intrinsic contrast agent, multiple vascular territories can be studied separately, and the study can be repeated as often as necessary because no contrast agent is injected. Disadvantage is that the method renders only maps of CBF and that multiple measurements are necessary to boost the signal-to-noise ratio, which lengthens the imaging time.

The combined use of DWI/DTI and PWI has proven to be beneficial especially in the diagnostic workup of children with an ischemic stroke. The typically irreversible core of infarction is characterized by an area of restricted diffusion on DWI/DTI, which matches a region of hypoperfusion on PWI. The surrounding ischemic penumbra which is believed to represent tissue at risk for infarct progression but which can potentially be salvaged with adequate treatment is characterized by a region of hypoperfusion without matching restricted diffusion.

Furthermore, PWI is helpful in the hemodynamic characterization of brain tumors and vascular malformations. Finally, PWI is being used in the preoperative diagnostic workup of children with chronic progressive vasculopathy such as in moyamoya disease.

7.6 ^{1}H-Magnetic Resonance Spectroscopy

^{1}H-MRS allows identification and quantification of various metabolites within the brain noninvasively. Various approaches are available including a semi-quantitative versus quantitative single or multivoxel technique. In the semi-quantitative technique, ratios between the various metabolites are being calculated. Typically, the metabolites are correlated against creatine, because this marker of energy metabolism is in most instances stable. In the quantitative approach, the exact concentration of the measured metabolite is determined. Typically, following metabolites are determined by ^{1}H-MRS: lactate (marker of anaerobic metabolism), N-acetyl aspartate (NAA; marker of neuronal density and integrity), creatine (marker of energy metabolism), and choline (marker of membrane turnover). In many disease processes, the ratios or concentrations of these major metabolites are altered. In ischemic stroke, lactate is typically elevated, while NAA is reduced; in highly malignant brain neoplasms, choline is elevated and NAA may be reduced. Furthermore, various additional metabolites (e.g., myo-inositol, glycine) may be detected or are significantly increased in their concentrations.

7.7 Functional MRI

fMRI allows study of functional processes within the brain noninvasively. fMRI relies on the blood-oxygen-level dependent (BOLD) technique. Areas of brain that are activated typically receive more oxygenated blood than necessary for the increased metabolic demands. This overshoot in oxygenated hemoglobin versus deoxygenated hemoglobin—the two different kinds of hemoglobin that have different magnetic susceptibility characteristics—results in a cortical activation–related decrease of MRI signal. Combining ultrafast fMRI sequences with conventional anatomical MRI sequences allows localization of functional centers within the brain. The function-related signal change is minimal (1–2% at 1.5-tesla field strength) but significant enough to give reliable data. This technique, however, requires robust and reproducible functional paradigms to study these functional centers. In pediatric neurosurgery, these techniques may be valuable to identify important functional centers in close proximity to surgical fields.

7.8 Digital Subtraction Angiography

Digital subtraction angiography (DSA) allows study of the vasculature of the central nervous system by selective injection of iodinated contrast agents into the vessels of interest via an endovascular catheter. By subtracting a "mask" image obtained prior to contrast injection from the contrast-injected images, the vessels are displayed in high detail, free of overlying or obscuring bony structures. Multiple images are collected at a rapid rate after injection in order to have multiple contrast phases including an arterial, venous, and late venous phase. Depending on the positioning of the catheter, selective or superselective vascular imaging is possible. DSA remains the gold standard of vascular imaging and can be combined with a subsequent endovascular intervention (e.g., aneurysm coiling, embolization of a vascular malformation, chemoembolization of a malignant tumor).

DSA in pediatric neuroimaging should be performed by an experienced angiography team. Frequently, the studies are performed in general anesthesia. Alternative angiographic imaging should always be pursued whenever possible. DSA may not be suitable for children with renal insufficiency because of the side effects of iodinated contrast agents. In addition, this technique relies on the use of ionizing radiation.

References

[1] Huisman TA, Tekes A. Advanced MR brain imaging. Why? Pediatr Radiol. 2008; 38 Suppl 3:S415–S432

[2] Huisman TA. Diffusion-weighted imaging: basic concepts and application in cerebral stroke and head trauma. Eur Radiol. 2003; 13(10):2283–2297

[3] Poretti A, Meoded A, Rossi A, Raybaud C, Huisman TA. Diffusion tensor imaging and fiber tractography in brain malformations. Pediatr Radiol. 2013; 43(1):28–54

[4] Huisman TA, Sorensen AG. Perfusion-weighted magnetic resonance imaging of the brain: techniques and application in children. Eur Radiol. 2004; 14(1):59–72

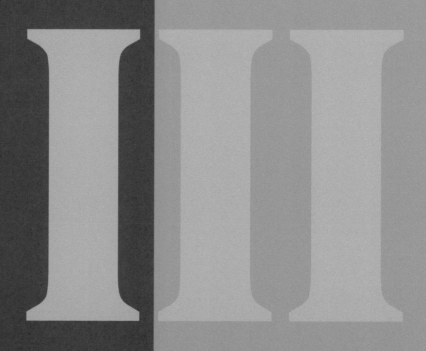

Section III

Neurology

8 The Neurological Examination of the Infant and Child

Neil R. Friedman

8.1 Introduction

A complete neurological assessment includes a meticulous, precise, and comprehensive history and detailed neurological examination. The goal of such an approach is to establish, and narrow, a differential diagnosis, thereby helping to direct further evaluation and investigations. This is particularly important given the breadth and extent of investigational studies, including metabolic, genetic, neurophysiology, and neuroimaging studies available to the practitioner. The old clinical adage that most diagnoses can be made on the basis of the history alone still holds true despite technological advances. The three fundamental questions to be addressed through the history and examination of a patient are the following: (1) Is the problem neurological? (2) If so, where within the neuroaxis can the problem be localized to? (3) What is the nature or pathophysiology of the problem?

There are fundamental differences between the neurological assessment of newborns, infants, and young children and that of adolescents or adults, given the rapidly developing and maturing brain, both structurally (e.g., maturation of myelin) and physiologically (e.g., the formation of neural networks), of newborn, infants, and young children. These developmental differences not only impact the history and examination, but also are subject to different pathophysiological processes and manifestations of disease states compared to those seen in a "mature" brain. Development, therefore, is an important variable in the evaluation of infants and young children, and delay in achieving age-specific developmental milestones and abnormal patterns of development are important indicators of underlying neurological disease.

One of the most important hallmarks of these developmental differences is white matter myelination in the brain. Progressive myelination occurs from early in the second trimester of pregnancy until well into childhood and adolescents. This is best reflected by brain magnetic resonant imaging studies, where white matter maturation on T2-weighted imaging does not reach a "mature pattern" until age 2. It is myelination of the corticospinal tracts in the first year of life that ultimately allows the infant to sit and subsequently to walk independently. Head growth, another reflection of brain development and maturation, on average is 12 cm during the first 2 years of life, compared with approximately 5 cm during the subsequent 16 years.

The age-dependent acquisition of gross motor, fine motor, speech and language, and social skills, inability of an infant or younger child to recount the history, and diverse nature of neurological conditions affecting children are fundamental differences between the pediatric and adult neurological assessment.

8.2 History

Know or listen to those who know.

Baltasar Gracián

Obtaining a good history is crucial to the neurological examination and requires a good rapport between the physician and the family. An accurate history also provides focus to the physical examination. While it is not always possible to obtain the history directly from the child, every effort should be made, when possible, to allow the child to express himself or herself in his or her own words in describing his or her symptoms. When the parent or guardian provides the history, it is important to distinguish the subjective interpretation of symptoms from direct observation of symptoms. Since the history is often a composite of the child's own words and third-party observation, every effort should be made to clarify the symptoms in simple, descriptive language rather than rely on medical jargon. The history should be informed by recognizing patterns of disease and disease processes, and as the history develops, directed questioning may be necessary to explore differential diagnostic possibilities. It is often helpful to consider this by taking into account the underlying pathophysiological basis of disease, namely:

- Congenital.
- Traumatic.
- Inflammatory.
- Infectious.

- Ischemic/vascular.
- Toxic/drug.
- Metabolic.
- Endocrine.
- Neoplastic.

8.2.1 History of Presenting Problem

A systematic approach to the history is important and begins with elucidating the nature of the presenting problem(s). This may involve a chronological or symptom-based approach. Important details include symptom onset (acute, subacute, chronic), duration of symptoms, temporal pattern of the problem (static, progressive, recurrent, diurnal variation, or regressive), potential modifying factors (exacerbation or relieving factors), and/or any associated symptoms. It is important to know what, if any, prior interventions have been tried and the results of these interventions, as this may impact the presentation of the current problem. Establishing a child's prior baseline functioning from current level of functioning helps in determining the severity and potential degenerative nature of an illness. The history should also help establish whether the symptoms can be localized to one region of the neuroaxis, or whether a combination of systems is involved. One distinguishing feature in the pediatric history is the frequent involvement of developmental concerns. Not only must one be aware of normal developmental milestones to know whether any deviation is abnormal, but also determining whether the developmental concern is global or limited to one or more of the four specific domains of development, that is, gross motor, fine motor, social, or speech/language, is crucial in generating a differential diagnosis and directing further testing. Genetic contribution to pediatric neurological disease is increasingly important, so knowing whether other family members are involved can narrow the differential diagnosis by considering potential X-linked or autosomal inheritance of a problem being addressed. When a metabolic disorder is suspected, parents should be asked whether the child's breath or urine has a strange odor, especially at times of illness. Marked decompensation at the time of illness, with vomiting, pallor, and delayed recovery, is suggestive of a disorder of intermediary energy metabolism or urea cycle defect. It is important to determine what prior testing or investigations have been undertaken so as to reduce unnecessary duplication of studies and potentially help eliminate certain diagnostic considerations.

8.2.2 Birth History

The birth history is an integral part of the neurological history of the infant and young child and may provide an etiological clue to the differential diagnosis in this age group. Many chronic neurological problems have their origins in the prenatal period at the time of prosencephalic development, migration, and maturation of the immature brain. Problems in the perinatal and peripartum period are also potentially important factors in subsequent neurological development. Genetic disorders, hypoxic-ischemic events, infection, drug use or abuse, toxins, trauma, and malnutrition all impact the developing brain and are important to inquire about in the history. More than one-half of the cases of cerebral palsy have an antenatal cause.

The birth history can best be considered in three discreet periods—the antenatal course, labor and delivery, and the postnatal period. Problems during these periods are not always mutually exclusive. For example, a child with an underlying neuromuscular or genetic disorder may not be as resilient in withstanding the process of labor and delivery, resulting in potential fetal distress.

Antenatal/Prenatal Period

There are a number of pertinent factors to inquire about during the antenatal period. This includes:
- Conception: It is important to determine if conception was natural or achieved through assisted reproductive technology (ART), as the latter has been associated with an increased risk for adverse neurological outcome. Whether the risk is related to the *indication* for ART, rather than the ART itself, is often unclear. Multiple births increase the risk for prematurity and unique situations such as twin-to-twin transfusion, thereby increasing the risk for brain injury.
- Maternal factors:
  - Age: Maternal age at both ends of the spectrum, namely, teenage years and woman over 40, has both been implicated in subsequent neurodevelopmental problems. In women over 40, there is also an increased risk for genetic abnormalities, the most common of which is Down's syndrome. Neurodevelopmental outcome of children born

to teenage mothers is confounded by other variables such as typically lower socioeconomic status. Increasingly, attention is being focused on paternal age and risk of neurodevelopmental disability.

- Maternal health: Pregnancy predisposes women to transient medical disease such as gestational diabetes or pregnancy-induced hypertension. Uncontrolled, this places the developing fetus at risk for neurological impairment and malformations, either directly or through risk factors such as prematurity and intrauterine growth retardation (IUGR). In addition to acquired medical problems during pregnancy, chronic medical illness, such as diabetes, thyroid disorders, malnutrition, obesity, and congenital heart disease, also places the fetus at risk for impaired neurological outcomes.

- Infection: Congenital infections, specifically the toxoplasmosis, rubella, cytomegalovirus, herpes simplex, and syphilis (TORCHS), lymphocytic choriomeningitis virus (LCMV), human parechovirus, and HIV infections are well-known causes of neurological impairment including cortical migration abnormalities, microcephaly, cognitive impairment, spastic quadriplegic cerebral palsy, and epilepsy. Almost any virus, however, may be implicated. These infections may be relatively silent in the mother.

- Drug or toxin exposure: It is important to ask about, and document, both illicit and prescription drug usage during pregnancy. Many prescription drugs, especially antiepileptic medications, are teratogenic and associated with well-established syndromes and phenotypes (e.g., phenytoin and fetal hydantoin syndrome, valproic acid and fetal valproate syndrome). Illicit drugs such as cocaine or "crack" may be associated with neonatal stroke or intracranial hemorrhage. Smoking and alcohol both affect fetal development. Cigarette smoking may result in IUGR and fetal distress at delivery. Alcohol abuse may result in fetal alcohol syndrome or fetal alcohol effects, which have neurological complications, especially impaired cognitive development and behavioral disturbances.

- Pregnancy factors: It is important to ask about the health of the pregnancy. Specific questions directed at fetal movement and amniotic fluid status may provide crucial clues to diagnosis. Diminished fetal movement, especially when abrupt, may be indicative of a fetus at risk or in distress, whereas decreased fetal movement throughout the pregnancy may be more indicative an underlying neuromuscular disorder. Excessive fetal movement, especially in short bursts, has been associated with in utero seizures. Oligohydramnios may result in diminished fetal movement and subsequent joint contractures (arthrogryposis), whereas impaired swallowing may result in oligohydramnios and provide a clue to an underlying brain/brainstem malformation or injury, or potential neuromuscular disorder. Prenatal ultrasound scans are now routine, and increasingly, fetal magnetic resonance imaging (MRI) is being done for better delineation of detected fetal central nervous system anomalies including brain malformations, hydrocephalus, ischemic or destructive brain injury, choroid plexus cysts, and spinal dysraphism.

Labor and Delivery

A number of factors during the peripartum period may potentially provide clues to subsequent neurological or neurodevelopmental problems in the child. Chief among this is the gestational age at the time of birth. A term pregnancy is 37 to 42 weeks of completed gestation, late preterm 34 to 36 weeks of completed gestation, and preterm < 34 weeks of gestation. The preterm brain is vulnerable to white matter hypoxic-ischemic injury and resultant periventricular leukomalacia (PVL) leading to typical spastic diplegic cerebral palsy. It is also susceptible to germinal matrix-intraventricular hemorrhage (IVH) with the potential consequence of obstructive hydrocephalus and/or hemiplegia in the case of a grade IV IVH or periventricular echodensity. Birth weight is relevant in so far as it relates to prematurity, with babies weighing < 1,500 g being at highest risk for PVL and IVH, and may also be indicative of IUGR, suggesting possible placental insufficiency. Other important factors to consider and document include Apgar score and the need for resuscitation, type of resuscitation, and the presence or absence of meconium, all of which may indicate potential fetal distress and/or perinatal depression. Mode of delivery may be of some relevance in that an emergency cesarean section *may* indicate concerns for fetal distress, whereas forceps delivery has been implicated in facial nerve palsy at birth.

Placental size and pathology, when available, may provide important clues to potential placental insufficiency, chorioamnionitis, placental calcifications, infarct(s), and/or prior placental abruption.

Chorioamnionitis is especially important as it is a frequent cause of preterm labor and has independently been implicated in IVH. It also increases the risk for cerebral palsy in the term infant through a number of pathophysiological processes, including sepsis resulting in shock, hypoxic-ischemic injury, or even meningitis. Identifying whether perinatal hypoxia and ischemia are primarily the result of a peripartum complication, versus the stress of labor exacerbating a preexisting condition, is crucial as the former situation does not require further neurological workup as to etiology, whereas with the latter situation further evaluation as to etiology may be necessary to consider a primary metabolic, genetic, or neuromuscular etiology.

Postnatal Course

Information regarding postnatal complications, newborn screen, and potential neurological studies should be asked about. Factors to consider include the need for mechanical ventilation, extracorporeal membrane oxygenation, whole-body or brain cooling, sepsis, hypoglycemia, and/or a history of neonatal seizures. Feeding difficulties, hypotonia, and neonatal encephalopathy are other important factors that may have relevance to the differential diagnostic consideration. Encephalopathy developing a few days after birth raises the concern and inborn error of metabolism or possible late-onset sepsis.

Neonatal seizures may be indicative of hypoxic-ischemic encephalopathy, especially when occurring within the first 24 hours after birth, and frequently within 12 hours of birth. Twelve to fifteen percent of all neonatal seizures occurring in term babies are secondary to a perinatal stroke. Other causes include electrolyte disturbances (hypoglycemia, hypocalcemia), metabolic disorders (such as nonketotic hyperglycinemia and neonatal adrenoleukodystrophy), malformations of cortical development, meningitis, and potential drug withdrawal effects. Determining the etiology of the seizures can be helpful when considering the differential diagnosis. History of a burst suppression electroencephalogram at birth is invariably associated with poor neurological outcome.

8.2.3 Developmental History

Development is a defining feature of childhood and differentiates the pediatric neurological history from that of the adult. The intellectual, social, and motor developments of the child follow predictable patterns and meeting these developmental milestones is an important indication of the maturation of the child's nervous system and neurological function. Delay in obtaining age-appropriate developmental milestones and abnormal patterns of development are therefore important indicators of underlying neurological disease. An appreciation of normal developmental milestones is critical when evaluating an infant or child. Assessing development is an essential part and core component of the pediatric neurological examination.

In assessing developmental delay, it is important to distinguish between four functional domains, namely, gross motor, fine motor, social, and speech and language arenas. Global developmental delays involving all four arenas should be distinguished from disorders affecting specific functional domains or specific patterns of delay, for example, pervasive developmental disorders. History should provide a sense of mild, moderate, or severe developmental delay based on deviation from normal. It is important to remember to correct for gestational age for the first 12 to 18 months in a child born prematurely. It is important to determine whether there is *regression* of skills in any arena, as this could indicate a neurodegenerative process (e.g., leukodystrophy) and focuses the differential diagnosis. As this history may not be evident on a child's initial evaluation, subsequent follow-up and observation are important.

A number of standardized developmental screening tests are available (e.g., the Denver developmental screening test, Gesell developmental test, and the Binet test). For school-aged children, information about cognitive functioning is often available from school proficiency tests or multifactorial evaluations that include psychometric and achievement tests. A strong hand preference in an infant younger than 12 to 18 months of age is always abnormal and suggests weakness or apraxia of the opposite hand and side of the body. Developmental speech and language delay, when associated with impairments of socialization, scripted behaviors, and repetitive and stereotyped behaviors, should raise the concern of a possible pervasive developmental disorder or autistic spectrum disorder. A history of true language regression raises the possibility of an acquired epileptic aphasia such as Landau–Kleffner syndrome.

8.2.4 Past Medical and Surgical History

The presenting problem must be viewed in the context of the patient's past medical and surgical history, as this often provides insights into the current problem. Pertinent aspects of the past history may provide additional clues or pattern recognition in generating a differential diagnosis; for example, in a child being investigated for proximal muscle and neck flexor weakness, a history of academic difficulties and hypertrophic cardiomyopathy should raise the diagnostic consideration of Danon's disease, and in a child with short stature, failure to thrive, hearing loss, and retinal dystrophy, being evaluated with microcephaly and developmental delay, a diagnosis of Cockayne's syndrome is considered.

Chronic underlying illness may also be a factor in considering treatment options (e.g., avoiding beta-blockers in patients with migraine headache who have asthma, diabetes mellitus, or depression).

All prior hospitalizations and surgeries should be noted.

8.2.5 Family and Social History

As genetic medicine is increasingly providing an etiological basis for many pediatric neurological diseases, obtaining a complete and accurate family history is increasingly important in establishing a possible autosomal, X-linked, or mitochondrial inheritance pattern for the problem under investigation. This may help in directing targeted gene testing or identifying a condition that might not otherwise be considered. Many other disorders are also clearly familial, even in the absence of an identified gene, for example, migraine headache, learning disability, epilepsy, and Tourette's syndrome, and their presence in a family may help with the differential diagnosis.

Social circumstances and environmental factors may also contribute toward and affect the expression of certain disorders. In adolescents, it is important to inquire about alcohol, tobacco, potential illicit drug use, and sexual history as it pertains to the presenting problem.

8.2.6 Review of Systems

A systematic review of all major organ systems should complete the medical history, and serves as a symptom checklist to assure that all important areas of the patient's physical and psychological health have been considered and not overlooked or forgotten. The review of systems may also help illuminate the diagnosis by eliciting information that the patient may not otherwise have perceived as being important or related to the presenting problem.

8.3 Examination

At its essence, the neurological examination of the infant and child is similar to the adult examination and incorporates the same elements. What is different, however, is the approach. Instead of a systematic systems approach, one needs to approach the child in a nonthreatening manner, and much of the examination involves "games" and the use of ancillary devices such as toys or puppets. Observation is key and many aspects of the neurological examination can be gleaned from watching the child play. Those parts of the examination that may be perceived by the child as threatening, for example, ophthalmological examination, should be deferred until the end of the examination so as to not destroy the trust between examiner and child. Observing the child at play, at rest, and interacting with his/her caregivers often reveals key elements of the examination such as interactions with their environment, behaviors, and asymmetries or abnormalities in posture or movement, for example, dystonia, posturing, tremor, or infantile spasms. In an older child and adolescent, a more traditional system approach to the child is possible.

8.3.1 General Examination

Three features of the general examination of the child that are important differentiating factors from the adult examination are attention to dysmorphology, neurocutaneous findings, and head size and shape. These areas should be addressed in all children, especially given the importance of genetic syndromes in pediatric neurological disease.

Dysmorphology

Many common genetic syndromes have neurological involvement as part of the syndrome, and many primary neurological conditions have a genetic basis as their etiology. More common examples of the former include trisomy 21 (Down's syndrome), Turner's syndrome, fragile X syndrome, Angelman's syndrome, Prader–Willi syndrome, Cornelia de Lange's syndrome, and velocardiofacial/DiGeorge's syndrome. Craniofacial and/or systemic dysmorphology usually give clues to these diagnoses and the phenotypic appearance is usually stereotyped. Midline defects such as cleft lip and/or palate, central incisors, and certain congenital heart defects may be associated with abnormalities of cortical migration, for example, cerebellar atrophy or polymicrogyria in q22 microdeletion syndromes, and a 30% incidence of major (agenesis of the corpus callosum, holoprosencephaly) or minor developmental brain anomalies in hypoplastic left heart syndrome.

Neurocutaneous Stigmata

The association between neurocutaneous lesions and central and/or peripheral nervous systems abnormalities is well established. The diversity of neurological symptoms is extensive and, as such, all children should have their skin closely examined as part of the neurological examination. Wood's lamp is usually more sensitive than visual inspection alone and should be utilized if there is any suspicion for birthmarks. The nature of the birthmark provides clues as to the specific neurocutaneous syndrome or phakomatoses (▶ Table 8.1). Eye involvement is a frequent accompaniment of these conditions.

Head Size and Shape

Measuring and plotting the head circumference is an important part of the pediatric neurological examination at all ages. Measurement should be in absolute terms as well as expressed as a centile for age. Relationship to weight and height centiles is also important as it may reflect a relative micro- or macrocephaly. Head size directly reflects intracranial contents and the most dramatic increase in brain volume occurs in the last trimester of pregnancy through the first two years after birth.

Microcephaly is present when head circumference is 2 standard deviations below the mean. It may be either primary, i.e., congenital or present from birth, or secondary/acquired. Differentiating the two can be helpful in establishing a differential diagnosis, for example, the acquired microcephaly seen in Rett's syndrome as opposed to microcephaly polycythemia (rubra) in which the microcephaly is present at birth. Microcephaly may be

Table 8.1 Neurocutaneous skin lesions and associated syndromes

Skin findings	Syndrome
Café-au-lait macule	Neurofibromatosis
	Legius' syndrome
	Tuberous sclerosis
	Hypomelanosis of Ito
	McCune–Albright syndrome
Hypopigmented macule	Tuberous sclerosis
	Hypomelanosis of Ito
Hyperpigmented macules (following lines of Blaschko)	Incontinentia pigmenti
Shagreen patch	Tuberous sclerosis
Adenoma sebaceum	Tuberous sclerosis
Nevus flammeus	Sturge–Weber syndrome
	Klippel–Trénaunay syndrome
Gottron's papules	Dermatomyositis
Unilateral linear nevus (usually face)	Linear sebaceous nevus syndrome
Papulovesicular lesions (following lines of Blaschko)	Incontinentia pigmenti
Telangiectasia	Ataxia-telangiectasia
	Xeroderma pigmentosum
Freckling	Neurofibromatosis (LEOPARD syndrome)
	Xeroderma pigmentosum
Axillary/inguinal freckling	Neurofibromatosis
Penile freckling	PTEN gene mutation
	Multiple lentigines syndrome (LEOPARD syndrome)

familial, so measurement of the parent's head circumference is important. Microcephaly may also be due to malformations of cortical development (e.g., schizencephaly, lissencephaly, and polymicrogyria), hypoxic-ischemic brain injury, congenital infections (e.g., cytomegalovirus, toxoplasmosis, and rubella), or premature fusion of the sutures (craniosynostosis).

Macrocephaly is defined as 2 standard deviations above the mean. In PTEN gene mutations, head circumference is typically 3 standard deviations above the mean. Macrocephaly is often a familial genetic trait inherited from one parents, so, when present, one should attempt to document the parents' head circumference measurements. Benign macrocrania of infancy (also known as benign external hydrocephalus) is another common cause of macrocephaly and is also often familial in nature. It has a distinctive radiographic appearance (increased extra-axial cerebrospinal fluid spaces predominantly over the frontal convexities and extending into the interhemispheric fissure) and may be associated with mild motor developmental delay. This needs to be distinguished from communicating or obstructive hydrocephalus, which may produce signs and symptoms of increased intracranial pressure (lethargy, vomiting, and "sun-setting" sign). Unlike benign macrocrania of infancy in which the head circumference follows its own appropriate centile, with hydrocephalus there is crossing of centile lines. Sequential measurement of head circumference is therefore important and may provide additional important information. Macrocephaly may occur in some of the neurocutaneous syndromes, especially neurofibromatosis type 1. Other rare causes of macrocephaly include Alexander's disease, Canavan's disease, glutaric aciduria type I, and thickening of the skull (e.g., myelodysplasias or sickle cell disease).

Abnormalities of skull shape should also be noted. Positional plagiocephaly is increasingly being encountered with the "back to sleep" policy for infants. Plagiocephaly may also occur secondary to torticollis or may be seen in children with developmental delay and decreased mobility due to hypotonia and/or weakness. Abnormal head shape may be seen in isolated craniosynostosis with premature fusion of one or more of the sutures, or as part of a craniofacial syndrome including Pfeiffer's syndrome (turribrachycephaly), Crouzon's disease (acrocephaly), Saethre–Chotzen syndrome (brachycephaly), and Apert's syndrome (brachycephaly).

The anterior fontanelle typically closes between 12 and 18 months of age, although this is variable and closure at 6 months may be normal. Premature closure may be associated with microcephaly or craniosynostosis. Persistence of the anterior fontanelle beyond 18 months, or a large anterior fontanelle, raises the suspicion of hypothyroidism. A large fontanelle may also be associated with increased intracranial pressure, although this is usually also associated with bulging of the fontanelle. The posterior fontanelle typically closes between 3 and 6 months of age.

8.3.2 Neurological Examination

Mental Status

The mental status examination in the newborn, infant, and child should include references to level of consciousness, cognition, behaviors, and age-based language ability. Identified deficits may require more specialized neuropsychometric or psychiatric testing, or completion of neurobehavioral or autism ratings scales. A child's awareness of their environment, alertness, and appropriateness of interaction with the examiner serves as a basis for level of consciousness. Altered awareness in an encephalopathic patient requires a more detailed assessment of level of consciousness, including whether the patient is confused or disoriented (time, place, or person), sedated (requiring external stimulus to maintain interaction), stuperose, or comatosed. It is very important to document the level of alertness when examining the newborn baby, as the examination may be very different depending on whether the baby is awake/alert, drowsy, light sleep, or in deep sleep.

A child's cognitive ability, and whether age appropriate or not, can usually be assessed from the examiner's direct interaction with the child and the child's ability to follow simple or more complex commands with or without need for visual or other clues. Poor eye contact may be indicative of an autistic spectrum disorder. With stranger anxiety, a young infant will typically turn to parents for reassurance when presented an object from a "stranger," whereas children with autistic spectrum disorders often do not display this phenomenon. Attention to task, impulsiveness, and motor hyperactivity are particularly important to note if academic difficulties or disorders of behavior are of concern. This should always be interpreted, however, in the context of the age of the child and with reasonable expectations, given the circumstances of a clinical examination. An assessment of mood may be important, particularly for patients with behavioral problems, chronic headache, or chronic pain syndromes. Language assessment should include age expressive and receptive language ability, fluency, and articulation. Awareness of age-related speech norms is important, such as cooing in infants less than 6 months of age, babbling with initial vowel sounds and then subsequently consonances and bisyllables between 6 and 12 months of age, cumulative word acquisition in the second year of life, and the joining of words or short phrases by 2 years of age.

A more detailed mental status examination is rarely necessary and should be dictated by the presenting symptoms and history. With older children and adolescents, a formal mini-mental assessment can be performed if necessary.

Cranial Nerves

Although examination of the cranial nerves in a child is similar to that of the adult, there are some notable exceptions.

Cranial nerve I (olfactory nerve): It is rarely tested in children except when anosmia is an important consideration (e.g., Kallmann's syndrome). As it requires differentiation of different smells, it is hard to test in very young children but can be tested by presenting the child with familiar smells (for age) and asking the child to identify it with his/her eyes closed.

Cranial nerve II (optic nerve): There are four components in the examination of the optic nerve, namely, visual acuity, visual fields, pupillary light reflex, and fundoscopic examination. In the newborn, the absence of a red reflex on direct ophthalmoscopic examination raises the concern of retinoblastoma. Confrontational visual field testing is not possible in a very young child, but a blink response to a threat provides a crude assessment of visual field integrity. In slightly older children, having them fixate on an object in the midline while bringing in a bright toy from the periphery will also provide an assessment of peripheral visual field based on when they recognize and turn toward the object. Visual acuity can be tested in the young child by using a Snellen eye chart or "E" chart.

Cranial nerve III, IV, and VI (oculomotor, trochlear, and abducens nerves): The extraocular muscles are tested by having the child look in the six cardinal directions of gaze, namely, horizontally, vertically, up and out to the left and right, and down and out to the left and right. Fluidity of movement and whether there are any saccadic intrusions into smooth pursuit should be noted. Although a very young infant will fix on and follow a face, "doll's head" movements (oculocephalic) are usually necessary for assessing extraocular movements during the neonatal period.

The use of a bright, colorful object is generally necessary in an infant or older child to sustain attention. Babies rarely begin to track until about 6 weeks of age. The trochlear nerve (IV nerve) innervates the superior oblique muscle of each eye, resulting in medial and downward deviation with intorsion of the eye. Paresis of the nerve results in an extorted eye and children often tilt their head toward the opposite side to accommodate for the double vision. A head tilt or torticollis in a child may therefore be the only clue to a fourth nerve palsy, because the child may not complain of diplopia. The abducens nerve (sixth nerve) innervates the lateral rectus muscle, which is responsible for abduction of the eye. Injury or paresis of the sixth nerve therefore results in adduction (medial deviation) of the eye and diplopia. This is often an accompanying sign and symptom in pseudotumor cerebri. The oculomotor nerve (III nerve) innervates the remainder of the eye muscles and also provides parasympathetic fiber innervation of the pupil responsible for pupillary constriction. Involvement of the third nerve results in the eye being in a "down and out" position, namely, laterally deviated and depressed, with a dilated pupil and ptosis. In the older child who can describe diplopia, the degree of diplopia will be greatest when he/she is looking toward the direction corresponding to the action of the impaired muscle. Ptosis and ophthalmoplegia raises the possibility of myasthenia gravis, mitochondrial cytopathy, or a myotubular myopathy. Exotropia and esotropia are frequently encountered in the infant and young child, and latent strabismus can be unmasked by the cover–uncover test. When these are detected, the child should be referred to an ophthalmologist for further evaluation and possible patching to allow for fusion and the development of binocular vision.

Cranial nerve V (trigeminal nerve): The trigeminal nerve is predominately a sensory nerve but does have a motor component that provides innervations to the muscles of mastication (temporalis and masseter muscles) and the muscle involved in keeping the jaw open (lateral pterygoid muscle). This can be assessed in younger children by having them chew a cookie and in older children by having them clench their teeth. The sensory distribution of the trigeminal nerve provides three distinct areas of facial innervation, namely, the ophthalmic branch (V1), maxillary branch (V2), and mandibular branch (V3). There branches can be individually tested for light touch, pinprick, and temperature, and when necessary vibration sense. The latter is most helpful when a psychogenic sensory disorder is suspected and the child or adolescent describes a "midline splitting" of vibration sense in the midline of the forehead, i.e., feeling the vibration up to the midline and then not feeling it as the midline is crossed. The rooting reflex in the newborn can provide a crude assessment of nerve function at birth. Examination of the sixth nerve also involves the corneal reflex as the afferent component of the corneal blink reflex is supplied from the V1 distribution of the corneal nerve. This is seldom part of the routine neurological examination in children, but is an important part of the examination if a brainstem injury is suspected, or in a comatose or brain dead patient.

Cranial nerve VII (facial nerve): The facial nerve supplies motor branches to the muscles of facial expression. There is also a sensory branch supplying the skin over part of the pinna, a patch of skin behind the ear, and the external surface of the tympanic membrane. In the newborn, the facial nerve is tested by direct observation of the baby feeding and crying, and watching the movement of the face. In an older child, asking them to make a "funny face," puff out their cheeks, smile or reveal their teeth, close their eyelids tightly against resistance, and raise their eyebrows or wrinkle up their forehead (if able to cooperate) allows a good assessment of facial nerve function. Taste is difficult to test in a young child and is generally unnecessary. An upper motor neuron lesion affecting the facial nerve causes contralateral weakness of the lower face, sparing the forehead (upper portions of the orbicularis oculi and the frontalis muscles) as the facial nuclei project bilaterally to the forehead muscles. In lower motor neuron lesions such as a Bell's palsy, the weakness involves the whole ipsilateral face, including forehead. In the newborn period, differentiating a lower motor neuron facial lesion from congenital absence or hypoplasia of the angularis oris muscle ("asymmetric smiling facies") is important. In the latter, there is failure to depress the corner of the mouth with smiling or crying while the rest of the facial muscles and nasolabial fold are normal and symmetric. Congenital absence or hypoplasia of the angularis oris muscle may occur in isolation and be familial (autosomal dominant inheritance), but may also be associated with Cayler's syndrome in which there may be associated congenital heart disease or central nervous system problems (including microcephaly, cognitive impairment, cerebral and cerebellar atrophy).

Cranial nerve VIII (vestibulocochlear or acoustic nerve): Examination of the eighth cranial nerve principally involves assessment of hearing (cochlear branch), although in select circumstances the assessment of inner ear vestibular function is important. In the first month of life, a neonate will alert and quieten to a bell presented at his/her ear, and by 5 or 6 months of age, he/she should turn and localize the source of sound. In an older child, gently rubbing one's fingers at the opening of the ear canal and asking the patient to identify the sound, and localize the side of the sound, can be utilized for screening hearing. If hearing loss is suspected, it is important to differentiate sensorineural hearing loss from conductive hearing loss. This can be clinically achieved with the use of a tuning fork. The Weber test involves placing a vibrating tuning fork over the vertex of the skull in the midline and having the patient identify which ear the vibrating tone is heard best. With normal hearing, this is equal in both ears. With sensorineural hearing loss, the tone is louder on the normal ear, whereas with conductive hearing loss the tone is louder on the deaf ear.

The Rinne test assesses the difference between bone conduction and air conduction. A vibrating tuning fork is held adjacent to each canal (air conduction) and is compared for intensity to the sound heard when placing the tuning fork handle on each mastoid process (bone conduction). In normal circumstances, air conduction is better appreciated than bone conduction. If bone conduction is louder than air conduction, this suggests a conduction hearing loss in the ipsilateral ear. In sensorineural hearing loss, however, air conduction is better than bone conduction in the affected ear. Vestibular testing may be necessary in select circumstances, such as in cases of vertigo to differentiate central from peripheral vertigo (Barany *or* Hallpike positional testing), or to assess ocular movements and intact brainstem function in comatose patients using the vestibulo-ocular reflex ("Doll's eye maneuver"). The vestibulo-ocular reflex utilizes stimulation of the afferent input from the vestibular apparatus (either cold caloric test or Doll's eye maneuver) with efferent outputs supplying the muscles involved with lateral eye movements.

Cranial nerve IX and X (glossopharyngeal and vagus nerve): Although the glossopharyngeal and vagus nerves have several branchial and visceral motor branches as well as sensory branches, from a practical perspective their integrity is assessed primarily through the gag reflex and palatal elevation. The gag reflex receives its afferent nerve supply from the glossopharyngeal nerve, while the efferent supply is mediated via the vagus nerve from the palate. Asking a child to say "AH" assesses palatal movement and symmetry. Gag reflex does not necessarily need to be routinely tested unless there is concern for impaired swallowing, oropharyngeal dysfunction, impaired consciousness, or suspected brainstem pathology. In the newborn baby or young infant, eliciting the gag response is often necessary to assess palatal function.

Cranial nerve XI (accessory nerve): The spinal accessory nerve innervates the trapezius and sternocleidomastoid muscles. These muscles are tested by having the child shrug their shoulders, and turn their head to the side in both directions against resistance. Formal testing of these muscles in the newborn or infant is difficult.

Cranial nerve XII (hypoglossal nerve): The hypoglossal nerve supplies motor innervation to the intrinsic and extrinsic muscles of the tongue. Paresis of the hypoglossal nerve results in ipsilateral deviation of the protruded tongue to the side of weakness and associated ipsilateral atrophy of the tongue. In the newborn or infant, tongue movement is best appreciated by placing a finger in the mouth and getting a sense of tongue movement as the child tries to manipulate the finger in its mouth. The older child should be asked to protrude the tongue midline (often achieved by visual mimicking of the examiner doing the action), and having them push their tongue into their cheek against the resistance of the examiner's fingers. Fasciculation of the tongue is indicative of anterior horn cell disease such as spinal muscular atrophy.

Motor Examination

The motor examination involves testing the integrity of the pyramidal, extrapyramidal, and cerebellar systems. The various components include assessment of muscle bulk and tone, and testing of strength, reflexes, coordination of movement, and gait. Reflexes, coordination of movement, and gait will be dealt with in separate sections below.

Muscle Bulk

Observe for asymmetry, atrophy, or hypertrophy of muscles. Pseudohypertrophy, particularly of calf muscles, is in several muscular dystrophies, including Duchenne's, Becker's, and limb-girdle muscular dystrophy. Generalized muscular hypertrophy is seen in myotonia congenita ("Hercules appearance"). Atrophy of muscle is seen in disuse, cachexia, neurogenic (e.g., Charcot–Marie–Tooth disease), or anterior horn cell disease (e.g., spinal muscular atrophy). Scapular winging due to weakness and wasting of the supraspinatus and infraspinatus muscles occurs in some forms of limb-girdle muscular dystrophy as well as in facioscapulohumeral muscular dystrophy. Fasciculation of the muscle are seen in anterior horn cell disease (e.g., spinal muscular atrophy, polio, Pompe's disease). Palpation of the muscles provides a sense of the underlying muscle mass and can elicit pain or discomfort. Muscle tenderness may suggest a myositis. A "doughy" feel to the muscles raises the suspicion of an underlying neuromuscular disorder. Percussion of muscle is not routinely performed but should be done when history suggests a possible myotonic muscle disorder. Percussion over the thenar eminence, tongue, or deltoid muscle may elicit a sustained muscle contraction (myotonia). Sustained grip or eye closure may result in difficulty opening the hand or eyes, respectively, confirming myotonia, and may be the only clue to the diagnosis in a young child.

Muscle Tone

Tone reflects the resistance of a limb to passive movement. It may be normal, increased (hypertonic), or decreased (hypotonic). When tone is increased, it is important to differentiate spasticity from rigidity. Spasticity results from damage to the descending corticospinal or pyramidal tracts, whereas rigidity results from damage to the basal ganglia. Spasticity is the hallmark of an upper motor neuron lesion (pyramidal tract injury) and results in a characteristic pattern of increased tone in the extremities—flexion of the upper extremities and extension of the lower extremities. It is velocity dependent and is assessed by quick flexion/extension of a joint giving rise to the so-called clasp knife phenomenon (initial resistance to passive movement of the joint, followed by sudden reduction in tone allowing the limb to move freely and unrestricted through the rest of the range of movement for that joint). Hyperreflexia, Babinski's response (extensor toe), and occasionally clonus are accompanying upper motor neuron signs to spasticity. Contractures result from muscle imbalance and reduced movement around the joint. An early sign of spasticity in the infant is extension of the legs with plantar flexion of the feet with vertical suspension. With more severe spasticity, scissoring of the legs occurs. Spasticity typically develops over the course of the first year of life in an infant as myelination of the white matter tracts occurs, and in the first few months of life, upper motor neuron lesion of the infant may result in hypotonia before hypertonia develops. Early hand preference (i.e., a strong hand preference before 12–18 months of age) is abnormal and is generally indicative of weakness or impairment of the opposite arm. Hypertonia or spasticity present at birth suggests an early prenatal brain insult, while the presence of contractures or arthrogryposis suggests in utero onset diminished fetal movement.

Another subtle sign of early brain insult or injury is obligatory fisting or the "cortical thumb" sign. This may be present even in the absence of hypertonia. An infant up to about 3 months of age may hold the hand fisted, with the thumbs adducted most of the time, but after 4 months of age, the hand should be open most of the time, and if not, it should raise concern of possible injury to the central nervous system. Damage to the basal ganglia (extrapyramidal injury) results in rigidity, dystonia, or extrapyramidal movements (see later). Rigidity results in increased tone in all directions of movement of the joint that is not velocity-dependent (so-called lead pipe rigidity). Resistance is present in both agonist and antagonist muscles. Cogwheel rigidity is present when there is a tremor superimposed on the rigidity, giving a "ratchet" feeling to the increased tone. Hypotonia or flaccidity is decreased or absent resistance of passive movement of a limb and is seen with lower motor neuron or cerebellar/cerebellar pathway lesions. Hyporeflexia/areflexia and hyperextensibility of the joint may be accompanying features. Muscle wasting or fasciculation may also be seen. Hypotonia frequently results in abnormal posture at rest, for example, the "frog leg" position and internal rotation of the shoulders seen in spinal muscular atrophy. A premature infant is hypotonic because flexor tone develops at about 32 weeks of gestation and is strongly established by term. Head lag on pull-to-sit and poor head and trunk posture with vertical suspension confirm axial hypotonia. By 3 months of age, an infant should be able to maintain the head in the horizontal midline position with ventral suspension, and after 4 months of age, an infant should be able to elevate and maintain the head above the midline. In certain conditions, a combination of central and peripheral nervous system involvement (peripheral neuropathy) may occur, for example, Krabbe's disease, metachromatic leukodystrophy, or mitochondrial cytopathy.

Muscle strength: One can reliably test strength in children as young as 4 or 5 years of age. Many different scales exist for testing manual strength, but the most commonly used is the Medical Research Council 5-point grade scale, with grade 0 representing complete paralysis of movement and grade 5 representing normal strength. Grade 1 represents a flicker or trace of movement, grade 2 represents active movement but with gravity eliminated, grade 3 represents a full range of antigravity movement for the joint, and grade 4 strength represents antigravity movement against varying degrees of resistance but with some weakness present. Grades 4 −, 4, 4 + are used to indicate the degree of force necessary to overcome the muscle strength being mild, moderate, or strong resistance, respectively. Strength in the lower extremities is best assessed with the patient supine. A Gowers sign is indicative of significant proximal pelvic girdle weakness and is elicited by having the child lie flat on his/her back and then attempting to stand as quickly as possible without the assistance of furniture. In the presence of weakness, the child will first roll over onto the stomach, adduct, and "lock" the legs at the knees, and then uses the arms to push off the floor and "walk" or climb up the legs by pushing on the knee. In the neonate/infant and young child, direct observation provides invaluable information about strength. In the newborn, spontaneous movements and/or gentle stimulation of the extremities can detect the presence of at least antigravity strength. Watching the child walk into the room, climbing onto and off a chair, reaching for toys, and jumping and hopping will readily identify marked weakness. Patterns of weakness should be documented because they provide useful clues about cause, for example, monoplegia or hemiplegia in focal cerebral injury or neonatal stroke, diplegia in injury to the premature brain, or quadriplegia in diffuse cortical or cerebral injury. A proximal-to-distal distribution of weakness or vice versa may be helpful in differentiating myopathy from neuropathy or distinguishing among the various myopathies.

Deep Tendon Reflexes

By convention, reflexes are graded using a 4-point scale, with 0 being absent, 1 + being reduced or present with reinforcement only, 2 + being normal, 3 + being increased/hyperactive without clonus, and 4 + being increased/hyperactive with clonus. Spreading of reflexes to other muscles not directly being tested and crossed adduction of the opposite leg when the medial aspect of the knee (medial epicondyle of the femur) is tapped ("cross adductor reflex") is suggestive of hyperreflexia. The crossed adductor reflex is normally present, however, for the first few months of life, but its presence after about 6 to 8 months of age should be regarded as pathological. Pathologically brisk reflexes are indicative of upper motor neuron dysfunction, whereas absent or depressed reflexes are indicative of a lower motor neuron lesion (e.g., anterior horn cell disease, peripheral neuropathy,

Table 8.2 Main deep tendon reflexes and root innervation

Reflex	Nerve/root innervation
Jaw jerk	Trigeminal nerve
Biceps	C5–C6
Brachioradialis	C5–C6
Triceps	C6–C7 (predominately C7)
Finger jerk	C8–T1
Knee/patellar jerk	L3–L4
Ankle jerk	S1
Superficial reflexes	
Corneal reflex	Afferent: V1 branch of trigeminal nerve (fifth cranial nerve) Efferent: facial nerve (seventh cranial nerve)
Abdominal reflex: above umbilicus	T8–T10
Abdominal reflex: below umbilicus	T10–T12
Cremasteric reflex	L1–L2
Anal reflex	S2–S4
Plantar reflex	L4–S2

Table 8.3 Primitive reflexes

Primitive reflex	Appearance of reflex	Disappearance of reflex
Moro	Birth	6 mo
Palmar and plantar grasp	32 wk	2 mo
Rooting and sucking	32 wk	4 mo
Stepping and placing	37 wk	Persists as voluntary standing
Tonic neck reflex	1 mo	6 mo
Neck righting reflex	4 mo	Persists voluntarily
Parachute	6–9 mo	Persists indefinitely

or myopathy) or cerebellar/cerebellar pathway dysfunction. Clonus is elicited by flexing the infant's or child's knee and rapidly dorsiflexing the ankle. Sustained clonus is always abnormal but a few beats of nonsustained clonus may occasionally occur in normal people, especially neonates. Nonpathological brisk reflexes may occasionally be seen in young people, especially adolescent females or children who are very anxious. Reinforcement maneuvers should be use when reflexes are difficult to elicit before concluding they are absent or reduced. These maneuvers include distraction by having the patient perform isometric contraction of muscles such as clenching of teeth or having patient clasp flexed fingers and pulling apart ("Jendrassik's maneuver"). The major reflexes tested in infants and children are the same as those tested in adults (▶ Table 8.2). Additional specific reflexes are evaluated as appropriate. A key difference between adults and children is the appearance and disappearance of certain primitive reflexes that serve as important indicators of the maturation and integrity of the nervous system (▶ Table 8.3). Asymmetries or persistence of these reflexes in certain instances is pathological. An obligate tonic reflex ("fencing posture") is always abnormal. Many of these reflexes (e.g., the grasp,

snout, and sucking reflexes) may also reappear in adults because of a loss of inhibition of the reflex that occurs in some neurodegenerative conditions.

The plantar response is a polysynaptic superficial reflex testing the integrity of the corticospinal tracts. It is elicited by stroking the lateral border of the foot with the thumb or blunt object from the heel toward the little toe and then moving medially toward the big (first) toe. A normal response is flexion of the toes, while an abnormal pathological response, indicative of an upper motor neuron lesion, involves extension of the big (first) toe with extension and fanning of the other toes (Babinski's sign). The Babinski method is the most reliable method of eliciting the plantar response, but other methods exist, including Chaddock's sign in which the stimulus is applied along the lateral aspect of the foot, below the external malleolus, and Oppenheim's reflex in which firm pressure is applied along the shin of the tibia from below the knee up to the level of the ankle. There is controversy as to whether a Babinski sign is abnormal during the first year of life. A unilateral Babinski response should, however, be regarded as pathological as should the presence of a Babinski response after a child starts walking. The Hoffman sign in the upper extremity is essentially the equivalent of the Babinski sign in the legs, its presence being abnormal and indicative of an upper motor neuron lesion. This sign is elicited by holding the child's middle finger loosely and rapidly flicking the fingernail downward, then allowing it to rebound slightly into extension. If the thumb flexes and adducts in response, Hoffmann's sign is present.

Coordination of Movement

Coordination of movement is a complex task and requires the integration of motor, sensory, and cerebellar systems. Dysfunction in any one of these systems may affect coordination, for example, proximal muscle weakness may resemble ataxia. The motor and sensory systems are generally tested separately, so tests of coordination predominately affect testing of the cerebellum and its pathways. The cerebellum is responsible for smooth, integrated, coordinated movement of the limb and gait, and disorders of the cerebellum therefore result in jerky, nonrhythmic movements or ataxia. Disorders or lesions of the cerebellar hemispheres result in ipsilateral appendicular ataxia, dysmetria (impaired judgment of distance with past pointing), and dysdiadochokinesia (abnormal or impaired rapid alternating movements). Midline lesions, on the other hand, produce gait and truncal ataxia. To be certain that the ataxia is of cerebellar origin, proprioceptive loss has to be excluded; however, proprioceptive testing is difficult to test reliably in a child younger than 5 or 6 years of age. Cerebellar testing can be very difficult to do in a young child and in the neonate where cooperation is limited. Often, careful observation of the child playing, undressing, and doing zippers or buttons provides useful information about dexterity, steadiness of reach, accuracy, and/or presence of abnormal involuntary movements. By 18 months of age, a child should know a number of body parts and, with the use of a doll, can be encouraged to go back and forward between a doll's nose and his or her own nose. Rapid alternating movement can be more difficult to test, but with patience, it is possible to get even a young child to mimic the action. More "traditional" finger–nose or heel–shin testing or rapid alternating movement testing is possible in the older child. Gently pushing down on the child's outstretched arms and then suddenly releasing the arms, causing the arm on the affected side suddenly to fly upward, can be used to demonstrate the phenomenon of limb rebound seen in cerebellar lesions. Romberg's testing is achieved by having the child stand with both feet touching one another and having him/her close the eyes. The test is positive if there is swaying and falling (to the side of the lesion). Postural stability is tested by having the child stand with his/her feet comfortably apart and then pulling back on the shoulders quickly while asking the child to maintain his/her balance (and remaining behind the child so he/she does not fall). Retropulsion is present if the child is unable to maintain his/her posture and steps or falls backward. This may be seen with cerebellar and/or extrapyramidal disorders. Tandem gait (walking a straight line with one foot in front of the other) is not reliably performed until a child is about 8 years old. With gait ataxia, the child tends to stand with the feet wide apart for stability and sways side to side with walking, often falling to the side of the lesion (if unilateral). Impairment of the visual pathways with resultant nystagmus (maximal toward side of lesion) and impairment of speech (scanning dysarthria and staccato speech) are often accompaniments to cerebellar lesions.

Gait: The gait is assessed by observing the child walk and run. A normal gait should be narrow based and steady with good, symmetric arm swing. Walking is typically achieved by 12 to 18 months of age with fast walking and running by 18 to 24 months of age. The toddler gait tends to be slightly wide based and unsteady. Watching the child stoop and recover, such as having them pick up a toy from the floor, provides useful information as to truncal stability. Classic abnormal gait patterns include hemiplegic, spastic/scissoring, ataxic, high steppage (footdrop or proprioceptive loss), waddling (proximal pelvic weakness), and antalgic patterns. Rarely, astasia-abasia or hysterical gait patterns may be found, with elaborate attempts to maintain balance. In the young child, toe walking requires further evaluation as it may represent early tightness or contractures of the Achilles tendon; if unilateral, it may represent a hemiplegia, and if bilateral, it may represent spastic diplegia or may be secondary to muscle weakness such as muscular dystrophy. Intermittent toe walking is often seen in the autistic-spectrum disorders and may occasionally be volitional in otherwise neurologically normal children. Over time, however, it may result in fixed contractures of the Achilles tendon. Even before a child can walk, dragging of a leg or arm when crawling may indicate hemiplegia. The appearance of asymmetric patterns of shoe wear may be seen even with mild hemiparesis.

Involuntary Movements

Damage or dysfunction of the basal ganglia results in involuntary movements (dyskinesias) that may be broadly classified into either an excess of movements (hyperkinesia) or a paucity of voluntary movements (hypokinesia) unrelated to weakness or spasticity. Collectively, these movements are known as extrapyramidal symptoms.

Hyperkinetic movements include:
- Chorea (fragmented, abrupt, jerky, involuntary movements of the limbs or face).

- Athetosis (a slow writhing-type movement).
- Tremors (rhythmic, involuntary, oscillatory movements); tremor may also arise from the cerebellum (cerebellar, "action," or "intention" tremor) due to dysfunction or injury of the ipsilateral cerebellar hemisphere.
- Ballismus (violent, large-amplitude movement involving flailing movements of the limbs).
- Dystonia (sustained or intermittent muscle contractions causing abnormal movements and posture of the limbs, trunk, or neck).
- Tics (brief, repetitive, nonrhythmical movements —motor or vocal; tendency to wax and wane over time).
- Myoclonus (sudden, brief, rapid involuntary jerking of a muscle or group of muscles; may be focal, multifocal, or generalized).

Hypokinetic movements include:
- Bradykinesia (slowness of movement).
- Akinesia (difficulty initiating and terminating movement).
- Rigidity (stiffness and/or inflexibility of a limb or trunk).

In general, movement disorders disappear during sleep and are exacerbated by pain, discomfort, anxiety, or agitation. In an infant, abnormal movements often need to be differentiated from a possible seizure. Dystonia with arching of the back and extension and rotation of the head is frequently a consequence of gastroesophageal reflux disease (Sandifer's syndrome). Chorea in childhood most commonly is due to rheumatic fever (Sydenham's chorea) or drugs (phenothiazines).

Juvenile Huntington's disease usually presents as stiffness rather than chorea in childhood. Choreoathetosis or dystonia may be a late sequela of cerebral palsy, occurring many years after the insult. Choreoathetosis also may occur with metabolic disorders or inborn errors of metabolism of childhood or with brain tumors affecting the basal ganglia or, rarely, as a complication of bypass surgery for congenital heart disease. Tics frequently are seen in children and adolescents as part of Tourette's syndrome (chronic vocal and motor tic disorder).

Sensory Examination

This is often the hardest part of the neurological examiantion in a child, and relies to a large extent on subjective reporting and interpretation. A rudimentary sensory examination is typiclly performed in children unless the history suggests a spinal cord lesion or peripheral nerve problem. Examination involves testing of primary and secondary (cortical sensory) sensory modalities. Primary sensory testing includes assessment of pain and temperature (spinothalamic tracts) and proprioception and vibration (dorsal columns). Light touch probably involves both spinothalamic and dorsal column tracts. Cortical sensory modalities include graphesthesia, two-point discrimination, and stereognosis. Discrimination and withdrawal to light touch and pain can be assessed readily even in a newborn, by watching the facial response and grimacing. In older children, sensory examination findings frequently are inconsistent, requiring repetition of the examination on multiple occasions.

9 Spinal Cord Tracts and Development

Micol Babini, Francesco Sala

9.1 Introduction

The spinal cord extends from the foramen magnum to the space between the first and second lumbar vertebrae. It is 40 to 50 cm long and 1 to 1.5 cm in diameter.

The spinal cord is divided into four different regions:
- Cervical.
- Thoracic.
- Lumbar.
- Sacral.

Two enlargements of the spinal cord can be identified:
- The cervical enlargement (from C3 to T1).
- The lumbar enlargement (from L1 to S2).

The cord is segmentally organized in 31 segments, defined by 31 pairs of nerves exiting the cord:
- Eight cervical.
- Twelve thoracic.
- Five lumbar.
- Five sacral.
- One coccygeal.

A transverse section of the spinal cord shows white matter in the periphery, gray matter inside, and a central canal filled with cerebrospinal fluid.

The gray matter mainly contains the cell bodies of neurons and glia, and is divided into four main columns:
- **Dorsal horn** comprises sensory nuclei that receive and process incoming somatosensory information. From there, ascending projections transmit the sensory information to brain.
- **Intermediate column and lateral horn** comprise autonomic neurons innervating visceral and pelvic organs.
- **Ventral horn** comprises motor neurons that innervate skeletal muscle.

Surrounding the gray matter is white matter containing nerve fibers that conduct information up (ascending) or down (descending) the cord (▶ Fig. 9.1).

The white matter is divided into:
- The **dorsal** column.
- The **lateral** column.
- The **ventral** column.

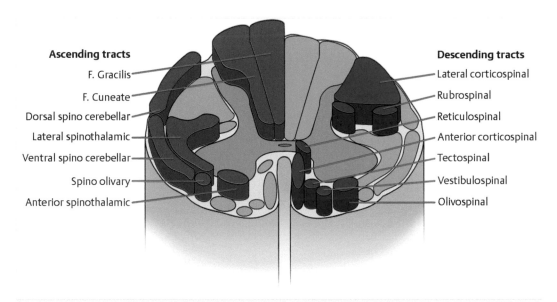

Ascending tracts
- F. Gracilis
- F. Cuneate
- Dorsal spino cerebellar
- Lateral spinothalamic
- Ventral spino cerebellar
- Spino olivary
- Anterior spinothalamic

Descending tracts
- Lateral corticospinal
- Rubrospinal
- Reticulospinal
- Anterior corticospinal
- Tectospinal
- Vestibulospinal
- Olivospinal

Fig. 9.1 Major ascending and descending tracts in a cross section of the spinal cord. (Reproduced with permission from Luka T. Ahčin, https://bellspalsycranialnerves.wordpress.com)

The spinal cord white matter contains ascending and descending tracts.

9.2 Ascending Tracts

The ascending tracts transmit sensory information from the sensory receptors to higher levels of the central nervous system (CNS).

The three major sensory tracts involve chains of neurons:
- First-order neuron: Delivers sensations to the CNS. The cell body is in the dorsal or cranial root ganglion.
- Second-order neuron: An interneuron with the cell body in the spinal cord or brain.
- Third-order neuron: Transmits information from the thalamus to the cerebral cortex.

Neurons in the sensory tracts are arranged according to three anatomical principles:
- Sensory modality: Fine touch sensations are carried in one sensory tract.
- Somatotopic: Ascending tracts are arranged according to the site of origin.
- Medial-lateral rule:
  - Sensory neurons that enter a low level of the spinal cord are more medial within the spinal cord.
  - Sensory neurons that enter at a higher level of the spinal cord are more lateral within the spinal cord.

The **dorsal column (medial lemniscal pathway)** is occupied by the gracile and cuneate fasciculi that carry information related to tactile, two-point discrimination of simultaneously applied pressure, vibration, position, and movement sense, and conscious proprioception. Within the medial lemniscal pathway, the afferents carrying discriminative touch information are kept separate from those carrying proprioceptive information up to the level of the cerebral cortex.

In the **lateral column**, the following are located:
- The neospinothalamic tract that carries pain, temperature, and crude touch information from somatic and visceral structures.
- The spinocerebellar tracts that carry unconscious proprioception information from muscles and joints of the lower extremity to the cerebellum.

In the **ventral column**, there are four prominent tracts:
- The paleospinothalamic tract (or anterior spinothalamic tract) carry pain, temperature, and information associated with touch.
- The spino-olivary tract carries information from Golgi tendon organs to the cerebellum.
- The spinoreticular tract.
- The spinotectal tract.

9.2.1 Posterior Column Tracts

It consists of:
- **Fasciculus gracilis**: Transmits information coming from areas inferior to T6.
- **Fasciculus cuneatus**: Transmits information coming from areas superior to T6.

First-order Neuron

- It arises from the sensory receptors of the body.
- Fibers enter the dorsal column and ascend to the medulla oblongata.
- It enters medulla oblongata.
- It ends in the gracile and cuneate nucleus.

Second-order Neuron

- It starts at the gracile and cuneate nucleus of the medulla oblongata.
- These fibers cross to the opposite side of the medulla oblongata.
- It ascends through the brainstem as flattened bundle medial lemniscus.
- It ends in the *ventral posterolateral nucleus* of the thalamus.

Third-order Neuron

- It arises from the thalamus.
- It passes through the internal capsule (medial aspect of the posterior limb of internal capsule).
- It reaches the postcentral gyrus and ends there.

9.2.2 Spinothalamic Tracts

- The **neospinothalamic tract (or lateral spinothalamic tract)** carries and processes sharp, pricking pain and dropping temperature (cool/cold) information from the body. The neospinothalamic pathway is also characterized

by somatotopic representation, which allows for accurate localization of the painful stimulus.
- The **anterior spinothalamic tract**.

First-order Neuron

- It arise from sensory receptors of the body.
- The fibers enter the white matter and end at the substantia gelatinosa.

Second-order Neuron

- The fibers of first-order neuron synapse with the second-order neuron at the substantia gelatinosa.
- These fibers then cross to the opposite side. Pain and temperature fibers enter the lateral spinothalamic tract. Light touch and pressure fibers enter the anterior spinothalamic tract.
- These tracts ascend to brainstem.
- It reaches the ventral posterolateral nucleus of the thalamus.
- It ends there.

Third-order Neuron

- The third-order neurons arise from the thalamus and pass through the internal capsule.
- Thalamocortical fibers pass through the medial part of the posterior limb of the internal capsule.
- They enter the postcentral gyrus.

9.2.3 Spinocerebellar Tracts

- The posterior spinocerebellar tract.
- The anterior spinocerebellar tract.

9.3 Descending Tracts

The descending tracts originate from different cortical areas and from brainstem nuclei. They carry information associated with maintenance of motor activities such as posture, balance, muscle tone, and visceral and somatic reflex activity.

Descending pathways are organized into two major groups:
- **Lateral pathways** control both proximal and distal muscles, and are responsible for most voluntary movements of arms and legs. They include:
  - The lateral corticospinal tract.
  - The rubrospinal tract.
- **Medial pathways** control axial muscles and are responsible for posture, balance, and coarse

control of axial and proximal muscles. They include:
  - The vestibulospinal tracts (both lateral and medial).
  - The reticulospinal tracts (both pontine and medullary).
  - The tectospinal tract.
  - The anterior corticospinal tract.

9.3.1 Corticospinal Tracts

The corticospinal tract originates in the motor cortex: the axons collect in the internal capsule, and then course through the crus cerebri (cerebral peduncle) in the midbrain.[1]

At the level of the caudal medulla, the corticospinal tract splits into two tracts:
- Approximately 90% of the axons cross over to the contralateral side at the pyramidal decussation, forming the **lateral corticospinal tract**. These axons continue to course through the lateral funiculus of the spinal cord, before synapsing either directly onto alpha motor neurons or onto interneurons in the ventral horn.
- The remaining 10% of the axons do not cross **the anterior corticospinal tract**, as they continue down the spinal cord in the anterior funiculus. When they reach the spinal segment at which they terminate, they cross over to the contralateral side through the anterior white commissure and innervate alpha motor neurons or interneurons in the anterior horn. Thus, both are crossed pathways.

The corticospinal tract is the primary pathway that carries the motor commands that underlie voluntary movement.

The lateral corticospinal tract is responsible for the control of the distal musculature and the anterior corticospinal tract is responsible for the control of the proximal musculature. A particularly important function of the lateral corticospinal tract is the fine control of the digits of the hand. In addition to the fine control of distal muscles, the corticospinal tract also plays a role in the voluntary control of axial muscles.

9.3.2 Rubrospinal Tract

The rubrospinal tract originates in the red nucleus of the midbrain: the axons immediately cross to the contralateral side of the brain, and they course through the brainstem and the lateral funiculus of the spinal cord.

The rubrospinal tract is an alternative by which voluntary motor commands can be sent to the spinal cord. Although it is a major pathway in many animals, it is relatively minor in humans. Activation of this tract causes excitation of flexor muscles and inhibition of extensor muscles.

9.3.3 Vestibulospinal Tracts

The two vestibulospinal tracts originate in two of the four vestibular nuclei.

- **The lateral vestibulospinal tract** originates in the lateral vestibular nucleus. It courses through the brainstem and through the anterior funiculus of the spinal cord on the ipsilateral side, before exiting ipsilaterally at all levels of the spinal cord.
- **The medial vestibulospinal tract** originates in the medial vestibular nucleus, splits immediately, and courses bilaterally through the brainstem via the medial longitudinal fasciculus and through the anterior funiculus of the spinal cord, before exiting at or above the T6 vertebra.

The vestibulospinal tracts mediate postural adjustments and head movements. They also help the body to maintain balance. The lateral vestibulospinal tract excites antigravity muscles in order to exert control over postural changes necessary to compensate for tilts and movements of the body. The medial vestibulospinal tract innervates neck muscles in order to stabilize head position. It is also important for the coordination of head and eye movements.

9.3.4 Reticulospinal Tracts

The two reticulospinal tracts originate in the brainstem reticular formation:

- **The pontine reticulospinal tract** originates in the pontine reticular formation, courses ipsilaterally through the medial longitudinal fasciculus and through the anterior funiculus of the spinal cord, and exits ipsilaterally at all spinal levels.
- **The medullary reticulospinal tract** originates in the medullary reticular formation, courses mainly ipsilaterally (although some fibers cross the midline) through the anterior funiculus of the spinal cord, and exits at all spinal levels.

The reticulospinal tracts are a major alternative to the corticospinal tract, by which cortical neurons can control motor function by their inputs onto reticular neurons. These tracts regulate the sensitivity of flexor responses to ensure that only noxious stimuli elicit these responses. The reticulospinal tracts are involved in many aspects of motor control, including the integration of sensory input to guide motor output.

9.3.5 Tectospinal Tract

The tectospinal tract originates in the deep layers of the superior colliculus and crosses the midline immediately. It then courses through the pons and medulla, just anterior to the medial longitudinal fasciculus. It courses through the anterior funiculus of the spinal cord, where the majority of the fibers terminate in the upper cervical levels.

9.4 Development

The nervous system develops from an area of embryonic ectoderm, called the neural plate which appears during the third week of gestational age. This area gives rise to

- The neural tube: that gives rise to the CNS.
- The neural crest: that gives rise to the peripheral nervous system.

The formation of the neural tube begins during the early part of week 4 (22–23 days) in the region of the fourth to sixth pairs of somites. The spinal cord is formed from the neural tube caudal to somites 4.

Once neurons have been generated, they move from their place of origin to their final place of destination in two different forms of migration. The migration peaks between the third and the fifth month of gestation and stops around 30-week postmenstrual age. The growth cones of the developing axon pathways navigate to their intermediate and final targets by responding to a variety of substrate-bound or diffusible molecular targets at near or long distance.

The development of the cerebral cortex can be divided into three periods:

- The embryonic.
- The fetal.
- The perinatal.

The corticospinal tract is the last of the major descending fiber systems to enter the spinal cord.[2]

Layer V neurons are among the first cortical neurons that reach their place in the cortical plate.[3,4] The first corticofugal projections originate in the embryonic period. They reach the pyramidal decussation at the end of the embryonic period.

The pyramidal decussation is complete by 17 weeks' postconceptional age (PCA).

Corticospinal axons reach the lower cervical spinal cord by 24 weeks PCA.[5,6] In a few weeks, they progressively innervate the gray matter, so before birth there is extensive innervation of spinal neurons, including motoneurons. By 40 weeks' PCA, corticospinal axons have begun to express neurofilaments and to undergo myelination.[6] Myelination of the pyramidal tract starts at the end of the second or the beginning of the third trimester, and it is not completed until the age of 2 to 3 years[7]; the cranial part is myelinated much earlier that its spinal part. Motor latencies decrease with age; in particular, a rapid decrease of the central motor conduction time happens during the first decade of life: and this corresponds to the maturation processes as myelination and axon growth.

In human, differently from subhuman primates, there is a prenatal establishment of functional corticospinal innervation.

During the final trimester of pregnancy, functional synaptic corticospinal projections to motoneurons and to interneurons are established.

At birth, the corticospinal tract is the least mature of the various tracts and undergoes dramatic changes during the first postnatal months. At birth, there is a significant bilateral innervation of spinal motoneuronal pool from each motor cortex. How-ever, in the first 15 to 18 months after birth, there is greater withdrawal of ipsilateral corticomotoneuronal projections than contralateral.[6,8,9]

References

[1] George TM, Adamson DC. Normal and abnormal development of the nervous system. In: Albright AL, Pollack IF, Adelson PD, eds. Principles and Practice of Pediatric Neurosurgery. 2nd ed. New York, NY: Thieme Medical Publishers; 2007:12–30

[2] Amiel-Tison C, Maillard F, Lebrun F, Bréart G, Papiernik E. Neurological and physical maturation in normal growth singletons from 37 to 41 weeks' gestation. Early Hum Dev. 1999; 54(2):145–156

[3] Martin JH, Friel KM, Salimi I, Chakrabarty S. Corticospinal development. In: Squire LR, ed. Encyclopedia of Neuroscience. Oxford: Academic Press; 2009:203–214

[4] ten Donkelaar HJ, Lammens M, Wesseling P, Hori A, Keyser A, Rotteveel J. Development and malformations of the human pyramidal tract. J Neurol. 2004; 251(12):1429–1442

[5] Eyre JA. Corticospinal tract development and its plasticity after perinatal injury. Neurosci Biobehav Rev. 2007; 31(8): 1136–1149

[6] Eyre JA. Development and plasticity of the corticospinal system in man. Neural Plast. 2003; 10(1–2):93–106

[7] Tanaka S, Mito T, Takashima S. Progress of myelination in the human fetal spinal nerve roots, spinal cord and brainstem with myelin basic protein immunohistochemistry. Early Hum Dev. 1995; 41(1):49–59

[8] Eyre JA, Taylor JP, Villagra F, Smith M, Miller S. Evidence of activity-dependent withdrawal of corticospinal projections during human development. Neurology. 2001; 57(9):1543–1554

[9] Müller K, Kass-Iliyya F, Reitz M. Ontogeny of ipsilateral corticospinal projections: a developmental study with transcranial magnetic stimulation. Ann Neurol. 1997; 42(5): 705–711

10 Migration Disorders

Gary Hsich

10.1 Introduction

The migrational disorders refers to a heterogenous group of disorders that share a similar pathogenesis. The neurons and glial cells are generated around the ventricles, the proliferative neuroepithelium. The first was of migrations results in the formation of the provisional cortex, the preplate. This is replaced by the permanent cortical plate. Migrating neurons are guided by adhesion molecules that are present on their membranes and are also neuronal and glial precursors.

These malformations are organized according to the underlying mechanism:
1. Abnormal cell proliferation
2. Abnormal neuronal migration
3. Abnormal cortical organization

10.2 Malformations

The following malformations are organized according to the timing of the insult during fetal central nervous system development, leading to the respective cortical migration disorders.

10.2.1 Anencephaly

Anencephaly is a condition in which major portions of the brain, skull, and scalp are absent. It occurs when the rostral (anterior) neuropore fails to close, which usually occurs between days 23 and 26 of gestation. About 1 in 1,000 pregnancies is affected by anencephaly, although most of the pregnancies result in miscarriage.[1] For fetuses that reach live birth, the rate is about 1 in 5,000 to 10,000; however, these infants do not survive longer than a few days. There is no treatment or surgical intervention indicated, except for comfort care and palliative measures. Management, therefore, has focused on preventive measures—folic acid supplementation has been shown to reduce the frequency of anencephaly by about 38%.[2]

10.2.2 Holoprosencephaly

Holoprosencephaly (▸ Fig. 10.1) is caused by failure of the prosencephalon to divide fully into two hemispheres during the third to fourth week of gestation. Definitive diagnosis is made by brain magnetic resonance imaging (MRI), and can show a spectrum of severity (in decreasing order of severity)[3]:
- **Alobar:** Single monoventricle, no separation of cerebral hemispheres.
- **Semilobar:** Left and right frontal and parietal lobes are fused, and the interhemispheric fissure is present only posteriorly.
- **Lobar:** Most of the right and left cerebral hemispheres and lateral ventricles are separated; but the frontal lobes are fused, especially ventrally.
- **Middle interhemispheric variant:** Posterior frontal and parietal lobes fail to separate, with varying lack of cleavage of the basal ganglia and

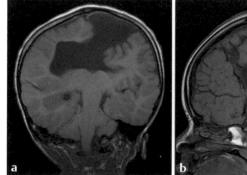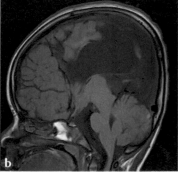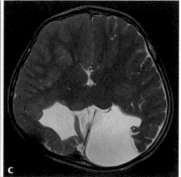

Fig. 10.1 Brain magnetic resonance imaging (MRI) of a 4-year-old child with holoprosencephaly. **(a)** Coronal, T1-weighted image. **(b)** Midline sagittal, T1-weighted image. **(c)** Axial, T2-weighted image. Note the fused thalami and single lateral ventricle.

thalami; absence of the body of the corpus callosum, but presence of the genu (anterior) and splenium (posterior) of the corpus callosum.

Likewise, clinically, there is a range of developmental disabilities; and affected children may have various craniofacial anomalies, such as cyclopia (one eye), proboscis (a noselike structure which may be located on the forehead), or cleft palate, or even normal facies. Seizures and pituitary dysfunction are common. Long-term prognosis depends on the severity of the malformation, with severely affected individuals surviving only a few years or less.

Approximately 25 to 50% of individuals have various causative chromosomal abnormalities; environmental causes, such as maternal diabetes, are also possible.[4]

Management is symptomatic, and may include shunting for hydrocephalus, anticonvulsant medication for seizures, hormone replacement for pituitary deficiencies, and interventions for feeding difficulties (gastrostomy tube, cleft palate repair).

10.2.3 Schizencephaly

Schizencephaly (▶ Fig. 10.2) is characterized by a cleft in the cerebral hemisphere, and this cleft is lined by gray matter. It is distinguished from porencephaly by the fact that porencephalic cysts are lined by white matter, while the disrupted cerebral cortex in schizencephaly is lined by gray matter. Schizencephaly can be classified as type I, in which the cleft is closed, or type II, in which the cleft is open and extends from the ventricle to the pia peripherally. Hydrocephalus is associated with about 50% of type II lesions.[5]

Schizencephaly is thought to be caused by a disruption in gray matter migration during the first trimester. The disruptive insult may be infarction, infection, a toxin, or genetic. Individuals with clefts in both hemispheres are typically quite impaired developmentally, while those with unilateral clefts may be of normal intelligence with unilateral weakness. Because of the presence of the heterotopic gray matter which lines the clefts, seizures are quite common.

10.2.4 Hydranencephaly

Hydranencephaly ("water brain") refers to a condition in which the cerebral hemispheres are replaced by cerebrospinal fluid (▶ Fig. 10.3). This malformation is thought to occur due to an insult (such as vascular or infection) during the late first or early second trimester, possibly in an anterior circulation distribution. The only remaining parts of the brain generally are the brainstem and the cerebellum. Because the brainstem is still intact, infants can appear and act normally for the first few months of life. They may have normal infant reflexes and behavior, such as sucking, swallowing, and crying. However, after a few weeks or months, these infants become irritable and spastic, and may develop hydrocephalus, seizures, and/or visual impairment. They do not achieve any significant developmental milestones, such as sitting,

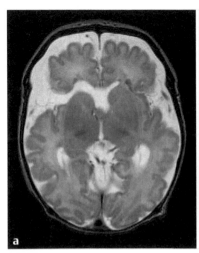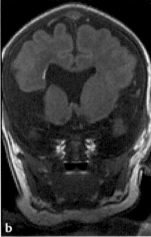

Fig. 10.2 Schizencephaly: brain MRI of newborn infant with schizencephaly, showing a gray matter–lined cleft in the right cerebral hemisphere. This cleft communicates with the right lateral ventricle. **(a)** Axial, T2-weighted image. **(b)** Coronal, T1-weighted image.

rolling, or speech production. Many children with this disorder die within the first few years of life, although some can live for several years or more with attentive care.

Differential diagnoses include severe hydrocephalus, alobar holoprosencephaly, and bilateral schizencephaly.

Treatment is symptomatic, and may include a palliative shunt for hydrocephalus. Gabapentin may be helpful for irritability, and baclofen is often used for spasticity.

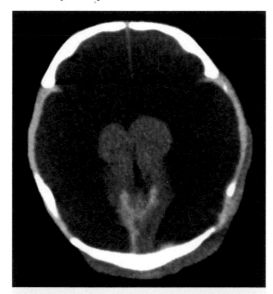

Fig. 10.3 Hydranencephaly: computed tomography (CT) scan of a newborn infant with hydranencephaly. The cerebral cortex has been almost entirely replaced with cerebrospinal fluid. The thalami, brainstem, and cerebellum are still present.

10.2.5 Lissencephaly and Pachygyria

Lissencephaly ("smooth brain") and pachygyria ("thick brain") are often considered variations along the same spectrum. The timing of the defect is thought to occur during the third to fourth month of gestation.[5] This cortical malformation is characterized by a lack of the normally folded gyri, such that the cerebral cortex is smooth with no folds (lissencephaly) or that the few existing folds are thickened and broad (▶ Fig. 10.4). Affected children have significant developmental impairments, do not learn to walk or speak, and almost always have seizures.

Lissencephaly can be classified into two different types.[5] In type I ("classic") lissencephaly, the cortex is smooth and underdeveloped, similar in appearance to that of a 12-week-old fetus. In type II lissencephaly, the meninges are thickened and adherent to the cortical surface. The resulting radiographic appearance has been described as "cobblestone lissencephaly," in which the cortex is composed of clusters and circular arrays of neurons. Type II lissencephaly is associated with a few specific syndromes, including Walker–Warburg, Fukuyama, and muscle-eye-brain disease.

A few notable syndromes and genes are associated with lissencephaly. Miller–Dieker syndrome is caused by microdeletions of chromosome 17p13.3, which includes the *LIS1* gene and additional telomeric genes.[6] The *LIS1* gene is also responsible for up to 50% of isolated lissencephaly sequence (ILS) cases, in which there is a smaller submicroscopic deletion, duplication, or mutation of *LIS1*. Neuropathological findings in *LIS1* gene mutations include not only lissencephaly but also subcortical band

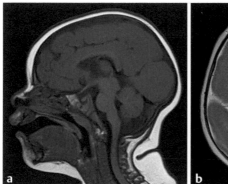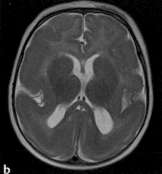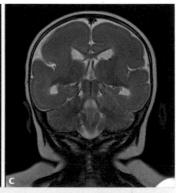

Fig. 10.4 Lissencephaly: brain MRI of 6-month-old child with lissencephaly due to *LIS1* gene mutation. (a) Midline sagittal, T1-weighted image. (b) Axial, T2-weighted image. (c) Coronal, T2-weighted image.

heterotopia (SBH). SBH refers to a band of heterotopic gray matter separated from overlying cortex by a thin zone of normal white matter. Subcortical bands restricted to the posterior lobes are more typically associated with *LIS1* mutations.

The *DCX* gene is responsible for about 10% of ILS cases.[7] *DCX* is inherited on the X chromosome. Males with *DCX* mutations have classic type I lissencephaly and severe global developmental impairment. Females with *DCX* mutations, however, are affected less severely, and tend to have an SBH pattern of neuropathology, rather than classic type I lissencephaly. Subcortical bands restricted to the frontal lobes are more typically associated with *DCX* mutations.

10.2.6 Corpus Callosum Abnormalities

Corpus callosum abnormalities can range from partial to complete absence, or manifest as various states of dysgenesis or hypoplasia. Disruption of callosal formation can occur anytime between the 5th and 16th week of gestation.[8] These abnormalities are best diagnosed by brain MRI, although head ultrasound or computed tomography (CT) of the head can also show the commonly associated parallel lateral ventricles. Callosal abnormalities may occur in isolation or in association with other CNS malformations, such as holoprosencephaly (discussed earlier), schizencephaly, or lissencephaly.[9] Some syndromes, such as Aicardi's syndrome, are defined by the presence of callosal abnormalities. Generally, most patients with callosal abnormalities have varying degrees of learning disabilities or developmental delays, including hypotonia, seizures, or autism. Rarely, an individual may be developmentally normal. No surgical intervention is indicated for the abnormality of the corpus callosum itself, although associated abnormalities, such as hydrocephalus, may need to be shunted.

10.2.7 Polymicrogyria

In polymicrogyria ("many small gyria"), the clinical severity is correlated with the extent and distribution of the malformation.[10] Mild, focal polymicrogyria may have minimal neurologic manifestations, whereas widespread, bilateral polymicrogyria invariably causes severe developmental impairment and refractory seizures.

The timing of the defect is thought to occur in the second trimester or later.[5] An insult during the stage of neuronal migration causes disruption of

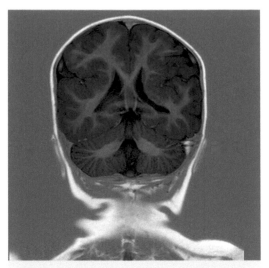

Fig. 10.5 Polymicrogyria: coronal, T1-weighted brain MRI of a 13-month-old boy with polymicrogyria.

formation of the six cortical layers, resulting in overfolded and aberrant gyri (▸ Fig. 10.5).

Polymicrogyria can be caused by either genetic or environmental causes. Genetic causes include Zellweger's/peroxisomal disorders or *GPR56* gene mutations. *GPR56* mutations are inherited in an autosomal recessive manner, and tend to cause a bilateral frontoparietal polymicrogyria.

Management is symptomatic. However, neurosurgery may be indicated if refractory seizures originate from a focal region of polymicrogyria.

10.2.8 Heterotopias

Heterotopias are foci of gray matter that are not located in their proper locations. Neuronal migration typically happens between 6 and 24 weeks of gestation.[11] In normal brain development, neural precursor cells originate in the subventricular zone, and then migrate peripherally toward the cortical surface to form the six cortical layers. However, when this process is disrupted, these neuronal precursors fail to migrate, and subsequently form aberrant clumps in the periventricular area. This heterotopic gray matter is then often an etiologic foci for seizures. Individuals may have normal intelligence or significant developmental disabilities, depending on the number and location of the heterotopic gray matter.

Many cases of periventricular heterotopia are caused by mutations in *FLNA*, an X-linked gene.[12]

Mutations are usually lethal in males, so most known affected individuals are female.

Neurosurgical intervention may be indicated if refractory seizures are isolated to certain heterotopic foci.

References

[1] Genetics Home Reference. Available at: http://ghr.nlm.nih.gov/condition/anencephaly. Published November 4, 2013. Accessed November 11, 2013

[2] De Wals P, Tairou F, Van Allen MI, et al. Reduction in neural-tube defects after folic acid fortification in Canada. N Engl J Med. 2007; 357(2):135–142

[3] Hahn JS, Barnes PD. Neuroimaging advances in holoprosencephaly: Refining the spectrum of the midline malformation. Am J Med Genet C Semin Med Genet. 2010; 154C (1):120–132

[4] Solomon BD, Gropman A, Muenke M. Holoprosencephaly overview. In: Pagon RA, Adam MP, Bird TD, et al., eds. GeneReviews® [Internet]. Seattle, WA: University of Washington; 1993–2013. Available at: http://www.ncbi.nlm.nih.gov/books/NBK1530/. Accessed November 12, 2013

[5] Volpe JJ. Neurology of the Newborn. Philadelphia, PA: W.B. Saunders Company; 2001:62–68

[6] Dobyns WB, Das S. LIS1-associated lissencephaly/subcortical band heterotopia. In: Pagon RA, Adam MP, Bird TD, et al., eds.

GeneReviews® [Internet]. Seattle, WA: University of Washington; 1993–2013. Available at: http://www.ncbi.nlm.nih.gov/books/NBK5189/. Accessed November 12, 2013

[7] Hehr U, Uyanik G, Aigner L, Couillard-Despres S, Winkler J. DCX-related disorders. In: Pagon RA, Adam MP, Bird TD, et al., eds. GeneReviews® [Internet]. Seattle, WA: University of Washington; 1993–2013. Available at: http://www.ncbi.nlm.nih.gov/books/NBK1185/. Accessed November 12, 2013

[8] Corpus Callosum Disorders. Available at: http://www.nodcc.org/index.php?option=com_content&task=view&id=12&Itemid=27. Retrieved November 13, 2013

[9] Medscape. Available at: http://emedicine.medscape.com/article/407730-overview. Published June 20, 2013. Accessed November 13, 2013

[10] Chang B, Walsh CA, Apse K, et al. Polymicrogyria overview. In: Pagon RA, Adam MP, Bird TD, et al., eds. GeneReviews® [Internet]. Seattle, WA: University of Washington; 1993–2013. Available at: http://www.ncbi.nlm.nih.gov/books/NBK1329/. Accessed November 12, 2013

[11] Genetics Home Reference. Available at: http://ghr.nlm.nih.gov/condition/periventricular-heterotopia. Published November 12, 2013. Accessed November 12, 2013

[12] Sheen VL, Bodell A, Walsh CA. X–linked periventricular heterotopia. In: Pagon RA, Adam MP, Bird TD, et al., eds. GeneReviews® [Internet]. Seattle, WA: University of Washington; 1993–2013. Available at: http://www.ncbi.nlm.nih.gov/books/NBK1213/. Accessed November 12, 2013

11 Neurofibromatosis Type 1

Ben Shofty, Liat Ben-Sira, Hagit Toledano-Alhadef, Felix Bokstein, Shlomi Constantini

11.1 Introduction

Neurofibromatosis type 1 (NF1) is a neurocutaneous, autosomal dominant disorder. Historically named *von Recklinghausen's disease*, it is now considered a "RASopathy" based on the intracellular signaling pathway that is hyperactivated. Because of the plethora of systems affected by the lack of *neurofibromin*, and the diversity of the clinical manifestations, NF1 patients should optimally be managed by a multidisciplinary team, including neurosurgical input, which is often required. NF1 affects approximately 1/2,700 newborns,[1] with variable presentation and disease severity. The main, disease-defining manifestations are café-au-lait macules (CALMs), neurofibromas, skin-fold freckling, iris hamartomas (Lisch's nodules), optic pathway gliomas (OPGs), and skeletal deformities. In addition, cognitive and behavioral impairments are noted in 50% of patients. Although considered benign, plexiform neurofibromas (PNs) and OPGs are a significant source of concern, and may cause disfigurement and blindness. Susceptibility to malignancies is the main reason for close, prolonged follow-up, as patients may develop malignant peripheral nerve sheath tumors (MPNSTs) and rarely high-grade gliomas.

11.2 Genetics and Cellular Biology

Neurofibromin is a giant intracellular protein (~320 kDa) that is encoded by the *NF1* tumor suppressor gene (chromosome 17q) and is nonfunctional in NF1 patients because of genetic alterations.[2,3] Normal neurofibromin acts as Ras-negative regulator (among its other, mostly unknown functions) by accelerating hydrolysis of Ras-bound GTP. When there is a lack of neurofibromin, Ras is constantly attached to GTP and the pathway is hyperactivated, leading to deregulated cellular proliferation and survival.[4] Upregulation of Ras triggers many downstream signaling pathways, including the mitogen-activated protein kinase (MAPK), RAF/MEK/ERK pathway, mammalian target of rapamycin (mTOR), and phosphatidylinositol 3-kinase (PI3K).[5]

NF1 is an autosomal dominant disease with 100% penetrance and highly variable clinical presentation.[6] Approximately 50% of NF1 patients have a familial disease,[7] and more than 80% of identified germline mutations are of the truncating type.[8,9] Deletion of the entire gene or large deletions are seen in approximately 5% of patients and are associated with a more severe phenotype.[10,11] Because of the 50% chance of inheriting the mutated gene, genetic counseling to known NF1 families should be offered. It is important to inform the patients that prenatal diagnosis using ultrasonography was reported for severe NF1 cases only.[12] For preimplementational diagnosis to be an option, the specific familial mutation needs to be mapped prior to pregnancy.[13,14,15]

11.3 Diagnosis and Clinical Presentation

Diagnosis of NF1 is based on clinical criteria established by the National Institutes of Health (NIH) in 1987 (▶ Table 11.1).[16] Two or more of these criteria are required for diagnosis of NF1. The sensitivity and specificity of this system is high; it is robust enough to diagnose 50% of affected children with no family history by the age of 1 year and 95% of affected children by the age of 8 years.[7,17,18] Because of the fact that some of major disease manifestations present slowly, young children with multiple (six or more) CALMs and no family history, or other major symptoms, should be followed carefully as 95% of them will eventually meet the criteria for NF1.[19] T2 hyperintensities (T2Hs) on brain magnetic resonance imaging (MRI) were suggested as a supplemental diagnostic criterion, but are seldom used for initial diagnosis because of the complexity in acquiring MRI data in young children and their lack of specificity.[20] CALMs and PNs may be present at birth, and can be noticed by the age of 1 to 3 years. Tibial dysplasias and skin-fold freckling typically present around the age of 1 to 2 years. Other manifestations, such as Lisch's nodules, OPGs, learning disabilities, and precocious puberty, usually present between the ages of 2 and 5 years. The last main manifestation of the disease to appear is cutaneous and subcutaneous neurofibromas, peaking at early adolescence.[21]

Table 11.1 Clinical diagnostic criteria for NF1,[16] and accessory diagnostic and clinical findings

Diagnostic criteria	Expected age of presentation	Percentage of patients
CALMs (six or more, larger than 15 mm in adults and 5 mm in children)	Birth to 2 y	>99%
Cutaneous neurofibromas (two or more)	5+y	>99%
One plexiform neurofibroma	Birth to 3 y	30–50%
Axillary or inguinal freckling	3–5 y	90%
Lisch's nodules (two or more)	5–10 y	90%
Optic pathway glioma	3–8 y	15–30%
Typical osseous lesion (SWD/long-bone cortical thinning, with or without pseudoarthrosis)	1–3 y	2% pseudoarthrosis 1% SWD
Family history of NF1 (first-degree relative)	–	50%
Additional common clinical findings (% of patients)	Required evaluation	
ADHD/memory and learning difficulties (50–75%)	Neuropsychological consultation	ADHD/memory and learning difficulties (50–75%)
T2 hyperintensities (60–70%)	None	T2 hyperintensities (60–70%)
Cardiovascular abnormalities (hypertension, renal artery stenosis, pulmonary artery stenosis, 2% each)	Yearly blood pressure monitoring and heart examination, echocardiography as needed	Cardiovascular abnormalities (hypertension, renal artery stenosis, pulmonary artery stenosis, 2% each)
Hormonal abnormalities/precocious puberty	Growth curves at every routine follow-up	Hormonal abnormalities/precocious puberty
Progressive scoliosis	Skeletal/bone evaluation	Progressive scoliosis
Neuropathy (~1%, usually distal and symmetrical)	Rule out other causes for neurological changes in NF1 patients (PNs, MPNSTs, etc.)	Neuropathy (~1%, usually distal and symmetrical)
Pheochromocytoma (2%)	24-h urinary excretion of catecholamines and their metabolites	Pheochromocytoma (2%)

Abbreviations: ADHD, attention-deficit/hyperactivity disorder; CALMs, café-au-lait macules; MPNSTs, malignant peripheral nerve sheath tumors; NF1, neurofibromatosis type 1; PNs, plexiform neurofibromas; SWD, sphenoid wing dysplasia.

11.4 Management

A multidisciplinary team at an NF1-dedicated center should optimally manage these complex patients. The team should include a pediatric neurologist, pediatric neurosurgeon, neuro-ophthalmologist, pediatric radiologist, social worker, neuropsychologist, geneticist, and a patient coordinator. Orthopedists, oncologists, head and neck surgeons, reconstructive surgeons, dermatologists, and other specialists should be consulted, depending on the issue at hand. This multidisciplinary approach will prevent management errors that may be made by physicians who are not familiar with the complexities and sensitivities of NF1 patients. Initial evaluation for a newly diagnosed pediatric NF1 patient should include a thorough physical and neurological examination with special emphasis on skin lesions, neuro-ophthalmological examination including fundus and,

if available, optical coherence tomography (OCT) for evaluation of retinal nerve fiber layer thickness, cardiovascular baseline (blood pressure and heart examination), neuropsychological test battery, and skeletal screening (yearly growth curves) to direct further workup.

11.5 Imaging

Imaging regimes for NF1 patients are controversial, and vary from center to center. MRI is the diagnostic tool of choice because of the nature of most of the pathologies involved. The high sensitivity of NF1 children to radiation should make the use of computed tomography (CT) minimal, reserved for occasional use only, essentially for skeletal pathologies. Screening MRIs in an asymptomatic patient at presentation are generally not recommended, but a high index of suspicion should nevertheless be kept. In patients who cannot be reliably assessed for functionality (visual exam, neurological signs, orthop-edic examination, etc.) or who cannot express complaints because of their young age (usually less than 1 year) or cognitive status, a baseline brain MRI at presentation should be considered.[22]

For patients presenting with a specific complaint or developing a specific symptom, an MRI of the relevant body part should be urgently acquired. When planning an MRI study in NF1 patients, one must take into account the different expected pathologies (cerebral, spinal, and peripheral) that correlate with the age of the patient and the nature of the signs and symptoms. A preliminary consultation with a pediatric radiologist with NF1 experience is advised in order to plan the imaging regime and protocol. A comprehensive study including pre- and postcontrast T1, T2, high-resolution 3D anatomical sequence, and orbit-oriented T1 and T2 with fat saturation is the minimal evaluation required for cerebral exam. For spinal and body imaging, a short T1 inversion recovery with fat saturation (such as short tau inversion recovery [STIR]) should be added in order to characterize and differentiate the PN from the surrounding fat and subcutaneous tissues. Whole-body MRI is a new, upcoming technique that should be considered in patients with a large disease burden.[23,24,25] More advanced sequences such as diffusion tensor imaging (DTI) and diffusion should be considered when attempting to assess functionality in OPG patients.[26,27,28] For long-term follow-up and monitoring of treatment efficacy, volumetric measurements are considered state of the art and are highly recommended for both cerebral lesions and PNs.[29,30,31,32,33]

Nonneoplastic abnormalities on MRI are relatively common in NF1, and should be carefully interpreted. T2Hs are perhaps the most common imaging abnormality, found in 60 to 70% of NF1 children. T2Hs are typically found in the basal ganglia, thalamus, cerebellum, brainstem, and cerebral white matter. These lesions are thought to represent foci of fluid accumulation within decompacted myelin sheath. T2Hs within the basal ganglia, thalamus, and brainstem tend to disappear with time, perhaps due to recycling of oligodendrocytes.[34] The presence of T2Hs, especially in the thalamus, is associated with cognitive impairment, although there is no clear-cut association between the cognitive phenotype and the number or size of the T2Hs.[35,36]

11.6 Cutaneous Manifestations

CALMs are the most common cutaneous manifestation of NF1, and can be observed in 95% of patients by the age of 3. Other common manifestations include freckling of skin folds (axillary and inguinal), found in the majority of the patients (Crowe's sign), and hypopigmented macules. All of the above findings are benign, and require no follow-up or intervention.[37]

Lisch's nodules are benign melanocytic iris hamartomas that appear between the ages of 5 and 10 years, and are best diagnosed on slit-lamp examination. They do not affect vision, nor should they be the cause for any clinical concern.

Cutaneous neurofibromas (CNs) are benign nerve sheath tumors comprised of neoplastic Schwann's cells nested within mast cells and fibroblast stroma. CNs arise from a single terminal nerve fascicle. These tumors can be sensed as subcutaneous pealike masses or small exophytic masses, and are not painful. The most common complaint associated with CNs is pruritus, which is unresponsive to antihistamines. CNs are not associated with malignant transformation or growth.[22] Cutaneous manifestations of NF1 may be treated cosmetically if causing distress; it is recommended to refer the patients to a plastic surgeon with NF1 experience or to a peripheral nerve surgeon in order to avoid neurological damage that may be associated with subcutaneous neurofibroma excision.

11.6.1 Plexiform Neurofibromas

PNs are the hallmark of neurofibromatosis, and one of the main causes of morbidity and mortality. Thirty percent of NF1 patients have visible PNs and 50% have PNs on imaging studies.[17] Hyperpigmentation or hypertrophy of the overlaying skin and patches of hair are often indicative of an underlying PN. Unlike CNs, PNs are diffuse tumors, which may involve multiple nerve branches or trunks and are often clinically described as a "bag of worms." PNs vary from tiny millimeter-diameter lesions to huge complex masses. PNs develop around the age of 7 and are prone to progression during pregnancy, since about 75% express progesterone receptors.[38] These tumors, although benign in nature, are infiltrative, often involving the surrounding structures. Growth pattern and natural history are unpredictable; periods of rapid growth (most common in early childhood or during the hormonal changes of puberty or during pregnancy) may be followed by long-term stability.

PNs have a typical MRI appearance: a hypointense T1 signal, high signal intensity in T2 with central areas of low signal, and hyperintensity in STIR sequences. No biopsy is needed in an NF1 patient with a typically appearing PN on MRI. The most common complications associated with PNs are local mass effect, bone deformity, spontaneous intratumoral bleed, and malignant transformation into an MPNST. PNs may progress and cause significant morbidity even without malignant transformation. Local mass effect or neurological deficits are considered indications for treatment.

Managing progressive PNs is extremely difficult because of the complexity of surgery and the lack of efficient medical treatment options. Early surgery, when possible, may spare complications later in life.[39] Radiotherapy is contraindicated because of the significant risk of malignant transformation. Many clinical trials for progressive PNs are being conducted; nevertheless, data in the literature are insufficient to support the use of any specific agent.[40]

11.6.2 Malignant Peripheral Nerve Sheath Tumor

MPNSTs are the most common malignant tumors associated with NF1, with 5-year survival of 34 to 58%.[41] These are highly aggressive tumors, occurring in 2 to 10% of the NF1 population and only in 0.001% of the general population.[42] MPNSTs occur mainly during the second and third decades of life, but diagnosis in patients as young as 5 years old has been reported.[43] MPNSTs often but do not exclusively arise from PNs, and are often metastatic at presentation. A high index of suspicion should be maintained in any NF1 patient with a "red flag" complaint. An NF1 patient with any of these complains should be urgently referred to an NF1 clinic, even in the absence of a known or visible PN, as MPNSTs often arise from hidden, central PNs (Box 11.1).

Box 11.1 "Red flags" warrant immediate workup for MPNSTs

Symptom
- Persistent pain that lasts more than a month/awakes from sleep.
- New or unexplained neurological deficit.
- Rapid increase in size of existing PN.
- Change in existing PN consistency.

Conventional MRI or positron emission tomography (PET; usually with FDG [fluorodeoxyglucose], or experimentally with F-thymidine) is the method of choice for evaluation of a de novo MPNST-suspected lesion or a suspected malignant transformation of an existing PN. Following multidisciplinary discussion, a Tru-Cut biopsy, preferably under imaging guidance, is recommended as the initial diagnostic method, obtaining multiple cores from the suspected area in the lesion. Excisional biopsies should only be considered for small superficial tumors, where clear margins are obtainable.[41] Aggressive surgical resection following biopsy is the preferred treatment method for nonmetastatic tumors, although because of the associated functional impairment, this approach should be thoroughly discussed with the patient and their families. Gross total resection with clear surgical margins significantly improves both overall survival and disease-free interval.[44]

Adjuvant radiation therapy and/or chemotherapy is indicated for incomplete excision, nonclear surgical margins, and large tumors.[41] Chemotherapy with either doxorubicin as a single agent or a combination of doxorubicin and ifosfamide may be considered in order to enable resection in nonresectable tumors or for metastatic tumors.[41]

11.7 Optic Pathway Gliomas

OPGs are low-grade glial neoplasms (WHO grade I) that originate from any location along the visual system, such as the optic nerve (ON), optic chiasm, optic tracts, and, rarely, the optic radiation. These lesions tend to have an erratic natural history, requiring careful follow-up and management by a multidisciplinary team. Patient age at presentation, histology, and molecular markers (such as BRAF fusion protein[45,46]) may be important factors in clinical behavior and in the practical individualized decision-making process. The subset of patients seen by the pediatric neurosurgeon may be biased toward the aggressive end of the spectrum, with a tendency to progress and require multiple treatment lines.

OPGs are relatively rare neoplasms, comprising approximately 1% of all central nervous system (CNS) neoplasms in the general population and approximately 5% of CNS neoplasms in children.[47] Eighty percent of all diagnosed patients are in the first decade of their lives, and 90% are in the first two decades. The mean age at diagnosis is 8.8 years in older series, ranging between 2.7 and

5.4 years in more recent series.[48,49,50] An estimated 37% of OPGs tend to progress.[51] There is no gender predisposition.

OPGs in NF1 patients tend to have a more benign course as compared to opposing sporadic OPGs.[51,52] In a recent series comparing NF1 OPGs to sporadic gliomas, children with NF1 had a significantly better clinical status at diagnosis, with less increase in intracranial pressure, less decrease in visual acuity (VA), and fewer abnormalities of fundus of the eye. Radiological progression, visual deterioration, and endocrinological damage were also less frequent in NF1 OPGs.[53] Historically, NF1 OPGs were considered relatively indolent tumors that do not tend to progress.

However, recently, several publications have described a more active clinical course, with progression of the tumor noted in up to 75% of NF1 patients, even in children older than 11 years old.[54] Recently, macrocephaly was also correlated with OPG incidence in NF1 patients.[55] In addition, in a genetic study targeting genotype–phenotype correlation done by Sharif et al, for an NF1 patient with OPG the odds ratio of a mutation being present in the 5' tertile end of the gene was 6.05, when compared to an NF1 patient with no OPG.[56]

Visual complaints are the mainstay of clinical symptoms and signs, although they may be hard to detect because of the young age of the patients. These include decreased VA, nystagmus, and proptosis, and are found at presentation in 46% of patients. To maximize diagnostic yield, MR protocols should be planned with the assistance of an experienced neuroradiologist and should include orbit-oriented scanning with fat suppression and contrast injection. Tumors may differ in MR appearance depending on their locations, but they are usually isointense on T1, hyperintense on T2, and receive variable enhancement patterns. Additional cystic as well as solid nonenhancing components are often present.

Isolated tumors of the ON proper usually do not have cystic changes, and are characterized by gross thickening of the nerve itself, with or without nerve sheath enlargement. The differential diagnosis for ON enlargement is broad, including meningioma, hemangioblastoma, and lymphoma.[57] ON sheath enlargement is also found in nonneoplastic diseases such as increased intracranial pressure, optic neuritis, Grave's disease, sarcoidosis, toxoplasmosis, central vein occlusion, idiopathic intracranial hypertension, and tuberculosis.[58,59] Posterior OPGs may appear as minimal chiasmal thickening or as large masses protruding into the third ventricle with apparent mass effect. Cystic changes are common in hypothalamic/chiasmatic tumors, and are a part of the natural history of the tumor. They may progress and enlarge with time, requiring treatment due to mass effect.

Neoplastic changes posteriorly to the lateral geniculate nucleus are rare and are difficult to differentiate from NF1 T2Hs. Because of the long follow-up required in these patients and the importance of early detection of changes in the tumor bulk or in its internal components, we recommend the use of volumetric measurements. These measurements, although time-consuming, may improve patient care by enabling more accurate decision-making.[29,30]

A decline in VA is often present at diagnosis and sometimes may be the reason for initial testing, even in the very young (e.g., an infant that starts bumping into objects or sitting closer to the television). In addition, color vision, visual field, eye movements, relative afferent pupillary defect, pupil size, and fundus should all be evaluated. Any progressive change should be considered seriously as a reason to initiate therapy. In very young children, a normal ophthalmological examination does not rule out visual impairment from an OPG. OCT has been shown to detect loss of retinal nerve fiber layer in children with OPG. This may prove to be an auxiliary tool in the diagnosis of visual damage in young children, as well as providing evidence regarding visual reserve and need for treatment.[60,61]

The follow-up and management of OPGs requires an experienced multidisciplinary team that provides individualized patient care. Only then can adequate therapeutic decisions be made. The goal of treatment is twofold: to prevent visual decline and to achieve long-term tumor control. In the presence of severe mass effect or hydrocephalus, immediate, life-saving neurosurgical procedures may be indicated. In most cases, however, OPGs are not a life-threatening tumor. The risk-to-benefit ratio of treatment must therefore be considered carefully for each patient.

The exact timing of treatment initiation is one of the major open questions in OPG management. In most cases, we recommend delaying treatment for as long as possible, unless a clear-cut radiological progression or visual decline is noted. Treating an asymptomatic or minimally symptomatic stable patient seems to offer no advantage over observation alone.[48,62,63] Thus, current guidelines suggest intervention only when there is a documented decline in vision or radiological progression.[51]

Treatment initiation dilemmas may be very relevant to a child, especially an infant, who presents for the first time with compromised vision. At the moment of presentation, progression cannot be defined. However, compromised reserve may be a relevant reason to start treatment earlier, rather than later.

We recommend imaging and neuro-ophthalmological examinations (including visual field and OCT if available) every 6 months. Patients with compromised reserve for whom a decision was taken not to treat should be clinically examined more frequently. If the tumor is chiasmatic/hypothalamic, a detailed endocrinological evaluation should be performed. If the patient has been stable for a period of 1 year and has no adverse prognostic factors, follow-ups may be scheduled on a yearly basis.

▶ Fig. 11.1 illustrates a suggested management algorithm for OPG. For tumors with characteristic MRI appearance that are epicentered on the optic pathway, no biopsy is required.[64] Biopsies are indicated if the tumor has an atypical appearance on MRI, for an unusual age group, or with unusual clinical characteristics (rapidly progressing or severe neurological deficits other than vision loss). Surgery is controversial and is reserved for tumors confined to the orbit in a blind or severely proptotic eye, and for shunt placement in patients with tumor-associated hydrocephalus. Total resection of hypothalamic/chiasmatic glioma in a patient with viable eyesight is usually not recommended.

Chemotherapy with vincristine and carboplatin is now considered an accepted first-line treatment. Other options (vinblastine, temozolomide, mTOR inhibitors) should be considered for second-line treatment. Cerebral irradiation for OPGs is relatively contraindicated in NF1 patients because of unacceptable adverse effects such as secondary malignancies and cognitive decline.

11.8 Other NF1 Brain Tumors

Brainstem gliomas (BSGs) are the most common CNS tumor seen in NF1 patients outside of the optic pathway.[65] These are usually low grade (pilocytic astrocytomas), and have a relatively indolent course. NF1-associated BSGs usually occur in patients 7 to 10 years of age, and are most commonly found in the medulla (not in the pons, typical of sporadic BSGs). Differentiating BSGs from T2Hs can be challenging at times, although T2Hs do not demonstrate mass effect.[22] Expectant management is recommended, as progression is usually rare and spontaneous regression has been reported.[66,67] Hydrocephalus is the main reason for concern in NF1 patients with brainstem (medullary or tectal) gliomas; endoscopic third ventriculostomy is the recommended method of treatment.[68] NF1 patients are prone to suffer from cerebral high-grade gliomas, although, as they do not differ genetically from sporadic high-grade gliomas, the treatment is the same.[22]

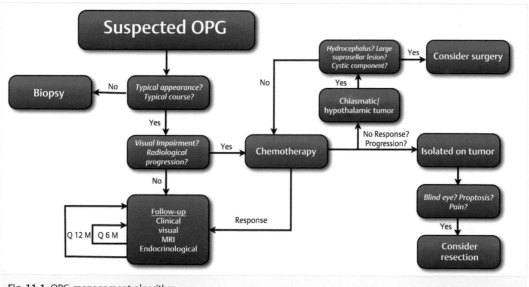

Fig. 11.1 OPG management algorithm.

11.9 NF1 Brain Function

Neurofibromin has a crucial role in normal development and function of the CNS. Besides being a tumor suppressor gene, it has many functions having to do with synaptic transmission, neuronal signaling, myelination, blood–brain barrier formation, and more. NF1 patients have a characteristic cognitive phenotype that is often a major cause for morbidity for patients and their families. NF1 patients typically have IQ in the low average range. Severe IQ deficit (< 70) is rare. Approximately 50 to 75% of NF1 patients suffer from learning and memory difficulties, attention-deficit/hyperactivity disorder, visuo-spatial coordination difficulties, and memory impairments.[69,70] Each patient should have an individualized treatment plan according to his/her specific issues and needs.

11.10 NF1 Skeletal Manifestations

Tibial or long-bone pseudoarthrosis and sphenoid wing dysplasia (SWD) are the two hallmark osseous lesions of NF1. Short stature occurs in 14% and scoliosis in approximately 20% of NF1 patients.[71,72,73,74,75] SWD may be a cause for enophthalmos and cerebral herniation into the orbit. Decreased bone density, cortical thinning, and dysplasias predispose NF1 patients to pathological fractures, and may worsen scoliosis. Early therapy with bisphosphonates is recommended in such cases usually seen in adult patients, as corrective surgery often has poor outcome and should be saved for a last resort.[73]

References

[1] Evans DG, Howard E, Giblin C, et al. Birth incidence and prevalence of tumor-prone syndromes: estimates from a UK family genetic register service. Am J Med Genet A. 2010; 152A(2):327–332

[2] Cawthon RM, Weiss R, Xu GF, et al. A major segment of the neurofibromatosis type 1 gene: cDNA sequence, genomic structure, and point mutations. Cell. 1990; 62(1):193–201

[3] Wallace MR, Marchuk DA, Andersen LB, et al. Type 1 neurofibromatosis gene: identification of a large transcript disrupted in three NF1 patients. Science. 1990; 249(4965): 181–186

[4] Trovó-Marqui AB, Tajara EH. Neurofibromin: a general outlook. Clin Genet. 2006; 70(1):1–13

[5] Denayer E, de Ravel T, Legius E. Clinical and molecular aspects of RAS related disorders. J Med Genet. 2008; 45(11): 695–703

[6] Pasmant E, Vidaud M, Vidaud D, Wolkenstein P. Neurofibromatosis type 1: from genotype to phenotype. J Med Genet. 2012; 49(8):483–489

[7] Huson SM, Harper PS, Compston DA. Von Recklinghausen neurofibromatosis. A clinical and population study in southeast Wales. Brain. 1988; 111(Pt 6):1355–1381

[8] Ars E, Kruyer H, Morell M, et al. Recurrent mutations in the NF1 gene are common among neurofibromatosis type 1 patients. J Med Genet. 2003; 40(6):e82

[9] Ars E, Serra E, García J, et al. Mutations affecting mRNA splicing are the most common molecular defects in patients with neurofibromatosis type 1. Hum Mol Genet. 2000; 9(2): 237–247

[10] Tonsgard JH, Yelavarthi KK, Cushner S, Short MP, Lindgren V. Do NF1 gene deletions result in a characteristic phenotype? Am J Med Genet. 1997; 73(1):80–86

[11] Kluwe L, Nguyen R, Vogt J, et al. Internal tumor burden in neurofibromatosis Type I patients with large NF1 deletions. Genes Chromosomes Cancer. 2012; 51(5):447–451

[12] McEwing RL, Joelle R, Mohlo M, Bernard JP, Hillion Y, Ville Y. Prenatal diagnosis of neurofibromatosis type 1: sonographic and MRI findings. Prenat Diagn. 2006; 26(12):1110–1114

[13] Spits C, De Rycke M, Van Ranst N, et al. Preimplantation genetic diagnosis for neurofibromatosis type 1. Mol Hum Reprod. 2005; 11(5):381–387

[14] Chen YL, Hung CC, Lin SY, et al. Successful application of the strategy of blastocyst biopsy, vitrification, whole genome amplification, and thawed embryo transfer for preimplantation genetic diagnosis of neurofibromatosis type 1. Taiwan J Obstet Gynecol. 2011; 50(1):74–78

[15] Abou-Sleiman PM, Apessos A, Harper JC, Serhal P, Winston RM, Delhanty JD. First application of preimplantation genetic diagnosis to neurofibromatosis type 2 (NF2). Prenat Diagn. 2002; 22(6):519–524

[16] NIH Consensus Development Conference. Neurofibromatosis. Conference statement. Arch Neurl. 1988; 45(5):575–578

[17] Ferner RE, Huson SM, Thomas N, et al. Guidelines for the diagnosis and management of individuals with neurofibromatosis 1. J Med Genet. 2007; 44(2):81–88

[18] DeBella K, Szudek J, Friedman JM. Use of the national institutes of health criteria for diagnosis of neurofibromatosis 1 in children. Pediatrics. 2000; 105(3, Pt 1):608–614

[19] Korf BR. Diagnostic outcome in children with multiple café au lait spots. Pediatrics. 1992; 90(6):924–927

[20] DeBella K, Poskitt K, Szudek J, Friedman JM. Use of "unidentified bright objects" on MRI for diagnosis of neurofibromatosis 1 in children. Neurology. 2000; 54(8):1646–1651

[21] Williams VC, Lucas J, Babcock MA, Gutmann DH, Korf B, Maria BL. Neurofibromatosis type 1 revisited. Pediatrics. 2009; 123(1):124–133

[22] Albers AC, Gutmann DH. Gliomas in patients with neurofibromatosis type 1. Expert Rev Neurother. 2009; 9(4): 535–539

[23] Nguyen R, Jett K, Harris GJ, Cai W, Friedman JM, Mautner VF. Benign whole body tumor volume is a risk factor for malignant peripheral nerve sheath tumors in neurofibromatosis type 1. J Neurooncol. 2014; 116(2):307–313

[24] Merker VL, Bredella MA, Cai W, et al. Relationship between whole-body tumor burden, clinical phenotype, and quality of life in patients with neurofibromatosis type 1. Am J Med Genet A. 2014; 164A(6):1431–1437

[25] Mautner VF, Asuagbor FA, Dombi E, et al. Assessment of benign tumor burden by whole-body MRI in patients with neurofibromatosis 1. Neuro-oncol. 2008; 10(4):593–598

[26] Jost SC, Ackerman JW, Garbow JR, Manwaring LP, Gutmann DH, McKinstry RC. Diffusion-weighted and dynamic contrast-enhanced imaging as markers of clinical behavior in children with optic pathway glioma. Pediatr Radiol. 2008; 38 (12):1293–1299

[27] de Blank PM, Berman JI, Liu GT, Roberts TP, Fisher MJ. Fractional anisotropy of the optic radiations is associated with visual acuity loss in optic pathway gliomas of neurofibromatosis type 1. Neuro-oncol. 2013; 15(8):1088–1095

[28] Filippi CG, Bos A, Nickerson JP, Salmela MB, Koski CJ, Cauley KA. Magnetic resonance diffusion tensor imaging (MRDTI) of the optic nerve and optic radiations at 3 T in children with neurofibromatosis type I (NF-1). Pediatr Radiol. 2012; 42(2):168–174

[29] Weizman L, Ben Sira L, Joskowicz L, et al. Automatic segmentation, internal classification, and follow-up of optic pathway gliomas in MRI. Med Image Anal. 2012; 16(1):177–188

[30] Shofty B, Weizman L, Joskowicz L, et al. MRI internal segmentation of optic pathway gliomas: clinical implementation of a novel algorithm. Childs Nerv Syst. 2011; 27(8):1265–1272

[31] Weizman L, Ben-Sira L, Joskowicz L, Precel R, Constantini S, Ben-Bashat D. Automatic segmentation and components classification of optic pathway gliomas in MRI. In: Jiang T, Navab N, Pluim JPW, Viergever MA, eds. Medical Image Computing and Computer-Assisted Intervention—MICCAI 2010. Lecture Notes in Computer Science, vol. 6361. Berlin: Springer; 2010:103–110

[32] Weizman L, Helfer D, Ben Bashat D, et al. PNist: interactive volumetric measurements of plexiform neurofibromas in MRI scans. Int J CARS. 2014; 9(4):683–693

[33] Weizman L, Ben-Sira L, Joskowicz L, et al. Prediction of brain MR scans in longitudinal tumor follow-up studies. In: Ayache N, Delingette H, Golland P, Mori K, eds. Medical Image Computing and Computer-Assisted Intervention—MICCAI 2012. Lecture Notes in Computer Science, vol. 7511. Berlin: Springer; 2012:179–187

[34] Hyman SL, Arthur Shores E, North KN. Learning disabilities in children with neurofibromatosis type 1: subtypes, cognitive profile, and attention-deficit-hyperactivity disorder. Dev Med Child Neurol. 2006; 48(12):973–977

[35] Payne JM, Pickering T, Porter M, et al. Longitudinal assessment of cognition and T2-hyperintensities in NF1: an 18-year study. Am J Med Genet A. 2014; 164A(3):661–665

[36] Hyman SL, Gill DS, Shores EA, Steinberg A, North KN. T2 hyperintensities in children with neurofibromatosis type 1 and their relationship to cognitive functioning. J Neurol Neurosurg Psychiatry. 2007; 78(10):1088–1091

[37] Korf BR. Clinical features and pathobiology of neurofibromatosis 1. J Child Neurol. 2002; 17(8):573–577, discussion 602–604, 646–651

[38] McLaughlin ME, Jacks T. Progesterone receptor expression in neurofibromas. Cancer Res. 2003; 63(4):752–755

[39] Friedrich RE, Schmelzle R, Hartmann M, Fünsterer C, Mautner VF. Resection of small plexiform neurofibromas in neurofibromatosis type 1 children. World J Surg Oncol. 2005; 3(1):6

[40] Packer RJ, Gutmann DH, Rubenstein A, et al. Plexiform neurofibromas in NF1: toward biologic-based therapy. Neurology. 2002; 58(10):1461–1470

[41] Ferner RE, Gutmann DH. International consensus statement on malignant peripheral nerve sheath tumors in neurofibromatosis. Cancer Res. 2002; 62(5):1573–1577

[42] Ducatman BS, Scheithauer BW, Piepgras DG, Reiman HM, Ilstrup DM. Malignant peripheral nerve sheath tumors. A clinicopathologic study of 120 cases. Cancer. 1986; 57(10):2006–2021

[43] Evans DG, Baser ME, McGaughran J, Sharif S, Howard E, Moran A. Malignant peripheral nerve sheath tumours in neurofibromatosis 1. J Med Genet. 2002; 39(5):311–314

[44] Dunn GP, Spiliopoulos K, Plotkin SR, et al. Role of resection of malignant peripheral nerve sheath tumors in patients with neurofibromatosis type 1. J Neurosurg. 2013; 118(1):142–148

[45] Tian Y, Rich BE, Vena N, et al. Detection of KIAA1549-BRAF fusion transcripts in formalin-fixed paraffin-embedded pediatric low-grade gliomas. J Mol Diagn. 2011; 13(6):669–677

[46] Hawkins C, Walker E, Mohamed N, et al. BRAF-KIAA1549 fusion predicts better clinical outcome in pediatric low-grade astrocytoma. Clin Cancer Res. 2011; 17(14):4790–4798

[47] Shamji MF, Benoit BG. Syndromic and sporadic pediatric optic pathway gliomas: review of clinical and histopathological differences and treatment implications. Neurosurg Focus. 2007; 23(5):E3

[48] Tow SL, Chandela S, Miller NR, Avellino AM. Long-term outcome in children with gliomas of the anterior visual pathway. Pediatr Neurol. 2003; 28(4):262–270

[49] Thiagalingam S, Flaherty M, Billson F, North K. Neurofibromatosis type 1 and optic pathway gliomas: follow-up of 54 patients. Ophthalmology. 2004; 111(3):568–577

[50] Grill J, Laithier V, Rodriguez D, Raquin MA, Pierre-Kahn A, Kalifa C. When do children with optic pathway tumours need treatment? An oncological perspective in 106 patients treated in a single centre. Eur J Pediatr. 2000; 159(9):692–696

[51] Listernick R, Ferner RE, Liu GT, Gutmann DH. Optic pathway gliomas in neurofibromatosis-1: controversies and recommendations. Ann Neurol. 2007; 61(3):189–198

[52] McClatchey AI. Neurofibromatosis. Annu Rev Pathol. 2007; 2:191–216

[53] Czyzyk E, Jóźwiak S, Roszkowski M, Schwartz RA. Optic pathway gliomas in children with and without neurofibromatosis 1. J Child Neurol. 2003; 18(7):471–478

[54] Hernáiz Driever P, von Hornstein S, Pietsch T, et al. Natural history and management of low-grade glioma in NF-1 children. J Neurooncol. 2010; 100(2):199–207

[55] Schindera C, Wingeier K, Goeggel Simonetti B, et al. Macrocephaly in neurofibromatosis type 1: a sign post for optic pathway gliomas? Childs Nerv Syst. 2011; 27(12):2107–2111

[56] Sharif S, Upadhyaya M, Ferner R, et al. A molecular analysis of individuals with neurofibromatosis type 1 (NF1) and optic pathway gliomas (OPGs), and an assessment of genotype-phenotype correlations. J Med Genet. 2011; 48(4):256–260

[57] Hollander MD, FitzPatrick M, O'Connor SG, Flanders AE, Tartaglino LM. Optic gliomas. Radiol Clin North Am. 1999; 37 (1):59–71, ix

[58] Peyster RG, Hoover ED, Hershey BL, Haskin ME. High-resolution CT of lesions of the optic nerve. AJR Am J Roentgenol. 1983; 140(5):869–874

[59] Shofty B, Ben-Sira L, Constantini S, Freedman S, Kesler A. Optic nerve sheath diameter on MR imaging: establishment of norms and comparison of pediatric patients with idiopathic intracranial hypertension with healthy controls. AJNR Am J Neuroradiol. 2012; 33(2):366–369

[60] Avery RA, Liu GT, Fisher MJ, et al. Retinal nerve fiber layer thickness in children with optic pathway gliomas. Am J Ophthalmol. 2011; 151(3):542–9.e2

[61] Chang L, El-Dairi MA, Frempong TA, et al. Optical coherence tomography in the evaluation of neurofibromatosis type-1 subjects with optic pathway gliomas. J AAPOS. 2010; 14(6):511–517

[62] Fouladi M, Wallace D, Langston JW, et al. Survival and functional outcome of children with hypothalamic/chiasmatic tumors. Cancer. 2003; 97(4):1084–1092

[63] Astrup J. Natural history and clinical management of optic pathway glioma. Br J Neurosurg. 2003; 17(4):327–335

[64] Leonard JR, Perry A, Rubin JB, King AA, Chicoine MR, Gutmann DH. The role of surgical biopsy in the diagnosis of glioma in individuals with neurofibromatosis-1. Neurology. 2006; 67(8):1509–1512

[65] Guillamo JS, Créange A, Kalifa C, et al. Réseau NF France. Prognostic factors of CNS tumours in Neurofibromatosis 1 (NF1): a retrospective study of 104 patients. Brain. 2003; 126(Pt 1):152–160

[66] Morris PW, Glasier CM, Smirniotopoulos JG, Allison JW. Disappearing enhancing brain lesion in a child with neurofibromatosis type I. Pediatr Radiol. 1997; 27(3):260–261

[67] Schmandt SM, Packer RJ, Vezina LG, Jane J. Spontaneous regression of low-grade astrocytomas in childhood. Pediatr Neurosurg. 2000; 32(3):132–136

[68] Al-Otibi M, Rutka JT. Neurosurgical implications of neurofibromatosis Type I in children. Neurosurg Focus. 2006; 20(1):E2

[69] North KN, Riccardi V, Samango-Sprouse C, et al. Cognitive function and academic performance in neurofibromatosis. 1: consensus statement from the NF1 Cognitive Disorders Task Force. Neurology. 1997; 48(4):1121–1127

[70] Hyman SL, Shores A, North KN. The nature and frequency of cognitive deficits in children with neurofibromatosis type 1. Neurology. 2005; 65(7):1037–1044

[71] Friedman JM. Neurofibromatosis 1: clinical manifestations and diagnostic criteria. J Child Neurol. 2002; 17(8):548–554, discussion 571–572, 646–651

[72] Alwan S, Armstrong L, Joe H, Birch PH, Szudek J, Friedman JM. Associations of osseous abnormalities in Neurofibromatosis 1. Am J Med Genet A. 2007; 143A(12):1326–1333

[73] Dulai S, Briody J, Schindeler A, North KN, Cowell CT, Little DG. Decreased bone mineral density in neurofibromatosis type 1: results from a pediatric cohort. J Pediatr Orthop. 2007; 27 (4):472–475

[74] Stevenson DA, Moyer-Mileur LJ, Murray M, et al. Bone mineral density in children and adolescents with neurofibromatosis type 1. J Pediatr. 2007; 150(1):83–88

[75] Yilmaz K, Ozmen M, Bora Goksan S, Eskiyurt N. Bone mineral density in children with neurofibromatosis 1. Acta Paediatr. 2007; 96(8):1220–1222

12 Medical Management for Epilepsy

Sarah A. Kelley, Adam L. Hartman

12.1 Introduction

Antiseizure medicines are used in the acute treatment of seizures and for seizure prophylaxis. Seizure prophylaxis is indicated when a patient has a diagnosis of epilepsy. Antiseizure medicines may be used for prophylaxis when a patient is at high risk for seizures, such as after a traumatic brain injury or after brain surgery.

In general, prophylactic medications to treat epilepsy are started after the second unprovoked seizure or in patients with a single seizure at high risk for further seizures (e.g., penetrating traumatic brain injury). The goal of medical management of epilepsy is to obtain good seizure control with as few side effects as possible, which operationally is a single agent at the lowest tolerated dose. There are now over 30 different antiseizure medications with varying mechanisms of action. The choice of medication is based on the patient's type of epilepsy (because some medicines can exacerbate certain types of seizures), comorbidities, and side effect profiles. However, even with trials of multiple medications, up to one-third of patients will not be seizure-free on medication.[1] If this occurs, then other treatment options including dietary therapy, seizure surgery, and vagus nerve stimulation are considered. Because neurosurgeons frequently encounter patients who are taking antiseizure medications, this chapter will focus on these medications and briefly discuss dietary therapy.

12.2 Treatment of Status Epilepticus

Status epilepticus is a neurologic emergency. Although the official definition is a seizure that continues for longer than 30 minutes, in fact it is thought that injury to the brain begins after 5 minutes of ongoing seizure activity.[2] It is therefore important to treat status epilepticus as soon as possible (▶ Table 12.1). The first dose of intravenous lorazepam, intravenous diazepam, or intramuscular midazolam should be given after 5 minutes of seizure activity. If seizure activity continues for 20 minutes, then treatment options include levetiracetam, valproate, or fosphenytoin.[3] If these medications do not stop the seizures, then subsequent medications can be tried and anesthetic agents used once the patient's airway has

Table 12.1 Treatment of status epilepticus

Times since seizure onset	Intervention
0–5 min	ABC, ECG, IV access, blood for CBC, CMP, AED levels, toxicology screen
5–20 min	Lorazepam IV 0.1 mg/kg (up to 4 mg) *or* Diazepam IV 0.2 mg/kg (up to 10 mg) May repeat dosing one time if needed *or* Midazolam IM (5 mg for 13-40 kg, 10 mg for > 40 kg) given once
20–40 min	Fosphenytoin/phenytoin 20 mg/kg IV, max 1500 mg/dose or Valproate 40 mg/kg IV, max 3000 mg/dose *or* Levetiracetam 60 mg/kg IV, max 4500 mg/dose
40–60 min	May repeat second-line therapy or general anesthesia with continuous EEG monitoring

Abbreviations: ABC, airway, breathing, and circulation; AED, antiepileptic drug; CBC, complete blood count; CMP, comprehensive metabolic panel; ECG, electrocardiogram; EEG, electroencephalogram; IV, intravenous.

been protected (▶ Table 12.2). While treating the seizures, the etiology of the status epilepticus should also be investigated (i.e., metabolic abnormalities, stroke, hemorrhage) and treated while monitoring breathing and circulation. It is important to note that in neonates, at the time of this writing, phenobarbital (PB) is the first drug of choice for treatment of status epilepticus followed by fosphenytoin and then lorazepam.

12.3 Specific Anticonvulsant Uses

Medications that can be given intravenously and therefore used for the treatment of *status epilepticus* or when medications cannot be taken enterally include lorazepam (or other benzodiazepines such as midazolam), fosphenytoin, phenobarbital, valproate, levetiracetam, or lacosamide.

- *Seizure prophylaxis* with phenytoin after traumatic brain injury has been studied and demonstrates that immediate use of this medicine prevents early (within the first 7 days) posttraumatic seizures but not late (that is, > 7 days) posttraumatic seizures.[4]

Table 12.2 Prophylactic medications for the treatment of epilepsy

Medication	Maintenance dose	Starting dose	Common side effects	Serious side effects	Other comments
Carbamazepine (Tegretol)	15 mg/kg divided twice a day to 30 mg/kg twice a day	7 mg/kg twice a day	Lethargy, ataxia, hyponatremia, hepatotoxicity	Stevens–Johnson syndrome	Focal seizures CYP inducer check HLA-B*1502 genetic status prior to use in patients of ancestry at high risk for adverse reactions
Oxcarbazepine (Trileptal)	15 mg/kg divided twice a day to 30 mg/kg twice a day	7 mg/kg twice a day	Lethargy, ataxia, hyponatremia		Focal seizures CYP inducer
Clobazam (Onfi)	5–40 mg/d (can divide doses BID)	5 mg daily	Sedation	Stevens–Johnson syndrome	Adjunctive treatment of seizures associated with Lennox Gastaut syndrome
Ethosuximide (Zarontin)	15–20 mg/kg/d to 40 mg/kg/d	3–6 y: 250 mg/d >6 y: 500 mg/d	Nausea, vomiting, GI upset	Aplastic anemia, rash	Childhood absence epilepsy (if no history of generalized tonic–clonic seizures)
Lacosamide (Vimpat)	4–16 y (11–30 kg): 3–6 mg/kg BID (max 200 mg BID) 4–16 y (30–50 kg): 2–4 mg/kg BID (max 200 mg BID) Older children: 200 mg BID	4–16 y (11–50 kg): 1 mg/kg BID 4–16 y (>50 kg): 50 mg BID	Nausea, ataxia, dizziness		Indication for focal seizures
Lamotrigine (Lamictal)	5–15 mg/kg/d divided twice a day Dosage depends on other drugs used (higher with enzyme inducers, lower with inhibitors, especially valproic acid)	2 mg/kg/d–very slow titration, which is even slower in combination with valproate	Rash, lethargy, tremor	Stevens–Johnson syndrome	Titrate very slowly Focal and generalized
Levetiracetam (Keppra)	20–60 mg/kg/d	10–20 mg/kg/d	Agitation, behavioral disinhibition	Suicide	Vitamin B6 may help with mood side effects. Focal and generalized
Phenobarbital	Neonates: 2–5 mg/kg/d Children: 3–7 mg/kg/d	2–3 mg/kg/d	Sedation, effect on cognition and behavior, coarsening of facial features		Often first line in neonates Focal and generalized seizures CYP inducer

Table 12.2 (Continued)

Medication	Maintenance dose	Starting dose	Common side effects	Serious side effects	Other comments
Phenytoin (Dilantin)	4–8 mg/kg/d	4–5 mg/kg/d	Hirsutism, gingival hyperplasia, dizziness, nystagmus, teratogen	Rash, purple glove	Focal and generalized tonic–clonic. CYP inducer. Maximum infusion rate for phenytoin: 50 mg/min
Topiramate (Topamax)	5–9 mg/kg/d divided twice a day	1–2 mg/kg/d (not to exceed 25 mg)	Cognitive slowing, anhydrosis, weight loss, kidney stones, metabolic acidosis, tingling in extremities	Rash	Focal and generalized CYP inducer at high doses
Valproate (Depakote, Depakene)	15–60 mg/kg/d divided twice to thrice a day	15 mg/kg divided twice to thrice a day	Tremor, weight gain, hair loss, cytopenias, increased serum transaminase, teratogen	Hemorrhagic pancreatitis, liver failure	Also used as a mood stabilizer and to treat headache. Focal and generalized. CYP inhibitor
Zonisamide (Zonegran)	>16 y: 100–600 mg/d	>16 y: 100 mg once a day	Somnolence, irritability, cognitive slowing, weight loss, oligohydrosis, renal stones	Rash	Focal and generalized

Abbreviations: CYP, cytochrome P450; GI gastrointestinal.

- *Infantile spasms treatment*: Adrenocorticotropic hormone (ACTH), prednisolone, vigabatrin.
- *Lennox–Gastaut syndrome*: felbamate, rufinamide, topiramate, clobazam, valproate, lamotrigine, zonisamide.
- *Medications used at home for repetitive seizures*:
  - Diazepam (Diastat): Rectal gel that can be used to abort a seizure or cluster of seizures. Dose per age and weight.
  - LZP/Diazepam Intensol solutions: Oral solution that can be placed in the side of the mouth (buccal administration) to abort a seizure or cluster of seizures. LZP Intensol needs to be refrigerated. LZP 2 mg/1 mL liquid, diazepam 5 mg/5 mL liquid.
  - LZP or clonazepam tablets may also be used for clusters of seizures.

12.4 Brief Overview of the Most Commonly Used Anticonvulsant Medications

12.4.1 Lorazepam (Ativan; LZP)

LZP is used primarily for acute treatment of seizures and status epilepticus. It is relatively short-acting and causes sedation. It is used first line in status epilepiticus[5] and the dose may be repeated once if seizures do not subside prior to moving on to a second agent. It also can be used orally as a rescue agent for seizure clusters.

12.4.2 Phenytoin/Fosphenytoin (Dilantin; PHT)

In children, these medications are used primarily for the treatment of status epilepticus. Historically, PHT was used widely for seizure prophylaxis after traumatic brain injury. They are difficult to use as seizure prophylaxis because of poor oral absorption (PHT), nonlinear kinetics requiring frequent blood draws and poor side effect profile leading to gum hyperplasia, hirsutism, and central nervous system side effects. For IV administration, fosphenytoin is preferred over PHT because of the less caustic nature of the compound, making it significantly less dangerous if it extravasates. Serum esterases metabolize fosphenytoin to PHT, so the onset of effect for the former may be slightly increased, compared to the latter.

12.4.3 Levetiracetam (Keppra; LEV)

LEV is one of the most commonly prescribed seizure medications due to its short half-life, good side effect profile, and availability in multiple forms. LEV may be used in focal or generalized epilepsy. It can be given intravenously and is therefore tried in status epilepticus. With chronic use, mood problems are the most common type of side effect and may be helped by B6 supplementation (25–100 mg/day depending on weight).

12.4.4 Valproate (Depakote; VPA)

It is effective in the treatment of all seizure types; however, VPA is not recommended for patients younger than 2 years due to the higher risk of liver and hematologic side effects. Rarely, it can cause liver disorders or hemorrhagic pancreatitis. More common side effects include weight gain, hair loss or thinning, abdominal pain, or sedation. VPA also may also cause a decrease in the number and/or function of platelets, leading to the potential for increased bleeding during surgery. VPA is teratogenic and can specifically cause neural tube malformations in the fetus.

12.4.5 Phenobarbital (Luminal; PB)

Used for treatment of focal and generalized seizures, PB is often the treatment of choice in neonatal seizures. PB is available in an IV formulation and may be loaded in status epilepticus. Uncommonly, it is used for maintenance therapy in older children or adults.

12.4.6 Lacosamide (Vimpat; LCM)

Generally used for treatment of focal seizures, LCM is available in an IV formulation (loading dose is 200–300 mg in an adult-size patient) in status epilepticus. The most common side effects for LCM include dizziness and loss of balance.

12.4.7 Carbamazepine (Tegretol; CBZ)

CBZ is effective in the treatment of focal seizures. It cannot be given intravenously or loaded. It is used for prophylaxis. Side effects include lowering serum sodium levels, hepatotoxicity, dizziness, and risk of Stevens–Johnson syndrome in certain populations. CBZ may exacerbate generalized seizure disorders.

12.4.8 Oxcarbazepine (Trileptal; OXC)

OXC is a newer ketone derivative of CBZ. It is effective in the treatment of focal seizures. It cannot be given intravenously. It is used for prophylaxis. Side effects include lowering serum sodium levels and dizziness. OXC may exacerbate generalized seizure disorders. OXC doses can be titrated once every 3 days.

12.4.9 Lamotrigine (Lamictal; LTG)

LTG is effective in the treatment of generalized and focal seizures. It has a good side effect profile, particularly with cognition. The biggest risk is rash that may evolve into Stevens–Johnson syndrome. This risk is greatly reduced by a slow titration schedule. LTG is well tolerated in all age groups.

12.4.10 Topiramate (Topamax; TPM)

TPM is used for generalized and focal seizures. Most common side effects include cognitive difficulty (difficulty thinking of words), acidosis, and decreased sweating. TPM carries and increased risk of kidney stones. Patients should stay well hydrated on this medication.

12.4.11 Zonisamide (Zonegran; ZNS)

ZNS is used for generalized and focal seizures. It has a similar side effect profile to TPM (above). One benefit is once daily dosing due to a long half-life.

12.4.12 Clobazam (Onfi; CLB)

CLB is a 1,5-benzodiazipine that has a longer half-life than other 1,4-benzodiazepines such as LZP and therefore has fewer side effects and less habituation. CLB is indicated in the treatment of seizures associated with Lennox-Gastaut syndrome. Recently, its manufacturer issued a warning about the risk of Stevens–Johnson syndrome.

12.4.13 Ethosuximide (Zarontin; ESM)

ESM is specifically used for the treatment of childhood absence epilepsy without generalized tonic-clonic seizures. Its side effects include abdominal pain and possible white count suppression.

12.4.14 Rufinamide (Banzel; RUF)

RUF is a newer drug indicated initially for Lennox–Gastaut syndrome. It is not available in IV form. Side effects may include somnolence and QTc shortening. It should not be stopped abruptly.

12.5 Medication Side Effects

All anticonvulsants virtually cause some central nervous system side effect, especially when first initiated. Most will cause sedation or fatigue. Some will cause dizziness or difficulty with balance and others will cause problems with cognition. These side effects can be seen even if the patient is not toxic on the medication. However, if a patient appears overly sedated, it is important to determine if she/he just had a seizure, is in subclinical status, or is sedated as a result of the medication. Ask about recent changes in medication, think about drug–drug interactions, and consider getting an electroencephalogram (EEG) if ongoing seizure activity is suspected. Levels may be checked for many anticonvulsant medications and compared to therapeutic ranges; however, there are some patients who tolerate high levels of medication without side effects.

12.6 Drug–Drug Interactions

Anticonvulsant medications that affect the cytochrome P450 (CYP) (cytochrome P450) system may interact with each other or other medications that the patient is taking. VPA and FBM are inhibitors and can slow the excretion of other medications. CBZ, PHT, OXC, and PB are inducers and can speed the metabolism of other medications including oral contraceptives.

12.7 Discontinuation of Anticonvulsant Therapy

Once a patient has been seizure-free on antiseizure medication for 2 years, it is reasonable to consider weaning off the medication. Successful discontinuation is more likely if seizures were easily controlled and the patient has a normal exam, a normal EEG, and magnetic resonance imaging (MRI), and in the setting of primary generalized epilepsy (other than juvenile myoclonic epilepsy) or a childhood epilepsy syndrome. Unsuccessful discontinuation is more likely if the patient has had multiple failed treatment attempts, previous unsuccessful withdrawal attempts, abnormal EEG prior to withdrawal, or a remote symptomatic epilepsy (e.g., known lesion).

After seizure surgery, most neurologists start weaning medicine after 6 months of seizure freedom. Weaning medication prior to the 6-month mark leads to an increased risk of recurrence.[6]

12.8 Treatment in the Setting of Comorbidities

Antiseizure medicines are also used in the treatment of other disorders. VPA and TPM are used in the treatment of migraine headaches. VPA, LTG, and CBZ are used for treatment of various mood disorders and/or anxiety. TPM and ZNS may lead to weight loss. Gabapentin, pregabalin, and CBZ are used in the treatment of pain syndromes.

During pregnancy, LTG and LEV have the best safety profile. VPA and PHT have known serious teratogenic potential. Many of the other antiseizure medicines have known risk in the setting of pregnancy as well.

12.9 Dietary Therapy

Diets, specifically the ketogenic diets and modified Atkins diet, are often used in patients when medications fail. These are high-fat, low-carbohydrate, and adequate-protein diets that are monitored closely by neurologists and nutritionists. Patients on these diets should not receive glucose in their fluids or medications mixed with solutions containing glucose unless this is medically necessary. If it is necessary to discontinue the diet due to another medical condition, it can be reinstituted once the patient has recovered.

12.10 Common Clinical Questions

1. In the treatment of a patient in status epilepticus, what are the first three medications you would use and what doses would you choose?

2. Which antiseizure medicine can cause metabolic acidosis?
3. Which medications could potentially exacerbate a generalized seizure disorder?
4. Why should valproate be avoided in young women if possible?

12.11 Answers to Common Clinical Questions

1. Lorazepam (0.1 mg/kg/dose up to 4 mg) can be given first and may be redosed one time if the patient continues to have seizures. Diazepam and midazolam are other options. Phenytoin/ fosphenytoin levetiracetam, or valproate would be the next line of treatment. Fosphenytoin is less likely to cause cutaneous injury if it extravagates and is therefore preferred.

2. Topiramate can cause metabolic acidosis as well as difficulty with word finding, tingling in the extremities, anhydrosis, and kidney stones.

3. Oxcarbazepine and carbamazepine, which are used to treat focal seizure disorders, may exacerbate generalized seizures.

4. Valproate is teratogenic and can cause spinal dysraphism and decreased IQ in the fetus. It can also cause weight gain, hair loss, and in rare cases hemorrhagic pancreatitis or liver failure.

References

[1] Kwan P, Brodie MJ. Early identification of refractory epilepsy. N Engl J Med. 2000; 342(5):314–319
[2] Lowenstein DH, Alldredge BK. Status epilepticus. N Engl J Med. 1998; 338(14):970–976
[3] Glauser T, Shinnar S, Gloss D, et al. Evidence-based guideline: treatment of convulsive status epilepticus in children and adults: report of the Guideline Committee of the American Epilepsy Society. Epilepsy Curr 2016;6(1):4861
[4] Temkin NR, Dikmen SS, Wilensky AJ, Keihm J, Chabal S, Winn HR. A randomized, double-blind study of phenytoin for the prevention of post-traumatic seizures. N Engl J Med. 1990; 323(8):497–502
[5] Brophy GM, Bell R, Claassen J, et al. Neurocritical Care Society Status Epilepticus Guideline Writing Committee. Guidelines for the evaluation and management of status epilepticus. Neurocrit Care. 2012; 17(1):3–23
[6] Lachhwani DK, Loddenkemper T, Holland KD, et al. Discontinuation of medications after successful epilepsy surgery in children. Pediatr Neurol. 2008; 38(5):340–344

IV

13 Pediatric Scalp and Skull Lesions

Rajiv R. Iyer, Lee S. Hwang, Jeffrey P. Mullin, Violette M.R. Recinos

13.1 Introduction

Pediatric neurosurgeons are frequently asked to evaluate children who present with various "lumps" and "bumps" on the head that come to attention in a multitude of ways. Often, such scalp and skull lesions are asymptomatic and incidentally discovered as general head swelling or a discreet mass on the scalp during infancy and childhood, identified by parents, teachers, or even hairdressers. Some lesions are preceded by trauma, while most are nontraumatic and idiopathic in nature. The majority of such lesions are benign, and some can be managed expectantly with serial monitoring. In other circumstances, when a diagnosis is sought, if the lesion is painful or bothersome to the patient, or for cosmetic reasons, surgical intervention can be considered. Broad heterogeneity exists in the types of scalp and skull lesions found in children, and the extent of soft tissue, calvarial, and intracranial involvement is variable. In many cases, the natural history of scalp and skull lesions is not well defined. Therefore, it is no surprise that thresholds to intervene surgically vary between surgeons. Nonetheless, when surgical intervention is pursued, it often represents a safe, durable treatment option.

Given the wide pathological variability of scalp and skull lesions, a structured diagnostic approach is important in the evaluation of infants and children. Frequently, a multidisciplinary approach allows for comprehensive treatment of these disorders, involving neurosurgeons, pediatricians, plastic surgeons, and dermatologists. Recognition of such lesions may begin with the general pediatrician or a dermatologist during general checkups. For the neurosurgeon, history and physical examination are important in delineating a time course for lesion growth or change, for determining head circumference, and for characterization of the lesion itself. Many times, physical examination alone can lead to a diagnosis. Imaging is obtained in some instances, and often includes ultrasound, plain radiographs, computed tomography (CT) and magnetic resonance (MR) imaging. CT imaging allows evaluation of the bony architecture surrounding, and possibly comprising, particular lesions. MR imaging allows for delineation of soft-tissue structures and may aid in determining the extent of intracranial and intradural involvement.

In some cases, vascular imaging can be helpful for those lesions that have robust blood supply, those that communicate with the dural venous sinuses, or those with have unique venous drainage. Reported incidences of each particular lesion vary considerably and may in part be due to varying referral patterns amongst institutions, in addition to the variety of medical subspecialties to which patients are referred.[1,2,3] Surgical intervention frequently involves a neurosurgeon and may also involve a plastic surgeon in situations where particular attention to wound healing is needed and in which primary scalp closure may pose a challenge.

In this chapter, we discuss some of the common scalp and skull lesions found in the pediatric population that come to the attention of a neurosurgeon.

13.2 Cephalohematoma

With the advent of improved obstetrical care and a decrease in the frequency of vacuum- and forceps-assisted vaginal delivery of neonates, the development of *cephalohematoma* is rare, occurring in approximately 1% of births. Such lesions are typically identified in the first days of life after particularly challenging deliveries, especially those involving abnormal fetal position, narrow birth canal, and vacuum and forceps assistance. After traumatic deliveries, a soft mass on the scalp, especially in the parietal regions, is suggestive of cephalohematoma formation (▶ Fig. 13.1). Because cephalohematomas arise between the skull and the pericranium, they are contained by the suture lines. This is in contrast to subgaleal hematomas, in which blood distributes above the pericranial space, and caput succedaneum, in which edema tracks below the skin and above the galea. Unlike cephalohematomas, both of these related phenomena share the ability to cross suture lines. In unstable neonates with expanding hematomas, it is essential to be aware that a large portion of the circulating blood volume can be lost in such lesions and that blood count monitoring may be necessary. In rare instances, hyperbilirubinemia or infection of the hematoma can also occur. The majority of cephalohematomas are managed expectantly with serial monitoring. Observation

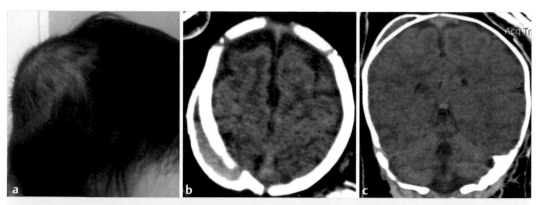

Fig. 13.1 Cephalohematoma. **(a)** Firm, expansile scalp lesion in the parietal region of an infant with a cephalohematoma at birth. **(b, c)** Computed tomography (CT) imaging demonstrating evolution of a cephalohematoma with an ossified rim.

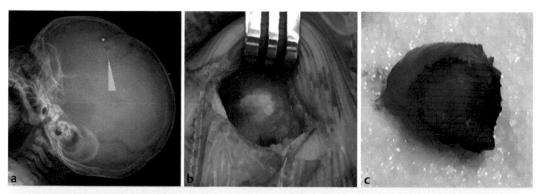

Fig. 13.2 Dermoid. **(a)** Plain radiograph demonstrating a lucent skull lesion (*arrowhead*) consistent with a dermoid. **(b, c)** A small scalp incision is utilized to visualize the raised dermoid attached to the calvarium **(b)** and its firm appearance grossly following en bloc excision **(c)**.

alone is often sufficient as these lesions frequently exhibit self-resolution. Rarely, initially malleable lesions ossify and can lead to morbidity from cosmetic deformity. In those instances, surgical intervention may be indicated and typically involves drilling the hematoma to the appropriate shape, or in severe cases, craniectomy and cranioplasty with split-thickness calvarial grafting may be required.

13.3 Epidermoids/Dermoids

The most frequently occurring pediatric skull lesions are *dermoid* and *epidermoid cysts*, which occur due to a failure of dysjunction during development, leading to intraosseous retention of epithelial and dermal elements. While epidermoids are often found in older children and adults in the intracranial space (especially the cerebellopontine angle and suprasellar region), dermoids have a preponderance for the midline scalp and skull, frequently located along the anterior fontanelle.[4] Cystic cavities containing keratin accumulation from desquamation is typical with epidermoids. Dermoids, on the other hand, contain skin elements in addition to dermal structures such as sebaceous glands and follicles. Physical examination typically reveals a firm, immobile lesion. Imaging is not always necessary, but may reveal a lytic skull lesion close to midline (▶ Fig. 13.2). Rarely, a dermoid sinus tract is associated and communicates with the intracranial space and, more unusually, the intradural space. These lesions have the propensity of becoming infected, which can thereby lead to infection of the subgaleal space and, theoretically, the intracranial space in communicating lesions. Surgical treatment often consists of excision using a curvilinear incision around the lesion. Ideally, removal would occur *en bloc* without lesion entry and potential seeding of the surrounding space. However, in some instances this is not possible and the resection cavity should be thoroughly inspected and expunged of suspected lesional tissue in order to prevent recurrence. While bony involvement is certainly possible, intradural exploration is typically unnecessary. Care must be taken for midline lesions, which may communicate with the sagittal sinus. In such instances, a tract entering the bone can be cauterized and ligated.

13.4 Langerhans Cell Histiocytosis

Langerhans cell histiocytosis is an umbrella term for a group of disorders that are characterized at the cellular level by proliferation of immune cells leading to a variety of clinical phenotypes, including lesions of the skeletal system, skin, and other organ systems. Some eponymous conditions such as Hand-Schüller-Christian and Letterer-Siwe disease are examples of multifocal Langerhans cell histiocytosis characterized by systemic features including hepatosplenomegaly and pancytopenia. In children, a common form of Langerhans cell histiocytosis that may come to the attention of a neurosurgeon is a solitary skull mass known as *eosinophilic granuloma*.[5] These lesions often present in children prior to puberty as gradually expanding skull masses that can be painful in nature. Imaging studies typically demonstrate an osteolytic skull lesion ("punched-out" appearance) with rare intracranial or intradural extension (▶ Fig. 13.3).

While the natural history of eosinophilic granulomas of the skull is not well defined, enlarging, painful lesions and the need for biopsy make surgical intervention the treatment of choice in many cases. The goal of surgery is complete resection, which can be performed with craniectomy surrounding the margins of the lesion, or with piecemeal curettage in cases when this is not feasible. Extensive, large skull lesions may require calvarial reconstruction following surgical excision. Thus, in preparation for extirpation of such bony lesions, calvarial donor sites may need to be prepped and accounted for during incision planning.

Recurrence rates following total resection of Langerhans cell histiocytosis of the skull are low. After surgery, children should be followed for some time by the neurosurgeon to monitor for recurrence. Radiographic skeletal surveys and radionuclide bone scans can be helpful in evaluating polyostotic disease. In lesions that are not surgically amenable, or for recurrent, aggressive lesions, alternative adjuvant therapy with chemotherapy or low-dose radiation is a possibility.

13.5 Fibrous Dysplasia

Fibrous dysplasia is a benign osseous condition characterized by the slow, abnormal deposition of collagen and fibrous tissue amongst a network of immature woven bone. Single and multiple areas of dysplasia are classified as monostotic and polyostotic, respectively. The underlying pathophysiology of this disorder is related to genetic mutations leading to constitutive activation of a G-protein-coupled receptor. McCune-Albright syndrome is a well-characterized syndrome consisting of a combination of polyostotic fibrous dysplasia, café-au-lait hyperpigmentation spots, and precocious puberty.

Because of the slow-growing nature of fibrous dysplasia, serial clinical monitoring is important in children and adolescents. Painless, progressive skull deformity is a possible for clinical presentation. High-resolution CT imaging provides information about the extent of bony involvement,

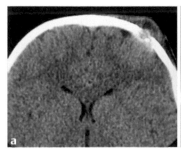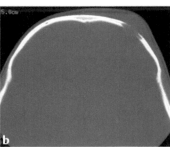

Fig. 13.3 Eosinophilic granuloma. **(a, b)** CT imaging demonstrating a punched out, lytic lesion consistent with an eosinophilic granuloma.

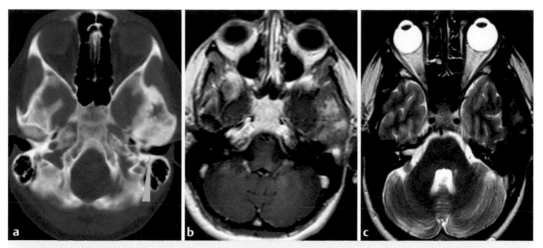

Fig. 13.4 Fibrous dysplasia. **(a)** CT imaging demonstrating ground-glass appearance of a left temporal lesion (*arrowhead*) consistent with fibrous dysplasia. **(b, c)** Magnetic resonance (MR) imaging demonstrating left temporal fibrous dysplasia on T1-weighted postcontrast imaging **(b)** T2-weighted imaging **(c)**.

including structures of the skull base. A typical appearance on CT imaging is of a ground-glass lesion that differentiates this from normal bone (▶ Fig. 13.4). Lesions can involve various aspects of the calvarium and skull base involvement can lead to narrowing of the natural corridors and foramina of the skull base, leading to cranial nerve dysfunction, vision loss from optic canal narrowing, proptosis, tinnitus, and other issues. A low risk of malignant transformation to osteosarcoma has been described, underlining the importance of clinical monitoring over time. Medical therapy with bisphosphonates may help slow bone turnover and reduce pain. Surgical intervention typically involves a multidisciplinary approach with skull base lesions in particular, often with combined efforts from neurosurgical, otolaryngology, and craniofacial experts, with the goal being decompression of normal neural structures, resection of all dysplastic bone, and cosmetic and functional reconstruction. In some cases, open craniofacial approaches are preferred, while in others endoscopic endonasal approaches can be used to achieve excellent outcomes.

13.6 Hemangiomas

Hemangiomas of the scalp and skull are rare occurrences in children and are often asymptomatic and incidentally found. Plain radiography in patients with hemangiomas will reveal a characteristic "honeycomb" appearance due to vascular channels interspersed with bony trabeculations. Typically, these lesions do not extend into the intracranial space. Some vascular supply may, however, emanate from the dura, although it is usually not involved. A theoretical risk of hemorrhage from trauma exists, but is unusual. Acceptable management of hemangiomas includes serial monitoring, but large or symptomatic lesions can be surgically excised en bloc with appropriate skull reconstruction, if needed, and primary scalp closure.

13.7 Sinus Pericranii

Soft, expansile, midline, or paramedian scalp lesions consisting of an abnormal communication between intracranial and extracranial veins are referred to as *sinus pericranii*. Typically in this condition, a slow-flow anastomosis exists between extracranial scalp veins and intracranial veins in proximity to the sagittal sinus, which extends through a calvarial defect to intercommunicate (▶ Fig. 13.5). While venous imaging can provide information regarding the abnormal venous networks associated with sinus pericranii, the diagnosis is usually clinically made. Soft, compressible lesions that enlarge and increase in prominence with recumbency or with Valsalva maneuvers differentiate sinus pericranii from other scalp lesions. Similar to hemangiomas, a theoretical risk of traumatic hemorrhage exists and thus, surgical intervention is often recommended. Intraoperatively, following induction with general anesthesia,

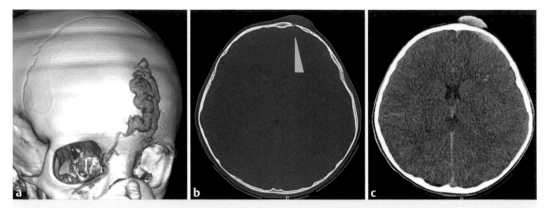

Fig. 13.5 Sinus pericranii. **(a)** Three-dimensional CT venogram reconstruction demonstrating scalp vein engorgement due to sinus pericranii. **(b)** CT imaging demonstrating calvarial defect (*arrowhead*) and scalp vein engorgement in communication with the superior sagittal sinus **(c)** in a patient with sinus pericranii.

Valsalva maneuvers can allow the surgeon to map out the pattern of scalp veins at the time of incision planning. This can be helpful in circumferentially excising the lesion with minimal blood loss, as each surrounding vein can be preemptively identified and controlled. Once circumferential dissection of the lesion is accomplished, a tract extending through a calvarial defect is typically isolated, ligated, and cut. Surgical intervention is well tolerated and often provides a durable solution.

13.8 Growing Skull Fracture

Growing skull fractures, also known as *leptomeningeal cysts*, are rare phenomena (~1%) in infants and young children, typically less than 5 years of age, who suffer from skull fractures. An occult dural tear occurring at the time of a skull fracture is typically the basis for this occurrence.[6,7] Weeks to months following the initial injury, normal brain growth can cause neural elements to herniate through the dural defect at the site of the fracture. This can lead to a soft, pulsatile lesion at the site of injury and its growth can result in neurological deficit or seizures.

Surgical intervention is the mainstay of therapy for growing skull fractures to prevent or treat neurological impairment or seizures. A wide-margin craniectomy is typically utilized to adequately surround the dural defect and herniating neural elements. This is necessary to encompass the entirety of the dural tear, which may extend beyond the elements of the skull fracture itself. Duraplasty with synthetic graft or autologous pericranium can be used to create a watertight dural closure, and depending on the quality of the fractured bone, it can be replaced and fixated, or cranioplasty can be performed, preferentially using split-thickness autologous grafting from a donor calvarial site.

13.9 Aneurysmal Bone Cyst

Aneurysmal bone cysts (ABCs) are osseous lesions that tend to expand in the diploic space of children, leading to the presentation of a variably painful, enlarging mass.[8] These lesions occur throughout the body in the long bones and spine, while only rarely involving the calvarium (3–6%). ABCs can form primarily due to unclear mechanisms and also secondarily due to the presence of an associated bone tumor, such as osteoblastomas, giant cell tumors, and others. Diagnostic imaging is critical for identification of the lesion, as CT imaging demonstrates expansion of cortical bone and MR imaging demonstrates a heterogenous, expansile lesion that may contain fluid–fluid levels and cystic components (▶ Fig. 13.6).

Treatment of ABCs is surgical resection, with good outcomes when gross resection is achieved. Due to the considerably vascular nature of these lesions, preoperative angiography and neurointerventional embolization may aid in hemostasis during resection. Surgical intervention with resection and curettage is the favored approach for these lesions, while cryotherapy, embolization, and radiation therapy serve as adjuvant therapeutic options.

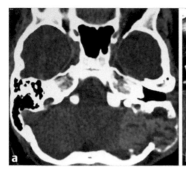
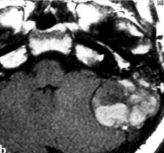

Fig. 13.6 Aneurysmal bone cyst. **(a)** CT and **(b)** MR imaging demonstrating cortical bone expansion and fluid–fluid levels in a posterior fossa lesion consistent with an aneurysmal bone cyst. Mass effect on the underlying can be seen, but the dura is typically not penetrated in such lesions.

13.10 Osteoma, Osteoblastoma, and Osteoid Osteoma

Three generally benign skull lesions that are rare in children include *osteomas, osteoblastomas*, and *osteoid osteomas.* Osteomas are hyperostotic skull lesions derived from mature cortical bone, arising from the inner or outer table. These lesions are rare in young children, occurring more commonly in young adults. Many times, osteomas are asymptomatic and without cosmetic significance. Their appearance on CT imaging is expansile and hyperdense, generally without evidence of bony destruction. Gardner's syndrome, an inheritable form of colonic polyposis, also features the development of osteomas throughout the body.

Osteoblastomas are comprised of immature osteoid material laced with osteoblasts, affecting the skull in approximately 10 to 20% of cases.[9] Their imaging appearance features more variable calcification, and malignant features resembling osteosarcoma are also possible.[10] These lesions may enlarge and become painful. Although benign, recurrence rates of osteoblastomas are higher than osteomas following resection, highlighting the importance of complete surgical removal. Malignant transformation has been reported, but is uncommon. Osteoid osteomas rarely occur in the skull and typically present with dull, throbbing pain that is worse at nighttime. Pain relief can be attained with aspirin and nonsteroidal anti-inflammatory drugs. Surgical resection for medically refractory cases can also alleviate pain.

13.11 Sarcoma and Neuroblastoma

Primary sarcomas of the skull are unusual, but can affect older children and young adults. Metastases to the skull are possible, including fibrosarcoma, osteosarcoma, or Ewing s sarcoma from the long bones. Postradiation sarcomas in children with a history of other tumors have also been described. On imaging, sarcomas often appear as osteolytic lesions with poorly defined margins on CT, and as infiltrative lesions on MR imaging. MR imaging plays an important role in determining intradural involvement, which is critical for preoperative planning. Preoperative angiography and embolization can be useful for particularly vascular lesions. Following resection, adjuvant radiation and chemotherapy are often used. Postresection skull reconstruction is often delayed until after chemoradiation in order to lessen the likelihood of wound complications.

Neuroblastoma is the most common extracranial solid tumor in children and is the most common tumor to metastasize to the skull in this age group. Focal skull enlargement, with a hair-on-end appearance with bony imaging, is common. The most important prognostic factor is pathological grade, with 5-year survival rates around 80% for low-grade lesions and 40% for high-grade lesions.[11] Maximal surgical resection is advocated if total or near-total resection is feasible. Along these lines, chemoradiation plays an important role in residual, recurrent, or inoperable disease.

References

[1] Yoon SH, Park SH. A study of 77 cases of surgically excised scalp and skull masses in pediatric patients. Childs Nerv Syst. 2008; 24(4):459–465

[2] Gibson SE, Prayson RA. Primary skull lesions in the pediatric population: a 25-year experience. Arch Pathol Lab Med. 2007; 131(5):761–766

[3] Ruge JR, Tomita T, Naidich TP, Hahn YS, McLone DG. Scalp and calvarial masses of infants and children. Neurosurgery. 1988; 22(6, Pt 1):1037–1042

[4] Hashiguchi K, Morioka T, Yokoyama N, Mihara F, Sasaki T. Subgaleal dermoid tumors at the anterior fontanelle. Pediatr Neurosurg. 2005; 41(1):54–57

[5] Lam S, Reddy GD, Mayer R, Lin Y, Jea A. Eosinophilic granuloma/Langerhans cell histiocytosis: pediatric neurosurgery update. Surg Neurol Int. 2015; 6 Suppl 17: S435–S439

[6] Singh I, Rohilla S, Siddiqui SA, Kumar P. Growing skull fractures: guidelines for early diagnosis and surgical management. Childs Nerv Syst. 2016; 32(6):1117–1122

[7] Muhonen MG, Piper JG, Menezes AH. Pathogenesis and treatment of growing skull fractures. Surg Neurol. 1995; 43 (4):367–372, discussion 372–373

[8] Gan YC, Hockley AD. Aneurysmal bone cysts of the cranium in children. Report of three cases and brief review of the literature. J Neurosurg. 2007; 106(5) Suppl:401–406

[9] McLeod RA, Dahlin DC, Beabout JW. The spectrum of osteoblastoma. AJR Am J Roentgenol 1976;126(2):321–325

[10] Aziz TZ, Neal JW, Cole G. Malignant osteoblastoma of the skull. Br J Neurosurg 1993;7(4):423–426

[11] Tsai EC, Santoreneos S, Rutka JT. Tumors of the skull base in children: review of tumor types and management strategies. Neurosurg Focus 2002;12(5):e1

14 Supratentorial Tumors

Eveline T. Hidalgo, Nir Shimony, Karl F. Kothbauer

14.1 Introduction

Supratentorial hemispheric tumors account for 17% of all central nervous system (CNS) tumors in children.[1] They are more common in children younger than 2 years; older children tend to have more infratentorial tumors. In adolescence, tumors of the sellar region are predominant.[1] An interdisciplinary approach and enrollment in studies is essential to achieve the best possible long-term outcome. Presentation at a tumor board is one of the first steps in the management of a child with this condition and should be planned before surgery to complete the diagnostic workup and to adjust the surgical approach if necessary. Surgical gross total resection (GTR) is the most important prognostic factor in most of these tumors; therefore, surgery should always be considered as the first-line treatment. Surgery is performed to obtain a diagnosis, to reverse neurologic deficit due to mass effect, to resect a seizure focus, and for cytoreduction as an oncologic objective.

The variety of tumors that may be encountered supratentorially range from benign types, which may be managed with surveillance, to highly malignant tumor types requiring adjuvant therapies.

14.2 Clinical Presentation

The clinical presentation depends on the location and size of the tumor. Age also plays an important role.

In children:
- Seizures—often first symptom, with and without neurologic deficit.
- Neurologic deficit—depends on site, location, and size of the lesion, often a late sign.
- Elevated intracranial pressure (ICP) manifests as:
  - Headache, vomiting, drowsiness.
  - Papilledema.

In infants:
- Developmental delay and failure to thrive.
- Elevated ICP manifests as:
  - Vomiting, bulging fontanels, and sunset sign.
  - Macrocephaly—head circumference curve should be used.
  - Ophthalmologic examination may reveal optic atrophy or papilledema.

The decision whether the patient should be admitted to the floor or the pediatric intensive care unit (PICU) depends on the clinical presentation (Box 14.1).

> ### Box 14.1 Indications to admit the patient to the PICU
>
> - Signs of elevated ICP.
> - Moderate to severe hydrocephalus.
> - Intratumoral hemorrhage.
> - First seizure.
> - GCS < 14.

14.2.1 Emergencies in Patients with Supratentorial Brain Tumors

If the child presents with clinical signs of elevated ICP, due to mass effect, hydrocephalus with trapped temporal horn, or trapped contralateral ventricle, and/or if Glasgow Coma Scale (GCS) < 13:
- Call anesthesiology and stabilize child (airways, breathing, and cardio).
- Perform computed tomography (CT) scan or preferably magnetic resonance imaging (MRI) if immediately available.
- Type and screen and order blood.
- Give steroids or mannitol if immediate surgery is considered.
- External ventricular drain (EVD) if hydrocephalus and/or consider urgent craniotomy for decompression and tumor resection.
- Make sure that parents are informed in an interdisciplinary fashion involving all required pediatric caregivers.

14.3 Clinical Evaluation

Evaluation should always be interdisciplinary, involving pediatricians, pediatric oncologists, and, in select cases, pediatric neurologists and the pediatric epilepsy team. Presentation at a multidisciplinary tumor board is useful prior to surgery to determine the strategy, including preoperative diagnostic evaluations, early inclusion in trials, surgical strategy, and, to a certain degree, anticipation of subsequent adjuvant treatment.

Potential inclusion in a clinical trial should be considered early and ongoing clinical trials as well as inclusion criteria may be found in:

- United States and worldwide: website of the National Cancer Institute at the National Institute of Health (www.clinicaltrials.gov).
- Europe: www.clinicaltrialsregister.eu

If the presenting symptom is longstanding epilepsy, it should be discussed prior to surgery with the epilepsy team to tailor the size of the resection. Invasive monitoring with subdural or depth electrodes before and/or after resection may be necessary to determine the epileptogenic zone. The epileptogenic zone may extend outside the radiographic lesion. Particularly in benign tumors (ganglioglioma, dysembryoplastic neuroepithelial tumor [DNET]), postoperative long-term seizure freedom is one of the goals of the surgery. Where the clinical evaluation of the patient occurs depends on the urgency of the presenting symptoms. It may be in an inpatient setting or in ambulatory care

The clinical evaluation includes:

- Thorough neurologic examination.
- Fundoscopy and/or ophthalmologic examination; in older children, the visual field should be examined with Goldmann perimetry.
- Electroencephalogram (EEG) if seizures are present or suspected and/or 24-hour video EEG (VEEG) to evaluate epileptic focus.
- Endocrinologic workup.
- Neuropsychological assessment—in older children and adolescents.
- Anesthesia consult—if the child suffers from any other medical condition.
- If a lumbar puncture is required for staging reasons, it should be performed only after imaging. Be aware of possible brain herniation due to mass effect. Send samples of cerebrospinal fluid (CSF) to cytology to evaluate for CSF dissemination. A diagnostic lumbar puncture is more often performed postoperatively, and should be delayed at least 14 days post-operative to avoid false-positive results.[2]

14.4 Imaging

The imaging of choice, if not in an emergency, is always MRI with and without contrast agent, including navigation, diffusion, and fluid-attenuated inversion recovery (FLAIR) images.

An MRI of the whole spine is necessary in almost all cases for staging reasons. If it cannot be obtained before surgery, it should be planned at least 14 days after surgery to reduce false-positive results.[2]

Functional MRI and diffusion tensor imaging (DTI), depending on location of tumor and age of child, can provide functional and structural information for surgical planning.

Positron emission tomography (PET) is a metabolic imaging modality that can be helpful in differentiating low-grade from high-grade lesions and for further differentiation of incidental supratentorial lesions.[3]

CT has almost no role in the evaluation of supratentorial hemispheric tumors, except in emergency situations. There is a small cumulative absolute risk reported for leukemia and brain tumors from numerous CT scans.[4]

Preoperative digital subtraction angiography and embolization may be useful in selected cases of highly vascularized tumors (meningioma, hemangioblastoma).[5]

Ultrasound is only a screening tool in infants, and it may be helpful in follow-up in CSF outflow obstructions.

14.5 Preoperative Management

- Extensive and thorough communication with parents/caregivers.
- The child should be informed in an age-appropriate fashion.
- Preoperative blood work (hemoglobin, electrolytes, coagulation, type and screen).
- Preoperative steroids plus omeprazole.
- Antiepileptic medication (AED) is indicated for suspected or diagnosed seizures.
- Neuroanesthesiologic evaluation.

If hydrocephalus is present, an EVD placement may be helpful to temporize until the time of surgery and avoid placement of a definitive shunt. Handling of an EVD needs special attention, particularly during transfers, as open drains may result in overdrainage and clamped drains may result in ICP elevation. There is generally no role for definitive placement of ventriculoperitoneal shunts prior to tumor surgery, as hydrocephalus often resolves with the tumor resection.

14.6 Perioperative Management

- Adequate temperature in the operating room.
- Antibiotics 30 to 60 minutes before incision.
- Have blood in the room before incision (especially in highly vascularized tumors such as atypical teratoid rhabdoid tumor [ATRT], meningiomas, and hemangioblastomas and in all infants).
- Apply SCD (sequential compression device) for children older than 12 years and/or beginning of puberty.
- Head shaving is contraindicated. Only minimal clipping on the site of incision is used; long hair is combed and braided away.
- Head fixation: In very young children and infants, headrests that do not require pins may be an option. In children older than 2 years, the head is fixed in a Sugita or Mayfield-type head holder. Appropriate pins and pressure must be used, depending on the patient's age. The six-pin Sugita head holder is optimal for smaller children.
- Neuronavigation is especially helpful in determining the location and size of the craniotomy and should be used in all cases. Intraoperative brain shift reduces its reliability.
- Intraoperative neurophysiological neuromonitoring—depending on the location of the tumor, this can help in performing a safer resection, for example, if the tumor is close to the central region. Somatosensory evoked potential and motor evoked potential as well as cortical stimulation mapping may be used.
- If one of the aims of the surgery is to resect the epileptogenic zone around the tumor, pre- or postresection invasive monitoring or intraoperative electrocorticography (ECoG) may be required.
- Ultrasonic aspirator is a useful and essential tool in the resection of supratentorial hemispheric tumors.
- Ultrasound is a real-time intraoperative imaging that provides information quickly and safely.
- Intraoperative MRI is a relative real-time tool only available in a few pediatric neurosurgery centers and only little data about its efficacy exist.
- Awake craniotomy with functional mapping can be used in selected cases where tumors are close to language areas and/or motor areas and only in older children, as cooperation of the patient is required.[6]
- Evaluate if 5-aminolevulinic acid (5-ALA) should be given as a surgical aid, but be aware that at the present time in most countries it is not approved for children and could only be given in the context of clinical trials. Convincing data exist for adults,[7] but little is known about its use in pediatric brain tumors. However, it appears to be useful in recurrent high-grade gliomas (HGGs) in children.[8]
- Repeated informing of the parents via telephone during surgery is very well received. It is an easy way to reduce stress for the family.
- Collect tissue for frozen section and definitive pathology in adequate container and storage media; evaluate if frozen samples for molecular analysis are necessary.

14.7 Postoperative Management

After elective surgery of supratentorial hemispheric tumors, all patients should be extubated in the operation room for immediate evaluation (Box 14.2).

> **Box 14.2 Management of postoperative drains**
>
> - If epidural/subgaleal/CSF drains are used, ensure that they are open and written orders regarding volumes and alarm triggers exist and are thoroughly communicated.
> - Soft silicone-type drains are preferable to all other types.
> - Never use strong vacuum bottle suction, as this carries a risk of low ICP and subsequent epidural hemorrhage even far from the original craniotomy site.
> - If CSF drainage is used, make sure it is on the correct drainage level and written orders about maximum drainage volume are provided.

All patients should be admitted to the ICU postoperatively:
- Head of bed elevation: approximately 30 degrees.
- Check every 30 minutes for GCS, pain score, neurologic deficits, and vital signs.
- Ensure sufficient analgesia (often underestimated).
- Continue steroids for 48 hours, then taper usually in 5 days.
- Check labs (hemoglobin and electrolytes) and fluid balance.

- Continue AED.
- Management of postoperative drains.
- Post-operative MRI within 24 hours should be considered a modern standard: it is essential to document the rate of resection/extent of residual tumor, hemorrhage, swelling, and postsurgical ischemia (include diffusion-weighted sequences!).
- Mobilization should be under instruction of physiotherapy as soon as possible, usually on the first postoperative day.
- Evaluate if the patient requires inpatient neurorehabilitation, physiotherapy, and speech therapy.
- Neuropathologic workup should include molecular diagnostics.
- Present the patient at the tumor board.
- Postoperative neuropsychological assessment—important to keep up with the child's school performance.

An appointment should be scheduled in an inpatient or outpatient setting to inform the parents/caregivers about the neuropathologic results and the recommendations of the tumor board. With a formal appointment, it can be ensured that all caregivers of the patient can be present and that sufficient time is available to answer all the questions.

If chemotherapy and radiation is indicated, it is usually started as soon as the surgical incision is healed. Patients should always be clinically seen by the surgeon and the healing incision must be inspected before starting radiation or chemotherapy.

14.8 Complications

14.8.1 Intraoperative Complications

- Hemorrhage: The risk of intraoperative hemorrhage can be reduced by careful planning, surgical technique, and checking the preoperative coagulation labs and evaluating the bleeding history.
- Swelling: General perioperative neurosurgical measures such as steroids at the beginning of the operation, keeping the Pco_2 at levels around 30 to 35 mm Hg, and making sure venous outflow is not obstructed can help in reducing swelling. Reverse Trendelenburg positioning and mannitol administration 0.5 to 1 mg/kg can be helpful as an acute measure.
- Seizures: Give AED the morning of the surgery and use cold ringer lactate irrigation. If seizures occur, have ice-cold ringer lactate in the room!

14.8.2 Postoperative Complications

- Postoperative hemorrhage: Asymptomatic hemorrhage in the resection cavity on postoperative MRI may be tolerated. If the size of the hemorrhage extends past the tumor size, or a drop in GCS and/or new onset of seizures occurs, consider reoperation. Epidural hematoma evacuation is indicated if symptomatic or if the width is greater than the skull diameter, or 1 cm. If a reoperation to evacuate hematoma is necessary, check for disturbances of coagulation and substitute if necessary. Evaluate if postoperative low-molecular-weight heparin administration should be postponed.
- Infection: Check wound and temperature daily; patients may have mildly increased temperature the first few days, usually not exceeding 37.9 °C. Check infection parameters on the first, second, and fifth postoperative day. An increase of C-reactive protein on the first and second postoperative day is physiologic; on the fifth day, it should have dropped to nearly normal levels. Leukocytosis can be expected postoperatively and in patients on steroids. As steroids are tapered, leucocyte counts decrease gradually.
- Wound healing: Check the wound daily. It would be preferable to leave the incision uncovered after the third day; however, draping may be required as children tend to scratch on the incision!
- Seizures: If a new seizure occurs and continues for more than 3 minutes, treat with benzodiazepines and evaluate intubation. Immediately perform CT to check for rebleeding or venous infarction. Consult pediatric epilepsy team for AED and start VEEG.

14.9 Low-Grade Gliomas (Diffuse, Juvenile Pilocytic Astrocytoma)

14.9.1 Key Features

- WHO classification I or II.
- Slow-growing tumors with comparatively favorable outcome.
- Better prognosis than in adults.
- Complete neurosurgical resection without adjuvant therapy is the treatment of choice.

14.9.2 Epidemiology

Gliomas account for approximately 53% of tumors in children 0 to 14 years of age and 36% in children 15 to 19 years of age.[1] Low-grade gliomas (LGGs) of the cerebral hemispheres account for approximately 24 to 40% of all low cerebral LGGs.[9,10]

14.9.3 Clinical Presentation

Approximately 40% of the tumors presents with seizures.[10] Other presentations are focal neurologic deficit and raised ICP.

14.9.4 Evaluation

EEG and epilepsy-surgery-specific evaluation are indicated if longstanding epilepsy is reported. Preoperative neuropsychological assessment is indicated in older children.

14.9.5 Imaging

- Diffuse astrocytomas are characterized by being homogeneously hyperintense on FLAIR imaging, hypointense on T1, and hyperintense on T2; also, they show no enhancement. No peritumoral edema; magnetic resonance spectroscopy (MRS) findings are nonspecific.[11]
- Pilocytic astrocytoma (PA) has in most cases the classic appearance of a cystic mass with an enhancing mural nodule. Less common appearances are quite nonspecific. Surrounding vasogenic edema is rarely present, and this feature provides a valuable clue to the correct diagnosis.[12]
- MRI navigation: Sequences should be obtained, and in nonenhancing tumors (LGGs excluding PA) MRI FLAIR sequences are mandatory to evaluate the size and margins of the tumor.

14.9.6 Pathology

LGGs encompass tumors of astrocytic, oligodendroglial, and mixed glial–neuronal histology. In children, juvenile pilocytic and fibrillary astrocytoma are the most common glial histological types.[13,14] Germline polymorphisms have been associated with high risk for gliomas.[15] BRAF duplications have been found in the majority of PA.[16] BRAF and CDKN2A alterations in childhood gliomas have been detected in LGGs, which transformed into secondary HGGs.[17] Pleomorphic xanthoastrocytoma (PXA), ganglioglioma, and a small subset of extracerebellar PA have BRAF V600E mutations.[18] Potential future treatment includes inhibition of the MAP kinase pathway, which regulates cell proliferation. Several signal transduction inhibitors are of potential clinical activity.

14.9.7 Treatment

GTR should be the goal when it can be achieved with an acceptable functional outcome.[9]

- Neuronavigation: If neuronavigation is used, FLAIR sequences should be fused with the T1 navigation sequences, as particularly GTR of diffuse LGGs means resection of the "FLAIRoma."
- Intraoperative imaging: Only high-resolution MRI would provide sufficient image quality to evaluate diffuse astrocytoma.
- Intraoperative neuromonitoring should be used in tumors close to eloquent regions.
- Consider awake surgery in children older than 12 years, with tumors near language areas.
- If there is a risk for intraoperative seizure, have cold irrigation in the operation room.
- Post-operative care: watch out for seizures and continue seizure medication.

Postoperative MRI should be obtained in the first 24 hours. Be aware that systematic and substantial overestimation of residual nonenhancing volume on MRI within 48 hours of resection compared with months postoperatively, in particular for FLAIR imaging, has been observed.[19]

14.9.8 Adjuvant Therapy

There is no role for adjuvant chemo- or radiotherapy if GTR was achieved in supratentorial hemispheric LGGs.

Radiotherapy and particularly chemotherapy may be indicated for unresectable or partially resected tumors.

Stereotactic radiotherapy or intensity-modulated radiotherapy can be applied; both provide local control for children with small, localized, low-grade glial tumors.[20,21] As always in children, the risk and benefit of radiation therapy must be strongly assessed vis-à-vis the risks of long-term effects of radiation in long-term tumor survivors.

14.9.9 Outcome

According to the data of the Children's Oncology Group, the overall 5-year progression-free survival (PFS) is 78% and 8-year PFS is 75% in hemispheric tumors. If GTR is achieved, 5-year PFS is 94%.

The 5- and 8-year overall survival (OS) rate is 96%.[9]

14.9.10 Follow-Up

Regular follow-up with sequential MRIs every 6 months for the first 2 years, and yearly thereafter.

14.10 High-Grade Gliomas

14.10.1 Key Features

- The most frequent entities in HGGs are glioblastoma multiforme (GBM; WHO grade IV) and anaplastic astrocytoma (AA; WHO grade III).
- As it is a relatively rare disease, enrollment in ongoing trials is crucial.
- GTR should be attempted.
- Highly aggressive and always needs adjuvant chemo- and radiotherapy.

14.10.2 Epidemiology

HGGs comprise approximately 17% of all brain and CNS tumors reported among 0 to 14 years old and 8% in children 15 to 19 years old.[1]

14.10.3 Clinical Presentation

HGGs often present with signs of raised ICP, and duration of symptoms is usually short as they are fast-growing tumors.

14.10.4 Evaluation

CT scan if emergency imaging is necessary, but MRI is the imaging of choice.

14.10.5 Imaging

MRI appearance: GBMs present as an aggressive-appearing, ill-defined, heterogeneous enhancing mass that may invade the corpus callosum. Necrosis and hemorrhage are the hallmarks of these tumors.[11,22] AAs are usually heterogenic hemispheric masses, with involvement and expansion to the cortex. They typically do not enhance and do not show necrosis or calcification. Anaplastic oligodendrogliomas can be differentiated from AAs by their high rates of calcification. MRS provides information about metabolic and biochemical activity of HGGs and decreased N-acetylaspartic acid (NAA), lactate peak, and elevated choline/creatinine ratio.[23]

14.10.6 Risk Factors

Prior radiation, Li–Fraumeni syndrome,[24] and neurofibromatosis type 1 (NF1).[25]

14.10.7 Pathology

According to the WHO classification, supratentorial HGGs are divided into AAs (WHO grade III), anaplastic oligodendrogliomas (WHO grade III), mixed astrocytic tumors, and GBM (WHO grade IV).[14] A subentity is identified as giant cell glioblastoma, which is reported to have a slightly better prognosis in the pediatric age group.[26]

14.10.8 Molecular Features

There are molecular differences between adult and pediatric HGGs; therefore, results from adult clinical trials cannot be extrapolated to children. Molecular markers overexpressed in pediatric HGGs include Platelet derived growth factor receptor alpha (PDGFRα) and p53. Amplification of epidermal growth factor receptor alpha (EGFRα) is observed, but to a lesser degree than in adult HGGs.[27] In pediatric GBM, broad chromosomal gains and losses, such as gain of chromosome 1q and broad losses of chromosome 10q, are common. The heterozygous K27 mutation on histone tail 3.1 and 3.3 and the G34 R/V mutations on the histone tail 3.3 have been found to be common in HGGs. Mutations of the p53 tumor suppressor gene play a key role in tumorigenesis in patients with Li–Fraumeni syndrome.[28]

14.10.9 Treatment

GTR should be achieved since the extent of tumor resection is also the strongest predictor of survival in pediatric glioblastoma.[27,29] GTR is significantly associated with OS in pediatric patients with glioblastoma excluding tumors located in the brainstem.[30] 5-ALA as off-label use for recurrent HGG is reported to be useful[8] and appears to be safe.

14.10.10 Chemotherapy

Chemotherapeutic agents such as temozolomide, bevacizumab, cisplatin, etoposide, vincristine, and ifosfamide are used, but there is no international standard protocol for children. Survival was significantly improved for patients with completely resected HGG when they were treated with the HIT-GBM-C chemotherapy.[31] The combination of bevacizumab and CPT-11 was reported to be fairly well tolerated, and most severe BVZ-related toxicities were rare, self-limiting, and manageable.[32] Molecular targeted therapies are not available yet, but promising results of preclinical data will lead to tailored therapies.

14.10.11 Radiation

Radiation therapy is the standard of care after surgical resection for children older than 3 years.[33] Treatment of children with glioblastoma with conformal radiation, temozolomide, and bevacizumab as adjuncts to surgical resection has shown promising results.[34]

14.10.12 Outcome

Glioblastoma survival is somewhat higher for children than adults; in children, the 5-year survival rate is 19%.[1] The higher survival rates may be due to more intensive chemotherapy protocols or due to the fact that pediatric HGGs differ biologically from HGGs in adults.[35] The prognosis is worse in very young children; this may be due to delayed radiotherapy.

14.10.13 Follow-Up

Follow-up should always be interdisciplinary and the children should be under the surveillance of the pediatric neuro-oncologists. If recurrence is suspected, there is a role for FDG-PET and MRS to distinguish between radiation necrosis and tumor recurrence.

14.11 Pleomorphic Xanthoastrocytomas

14.11.1 Key Features

- WHO grade II, but worse outcome than LGG.
- GTR is the primary goal; unclear role of adjuvant therapy.
- PXAs with anaplastic features have been described and tend to have worse outcome.
- Older children and seizures as first presentation.

14.11.2 Epidemiology

Very rare, approximately 1% of all pediatric brain tumors.

14.11.3 Presentation

May present with a longstanding history of seizures.

14.11.4 Evaluation

MRI appearance: peripheral or cortical mass composed of cystic and solid components and heterogeneous enhancement.[11]

Staging with MRI neuroaxis is mandatory, as CSF dissemination has been reported.[36,37]

14.11.5 Pathology

PXAs demonstrate immunoreactivity for neuronal markers like S100 and GFAP. P53 immunolabeling is usually weak or negative, but CD34 labeling is frequent. PXAs can have anaplastic features but little is known regarding clinicopathologic and molecular features.

14.11.6 Molecular

PXAs have been found to have the highest frequency of BRAF V600E mutations out of all CNS neoplasms.[18]

14.11.7 Treatment

GTR is the primary goal as it is a strong predictor of PFS. The role of adjuvant treatment is not well established, and both chemotherapy and radiation therapy have been used with reports of a good response. However, since radiation has been reported as a negative predictor for long-term OS in LGG,[38] this therapy should be spared for tumors with anaplastic features.

14.11.8 Outcome

PXAs have very variable outcome. Five-year PFS is reported to be 40 to 68% and 5-year OS rate is 76 to 87%.[39,40,41] Ten-year OS rate is reported to be about 43%.[38] There has been no difference in pediatric PXA with and without anaplastic features regarding outcome. Prognosis is overall worse in children than in adults.[41]

14.12 Primitive Neuroectodermal Tumors

14.12.1 Key Features

- Heterogeneous group of tumors.
- Young age, aggressive tumor.
- Histology similar to medulloblastomas, but worse outcome.
- All patients should be treated on a clinical trial.
- Adjuvant chemo- and radiotherapy show increased survival.[42]

14.12.2 Epidemiology

Supratentorial primitive neuroectodermal tumors (SPNETs) account for approximately 2.5% of all pediatric brain tumors.[43]

14.12.3 Clinical Presentation

As it is a rapidly growing tumor, it often presents with increased ICP. Focal neurologic deficits and seizures are described as well.

14.12.4 Clinical Evaluation

Patients should have a staging workup to assess the extent of disease. Preoperative MRI of the brain, MRI of the spinal axis, and lumbar CSF sampling for cytological examination (lumbar and intraoperatively) is mandatory. Discordance between the results of neuroaxis MRI imaging and lumbar and intracranial CSF cytology in perioperative detection of tumor dissemination has been reported for pediatric SPNETs.[44]

14.12.5 Imaging

MRI appearance: SPNETs are heterogeneous; no specific distinct pattern characterizes them. The solid component of PNETs usually has avid heterogeneous enhancement with minimal surrounding edema.[22] Necrosis and hemorrhage are common and are seen as restriction on diffusion-weighted imaging (DWI).[11]

14.12.6 Pathology

Definition of the WHO Working Group[14]: heterogeneous embryonal tumor composed of undifferentiated or poorly differentiated neuroepithelial cells which have the capacity for or display divergent differentiation along neuronal, astrocytic, and ependymal lines.

- Cerebral neuroblastomas—only neuronal differentiation.
- Ganglioneuroblastomas—neuronal differentiation and ganglion cells.
- Medulloepitheliomas—features of neural tube formation.
- Ependymoblastomas—ependymoblastic rosettes.

14.12.7 Molecular

CNS PNETs have complex genomic alterations.[45] Oncogenes located on chromosome 2p are involved in initiating and sustaining CNS PNET.

14.12.8 Treatment

Blood should be in the operation room before skin incision. This tumor is often highly vascularized, so hypervolemia due to blood loss is a common complication.

Be aware of brain collapse; occasionally, a shunt is needed due to hydrocephalus. Surgical resection of tumor should be done only if additional permanent neurologic deficits can be spared. The role of GTR is controversial.

14.12.9 Chemotherapy

All patients are treated with chemotherapy. The specific protocol should be discussed in tumor board. Chemotherapy combined with radiation therapy has been associated with a significant increase in survival.[42]

14.12.10 Radiation Therapy

Radiation of neuroaxis with focal beam on tumor location is included in most protocols. Whole-spine radiation is indicated for spinal metastasis. There are promising data about favorable local control and low rates of acute radiation-induced toxicity for proton radiation therapy.[46]

14.12.11 Outcome

Despite adjuvant chemo- and radiotherapy, the outcome is relatively poor. One-year survival rate is 76.4% and 5-year survival is 49.5%.[1] Children younger than 2 years have a worse prognosis.[47] The outcome for children with SPNET generally has been reported to be poor and worse than medulloblastomas.[48,49]

14.12.12 Follow-Up

Interdisciplinary follow-up under the lead of pediatric neuro-oncology is indicated.

14.13 Atypical Teratoid Rhabdoid Tumors

14.13.1 Key Features

- Highly malignant.
- Mostly in infants.
- SMARCB1 is a specific marker.

14.13.2 Epidemiology

Around 80% of the patients diagnosed with ATRT are children younger than 3 years. There is a slight male predominance of 58%.[50] About 50% are supratentorial and 50% infratentorial.[51] Rhabdoid tumor predisposition syndrome is a risk factor for ATRT.

14.13.3 Clinical Presentation

As most of the tumors arise in infants, symptoms of elevated ICP such as macrocephaly, bulging fontanels, and vomiting are the presenting symptoms.

14.13.4 Evaluation

MRI: A supratentorial tumor with a thick, wavy (irregular) heterogeneously enhancing wall surrounding a central cystic region is suggestive of ATRT,[52] as it is a distinctive and unusual pattern. It is present in approximately 40% of ATRT.[53]

MRI spectroscopy may be helpful to distinguish them from other brain tumors. The combination of prominent choline and lactate and lipid peaks and generally absent NAA and myo-inositol peaks provide a metabolite profile typically distinct from other malignant pediatric brain tumors.[54]

MRI of the neuroaxis for staging reasons is mandatory, especially in young children, as 13% present with metastatic disease.[50] If possible, a lumbar puncture should be done as well, but be aware of the risks described in the introduction chapter.

14.13.5 Risk Factors

In older children, ATRT can occur as secondary tumor after whole-brain irradiation.[55]

14.13.6 Pathology

ATRTs, Medulloblastomas, and cerebral PNETs form the group of embryonal tumors. The main histologic characteristics of rhabdoid tumor cells are abundant cytoplasm with juxtanuclear eosinophilic inclusions and nuclei that display a single, prominent nucleolus in clear, uncondensed chromatin.[14] A defect in the INI 1 gene (*SMARCB1*) leading to loss of expression is associated with rhabdoid tumors and is used for diagnosis. SMARCB1 gene abnormalities are found in 76 to 95% of ATRT patients.[56,57]

14.13.7 Treatment

Improved OS and PFS have been reported with maximal primary tumor resection,[58] but an association between the extent of resection and OS is still controversial.[50]

14.13.8 Chemotherapy

No standard therapeutic approach has been established given the rarity of ATRTs and the variety of treatment regimens used to date. High-dose chemotherapy regimens seem to provide good results and increase survival.[51] Intrathecal therapy is widely used as it has shown significantly higher survival rates.[59]

14.13.9 Radiotherapy

In children younger than 3 years, the strategy is usually to avoid or delay radiation. Given the poor prognosis of ATRT, delayed risks of neurocognitive developmental problems should be balanced with potential survival benefit derived from adjuvant radiotherapy.[50] If radiotherapy is indicated, it should be started as soon as the incision is well healed. There has been a search for treatments avoiding irradiation to healthy tissue. Initial clinical outcomes with proton therapy show favorable results. The advantages of proton therapy are particularly suited to the treatment of ATRT, since the disease often requires radiation treatment at an early age.[60]

14.13.10 Outcome

One-year survival is 48% and 5-year survival is 28%.[1] The median OS is about 10 months and metastatic disease correlates with a worse prognosis.[50] Age less than 2 years, metastasis at diagnosis, and strong claudin-6 positivity appear to be independent prognostic factors for outcome.[61]

14.13.11 Follow-Up

Interdisciplinary follow-up under the lead of pediatric neuro-oncology is indicated, similar to CNS PNET. Several long-term complications have been reported, such as peritoneal metastasis from seeding through a ventriculoperitoneal shunt in pineal and ventricular ATRT[62,63] and multifocal necrotizing leukoencephalopathy as a treatment-related morbidity.[64]

14.14 Desmoplastic Neuroepithelial Tumors

14.14.1 Key Features

- The presenting symptom is often seizures; characteristically, it causes intractable partial seizures.
- First described in 1988, WHO classified in 1993.

14.14.2 Epidemiology

DNET belongs to the neuronal–glial tumors, which together with the neuronal tumors comprise 6.5 to 7.9% of CNS tumors in children.[1]

14.14.3 Pathology

DNET is a grade I glioneuronal tumor in the WHO classification[14] and shows no IDH1 mutations. The genetic basis of DNET is not well known or well defined. Somatic FGFRI alterations and MAP kinase pathway activation are events that both cause DNETs to develop. Gains of chromosomes 5 and 7 and loss of chromosomes 1p, 10q, and 19q have been observed and are associated with DNETs.[65]

14.14.4 Clinical Evaluation

Preoperative evaluation must always include consultation with the epilepsy service. Children with epilepsy and AED may have coagulation abnormalities, so preoperative hematology consultation may be indicated.

14.14.5 Imaging

MRI appearance: DNETs are characterized as having a "bubbly" appearance, are multilobulated, are hypointense on T1 in a wedge-shaped configuration, and hyperintense on T2-weighted images. FLAIR imaging shows a characteristic bright rim. DNETs have one of the highest apparent diffusion coefficient values among benign tumors. MRS is nonspecific.[11]

14.14.6 Treatment

Surgery is curative if the tumor can be completely resected. DNETs in the temporal lobe are often resected by temporal lobectomy (with or without hippocampectomy), and in select cases, intraoperative ECoG and pre- and/or postoperative invasive monitoring may be indicated.

14.14.7 Outcome

DNETs have a very good outcome from an oncologic standpoint, similar to LGGs. Long-term seizure freedom can be achieved in 86%.[66]

14.14.8 Follow-Up

Interdisciplinary follow-up under the lead of the pediatric epilepsy team is indicated.

14.15 Gangliogliomas

14.15.1 Key Features

- Seizures are the most common presentation.
- Two different cell types (combination of neuronal and glial cell).
- WHO I, rarely anaplastic.
- Very good prognosis with GTR.

14.15.2 Epidemiology

The majority of gangliogliomas are localized in the temporal lobe, but can occur throughout the CNS.[14] Most of the supratentorial cases are temporal and frontal.

14.15.3 Clinical Presentation

Seizures are the most frequent presentation, and gangliogliomas are the most common tumor to cause intractable, chronic pediatric epilepsy.[67]

14.15.4 Imaging

MRI shows a circumscribed mass and enhancement varies; a mural nodule with a cyst is also described. In CT, calcifications may be visible.

14.15.5 Pathology

Well-differentiated, slow-growing neuroepithelial tumor composed of neoplastic, mature ganglion cells alone (gangliocytoma) or in combination with neoplastic glial cells (ganglioglioma). Polymorphisms of the *TSC1* and *TSC2* genes have been common in patients with gangliogliomas.[68] Anaplastic gangliogliomas are rare.

14.15.6 Treatment

It is very important to identify pre- and intraoperatively the epilepsy focus and to perform a complete lesionectomy. The use of intraoperative neuromonitoring is indicated. GTR should be performed safely whenever possible and does not require postoperative irradiation. If only a subtotal resection is achieved, then radio therapy may improve long-term tumor control of both low-grade and high-grade tumors and, thus, should be considered.[69]

14.15.7 Post-operative Care

Continue AED.

14.15.8 Outcome

Overall, outcome is favorable. Five-year PFS rate is 81.2% and the OS rate is 97.4%.[70] The 15-year OS rate is reported to be 94%. PFS is affected by the extent of initial resection, so GTR should be achieved.[71]

For tumors located in the cerebral hemispheres, the achievement of total resection and seizures at presentation were associated with prolonged PFS.[70]

14.15.9 Follow-Up

Interdisciplinary follow-up with the pediatric epilepsy team and neuro-oncology is indicated.

14.16 Ependymomas
14.16.1 Key Features

- GTR is the most important prognostic factor.
- Recent molecular classification of ependymomas identified nine different subgroups in the CNS, two of which are in pediatric supratentorial tumors.

14.16.2 Epidemiology

A total of 5.4% of all tumors in childhood are ependymomas.[1] One-third of all pediatric ependymomas are supratentorial.[72]

14.16.3 Clinical Presentation

In most of the cases, they present with elevated ICP.[73]

14.16.4 Imaging

MRI of the neuroaxis and CSF analysis for cytology for staging are indicated.

14.16.5 Pathology

Ependymomas are classified according to the WHO grading system. The WHO classification system separates ependymomas into three groups based on histopathological criteria[14]: grade I (myxopapillary); grade II, which is further subdivided into four subtypes (cellular, papillary, clear-cell, and tanycytic); and grade III (anaplastic). Germline mutations on the tumor suppressor gene NF2 on chromosome 22q are associated with ependymomas. Loss of chromosome 1p and gain of chromosome 1q are genetic abnormalities highly linked to ependymomas. Recent molecular classification of ependymomas identified nine different subgroups in the CNS, with three subgroups in the supratentorial location. Two supratentorial subgroups are in the pediatric population and are characterized by prototypic fusion genes involving RELA and YAP1, respectively.[74]

14.16.6 Treatment

Ependymoma remains a "surgical disease."[75] Surgical considerations aim for GTR, as it is the most important prognostic factor. For supratentorial pediatric tumors, the GTR and GTR combined with external beam radiation therapy results in the longest time to recurrence/progression. Subtotal resection is correlated with inferior outcome.[72] Perioperative considerations are similar to those in astrocytomas.

Young age at diagnosis and the proximity of critical structures in patients with ependymoma make proton radiation therapy a possible radiation modality.[76]

14.16.7 Outcome

Favorable outcome is reported with a 5-year OS rate of 72 to 85%.[77,78]

There are case reports of grade II ependymomas with GTR without adjuvant therapy and long-term survival.[79]

It is controversial if classical grading plays a contributing role in predicting outcome. In a report of 40 pediatric patients, the Children's Cancer Group found no differences in PFS across WHO grades.[80]

14.16.8 Follow-Up

Follow-up should be continued with MRI scans after 3 and 6 months, and yearly in stable situations with or without residual disease.

14.17 Meningiomas

14.17.1 Key Features

- Meningiomas are much rarer in children than in adults.
- Believed to be more aggressive than in adults, but this may be just a matter of a larger variety of outcomes.
- Strong association with prior radiation treatment[81] and with neurofibromatosis.[82]

14.17.2 Epidemiology

Only about 2.5% of all primary pediatric CNS tumors are meningeal in origin. The incidence rises with age.[1]

14.17.3 Evaluation

A history of prior radiation treatment should be actively inquired. Approximately 40% of children with meningiomas have NF2.[83] After vestibular schwannoma, the next most common tumor type in NF2 is meningioma, which is encountered in roughly half of the cases.[84]

14.17.4 Imaging

MRI is also the imaging modality of choice and optimally shows extent and vascularity. Childhood meningiomas may more frequently lack any dural attachment.[82]

14.17.5 Pathology

A large fraction of pediatric meningiomas are WHO grade II or III (60%) and commonly demonstrate aggressive variant morphology, brain invasion, an increased mitotic index, and frequent deletions of 1p and 14q. About half of these children have significantly shortened PFS and OS.[85] Even metastatic meningioma is reported.[86]

14.17.6 Treatment

Preoperative embolization should be considered in extensive, highly vascularized tumors, particularly in small children. Blood in the room before incision is mandatory, since intraoperative mortality due to blood loss has been reported.[82]

Because of very small numbers and lack of standardized adjuvant treatment options, the management has to be tailored to the individual situation.

14.17.7 Outcome and Adjuvant Treatment

The 5-year survival is 83.9%, suggesting that the biological behavior of pediatric meningiomas is more aggressive than that of its adult counterparts.[87,88]

14.17.8 Follow-Up

As children more frequently have higher grade tumors, the clinical and imaging follow-up should be in rather short intervals of initially 3 to 6 months.

14.18 Surgical Pearls

- Supratentorial tumors in children are less common than posterior fossa tumors but occur in a much greater variety.
- Each entity requires extensive resection.
- Outcomes vary from "cure" with surgery only to very short intervals to recurrence and death in spite of extensive adjuvant treatment.
- These tumors may be large and vascular, so "have blood in the room."

14.19 Common Clinical Questions

1. What is the best treatment for a supratentorial LGG?
2. Is there a role for "watchful waiting" or for stereotactic biopsy in supratentorial LGG?
3. What is the outcome of LGGs that underwent GTR?
4. Is the outcome of pediatric PXAs similar to LGGs?
5. What is the perioperative strategy in patients with chronic epilepsy and suspected DNETs or gangliogliomas?

14.20 Answers to Clinical Questions

1. The aim of surgery in supratentorial hemispheric LGGs is GTR. This can be achieved with the aid of pre- and perioperative tools such as navigation, neuromonitoring, and awake craniotomy. If GTR cannot be achieved, further surveillance is indicated, as residual disease can be stable (progression-free disease) in up to 55%.[9]
2. Wait and see has a role in asymptomatic small tumors, but the risk of surgery and progression of the tumor must be constantly evaluated. Stereotactic biopsy usually has only a limited role. GTR remains the goal and can be achieved safely in the majority of cases. The role of stereotactic biopsy is limited to the rare cases where no oncologically meaningful, if still partial, resection is possible due to localization and/or diffuse nature of the tumor.
3. Outcome data from the Children's Cancer Group (CCG) and Pediatric Oncology Group (POG) study of primary surgery in LGGs indicate 5-year PFS in 92% of children after GTR, ranging from 95 to 100% for juvenile pilocytic astrocytomas and gangliogliomas to 80% for grade II diffuse astrocytomas in this age group.[9]
4. No, the outcome of pediatric PXA is more variable and typically worse than LGGs. The 5-year PFS in PXA is reported to be 40 to 68% and the 5-year OS rate is 76 to 87%.[39,40,41] The 5-year PFS in LGG is 78% and the 5-year OS rate is 96%.[9]
5. The perioperative strategy of DNETs and gangliogliomas is preoperative presentation at a multidisciplinary epilepsy surgery conference. The preoperative evaluation of the patient should include VEEG and MRI in all cases, and when indicated, fMRI (functional MRI), SPECT (single-photon emission computed tomography), PET, and neuropsychological testing. To detect more precisely the extension of the epileptogenic zone in order to achieve a more complete resection and better outcome, pre- and/or postoperative invasive monitoring may be indicated. AED should be continued postoperatively and should be reduced gradually in collaboration with the epilepsy team.

References

[1] Ostrom QT, Gittleman H, Farah P, et al. CBTRUS statistical report: Primary brain and central nervous system tumors diagnosed in the United States in 2006–2010. Neuro-oncol. 2013; 15 Suppl 2:ii1–ii56

[2] Meyers SP, Wildenhain SL, Chang JK, et al. Postoperative evaluation for disseminated medulloblastoma involving the spine: contrast-enhanced MR findings, CSF cytologic analysis, timing of disease occurrence, and patient outcomes. AJNR Am J Neuroradiol. 2000; 21(9):1757–1765

[3] Pirotte BJ, Lubansu A, Massager N, et al. Clinical interest of integrating positron emission tomography imaging in the workup of 55 children with incidentally diagnosed brain lesions. J Neurosurg Pediatr. 2010; 5(5):479–485

[4] Pearce MS, Salotti JA, Little MP, et al. Radiation exposure from CT scans in childhood and subsequent risk of leukaemia and brain tumours: a retrospective cohort study. Lancet. 2012; 380(9840):499–505

[5] Wang HH, Luo CB, Guo WY, et al. Preoperative embolization of hypervascular pediatric brain tumors: evaluation of technical safety and outcome. Childs Nerv Syst. 2013; 29(11): 2043–2049

[6] Duffau H, Lopes M, Arthuis F, et al. Contribution of intraoperative electrical stimulations in surgery of low grade gliomas: a comparative study between two series without (1985–96) and with (1996–2003) functional mapping in the same institution. J Neurol Neurosurg Psychiatry. 2005; 76(6): 845–851

[7] Stummer W, Pichlmeier U, Meinel T, Wiestler OD, Zanella F, Reulen HJ, ALA-Glioma Study Group. Fluorescence-guided surgery with 5-aminolevulinic acid for resection of malignant glioma: a randomised controlled multicentre phase III trial. Lancet Oncol. 2006; 7(5):392–401

[8] Preuß M, Renner C, Krupp W, et al. The use of 5-aminolevulinic acid fluorescence guidance in resection of pediatric brain tumors. Childs Nerv Syst. 2013; 29(8):1263–1267

[9] Wisoff JH, Sanford RA, Heier LA, et al. Primary neurosurgery for pediatric low-grade gliomas: a prospective multi-institutional study from the Children's Oncology Group. Neurosurgery. 2011; 68(6):1548–1554, discussion 1554–1555

[10] Youland RS, Khwaja SS, Schomas DA, Keating GF, Wetjen NM, Laack NN. Prognostic factors and survival patterns in pediatric low-grade gliomas over 4 decades. J Pediatr Hematol Oncol. 2013; 35(3):197–205

[11] Borja MJ, Plaza MJ, Altman N, Saigal G. Conventional and advanced MRI features of pediatric intracranial tumors: supratentorial tumors. AJR Am J Roentgenol. 2013; 200(5): W483–503

[12] Koeller KK, Rushing EJ. From the archives of the AFIP: pilocytic astrocytoma: radiologic-pathologic correlation. Radiographics. 2004; 24(6):1693–1708

[13] Burger PC, Scheithauer BW, Vogel FS. Surgical Pathology of the Nervous System and Its Coverings. 4th ed. New York, NY: Churchill Livingstone; 2002

[14] Louis DN, International Agency for Research on Cancer. World Health Organization. WHO Classification of Tumours of the Central Nervous System. 4th ed. Lyon: International Agency for Research on Cancer; 2007

[15] Jenkins RB, Xiao Y, Sicotte H, et al. A low-frequency variant at 8q24.21 is strongly associated with risk of oligodendroglial tumors and astrocytomas with IDH1 or IDH2 mutation. Nat Genet. 2012; 44(10):1122–1125

[16] Jones DT, Kocialkowski S, Liu L, et al. Tandem duplication producing a novel oncogenic BRAF fusion gene defines the majority of pilocytic astrocytomas. Cancer Res. 2008; 68(21): 8673–8677

[17] Mistry M, Zhukova N, Merico D, et al. BRAF mutation and CDKN2A deletion define a clinically distinct subgroup of childhood secondary high-grade glioma. J Clin Oncol. 2015; 33(9):1015–1022

[18] Schindler G, Capper D, Meyer J, et al. Analysis of BRAF V600E mutation in 1,320 nervous system tumors reveals high mutation frequencies in pleomorphic xanthoastrocytoma, ganglioglioma and extra-cerebellar pilocytic astrocytoma. Acta Neuropathol. 2011; 121(3):397–405

[19] Belhawi SM, Hoefnagels FW, Baaijen JC, et al. Early postoperative MRI overestimates residual tumour after resection of gliomas with no or minimal enhancement. Eur Radiol. 2011; 21(7):1526–1534

[20] Paulino AC, Mazloom A, Terashima K, et al. Intensity-modulated radiotherapy (IMRT) in pediatric low-grade glioma. Cancer. 2013; 119(14):2654–2659

[21] Marcus KJ, Goumnerova L, Billett AL, et al. Stereotactic radiotherapy for localized low-grade gliomas in children: final results of a prospective trial. Int J Radiat Oncol Biol Phys. 2005; 61(2):374–379

[22] Poussaint TY. Magnetic resonance imaging of pediatric brain tumors: state of the art. Top Magn Reson Imaging. 2001; 12 (6):411–433

[23] Howe FA, Opstad KS. 1 H MR spectroscopy of brain tumours and masses. NMR Biomed. 2003; 16(3):123–131

[24] Li FP, Fraumeni JF, Jr, Mulvihill JJ, et al. A cancer family syndrome in twenty-four kindreds. Cancer Res. 1988; 48 (18):5358–5362

[25] Rosenfeld A, Listernick R, Charrow J, Goldman S. Neurofibromatosis type 1 and high-grade tumors of the central nervous system. Childs Nerv Syst. 2010; 26(5):663–667

[26] Borkar SA, Lakshmiprasad G, Subbarao KC, Sharma MC, Mahapatra AK. Giant cell glioblastoma in the pediatric age group: report of two cases. J Pediatr Neurosci. 2013; 8(1):38–40

[27] MacDonald TJ, Aguilera D, Kramm CM. Treatment of high-grade glioma in children and adolescents. Neuro-oncol. 2011; 13(10):1049–1058

[28] Varley JM. Germline TP53 mutations and Li-Fraumeni syndrome. Hum Mutat. 2003; 21(3):313–320

[29] Das KK, Mehrotra A, Nair AP, et al. Pediatric glioblastoma: clinico-radiological profile and factors affecting the outcome. Childs Nerv Syst. 2012; 28(12):2055–2062

[30] Yang T, Temkin N, Barber J, et al. Gross total resection correlates with long-term survival in pediatric patients with glioblastoma. World Neurosurg. 2013; 79(3–4):537–544

[31] Wolff JE, Driever PH, Erdlenbruch B, et al. Intensive chemotherapy improves survival in pediatric high-grade glioma after gross total resection: results of the HIT-GBM-C protocol. Cancer. 2010; 116(3):705–712

[32] Fangusaro J, Gururangan S, Poussaint TY, et al. Bevacizumab (BVZ)-associated toxicities in children with recurrent central nervous system tumors treated with BVZ and irinotecan (CPT-11): a Pediatric Brain Tumor Consortium Study (PBTC-022). Cancer. 2013; 119(23):4180–4187

[33] Cage TA, Mueller S, Haas-Kogan D, Gupta N. High-grade gliomas in children. Neurosurg Clin N Am. 2012; 23(3):515–523

[34] Friedman GK, Spiller SE, Harrison DK, Fiveash JB, Reddy AT. Treatment of children with glioblastoma with conformal radiation, temozolomide, and bevacizumab as adjuncts to surgical resection. J Pediatr Hematol Oncol. 2013; 35(3): e123–e126

[35] Pollack IF, Finkelstein SD, Woods J, et al. Children's Cancer Group. Expression of p53 and prognosis in children with malignant gliomas. N Engl J Med. 2002; 346(6):420–427

[36] Nern C, Hench J, Fischmann A. Spinal imaging in intracranial primary pleomorphic xanthoastrocytoma with anaplastic features. J Clin Neurosci. 2012; 19(9):1299–1301

[37] Okazaki T, Kageji T, Matsuzaki K, et al. Primary anaplastic pleomorphic xanthoastrocytoma with widespread neuroaxis dissemination at diagnosis–a pediatric case report and review of the literature. J Neurooncol. 2009; 94(3):431–437

[38] Krishnatry R, Zhukova N, Guerreiro Stucklin AS, et al. Clinical and treatment factors determining long-term outcomes for adult survivors of childhood low-grade glioma: a population-based study. Cancer. 2016; 122(8):1261–1269

[39] Rao AA, Laack NN, Giannini C, Wetmore C. Pleomorphic xanthoastrocytoma in children and adolescents. Pediatr Blood Cancer. 2010; 55(2):290–294

[40] Dodgshun AJ, Sexton-Oates A, Saffery R, MacGregor D, Sullivan MJ. Pediatric pleomorphic xanthoastrocytoma treated with surgical resection alone: clinicopathologic features. J Pediatr Hematol Oncol. 2016; 38(7):e202–e206

[41] Ida CM, Rodriguez FJ, Burger PC, et al. Pleomorphic xanthoastrocytoma: natural history and long-term follow-up. Brain Pathol. 2015; 25(5):575–586

[42] Johnston DL, Keene DL, Lafay-Cousin L, et al. Supratentorial primitive neuroectodermal tumors: a Canadian pediatric brain tumor consortium report. J Neurooncol. 2008; 86(1): 101–108

[43] Gaffney CC, Sloane JP, Bradley NJ, Bloom HJ. Primitive neuroectodermal tumours of the cerebrum. Pathology and treatment. J Neurooncol. 1985; 3(1):23–33

[44] Terterov S, Krieger MD, Bowen I, McComb JG. Evaluation of intracranial cerebrospinal fluid cytology in staging pediatric medulloblastomas, supratentorial primitive neuroectodermal tumors, and ependymomas. J Neurosurg Pediatr. 2010; 6(2): 131–136

[45] Miller S, Rogers HA, Lyon P, et al. Genome-wide molecular characterization of central nervous system primitive neuroectodermal tumor and pineoblastoma. Neuro-oncol. 2011; 13(8):866–879

[46] Jimenez RB, Sethi R, Depauw N, et al. Proton radiation therapy for pediatric medulloblastoma and supratentorial primitive neuroectodermal tumors: outcomes for very young children treated with upfront chemotherapy. Int J Radiat Oncol Biol Phys. 2013; 87(1):120–126

[47] Geyer JR, Zeltzer PM, Boyett JM, et al. Survival of infants with primitive neuroectodermal tumors or malignant ependymomas of the CNS treated with eight drugs in 1 day: a report from the Childrens Cancer Group. J Clin Oncol. 1994; 12(8):1607–1615

[48] Dirks PB, Harris L, Hoffman HJ, Humphreys RP, Drake JM, Rutka JT. Supratentorial primitive neuroectodermal tumors in children. J Neurooncol. 1996; 29(1):75–84

[49] Reddy AT, Janss AJ, Phillips PC, Weiss HL, Packer RJ. Outcome for children with supratentorial primitive neuroectodermal tumors treated with surgery, radiation, and chemotherapy. Cancer. 2000; 88(9):2189–2193

[50] Buscariollo DL, Park HS, Roberts KB, Yu JB. Survival outcomes in atypical teratoid rhabdoid tumor for patients undergoing radiotherapy in a Surveillance, Epidemiology, and End Results analysis. Cancer. 2012; 118(17):4212–4219

[51] Lafay-Cousin L, Hawkins C, Carret AS, et al. Central nervous system atypical teratoid rhabdoid tumours: the Canadian Paediatric Brain Tumour Consortium experience. Eur J Cancer. 2012; 48(3):353–359

[52] Au Yong KJ, Jaremko JL, Jans L, et al. How specific is the MRI appearance of supratentorial atypical teratoid rhabdoid tumors? Pediatr Radiol. 2013; 43(3):347–354

[53] Warmuth-Metz M, Bison B, Dannemann-Stern E, Kortmann R, Rutkowski S, Pietsch T. CT and MR imaging in atypical teratoid/rhabdoid tumors of the central nervous system. Neuroradiology. 2008; 50(5):447–452

[54] Bruggers CS, Moore K. Magnetic resonance imaging spectroscopy in pediatric atypical teratoid rhabdoid tumors of the brain. J Pediatr Hematol Oncol. 2014; 36(6):e341–e345

[55] De Padua M, Reddy V, Reddy M. Cerebral atypical teratoid rhabdoid tumour arising in a child treated for acute lymphoblastic leukaemia. BMJ Case Rep. 2009; 2009

[56] Biegel JA. Molecular genetics of atypical teratoid/rhabdoid tumor. Neurosurg Focus. 2006; 20(1):E11

[57] Tekautz TM, Fuller CE, Blaney S, et al. Atypical teratoid/rhabdoid tumors (ATRT): improved survival in children 3 years of age and older with radiation therapy and high-dose alkylator-based chemotherapy. J Clin Oncol. 2005; 23(7):1491–1499

[58] von Hoff K, Hinkes B, Dannenmann-Stern E, et al. Frequency, risk-factors and survival of children with atypical teratoid rhabdoid tumors (AT/RT) of the CNS diagnosed between 1988 and 2004, and registered to the German HIT database. Pediatr Blood Cancer. 2011; 57(6):978–985

[59] Athale UH, Duckworth J, Odame I, Barr R. Childhood atypical teratoid rhabdoid tumor of the central nervous system: a meta-analysis of observational studies. J Pediatr Hematol Oncol. 2009; 31(9):651–663

[60] De Amorim Bernstein K, Sethi R, Trofimov A, et al. Early clinical outcomes using proton radiation for children with central nervous system atypical teratoid rhabdoid tumors. Int J Radiat Oncol Biol Phys. 2013; 86(1):114–120

[61] Dufour C, Beaugrand A, Le Deley MC, et al. Clinicopathologic prognostic factors in childhood atypical teratoid and rhabdoid tumor of the central nervous system: a multicenter study. Cancer. 2012; 118(15):3812–3821

[62] Ingold B, Moschopulos M, Hutter G, et al. Abdominal seeding of an atypical teratoid/rhabdoid tumor of the pineal gland along a ventriculoperitoneal shunt catheter. Acta Neuropathol. 2006; 111(1):56–59

[63] Han YP, Zhao Y, He XG, Ma J. Peritoneal metastasis of third ventricular atypical teratoid/rhabdoid tumor after VP shunt implantation for unexplained hydrocephalus. World J Pediatr. 2012; 8(4):367–370

[64] Hasan A, Palumbo M, Atkinson J, et al. Treatment-related morbidity in atypical teratoid/rhabdoid tumor: multifocal necrotizing leukoencephalopathy. Pediatr Neurosurg. 2011; 47(1):7–14

[65] Rivera B, Gayden T, Carrot-Zhang J, et al. Germline and somatic FGFR1 abnormalities in dysembryoplastic neuroepithelial tumors. Acta Neuropathol. 2016; 131(6):847–863

[66] Ranger A, Diosy D. Seizures in children with dysembryoplastic neuroepithelial tumors of the brain–a review of surgical outcomes across several studies. Childs Nerv Syst. 2015; 31(6):847–855

[67] Prayson RA. Tumours arising in the setting of paediatric chronic epilepsy. Pathology. 2010; 42(5):426–431

[68] Becker AJ, Löbach M, Klein H, et al. Mutational analysis of TSC1 and TSC2 genes in gangliogliomas. Neuropathol Appl Neurobiol. 2001; 27(2):105–114

[69] Rades D, Zwick L, Leppert J, et al. The role of postoperative radiotherapy for the treatment of gangliogliomas. Cancer. 2010; 116(2):432–442

[70] El Khashab M, Gargan L, Margraf L, et al. Predictors of tumor progression among children with gangliogliomas. Clinical article. J Neurosurg Pediatr. 2009; 3(6):461–466

[71] Compton JJ, Laack NN, Eckel LJ, Schomas DA, Giannini C, Meyer FB. Long-term outcomes for low-grade intracranial ganglioglioma: 30-year experience from the Mayo Clinic. J Neurosurg. 2012; 117(5):825–830

[72] Cage TA, Clark AJ, Aranda D, et al. A systematic review of treatment outcomes in pediatric patients with intracranial ependymomas. J Neurosurg Pediatr. 2013; 11(6):673–681

[73] Vinchon M, Soto-Ares G, Riffaud L, Ruchoux MM, Dhellemmes P. Supratentorial ependymoma in children. Pediatr Neurosurg. 2001; 34(2):77–87

[74] Pajtler KW, Witt H, Sill M, et al. Molecular classification of ependymal tumors across all CNS compartments, histopathological grades, and age groups. Cancer Cell. 2015; 27(5):728–743

[75] Bouffet E, Perilongo G, Canete A, Massimino M. Intracranial ependymomas in children: a critical review of prognostic factors and a plea for cooperation. Med Pediatr Oncol. 1998; 30(6):319–329, discussion 329–331

[76] Macdonald SM, Sethi R, Lavally B, et al. Proton radiotherapy for pediatric central nervous system ependymoma: clinical outcomes for 70 patients. Neuro-oncol. 2013; 15(11):1552–1559

[77] Merchant TE, Li C, Xiong X, Kun LE, Boop FA, Sanford RA. Conformal radiotherapy after surgery for paediatric ependymoma: a prospective study. Lancet Oncol. 2009; 10(3):258–266

[78] Landau E, Boop FA, Conklin HM, Wu S, Xiong X, Merchant TE. Supratentorial ependymoma: disease control, complications, and functional outcomes after irradiation. Int J Radiat Oncol Biol Phys. 2013; 85(4):e193–e199

[79] Tanaka T, Kato N, Hasegawa Y, Nonaka Y, Abe T. Long-term survival following gross total resection of pediatric supratentorial ependymomas without adjuvant therapy. Pediatr Neurosurg. 2012; 48(6):379–384

[80] Robertson PL, Zeltzer PM, Boyett JM, et al. Survival and prognostic factors following radiation therapy and chemotherapy for ependymomas in children: a report of the Children's Cancer Group. J Neurosurg. 1998; 88(4):695–703

[81] Sadetzki S, Flint-Richter P, Ben-Tal T, Nass D. Radiation-induced meningioma: a descriptive study of 253 cases. J Neurosurg. 2002; 97(5):1078–1082

[82] Erdinçler P, Lena G, Sarioğlu AC, Kuday C, Choux M. Intracranial meningiomas in children: review of 29 cases. Surg Neurol. 1998; 49(2):136–140, discussion 140–141

[83] Perry A, Dehner LP. Meningeal tumors of childhood and infancy. An update and literature review. Brain Pathol. 2003; 13(3):386–408

[84] Evans DG. Neurofibromatosis type 2 (NF2): a clinical and molecular review. Orphanet J Rare Dis. 2009; 4:16

[85] Perry A, Giannini C, Raghavan R, et al. Aggressive phenotypic and genotypic features in pediatric and NF2-associated meningiomas: a clinicopathologic study of 53 cases. J Neuropathol Exp Neurol. 2001; 60(10):994–1003

[86] Doxtader EE, Butts SC, Holsapple JW, Fuller CE. Aggressive pediatric meningioma with soft tissue and lymph node metastases: a case report. Pediatr Dev Pathol. 2009; 12(3): 244–248

[87] Thuijs NB, Uitdehaag BM, Van Ouwerkerk WJ, van der Valk P, Vandertop WP, Peerdeman SM. Pediatric meningiomas in the Netherlands 1974–2010: a descriptive epidemiological case study. Childs Nerv Syst. 2012; 28(7):1009–1015

[88] Di Rocco C, Di Rienzo A. Meningiomas in childhood. Crit Rev Neurosurg. 1999; 9(3):180–188

15 Hypothalamic and Optic Pathway Tumors

Rajiv R. Iyer, Nir Shimony, George I. Jallo

15.1 Introduction/ Epidemiology

Optic pathway and hypothalamic gliomas (OP-HGs) are rare, representing about 5% of all central nervous system tumors in children. Many OP-HGs arise within the first 5 years of life, with no gender predilection and an incidence of approximately 1/100,000. OP-HGs represent a group of tumors with variable location along the visual pathways, including optic nerve lesions isolated to the orbit, chiasmatic tumors, optic tract lesions, those that extend laterally into the hypothalamus or superiorly into the suprasellar space, and those that extend beyond the thalamus posteriorly into the optic radiations. Given the spectrum of anatomic locations within which this disorder occurs, it is not surprising that the clinical manifestations are variable and that the natural history is not well understood. Nonetheless, given the histopathological similarity and overall indolent biological nature of these tumors, they are considered together as a disease process.

The majority of OP-HGs are low-grade gliomas and are most frequently pilocytic astrocytomas. Fibrillary astrocytomas can also be found, while pilomyxoid astrocytomas, gangliogliomas, and meningiomas are more unusual in these locations, but should be considered on the differential diagnosis.

A well-known association exists between OP-HGs and neurofibromatosis type 1 (NF1), a predominantly inherited, autosomal dominant disorder caused by mutation of the *NF1* gene on the long arm of chromosome 17. Along the same lines, the presence of an optic pathway tumor is part of the clinical diagnostic criteria for the NF1 syndrome. The presence of bilateral OP-HGs is a nearly exclusive feature of patients with NF1. Incidences of OP-HGs in patients with NF1 vary widely and have been reported to be between 4 and 20%, although only half of these patients exhibit symptoms. Patients found to have OP-HGs share features of NF1 upward of 30% of the time. In NF1 patients, OP-HGs most frequently arise within the first decade of life. In contrast to sporadically occurring OP-HGs, these tumors are more likely to be clinically silent, and are serially monitored over time without intervention. This is especially true for children with tumors arising from the prechiasmatic optic apparatus. While there is no official consensus on the frequency with which NF1 patients should be monitored for the presence of OP-HGs, the general recommendation is that these children should undergo annual ophthalmologic evaluation, especially during the first 5 to 7 years of life. Although the incidence of development of a symptomatic OP-HG is higher earlier in life, children are frequently monitored until adolescence and even into adulthood. If a suspected change in visual status is discovered, repeat diagnostic imaging, typically with magnetic resonance imaging (MRI), can be pursued.

15.2 Clinical Presentation

Although many times patients with OP-HGs are asymptomatic, given the anatomic variability of these tumors and the critical elements they encompass and surround, clinical symptoms may occur and presentation is heterogeneous. With OP-HGs, lesion size and location does not always predict symptomatology. Typical clinical manifestations arise in the form of visual disturbances, endocrine dysfunction, and—in large, exophytic tumors—obstructive hydrocephalus. Visual abnormalities are most common and can involve diminished acuity, altered visual fields, nystagmus, and proptosis. Unfortunately, poor correlation exists between the pattern of visual loss and imaging characteristics of these lesions using MRI.[1] Ophthalmological evaluation is critical and may demonstrate signs of optic nerve pallor or atrophy, or an afferent pupillary defect. OP-HGs can also affect the hypothalamic–pituitary axis, and endocrine dysfunction is present in approximately 20 to 50% of patients at diagnosis, manifesting in various ways, such as growth hormone deficiency, failure to thrive, precocious puberty, hypopituitarism, metabolic deficits, obesity, and, in severe cases, diencephalic syndrome.[2,3] Other symptoms include headaches that may be related to elevated intracranial pressure and obstructive hydrocephalus, which may ultimately require cerebrospinal fluid (CSF) diversion.

15.3 Diagnostic Imaging

The gold standard diagnostic imaging modality for OP-HG detection and monitoring is MRI. Although computed tomography (CT) imaging has an adjunct role in delineating tumor-associated calcifications and cysts, as well as the ventricular system, serial monitoring of the tumor substance itself preferably utilizes MRI. Imaging typically includes the entire cerebrum as well as focused views of the orbits to evaluate the optic nerves. Frequently, OP-HGs are hypointense or isointense on T1-weighted imaging and hyperintense on T2-weighted imaging. Gadolinium contrast administration will demonstrate a variable enhancement pattern for these tumors. A varying degree of solid and cystic components may also be seen. Generally, OP-HGs isolated to the optic nerves will demonstrate nerve expansion as well as increased nerve tortuosity or optic nerve sheath enlargement (▶ Fig. 15.1). Importantly, the finding of nerve sheath enlargement in and of itself may be present in other conditions in which elevated intracranial pressure is present. Tumors extending posteriorly into the optic chiasm may also demonstrate enlargement of this structure (▶ Fig. 15.1). Expansion of these neural structures is demonstrative of the diffuse properties of OP-HGs; however, in some cases, significant exophytic components may extend into the suprasellar space, causing obstructive hydrocephalus due to third ventricular compression (▶ Fig. 15.2). In addition to bulky exophytic lesions, tumor-associated cysts can cause a similar obstructive process, necessitating cyst drainage and aspiration in some cases. In some instances, especially during presurgical planning stages, vascular imaging with MR or CT

angiography can be helpful in demarcating critical vascular structures that may be encompassed by tumor.

Various classification systems have been used to describe optic pathway tumors. Although these categorization schemes may be useful for research purposes, they play less of a role in the clinical management and prognostication of OP-HGs. For example, the Dodge classification system (▶ Fig. 15.3) differentiates tumors between three categories based on anatomic location, whether there is involvement of the optic nerve (Dodge I), optic chiasm (Dodge II), or postchiasmatic (Dodge III). More detailed anatomical classification systems, such as the modified Dodge system, are also available.

15.4 Treatment

Unfortunately, given the lack of a well-defined natural history of OP-HGs and the heterogeneity present within this disease process, treatment options must be tailored to each individual patient based on age, comorbidities, presentation, duration of symptoms, anatomy, and other factors. In most cases, asymptomatic or incidentally discovered lesions are serially monitored over time. However, in cases with progressive symptomatology and lesion growth, surgery, chemotherapy, radiation therapy (RT), or a combination of these interventions should be considered. In the majority of cases, treating physicians are part of a

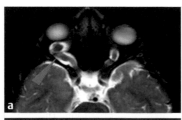
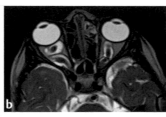
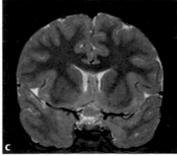

Fig. 15.1 Optic pathway tumor in a patient with neurofibromatosis type 1 (NF1). (a,b) Axial T2-weighted magnetic resonance (MR) imaging demonstrating right optic nerve enlargement (*arrowhead*), increased nerve tortuosity, and a dilated right optic nerve sheath, consistent with an optic pathway glioma. (c) Coronal T2-weighted MR image demonstrating expansion of the optic chiasm (*arrowhead*), indicative of tumor extension into this structure.

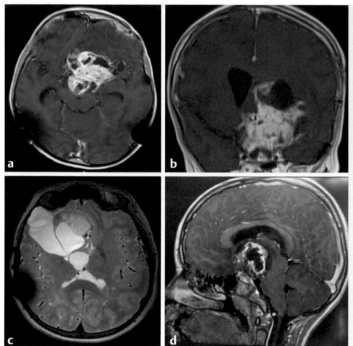

Fig. 15.2 Suprasellar extension of optic pathway tumor. **(a)** Axial and **(b)** coronal T1-weighted with contrast MR images demonstrating lobulated, cystic suprasellar extension of an optic pathway tumor. **(c)** Axial T2-weighted MR image demonstrating loculated cystic components of an optic pathway tumor causing mass effect in a child with NF1. **(d)** Sagittal T1-weighted MR with contrast demonstrating suprasellar extension of optic pathway tumor causing third ventricular effacement and obstruction.

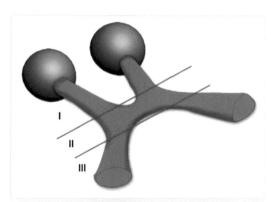

Fig. 15.3 Dodge classification system. Illustration depicting optic pathways and classification zones based on the region of tumor expansion. (Reproduced with permission from Thieme eNeurosurgery, 2016.)

multidisciplinary group that includes neurosurgeons, neuro-ophthalmologists, oncologists, endocrinologists, and others.

15.4.1 Surgery

Compared to other neurosurgical diseases, the role of surgery for OP-HGs is limited. For example, even diagnostic biopsy is unnecessary when a classically appearing lesion isolated to the optic nerve is identified in a patient with NF1. In many such cases, chemotherapy may be initiated in symptomatic patients without a tissue diagnosis. Especially relevant to the limited surgical role in this disease are the critical surrounding structures of these lesions. Given the critical structures surrounding such tumors and the neural structures within which they arise, the risks of surgical intervention must be weighed strongly against alternate treatment modalities or, simply, serial monitoring.

As mentioned, identification of a classically appearing OP-HG radiographically may not necessitate tissue diagnosis with surgical biopsy. Certain features, however, such as rapid tumor growth or symptom progression, or worsening hydrocephalus, may warrant surgical intervention. The benefits of surgical debulking include facilitation of chemotherapeutic intervention as well as relief of obstructive hydrocephalus. Given the indolent nature of OP-HGs, emergent intervention is rarely necessary. In some instances, urgent CSF diversion is needed to treat obstructive hydrocephalus, or malfunction of already shunted patients may warrant immediate intervention. Other indications for surgery include the need for a diagnosis, especially in those with atypical imaging features or in older children with rapid neurological decline. A tailored, individualized treatment approach should be created for each patient. Growing, exophytic lesions are more easily debulked than diffuse, expansile lesions of the optic pathways. In children with growing tumors isolated to an orbit in which there is no preserved vision, surgical intervention can prevent tumor invasion of the optic chiasm, which could prevent deterioration of vision in the contralateral, functional eye. This treatment plan may be especially relevant in patients who have already failed a trial of chemotherapy who also demonstrate evidence of tumor progression toward the chiasm. In a child with severely affected vision and an optic nerve tumor causing pain or proptosis, surgical treatment may aid in alleviating disfiguration and pain.

Surgical approaches include a standard pterional craniotomy in order to obtain access to the anterior skull base and orbital roof, with or without use of an orbital unroofing procedure. The optic nerve is removed close to but not directly at the chiasm so as to not injure crossing fibers from the contralateral eye. Alternative or ancillary approaches include an orbital approach alone, which may be warranted when the goal of surgery is enucleation. As many tumors are infiltrative and expansile within normal neural structures, gross total resection can pose a threat to remaining visual function and thus is not frequently the surgical goal. For example, cytoreductive debulking can alleviate CSF obstruction and restore ventricular flow. Lesions of the suprasellar space can also be reached through a frontotemporal craniotomy using a subfrontal or transsylvian approach, as well as transcortical, transventricular, or interhemispheric approaches.

15.4.2 Chemotherapy

The current mainstay of treatment for OP-HGs is with chemotherapy. Given the potential morbidity of surgical intervention and the unlikelihood of achieving total tumor extirpation without causing visual harm or other adverse events, as well as the unwanted risks of RT in the developing child, the primary modality for intervention is with chemotherapy.

Several studies have evaluated the role of chemotherapy in children with low-grade tumors and OP-HGs. Packer and colleagues determined that a combination of vincristine and carboplatin resulted in a progression-free survival (PFS) of around 75% at 2-year follow-up in children with low-grade gliomas.[4] Other studies evaluating platinum-based therapy demonstrated good response

rates to this treatment, with toxicity occurring in the form of transient neutropenia and thrombocytopenia, as well as rare allergic reactions.[5,6] Other regimens include weekly vinblastine treatment for low-grade pediatric gliomas, with close to 95% 5-year overall survival (OS) and 53% PFS, with treatment being well tolerated and demonstrating increased PFS in NF1 patients compared to non-NF1 patients.[7,8] Such treatments may be especially useful as second-line therapy after prior chemotherapeutic agents have been attempted.

Other studies have also compared the effectiveness of carboplatin and vincristine to a combination of thioguanine, procarbazine, lomustine, and vincristine (TPCV) in pediatric low-grade gliomas, demonstrating an OS between the groups of 86% and similar event-free survival (EFS), but with a trend toward improved EFS in the TPCV group.[9] While the majority of chemotherapeutic interventions have only a modest, if any, effect on visual outcomes, recent evidence has suggested that bevacizumab therapy may result in a more robust response in improved visual outcomes in patients with OP-HGs.[10] Examples of targeted therapy, such as BRAF inhibitors, have demonstrated some efficacy in children with low-grade gliomas, and their utility in children with OP-HGs remains to be evaluated.

15.4.3 Radiation Therapy

As we have entered the chemotherapy era of treatment for OP-HGs, the role of RT has been limited. In fact, typical treatment models would attempt various forms of chemotherapy prior to the initiation of RT in an attempt to delay its potential adverse effects. For example, optic neuritis, vasculopathy, neurocognitive delay, and endocrine and hypothalamic disturbances are all risks associated with RT, especially in young, developing children. Additionally, the possibility of secondary neoplasia exists with RT, especially in NF1 patients.[11]

In the prechemotherapy era, RT was utilized more frequently as an adjunct treatment for nonresectable OP-HGs. Reported 10-year OS and PFS vary, from 80 to 94% and 65 to 100%, respectively.[12,13,14] Tumor response rates varied, but a modest probability of radiographic response (25–50%) has been shown in the first 24 to 60 months following RT. Although radiographic response and some improvement in vision was demonstrated in these studies, long-term sequelae of RT included significant endocrine and neurological abnormalities. Overall, current treatment algorithms would categorize RT as a last resort option in children with OP-HGs, after surgical and chemotherapeutic intervention were first attempted.

15.5 Summary

Regardless of the need for intervention, overall outcomes for children with OP-HGs are favorable. Higher-grade lesions arising from the optic nerves and pathways are extremely unusual in the pediatric population and, when encountered, rapid symptom onset and progression to death occur. Given the variability of OP-HGs of low grade, the natural history lacks concrete definition and thresholds for treatment vary from institution to institution. Treatment is often initiated when there is tumor growth and progression of visual symptoms. Those with NF1 tend to demonstrate improved outcomes in comparison to their non-NF1 counterparts. OS for OP-HGs is greater than 90%, and surgery is often well tolerated when a judicious approach is taken so as to not harm normal neural structures.

Overall, OP-HGs represent a heterogeneous population of tumors occurring in both NF1 and non-NF1 patients that require a patient-centric, individualized management approach. A multidisciplinary team should serially evaluate patients clinically and radiographically in order to maximize neurological function, while minimizing adverse effects of intervention.

References

[1] Aquilina K, Daniels DJ, Spoudeas H, Phipps K, Gan HW, Boop FA. Optic pathway glioma in children: does visual deficit correlate with radiology in focal exophytic lesions? Childs Nerv Syst. 2015; 31(11):2041–2049

[2] El Beltagy MA, Reda M, Enayet A, et al. Treatment and outcome in 65 children with optic pathway gliomas. World Neurosurg. 2016; 89:525–534

[3] Gan HW, Phipps K, Aquilina K, Gaze MN, Hayward R, Spoudeas HA. Neuroendocrine morbidity after pediatric optic gliomas: a longitudinal analysis of 166 children over 30 years. J Clin Endocrinol Metab. 2015; 100(10):3787–3799

[4] Packer RJ, Ater J, Allen J, et al. Carboplatin and vincristine chemotherapy for children with newly diagnosed progressive low-grade gliomas. J Neurosurg. 1997; 86(5):747–754

[5] Listernick R, Charrow J, Tomita T, Goldman S. Carboplatin therapy for optic pathway tumors in children with neurofibromatosis type-1. J Neurooncol. 1999; 45(2):185–190

[6] Mahoney DH, Jr, Cohen ME, Friedman HS, et al. Carboplatin is effective therapy for young children with progressive optic pathway tumors: a Pediatric Oncology Group phase II study. Neuro-oncol. 2000; 2(4):213–220

[7] Bouffet E, Jakacki R, Goldman S, et al. Phase II study of weekly vinblastine in recurrent or refractory pediatric low-grade glioma. J Clin Oncol. 2012; 30(12):1358–1363

[8] Lassaletta A, Scheinemann K, Zelcer SM, et al. Phase II weekly vinblastine for chemotherapy-naïve children with progressive low-grade glioma: A Canadian Pediatric Brain Tumor Consortium Study. J Clin Oncol. 2016; 34(29):3537–3543

[9] Ater JL, Zhou T, Holmes E, et al. Randomized study of two chemotherapy regimens for treatment of low-grade glioma in young children: a report from the Children's Oncology Group. J Clin Oncol. 2012; 30(21):2641–2647

[10] Avery RA, Hwang EI, Jakacki RI, Packer RJ. Marked recovery of vision in children with optic pathway gliomas treated with bevacizumab. JAMA Ophthalmol. 2014; 132(1):111–114

[11] Sharif S, Ferner R, Birch JM, et al. Second primary tumors in neurofibromatosis 1 patients treated for optic glioma: substantial risks after radiotherapy. J Clin Oncol. 2006; 24 (16):2570–2575

[12] Cappelli C, Grill J, Raquin M, et al. Long-term follow up of 69 patients treated for optic pathway tumours before the chemotherapy era. Arch Dis Child. 1998; 79(4):334–338

[13] Grabenbauer GG, Schuchardt U, Buchfelder M, et al. Radiation therapy of optico-hypothalamic gliomas (OHG)–radiographic response, vision and late toxicity. Radiother Oncol. 2000; 54(3):239–245

[14] Tao ML, Barnes PD, Billett AL, et al. Childhood optic chiasm gliomas: radiographic response following radiotherapy and long-term clinical outcome. Int J Radiat Oncol Biol Phys. 1997; 39(3):579–587

16 Craniopharyngiomas and Other Sellar Tumors

David S. Hersh, Rafael U. Cardenas, Nir Shimony, and Mari L. Groves

16.1 Introduction

Primary tumors of the sellar and parasellar region constitute 10% of all primary brain tumors in children.[1,2] Craniopharyngiomas are the most common tumor found in this region, constituting 90% of pediatric sellar and parasellar tumors. The remaining 10% are comprised mainly of Rathke's cleft cysts and pituitary adenomas, although, rarely, germinomas, hamartomas, lipomas, teratomas, dermoid cysts, and epidermoid cysts may be found as well.[3,4]

16.2 Craniopharyngiomas

- Incidence: 0.5 to 2 cases per million per year.[5]
- Bimodal age distribution, with peaks during the first and second decades of life (typically between the ages of 5 and 14 years) as well as the fifth decade of life.[6,7]
- Approximately 30 to 50% of craniopharyngiomas occur in pediatric patients.
- Craniopharyngiomas comprise up to 5% of pediatric intracranial masses and up to 10% of pediatric brain tumors.[7,8]

16.3 Rathke's Cleft Cysts

- Rathke's cleft cysts are most commonly found as incidental lesions, and are found in 11 to 33% of autopsies.[5,9,10]
- Asymptomatic cystic sellar or parasellar lesions are found in 1.2% of children who undergo magnetic resonance imaging (MRI).[11]
- Rathke's cleft cysts account for only 9 to 10% of sellar lesions that require surgical treatment.[12]

16.4 Pituitary Adenomas

- Incidence: 0.1 cases per million children per year.[6]
- Pituitary adenomas account for approximately 4% of pediatric intracranial tumors.[13]
- Pituitary adenomas are more common in females.
- Macroadenomas occur more commonly than microadenomas.
- Pituitary adenoma subtypes:
  - Prolactinomas occur most frequently (30–50% of pediatric pituitary adenomas), particularly during and after puberty.
  - They are followed by adrenocorticotropic hormone (ACTH)–secreting tumors, which are more common prior to the onset of puberty, and growth hormone (GH)–secreting adenomas, which comprise 10 to 15% of pediatric adenomas and occur most commonly in infants.
  - Only about 5% of pediatric adenomas are nonfunctioning pituitary adenomas (which, in contrast, constitute one-third of adenomas in the adult population).[6,14]

16.5 Embryology and Pathology

Rathke's cleft cysts and craniopharyngiomas have been described as similarly derived lesions that likely represent different ends of the spectrum of pathological progression.[2] Rathke's cleft cysts are nonneoplastic cystic remnants of the Rathke pouch that form in the region of the pars intermedia, and are characterized by columnar or cuboidal epithelial walls surrounding mucoid material. Craniopharyngiomas, too, are nonglial, extra-axial tumors that develop from epithelial remnants of the Rathke pouch or the craniopharyngeal duct. Despite benign histological features, craniopharyngiomas are typically aggressive tumors that produce significant neurological morbidity.[7] Craniopharyngiomas are characterized by two histopathological subtypes: adamantinomatous and papillary (▶ Fig. 16.1).

16.5.1 Adamantinomatous Craniopharyngiomas

- Adamantinomatous tumors are the most common subtype, particularly in the pediatric population.
- These tumors are characterized by keratinized cells that face a cyst lumen, and "wet" keratin nodules consisting of desquamated epithelial cells. The nodules may become calcified over time.
- The cystic regions of adamantinomatous craniopharyngiomas contain fluid with a "motor oil" consistency, rich in cholesterol.

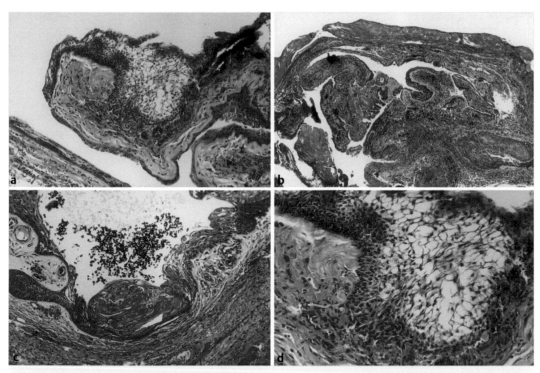

Fig. 16.1 **(a)** Adamantinomatous craniopharyngioma with a highly distinctive pattern of epithelial maturation. **(b)** On low-power view, the tumor consists of both solid and cystic epithelial components associated with chronically inflamed fibrous stroma. **(c)** Another characteristic feature of adamantinomatous craniopharyngioma is the presence of nodules of plump eosinophilic keratinized cells with ghosted nuclei. **(d)** On higher power view, tumor cells abutting the stroma are palisaded, whereas centrally they readily dehisce to create a loose "stellate reticulum." (Reproduced with permission from Couldwell W. Craniopharyngiomas. In: Bernstein M, Berger MS, eds. Neuro-oncology: The Essentials. New York, NY: Thieme; 2015:Fig. 35.1a–d.)

16.6 Papillary Craniopharyngiomas

- Squamous papillary tumors occur primarily in adults, and are rarely found in the pediatric population.
- These tumors are characterized by a solid, papillary architecture with minimal cysts.[4]
- Papillary craniopharyngiomas rarely undergo calcification.

16.7 Clinical Presentation

Pediatric sellar and parasellar tumors present with symptoms that reflect their relationship to critical surrounding structures, including the pituitary gland, infundibulum, hypothalamus, optic pathways, third ventricle, and cerebral vasculature.[15] As a result, symptoms associated with the endocrine, limbic, and visual systems tend to predominate. The anatomical relationship between the tumor and adjacent structures is dictated by the degree of intrasellar and/or suprasellar involvement, which, in turn, determines the clinical presentation.

16.8 Craniopharyngiomas

- Approximately 95% of craniopharyngiomas have a suprasellar component, while 30% also extend into the anterior and middle cranial fossae.[4]
- The most common complaints related to craniopharyngiomas are nonspecific symptoms of intracranial hypertension, particularly headaches and nausea.
- Visual deficits occur in over half of patients, although this tends to be well tolerated in children.

- Over half of patients also have signs and symptoms of endocrine deficiency at the time of presentation.
  - GH is most commonly affected, with low levels found in 75% of patients. Gonadotropins—follicle-stimulating hormone (FSH) and luteinizing hormone (LH)—are deficient in 40% of patients. ACTH- and thyroid-stimulating hormone (TSH) are affected in 25% of patients.[6,16]
  - Possible findings include growth failure, delayed puberty, weight gain, and diabetes insipidus.
- Frontal lobe dysfunction, memory deficits, and obstructive hydrocephalus may occur as well.

16.9 Rathke's Cleft Cysts

- Rathke's cleft cysts are typically intrasellar cysts, although the majority demonstrate suprasellar extension as well.[5]
- Many Rathke's cleft cysts are asymptomatic and present as "incidentalomas"—lesions that are identified during imaging that is performed for unrelated reasons.
- Symptomatic Rathke's cleft cysts typically present with headaches, visual loss, and/or endocrine insufficiency due to mass effect.[17]
- In the pediatric population, Rathke's cleft cysts may also present with a variety of endocrine signs and symptoms including delayed or precocious puberty, amenorrhea, galactorrhea, hypogonadism, growth retardation, and weight gain.[18]

16.10 Pituitary Adenomas

- Pituitary adenomas are predominantly intrasellar, and typically present with endocrine symptoms.
- The particular presentation depends on the adenoma subtype.
- Prolactinomas:
  - In females, prolactinomas commonly present with primary or secondary amenorrhea (depending on the age of presentation), with or without galactorrhea.[6]
  - In males, macroadenomas occur more frequently, resulting in headaches and visual deficits.
  - Growth arrest may occur in children and adolescents regardless of gender.[19]

- ACTH-secreting adenomas:
  - Growth failure is commonly the initial presenting symptom, often resulting in a delayed diagnosis.[6]
  - Other features of Cushing's disease subsequently appear, including facial plethora, striae of the abdomen and extremities, osteoporosis, and impaired carbohydrate tolerance. Muscular weakness, hypertension, acne, hair growth, precocious puberty, or, alternatively, pubertal delay may be seen as well.[6]
- GH-secreting adenomas:
  - Although GH-secreting adenomas typically present with acromegaly (due to hyperostosis) in adults, pediatric patients may present with gigantism due to delayed epiphyseal closure.[6]

16.11 Examination and Diagnostic Workup

Patients with sellar or parasellar masses should undergo a thorough evaluation prior to surgical intervention. Neuroimaging, formal ophthalmological studies, and a complete endocrine workup are integral for medical and operative decision-making, as well as to serve as a baseline for postoperative evaluations. In patients with suprasellar and/or frontal lobe involvement, a preoperative neuropsychiatric evaluation should be considered, as well.

16.12 Neuroimaging

- Patients should undergo a head computed tomography (CT) without contrast to assess for calcification within the mass. Thin slices through the sinuses and skull base may be indicated for surgical planning if a transsphenoidal approach is planned (▶ Fig. 16.2).
- A magnetic resonance imaging (MRI) of the brain with and without gadolinium is useful for both diagnostic purposes and assessing the relationship of the mass to its surrounding structures. Dedicated pituitary protocols focus on the sellar and parasellar regions and are helpful in providing enhanced detail (▶ Fig. 16.3).
- Vascular imaging (either CT angiography or MR angiography) is particularly helpful in cases of craniopharyngiomas in order to map their relationship with the adjacent circle of Willis.

- Imaging pearls and pitfalls:
  - During the first 6 to 8 weeks of life, the adenohypophysis is globular and hyperintense on T1-weighted imaging. It is only subsequently that it flattens and becomes isointense, while the neurohypophysis remains hyperintense on T1-weighted imaging.[4]
  - Physiological pituitary hyperplasia may occur, particularly in pubertal females. During puberty, the pituitary gland may reach 10 mm in height.[4] This should not be mistaken for a pituitary adenoma.
  - In contrast to craniopharyngiomas and pituitary adenomas, Rathke's cleft cysts typically do not demonstrate enhancement. However, *pseudoenhancement* may occur secondary to the normal enhancement of the pituitary gland when the gland is stretched around the cyst.[4,18]

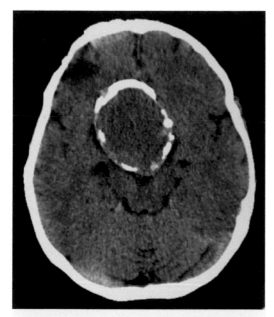

Fig. 16.2 Imaging of a 48-year-old patient who had a subtotal resection of a craniopharyngioma at age 5 and 43 years later experienced increasing headaches and decline in vision. Computed tomography demonstrated a suprasellar lesion with a calcified rim. (Reproduced with permission from Couldwell W. Craniopharyngiomas. In: Bernstein M, Berger MS, eds. Neuro-oncology: The Essentials. New York, NY: Thieme; 2015:Fig. 35.2.)

16.13 Ophthalmological Evaluation

- A full ophthalmological examination, including formal visual field testing, should be performed.
- While younger children may not complain of gradually progressive visual deficits, subtle findings are often found on examination.

16.14 Endocrine Workup

- Laboratory studies should include a full endocrine panel, including serum prolactin, TSH, free thyroxine (T4), ACTH, morning fasting cortisol, GH, insulinlike growth factor-1, FSH/LH in females, and free testosterone in males. A basic metabolic panel, serum osmolarity, and

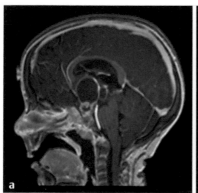
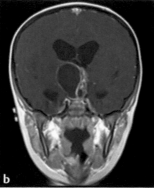
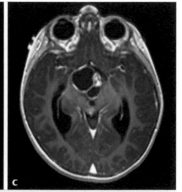

Fig. 16.3 T1 gadolinium-enhanced MRI shows a cystic craniopharyngioma on sagittal (a), coronal (b), and axial (c) imaging.

urine specific gravity should be sent to assess for diabetes insipidus.[20]

- A diluted prolactin level should be obtained due to the hook effect, which produces falsely low levels in undiluted samples.
- If the morning fasting cortisol level is elevated, a dexamethasone suppression test should be performed. In patients with Cushing's syndrome, low-dose dexamethasone administered at midnight does not suppress the serum cortisol concentration the next morning. High-dose dexamethasone administered at midnight suppresses the morning cortisol level by more than 50% in cases of Cushing's disease, but not in patients with ectopic ACTH-secreting masses.
- In patients with cortisol deficiency, an ACTH stimulation test should be performed. Following a baseline, fasting serum cortisol level obtained in the morning, a synthetic form of ACTH—cosyntropin—is administered. Serum cortisol levels are then obtained 30 and 60 minutes later. Cortisol levels rise significantly in patients with secondary adrenal insufficiency (i.e., a sellar mass causing hypopituitarism), but not in patients with primary adrenal insufficiency (i.e., Addison's disease).
- In patients with elevated GH levels, an oral glucose tolerance test may be performed. Failure to suppress GH levels, or alternatively a further increase in GH levels, are associated with GH-secreting pituitary adenomas.[21]

16.15 Classification Systems

- Several functional classification systems have been developed to describe patients with craniopharyngiomas. These classification systems may be applied both pre- and postoperatively.
- One of the simpler systems[22] classifies patients as:
  - Class I: independent, with only mild hormonal deficiencies.
  - Class II: independent, with panhypopituitarism, mild/moderate visual compromise, mild neurological/cranial nerve deficits, and mild psychological dysfunction.
  - Class III: partially dependent, with serious visual compromise, serious deficits, and learning disorders.
  - Class IV: fully dependent.
- A more recent, comprehensive classification system, the Craniopharyngioma Clinical Status

Scale, assigns a score of 1 to 4 (ranging from normal to extremely abnormal) across five domains: neurological status, vision, pituitary function, hypothalamic function, and educational status.[15]

16.16 Nonsurgical Management

- Many Rathke's cleft cysts are "incidentalomas"—asymptomatic lesions found on imaging.
  - Patients with small (less than 10 mm), asymptomatic Rathke's cleft cysts, a normal visual examination, and normal endocrine findings are typically managed nonoperatively. Such patients undergo observation with yearly MRIs and clinical examinations.
  - In some situations, asymptomatic patients with larger lesions (greater than 10 mm) may also undergo close observation, including serial visual field testing.[20]
  - Headache in the absence of visual or endocrine symptoms is typically *not* considered to be an indication for surgical resection.[18]
- Prolactinomas are typically treated medically, with therapy consisting of dopamine agonists.
  - Most prolactinomas respond well to dopamine agonists including bromocriptine and cabergoline—prolactin levels normalize and the tumor shrinks in response to treatment.
  - Cabergoline has a longer half-life than bromocriptine, allowing it to be administered once a week, which is particularly useful in the pediatric population.[23]
  - Patients who cannot tolerate medical therapy, or whose tumors are refractory to medication, are subsequently referred for surgical resection.[6]
- In adults with GH-secreting adenomas, somatostatin analogues such as octreotide and lanreotide have been applied as options for medical therapy. However, surgical resection remains the primary form of treatment, particularly in children, in whom there is little experience with somatostatin analogues.[6,23]

16.17 Surgical Approaches

Sellar and parasellar masses may be accessed via a craniotomy, a transsphenoidal approach, or both. Traditionally, the transsphenoidal approach has been utilized for intrasellar lesions, while a craniotomy is reserved for suprasellar masses. As a result, Rathke's cleft cysts and pituitary adenomas are typically approached via the transsphenoidal route. Conversely, the majority of craniopharyngiomas arise from the tuber cinereum in the suprasellar region, and are therefore approached via a craniotomy. However, up to 30% of pediatric craniopharyngiomas have a sellar component, and as many as 15% have an infradiaphragmatic intrasellar origin (suggested by sellar expansion on preoperative imaging), with the diaphragma sellae serving as a barrier that separates the tumor from the overlying suprasellar structures including the optic chiasm, hypothalamus, and circle of Willis. Infradiaphragmatic craniopharyngiomas are therefore suitable for transsphenoidal resection.[23,24] In contrast, supradiaphragmatic masses, or those that cross the diaphragma, are adherent to the adjacent neurological structures, which increases the risks associated with placing traction on the tumor from below.[12] However, extended transsphenoidal approaches, such as those that involve removal of the tuberculum sellae, are being adopted in order to access suprasellar locations, as well.[3]

- The transsphenoidal route may be reached via a sublabial or endonasal approach.
  - The sublabial approach is associated with increased patient discomfort, including upper lip and incisor paresthesias.[3]
  - The endonasal approach is gaining broader acceptance, despite initial hesitation due to the small nostril and nasal cavity size of pediatric patients.
- Transsphenoidal surgery may be accomplished with the operative microscope, an endoscope, or both.
  - The microscope offers the advantage of depth perception by providing the surgeon with a stereoscopic three-dimensional field.[3]
  - The endoscope, on the other hand, provides a wider field of view. Angled endoscopes also allow the closer examination of difficult angles.[3,23] Newer three-dimensional endoscopes offer improvements in depth perception, as well.
- The transsphenoidal approach has a number of advantages, including:
  - Minimal brain retraction.
  - Early decompression of the optic apparatus while avoiding manipulation of the optic nerves and chiasm.
  - Less tissue trauma, less postoperative pain, and shorter hospital stays.

- Prior to performing a transsphenoidal resection in a pediatric patient, the degree of pneumatization of the sphenoid sinus should be assessed.[12]
- Craniopharyngiomas treated via the transsphenoidal approach tend to be smaller than those resected via a craniotomy.[12]
- Significant suprasellar calcification and tumor extension lateral to the carotid arteries have been suggested as relative contraindications to the transsphenoidal approach. When the goal of surgery is gross total resection, adhesivity to the adjacent structures and an increased risk of vascular injury are challenging to manage through the limited field of view afforded by the transsphenoidal route.[12] However, micro-Doppler probes offer some degree of protection against vascular injury.
- The transsphenoidal approach is associated with a higher risk of cerebrospinal fluid (CSF) leak and meningitis postoperatively. However, the rate of CSF leak has gradually decreased with the development of reconstructive skull base techniques including but not limited to multilayered closures and pedicled flaps (both pericranial and nasoseptal).[12]

16.18 Surgical Technique

16.18.1 Transsphenoidal Approach (▶ Fig. 16.4)[3,12,20,23,24,25]

- Setup and equipment:
  - A right-sided approach is used for right-handed surgeons and/or for lesions that are to the left of the midline.
  - If an endoscope is used, a table-mounted pneumatic arm may be used to hold the scope.
  - Either fluoroscopy or neuronavigation, or both, may be used in order to assist in identifying the sphenoid ostia and guiding the surgical trajectory.
  - Micro-Doppler probes may be used in order to identify the carotid arteries, in order to minimize the risk of vascular injury.
  - A lumbar drain may or may not be placed preoperatively, depending on surgeon preference. If used, the drain is generally removed at the end of the case if a CSF leak is not encountered.
- The nasal cavities are prepped with Betadine.
- An area of the abdomen is prepared in the event a fat graft is needed.

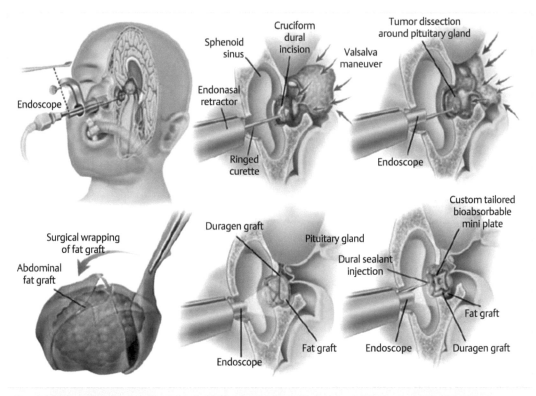

Fig. 16.4 Schematics of an endonasal transsphenoidal resection of a pituitary adenoma in a pediatric patient. (Reproduced with permission from Chaichana KL, Jusue-Torres I, Jallo GI. Tumors of the skull base and orbit. In: Cohen AR, ed. Pediatric Neurosurgery. New York, NY: Thieme; 2016.)

- Oxymetazoline (Afrin)-soaked cotton pledgets are placed in the nares bilaterally for 5 to 10 minutes.
- Using a handheld pediatric intranasal speculum and a #2 Penfield, the middle turbinate may be mobilized laterally. Some surgeons prefer to resect the middle turbinate for additional exposure.
  - A more aggressive "two-nostrils-four-hands" technique involves bilateral maxillary antrostomy, bilateral total sphenoethmoidectomy, a posterior partial septectomy, and a right partial middle turbinate resection for maximal exposure when the pathology is suprasellar.[25]
- The sphenoid ostia are identified and using the #2 Penfield, Kerrison punches, and pituitary rongeurs, the anterior wall of the sphenoid sinus is opened.
- A pneumatic drill with a 3-mm diamond drill bit is used to remove the anterior wall of the sellae.

- A significant amount of drilling may be required in patients with incompletely pneumatized sphenoid sinuses.
- An irrigating drill may be used to reduce the risk of thermal injury to the adjacent structures.
- Extended transsphenoidal approaches are necessary to reach suprasellar and parasellar pathology.
  - Transtuberculum and/or transplanum approach for suprasellar lesions.
  - Transclival approach for retrosellar lesions.
- The dura is opened with an 11-blade scalpel, and ringed curettes are used for tumor removal. Bipolar coagulation and sharp dissection have been described for the resection of craniopharyngiomas, as well.
  - A Valsalva maneuver may be used to force suprasellar portions of the tumor into the sella and into the field of view.
  - For Rathke's cleft cysts, cyst drainage and biopsy of the cyst wall is recommended, given

the comparable recurrence rate and lower morbidity compared to complete resection of the cyst wall.[5,9] Biopsy of the anterior cyst wall should be performed before substantial drainage has taken place. Large dural openings may promote continued drainage and reduce the recurrence rate of Rathke's cleft cysts.

- Reconstruction of the skull base depends on surgeon preference as well as the degree of suspicion for CSF leak. Options include one or a combination of the following: abdominal fat grafts, dural substitutes, various forms of biodegradable glue, bioabsorbable miniplates, and pedicled flaps.

16.18.2 Transcranial Approach (▶ Fig. 16.5)[23,26,27]

- A pterional exposure is typically reserved for large craniopharyngiomas and is used to access

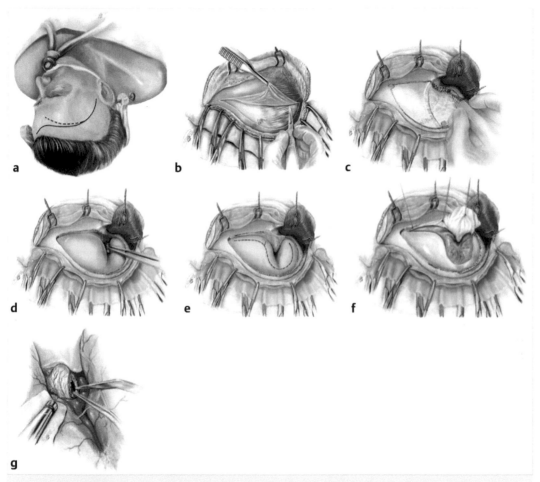

Fig. 16.5 Pterional approach for craniopharyngiomas. **(a)** The head position for the pterional approach. Also seen are the curvilinear incision (*dotted line*) for the classic pterional approach and the bicoronal incision (*solid line*) for the craniotomy with medial extension. **(b)** The skin flap reflected and the pericranial dissection. **(c)** The temporalis muscle cut and reflected. Also seen are burr holes and the craniotomy flap. Note the frontal burr hole placed medially in the frontal region. **(d)** The bone flap elevated, the dura exposed, and the sphenoid wing being removed. **(e)** The dural incision (*dotted line*). Note the wide space achieved at the frontal–temporal junction after drilling the sphenoid wing. **(f)** The dura opened and reflected over the sylvian fissure. **(g)** The transsylvian approach to the craniopharyngioma through the opticocarotid space. Note the visualization of the carotid bifurcation that is achieved after splitting the sylvian fissure. (Reproduced with permission from Yasargil MG. Microneurosurgery. Vol 4B. New York, NY: Thieme; 1994; and Krisht AF, Türe U. Surgical approaches to craniopharyngiomas. In: Behnam B, ed. Neurosurgical Operative Atlas: Neuro-Oncology. New York, NY: Thieme; 2007:Fig. 2-2.)

the suprasellar region with minimal frontal and temporal lobe retraction. This approach allows for early visualization of the carotid arteries and optic chiasm, facilitating the protection of these structures.

- A frontotemporal craniotomy is performed.
  - Removal of the sphenoid wing and/or orbital rim may be used to maximize the exposure.
- The dura is opened. Mannitol, hyperventilation, and release of CSF from the subarachnoid cisterns may be used to facilitate brain relaxation and minimize retraction.
- The sylvian fissure is opened widely and the carotid arteries and optic apparatus are identified.
- An arachnoidal plane is developed between the tumor and the ipsilateral cerebral vasculature.
- Cystic portions of the tumor are then aspirated, and solid components of the tumor are debulked while preserving the tumor capsule.
  - Premature aspiration of the cyst makes further dissection of the arachnoid difficult, and should only be performed once the vascular anatomy has been clearly identified.
- The goal of surgery—debulking versus gross total resection—remains controversial. The following steps may be adapted depending on surgeon preference.
- An arachnoidal plane is developed between the tumor and the optic apparatus as well as the contralateral cerebral vasculature.
- Whenever possible, the pituitary stalk is preserved. When it is adherent to the tumor and the surgical goal is gross total resection, the pituitary stalk may sectioned, given the high rate of diabetes insipidus following radical resection regardless of whether the stalk is intact.
  - The stalk should be sectioned as distally to the hypothalamus as possible in order to prevent traction on the hypothalamus.
- When gross total resection is desired, the tumor is bluntly dissected away from its attachment to the hypothalamus, which is typically located at the tuber cinereum.
- When there is significant extension into the third ventricle or into the retrochiasmatic space, the lamina terminalis may be fenestrated.
- When there is extension of the tumor into the sella, the posterior planum sphenoidale and tuberculum sellae may be removed.
- A micromirror or an angled endoscope may be used to inspect the surgical bed for residual tumor.

16.18.3 Complications

The surgical complications that are encountered depend largely on the precise location of the mass (sellar vs. suprasellar) and whether a transsphenoidal approach or a craniotomy is performed. Injury to the adjacent structures may include hypothalamic damage, pituitary dysfunction, injury to the optic apparatus, and vascular injury. Large, invasive tumors are naturally associated with greater morbidity.[6] Surgical morbidity and patient outcomes are also dependent on surgeon experience.[28]

- Hypothalamic dysfunction is associated with a variety of signs and symptoms that have a major impact on quality of life, including[15]:
  - Hyperphagia and obesity.
  - Memory deficits.
  - Emotional lability.
  - Inability to regulate body temperature.
  - Disturbance of the circadian rhythm.
- Although some degree of hypothalamic dysfunction is found in up to 35% of pediatric patients with craniopharyngiomas, surgical treatment has been associated with higher postoperative rates of hypothalamic dysfunction.
  - Obesity, in particular, increases during the first 6 to 12 months following treatment.[16]
- A grading scale was designed by De Vile et al[29] to predict hypothalamic dysfunction in order to help guide the intended extent of surgical resection. This remains a controversial area.
  - Some surgeons propose incomplete resection followed by radiotherapy in order to minimize acute postoperative morbidity, while others point to the risk of delayed hypopituitarism associated with radiotherapy, therefore arguing for gross total resection at the time of initial presentation.[6]
- Craniopharyngioma resection is associated with high rates of postoperative hypopituitarism and diabetes insipidus in particular. GH deficiency is also commonly found postoperatively, although most patients respond well to exogenous GH. Patients and their families should be counseled about the risk of pituitary dysfunction and the need for close endocrinologic follow-up and hormone supplementation.[16]
  - The transsphenoidal approach is associated with a lower rate of diabetes insipidus than the transcranial approach. This may be secondary to superior visualization of the infundibulum. Alternatively, intrasellar tumors involve the infundibulum distally, while suprasellar

tumors requiring a transcranial approach tend to involve the infundibulum proximally, where surgical manipulation is more likely to result in diabetes insipidus.[12]

- Following surgical treatment of craniopharyngiomas, vision tends to improve in over half of cases. However, visual deterioration does occur in some patients, although this is less common with the transsphenoidal approach.[15]

16.19 Postoperative Care

Following an endonasal transsphenoidal approach, patients should avoid inserting anything into the nares, including nasal cannula for oxygen supplementation. Straws, nasogastric tubes, oral temperature probes, Valsalva's maneuvers, and nose blowing should be strictly avoided.

Postoperatively, a full endocrine panel should be sent to assess for signs of new or worsening pituitary dysfunction. In particular, patients should be monitored closely for signs of diabetes insipidus. In the setting of diabetes insipidus, patients should be encouraged to maintain their fluid status orally if possible; if this is not possible, intravenous supplementation may be necessary. The serum sodium level, osmolarity, and urine specific gravity should be followed. Patients are also typically placed on hydrocortisone postoperatively and the dose is tapered in coordination with endocrine specialists.

16.20 Adjuvant Treatment

Given the aggressive and recurrent nature of craniopharyngiomas, a variety of adjuvant treatments have been explored, especially for patients in whom a gross total resection cannot be achieved. Radiation treatment, in particular, plays a prominent role in the adjuvant treatment of craniopharyngiomas. Various methods for delivering radiation—including fractionated radiation, stereotactic radiosurgery, and intracavitary radiation therapy—have been studied.

- Fractionated focal radiation therapy to the sellar and parasellar region typically involves doses of 50 to 60 Gy delivered in 2-Gy fractions.[7]
- Following incomplete resection of a craniopharyngioma, adjuvant radiotherapy decreases the rate of progression from about 70–90% to about 20%.[16,30]
  - However, those tumors that do progress following failed radiotherapy are associated with increased morbidity and mortality, and are more challenging to re-resect.[15]

- Fractionated radiation also carries a number of risks[7]:
  - In a similar manner as surgical resection, radiation-induced injury to the adjacent structures may result in hypothalamic dysfunction (including obesity and/or disruption of the sleep–wake cycle), hypopituitarism, and diabetes insipidus.
  - There is a 3% risk of optic neuropathy associated with fractionated radiation.
  - Radiation may have deleterious cognitive effects and is associated with delayed secondary malignancies, both of which are particularly concerning in the pediatric population.
- Immediate postoperative radiation and "progression-contingent radiation" have similar rates of overall survival, although the latter delays the negative effects of radiation on neurological development.[16]
- Single-session stereotactic radiosurgery is typically limited to craniopharyngiomas that are less than or equal to 3 cm in diameter and are 3 to 5 mm away from the optic apparatus.[7]
  - Exposure of the optic chiasm to doses higher than 8 to 10 Gy per session results in an elevated risk of optic neuropathy.
  - Multisession stereotactic radiosurgery has been proposed as a technique for treating craniopharyngiomas that are even closer to the optic nerves and chiasm.
- Cystic craniopharyngiomas may be treated via the stereotactic placement of an intracystic catheter with a subcutaneous reservoir. Percutaneous decompression of the cyst may be performed. Alternatively, the catheter may be used to instill radioisotopes (beta emitters such as Re-186, P-32, Au-198, or Y-90) or sclerosing agents (e.g., bleomycin). Despite encouraging response rates to intracavitary radiation, neurotoxicity resulting from leakage into the CSF remains a limiting factor.[6,7,16]

16.21 Outcomes

The treatment of craniopharyngiomas and other sellar and parasellar lesions is associated with high rates of survival (as high as 95%).[5] As a result, the success of treatment is now measured in terms of the recurrence rate as well as by the quality of life experienced by the patient. The latter, in particular, is critically affected by the hypothalamic, endocrine, and visual function of the patient following treatment. Several variables have been correlated with patient outcomes—younger age at diagnosis, larger tumor size, and worse preoperative functional status are all associated with worse outcomes, while surgeon experience is associated with improved outcomes.[15,28]

16.21.1 Craniopharyngiomas

- Postoperative imaging is performed within 48 hours of craniopharyngioma resection and residual tumor is graded by the Hoffman scale,[31] which ranges from grade 1 (no residual tumor or calcification) to grade 5 (contrast enhancing mass).[1,5]
- Gross total resection reduces the recurrence rate of pediatric craniopharyngiomas by more than half (18–28% following incomplete resection vs. 0–13% following gross total resection).[24]
- Although the transsphenoidal approach appears to offer higher rates of gross total resection than the transcranial approach, this is likely due to selection bias—transsphenoidal resection is typically chosen for small tumors confined to the sella. Larger tumors are associated with lower rates of gross total resection and higher rates of recurrence.[12]
- Adjuvant radiotherapy following incomplete surgical resection dramatically reduces the risk for progression of a craniopharyngioma.[7]
- Gross total resection of a craniopharyngioma and limited resection followed by adjuvant radiation are both associated with similar rates of tumor control and overall survival. Controversy arises as to which approach affords a better functional outcome and higher quality of life.[15]
- De Vile et al[29] and Puget et al[32] developed classification systems that could be used to predict the risk of hypothalamic dysfunction following surgical resection of a craniopharyngioma.
- The transsphenoidal approach is associated with higher rates of visual improvement, and less visual deterioration postoperatively, relative to the transcranial approach.[12]
  - This is most likely due to the opportunity afforded by the transsphenoidal approach to perform an early decompression of the optic apparatus with minimal manipulation.

16.21.2 Rathke's Cleft Cysts

- Headaches and visual function tend to improve following surgical drainage.

- In general, resolution of hormonal deficits occurs in only 14 to 20% of patients. Hyperprolactinemia resolves in over half of patients following drainage.[18]
- Recurrence occurs in 14 to 18% of patients in spite of gross total resection of the cyst wall. However, aggressive resection is associated with increased morbidity, including permanent diabetes insipidus.[17,18,20]
  - Recurrence has been associated with the presence of squamous metaplasia.[20]
- Following surgical drainage, close clinical and radiographic follow-up is warranted for at least 5 years, followed by further imaging every 2 to 3 years for an additional 5 years.[20]

16.21.3 Pituitary Adenomas

- Prolactinomas: Medical therapy is widely effective. Those who cannot tolerate the medication or patients in whom the tumor is refractory to medication are referred for surgical resection.
- Cushing's disease: Surgical resection results in high remission rates (70–98%) in the short term, but many tumors recur if followed for more than 5 years.[6]
  - Hydrocortisone replacement is typically required for 6 to 12 months following surgery due to transient adrenal insufficiency.
  - Normal growth resumes once the cortisol level normalizes.
  - ACTH and cortisol levels may be monitored for early signs of recurrence.
- GH-secreting adenomas: GH levels frequently remain elevated postoperatively, and normalize in only 60% of patients.[6]

16.22 Clinical Pearls

- Reconstruction is generally not performed for Rathke's cleft cysts in the absence of a CSF leak, in order to facilitate continued cyst drainage.
- During craniopharyngioma resection, the normal pituitary gland is often identified ventral and anterior to the tumor. In order to reach the dorsally located tumor from a transsphenoidal approach, a vertical incision may be used to mobilize the pituitary gland. This maneuver is associated with low rates of iatrogenic endocrine deficits.
- When gross total resection of a craniopharyngioma is the goal, resection of the diaphragma sellae may be necessary if it is

adherent to the tumor capsule. A CSF leak should be expected and careful skull base reconstruction should be performed.

- A Valsalva maneuver may be used to force suprasellar portions of the tumor into the sella and into the field of view.
  - The right lower quadrant is not used in pediatric patients so that the incision is not confused with an appendectomy scar in the future.

16.23 Common Clinical Questions

1. How do pediatric craniopharyngiomas most commonly present?
2. How is Cushing's disease identified preoperatively?
3. Craniopharyngiomas in which location are most suitable for the transsphenoidal approach?
4. Describe the options for adjuvant radiotherapy following surgical resection of a craniopharyngioma.

16.24 Answers to Common Clinical Questions

1. Craniopharyngiomas most commonly present with nonspecific symptoms of raised intracranial pressure, such as headaches and nausea. Many patients also have at least some level of endocrine dysfunction at the time of presentation. GH is most commonly affected, resulting in growth failure. Patients may also show signs of delayed puberty, weight gain, and diabetes insipidus. Visual deficits, although frequently found in patients, tends to be well tolerated by the pediatric population.
2. Upon identification of a sellar or parasellar mass on neuroimaging, a full endocrine workup should be performed. Cushing's disease is associated with elevated serum ACTH and cortisol levels. Low-dose dexamethasone administered at midnight does not suppress the production of cortisol (measured the next morning), although cortisol production is indeed suppressed by high-dose dexamethasone. In contrast, ectopic ACTH-secreting tumors result in elevated cortisol levels that are suppressed by neither low- nor high-dose dexamethasone.
3. The transsphenoidal approach is most appropriate for intrasellar pathology (unless an extended transsphenoidal approach is utilized, in which case the suprasellar region may be reached as well). Craniopharyngiomas with an infradiaphragmatic intrasellar origin may be safely resected via the transsphenoidal approach, as the diaphragma sellae drapes over the tumor and separates it from suprasellar structures such as the optic chiasm, hypothalamus, and circle of Willis.
4. Various strategies for delivering adjuvant radiotherapy have been described, including fractionated radiation (50–60 Gy delivered in 2-Gy fractions), single or multi-session stereotactic radiosurgery, and intracystic radioisotopes delivered via a stereotactically implanted catheter. Radiosensitivity of adjacent structures—in particular the optic apparatus—remains a key limiting factor in the dosing of adjuvant radiotherapy.

References

[1] Surawicz TS, McCarthy BJ, Kupelian V, Jukich PJ, Bruner JM, Davis FG. Descriptive epidemiology of primary brain and CNS tumors: results from the Central Brain Tumor Registry of the United States, 1990–1994. Neuro-oncol. 1999; 1(1):14–25

[2] Zada G, Lin N, Ojerholm E, Ramkissoon S, Laws ER. Craniopharyngioma and other cystic epithelial lesions of the sellar region: a review of clinical, imaging, and histopathological relationships. Neurosurg Focus. 2010; 28(4):E4

[3] Frazier JL, Chaichana K, Jallo GI, Quiñones-Hinojosa A. Combined endoscopic and microscopic management of pediatric pituitary region tumors through one nostril: technical note with case illustrations. Childs Nerv Syst. 2008; 24(12):1469–1478

[4] Schroeder JW, Vezina LG. Pediatric sellar and suprasellar lesions. Pediatr Radiol. 2011; 41(3):287–298, quiz 404–405

[5] Müller HL, Gebhardt U, Faldum A, et al. Kraniopharyngeom 2000 Study Committee. Xanthogranuloma, Rathke's cyst, and childhood craniopharyngioma: results of prospective multinational studies of children and adolescents with rare sellar malformations. J Clin Endocrinol Metab. 2012; 97(11): 3935–3943

[6] Jagannathan J, Dumont AS, Jane JA, Jr, Laws ER, Jr. Pediatric sellar tumors: diagnostic procedures and management. Neurosurg Focus. 2005; 18 6A:E6

[7] Veeravagu A, Lee M, Jiang B, Chang SD. The role of radiosurgery in the treatment of craniopharyngiomas. Neurosurg Focus. 2010; 28(4):E11

[8] Bunin GR, Surawicz TS, Witman PA, Preston-Martin S, Davis F, Bruner JM. The descriptive epidemiology of craniopharyngioma. J Neurosurg. 1998; 89(4):547–551

[9] Jahangiri A, Molinaro AM, Tarapore PE, et al. Rathke cleft cysts in pediatric patients: presentation, surgical management, and postoperative outcomes. Neurosurg Focus. 2011; 31(1): E3

[10] Teramoto A, Hirakawa K, Sanno N, Osamura Y. Incidental pituitary lesions in 1,000 unselected autopsy specimens. Radiology. 1994; 193(1):161–164

[11] Takanashi J, Tada H, Barkovich AJ, Saeki N, Kohno Y. Pituitary cysts in childhood evaluated by MR imaging. AJNR Am J Neuroradiol. 2005; 26(8):2144–2147

[12] Elliott RE, Jane JA, Jr, Wisoff JH. Surgical management of craniopharyngiomas in children: meta-analysis and comparison of transcranial and transsphenoidal approaches. Neurosurgery. 2011; 69(3):630–643, discussion 643

[13] Webb C, Prayson RA. Pediatric pituitary adenomas. Arch Pathol Lab Med. 2008; 132(1):77–80

[14] Abe T, Lüdecke DK, Saeger W. Clinically nonsecreting pituitary adenomas in childhood and adolescence. Neurosurgery. 1998; 42(4):744–750, discussion 750–751

[15] Elliott RE, Sands SA, Strom RG, Wisoff JH. Craniopharyngioma Clinical Status Scale: a standardized metric of preoperative function and posttreatment outcome. Neurosurg Focus. 2010; 28(4):E2

[16] Müller HL. Childhood craniopharyngioma: treatment strategies and outcomes. Expert Rev Neurother. 2014; 14(2): 187–197

[17] Higgins DM, Van Gompel JJ, Nippoldt TB, Meyer FB. Symptomatic Rathke cleft cysts: extent of resection and surgical complications. Neurosurg Focus. 2011; 31(1):E2

[18] Zada G, Ditty B, McNatt SA, McComb JG, Krieger MD. Surgical treatment of rathke cleft cysts in children. Neurosurgery. 2009; 64(6):1132–1137, author reply 1037–1038

[19] Keil MF, Stratakis CA. Pituitary tumors in childhood: update of diagnosis, treatment and molecular genetics. Expert Rev Neurother. 2008; 8(4):563–574

[20] Zada G. Rathke cleft cysts: a review of clinical and surgical management. Neurosurg Focus. 2011; 31(1):E1

[21] Samii M, Tatagiba M. Craniopharyngioma. In: Kaye A, Laws E, eds. Brain Tumors. New York, NY: Churchill Livingstone; 1995:873–94

[22] Wen BC, Hussey DH, Staples J, et al. A comparison of the roles of surgery and radiation therapy in the management of craniopharyngiomas. Int J Radiat Oncol Biol Phys. 1989; 16(1):17–24

[23] Wisoff J, Donahue B. Craniopharyngiomas. In: Albright A, Pollack I, Adelson P, eds. Principles and Practice of Pediatric Neurosurgery. New York, NY: Thieme; 2015:483–502

[24] Jane JA, Jr, Prevedello DM, Alden TD, Laws ER, Jr. The transsphenoidal resection of pediatric craniopharyngiomas: a case series. J Neurosurg Pediatr. 2010; 5(1):49–60

[25] Ali ZS, Lang SS, Kamat AR, et al. Suprasellar pediatric craniopharyngioma resection via endonasal endoscopic approach. Childs Nerv Syst. 2013; 29(11):2065–2070

[26] Elliott RE, Hsieh K, Hochm T, Belitskaya-Levy I, Wisoff J, Wisoff JH. Efficacy and safety of radical resection of primary and recurrent craniopharyngiomas in 86 children. J Neurosurg Pediatr. 2010; 5(1):30–48

[27] Sands SA, Milner JS, Goldberg J, et al. Quality of life and behavioral follow-up study of pediatric survivors of craniopharyngioma. J Neurosurg. 2005; 103(4) Suppl:302–311

[28] Sanford RA. Craniopharyngioma: results of survey of the American Society of Pediatric Neurosurgery. Pediatr Neurosurg. 1994; 21 Suppl 1:39–43

[29] De Vile CJ, Grant DB, Kendall BE, et al. Management of childhood craniopharyngioma: can the morbidity of radical surgery be predicted? J Neurosurg. 1996; 85(1):73–81

[30] Becker G, Kortmann RD, Skalej M, Bamberg M. The role of radiotherapy in the treatment of craniopharyngioma–indications, results, side effects. Front Radiat Ther Oncol. 1999; 33:100–113

[31] Hoffman HJ. Craniopharyngiomas. Can J Neurol Sci. 1985; 12 (4):348–352

[32] Puget S, Garnett M, Wray A, et al. Pediatric craniopharyngiomas: classification and treatment according to the degree of hypothalamic involvement. J Neurosurg. 2007; 106(1) Suppl:3–12

17 Germ Cell Tumors

Gerald F. Tuite, Stacie Stapleton

17.1 Introduction

All germ cell tumors (GCTs) are thought to have a common cell of origin, the primordial germ cell. GCTs are divided into gonadal and extragonadal tumors. Approximately half of GCTs are extragonadal, and most of these occur intracranially.[1]

GCTs account for only a small proportion of all cancers in children, and the incidence and location vary significantly with age and gender.

17.2 Epidemiology Factors

17.2.1 Extracranial Germ Cell Tumors

- GCTs have a bimodal distribution: a peak in infancy and a second peak after the onset of puberty.[2]
- Newborns more commonly have teratomas and yolk sac tumors, but tumors in the peripubertal period have a wider range of histologies.[2]
- Sacrococcygeal teratomas are the most common GCT of childhood, accounting for 40% all GCTs and 78% of extragonadal GCTs.[3] Prior to age 5, 42% of GCTs are sacrococcygeal teratomas.[4]
- Malignant GCTs are rarely diagnosed in early childhood but the incidence begins to rise during the onset of puberty in boys and girls.[2]
- During adolescence, GCTs make up a much larger proportion of all cancer: for patients younger than 15 years, GCTs make up only 2 to 4% of all cancer diagnoses, but they account for 16% of all cancers in adolescent between 15 and 19 years of age.[2,5,6] Overall, there is a higher incidence in males[5]; however, GCTs are more common in females in the neonatal period and during the peripubertal period.[2,5]
- Gonadal tumors are more common than extragonadal tumors, but females have a higher proportion of extragonadal tumors (33%) than males (15%).[2,5] In the first year of life, males have an equal proportion of gonadal and extragonadal tumors, but females have a higher proportion of extragonadal tumors than ovarian tumors. Rates of all GCTs remain low in both genders during childhood, but the rates increase significantly in both girls and boys with the onset of puberty. In puberty and the peripubertal periods, rates of extragonadal tumors increase somewhat but the incidence of gonadal tumors has a dramatic increase, much more so in males than females.[4]

17.2.2 Intracranial Germ Cell Tumors

Overall, intracranial GCTs represent a small proportion of all pediatric brain tumors.[2,5] The incidence varies significantly according to geography. In western countries, intracranial GCTs represent 0.4 to 3.4% of all pediatric central nervous system (CNS) tumors,[7,8] while in Japan and other Asian countries, intracranial GCTs represent up to 11% of all pediatric CNS tumors.[9,10]

- The most common primary sites in the brain are the pineal gland (56%) and the suprasellar region (28%). The basal ganglia, thalamus, corpus callosum, cerebellum, and spinal cord are much less common.[11]
- CNS GCTs predominate in the young population, with more than 90% of CNS GCTs diagnosed before the age of 20 years,[8] with the peak age at diagnosis being 10 to 12 years.[12]
- Nongerminomatous germ cell tumors (NGGCTs) predominate in younger children and germinomas are more common in older children.[7,8]
- Gender differences are marked. In males, 70% of GCTs occur in pineal region, and in females, 75% of GCTs are suprasellar. For NGGCTs, the male-to-female ratio is 3:1, but in germinomas it is 1.8:1.[7,8]

17.3 Predisposing Factors

17.3.1 Extracranial Germ Cell Tumors

There has been a doubling of the worldwide rate of testicular cancer in the past 30 years as well as a general rise in the incidence of pediatric GCTs.[2]

Prenatal exposure to high levels of maternal estrogens (diethylstilbestrol or oral contraceptives) may be a possible environmental cause, which has been linked to increased GCTs in animal experiments; however, these links have not been supported in clinical epidemiological studies.[2] Predisposing syndromes include: cryptorchidism—relative risk of testicular cancer of 2.1 to 17.6%[13]; Turner's syndrome (45, X, loss of X chromosome)—increased risk of gonadoblastoma[2]; Klinefelter's syndrome (47, XXY)—increased risk of mediastinal GCT but not increased risk of testicular cancer[2]; and androgen insensitivity syndromes (X,Y)—cryptorchid testes are at high risk for GCT.[2]

17.3.2 Intracranial Germ Cell Tumors

The only known predisposing factor is Japanese or other Asian ancestry. In western countries, intracranial GCTs account for only 0.4 to 3.4% of all pediatric CNS tumors; in Japan and other Asian countries, intracranial GCTs account for up to 11% of all pediatric CNS tumors.[8] Peripubertal individuals are predisposed for GCTs. Circulating gonadotropin levels may be a factor in tumor development.[14] There are no known environmental risk factors.

17.4 Pathophysiology

GCTs arise from cells of the germline, cells that are destined to become either the egg or the sperm.[2] Different GCTs may represent the malignant forms of different stages of normal embryonic development. Primordial germ cells may result in germinomas, embryonic differentiation may give rise to teratomas and embryonal carcinomas, extraembryonic yolk sac cells may give rise to endodermal sinus tumors, and derivatives of the trophoblast may give rise to choriocarcinomas.[1]

There are multiple theories for the development of GCTs in the brain:

- The "germ cell theory" states that primordial germ cells, which normally develop from the extraembryonic yolk sac endoderm and migrate to the gonadal folds, have abnormal migration and end up in brain; then, these cells undergo malignant transformation.[2,15]
- The "embryonic cell theory" suggests there is mismigration of pluripotent embryonic cells, which give rise to GCTs.[2,8]
- Another theory proposes that germinomas are the only GCTs that arise from germ cells. and that other GCTs develop secondary to misfolding and misplacement of embryonic cells into the lateral mesoderm, resulting in entrapment in different brain regions.[8,16,17]

17.5 Pathology

The pathologic classification of intracranial GCTs is based primarily on the tumor's histopathology and tumor markers (▶ Table 17.1)

17.5.1 Germinoma (Pure Germinoma)

- Histologically indistinguishable from tumors in extracranial locations such as gonads or mediastinum.
- Key features include large round blue cells, with abundant clear cytoplasm arranged in nests around bands of connective tissue, focal microvilli.
- Negative for alpha-fetoprotein (AFP), may be positive for beta-human chorionic gonadotropin (b-HCG) if syncytiotrophoblastic cells are present, may have elevation of placental alkaline phosphatase (PLAP), and c-kit is typically elevated.[7,18,19]

Table 17.1 Tumor markers in germ cell tumors

Type of germ cell tumor	AFP	b-HCG	PLAP	c-kit
Germinoma	–	–1	+/–	+
Embryonal carcinoma	–	–	+	–
Endodermal sinus (yolk sac) tumor	+++	–	+/–	–
Choriocarcinoma	–	+++	+/–	–
Mixed germ cell tumor	+/–	+/–	+/–	+/–
Teratoma	–2	–2	–	–2

Abbreviations: AFP, alpha-fetoprotein; b-HCG, beta-human chorionic gonadotropin; PLAP, placental alkaline phosphatase.
Source: Data from Louis et al.[18]
Note: 1, positive if syncytiotrophoblastic; 2, positive if immature.

17.5.2 Nongerminomatous Germ Cell Tumors

Embryonal Carcinoma

- Cuboidal-columnar cells in sheets and cords, large nuclei and large prominent nucleoli, very little lymphocytic infiltration.
- PLAP positive, AFP, and b-HCG.[7,18,19]

Endodermal Sinus Tumor (Yolk Sac Tumor)

- Differentiation of yolk sac noted, Schiller–Duval bodies are pathognomonic (glomeruloid structures), invaginated vascular pedicle lined by a single layer of tumor cells.
- AFP positive, PLAP may or may not be elevated.[7,18,19]

Choriocarcinoma

- Differentiated trophoblasts, bilaminar cytotrophoblasts/syncytiotrophoblasts, hypervascular, intratumoral hemorrhage common.
- b-HCG positive, PLAP may or may not be elevated.[7,18,19]

Mixed Germ Cell Tumor

- May contain a mixture of multiple elements including germinoma elements.
- May demonstrate any variation of tumor markers.

Teratoma

- Key characteristic is presence of all three germ layers.
- Immature teratoma versus mature teratoma based on degree of differentiation.
- Teratoma with malignant transformation is a designation for teratomas that contain an additional malignant component such as sarcoma or carcinoma.[20]
- Solid or cystic foci of squamous epithelium, cartilage, or glandular elements.[7,18,19]
- Mature teratomas are negative for tumor markers, although immature teratomas may have AFP or b-HCG if certain components are present.

17.6 Molecular Biology

The molecular biology of GCTs is an evolving field of uncertain clinical significance, and additional work is needed in this area. Interesting data are mentioned here:

- One study demonstrated 92% of intracranial GCTs had an extra X chromosome and that 81% of those were hypomethylated. In addition, 20% had increased copy numbers of 12p.[21]
- Compared with astrocytomas, *p53* mutation is rare (5%) in GCTs, but *mdm2* amplification (19%) and homozygous deletion or frameshift mutation of *INK4a/ARF* (71%) are frequent.[22,23]
- Various mutations of *c-kit* have been noted with up to three different mutations in a single tumor.[22]

17.7 Radiographic Findings of Intracranial Germ Cell Tumors

Most intracranial GCTs originate in the vicinity of the third ventricle, with most tumors localized to the pineal region or the suprasellar cistern.[1] Pineal region GCTs outnumber those occurring in the suprasellar cistern by a ratio of approximately 2:1.[7] So-called synchronous GCTs, occurring in both the pineal and suprasellar locations, occur in approximately 5 to 10% of cases.[7] Germinomas more commonly occur in the pineal region in males, whereas females are more likely to have lesions in the suprasellar region.[7] GCTs have a predilection to metastasize along the entire neural axis but they have also been reported to originate at various areas outside the third ventricle, including the basal ganglia, thalamus, lateral and fourth ventricles, medulla, cerebellum, optic nerves, and spinal cord.

MRI with and without intravenous contrast is the imaging modality of choice, but computed tomography (CT) scanning can help delineate the degree of calcification. Historically, GCTs were suspected when calcifications were seen in the pineal region on skull radiographs. When a GCT is considered, brain and total spine MRI with and without contrast are recommended to delineate the extent of disease.[8] Angiography is rarely indicated, unless other imaging modalities suggest a primary vascular malformation.

The radiographic characteristics of all GCTs are very similar: enhancing, sometimes calcified and/

or cystic lesion within the pineal or suprasellar area. Because the imaging characteristics of most GCTs are so similar, a precise and reliable histologic diagnosis cannot be made based on radiographs alone.[8] There is also significant overlap in the radiographic characteristics of several other tumor types that occur in these location, including pineoblastoma, trilateral retinoblastoma, pineocytoma, glioma, meningioma, lymphoma, cyst, and vascular abnormalities. However, certain imaging characteristics of GCTs tend to follow the following trends:

- Synchronous third ventricular lesions, within the pineal and suprasellar areas, occur more often with germinoma than with NGGCTs.[8]
- Germinomas tend to diffusely and homogenously enhance. NGGCTs and very large germinomas have a more heterogeneous enhancement pattern.[1]
- Choriocarcinoma is the most common GCT associated with hemorrhage. In general, NGGCTs are more likely to hemorrhage than germinomas.[1]
- Mature teratomas have a very heterogeneous appearance with predominant cysts and calcifications. Immature teratomas tend to have less cysts and calcifications.
- A calcified, benign-appearing pineal cyst seen on CT warrants an MRI scan to rule out tumor.[24]

17.8 Presenting Signs and Symptoms

The clinical presentation of intracranial GCTs depends on the patient age, tumor location, and size of the tumor.

17.8.1 Suprasellar GCTs

- Rarely present with signs of raised intracranial pressure (ICP).
- Usually present with dysfunction of the pituitary/hypothalamic axis: diabetes insipidus, delayed sexual development, hypopituitarism, isolated growth hormone deficiency, precocious puberty.
- Ophthalmic abnormalities such as visual field deficits or bitemporal hemianopsia.

17.8.2 Pineal GCTs

- Usually present with signs of raised ICP related to obstructive hydrocephalus—somnolence, vomiting, headaches.

- Ophthalmologic findings are present in 25 to 50% of patients with pineal region tumors and include papilledema or Parinaud's syndrome (paralysis of upward gaze, impaired accommodation, and convergence-retraction nystagmus).[8]
- Ataxia, seizures, and behavioral changes in approximately 25%.
- Endocrinopathies are less common than with suprasellar tumors. However, the presence of diabetes insipidus with a pineal region tumor, even without radiographic abnormality in the suprasellar area, may be an indication of suprasellar tumor involvement.[15]

17.9 Laboratory Evaluation

Because radiographs are not always diagnostic, b-HCG and AFP should be measured in the cerebrospinal fluid (CSF) and serum. Tumor markers may frequently be negative or only show mild levels of elevation, but radiographs in combination with tumor markers can often narrow the diagnostic possibilities substantially. U.S. and European groups have traditionally classified tumors as "secreting" if the serum and/or CSF AFP is ≥ 10 ng/dL and the b-HCG is ≥ 50 IU/L.[15] Elevation in PLAP and c-kit have shown association with pure germinomas, but these are not routinely used in diagnostic decision-making. These tumor markers may not always be readily available in all hospitals and may require submission to a reference lab, which may delay time to diagnosis.[25,26]

- Pure germinomas, mature teratomas, and embryonal carcinomas typically have negative AFP and b-HCG. However, syncytiotrophoblastic germinomas may have modest elevations in b-HCG of up to 50 IU/L.[15]
- Choriocarcinoma characteristically has a very high b-HCG level.[27]
- Endodermal sinus tumors (yolk sac tumors) typically have an isolated elevated AFP.
- Immature teratomas and mixed GCTs have variable expressions of AFP and b-HCG.
- Pure germinomas tend to be negative for b-HCG and AFP.
- Some patients with germinoma can have a modest elevation of b-HCG, which can confuse the diagnostic picture. However, current convention has accepted levels of 50 to 100 mIU/mL for diagnosis as a pure germinoma and higher levels to recommend diagnosis as a mixed GCT.[28,29]

17.10 Nonsurgical Management

Although there is a broad differential diagnosis for pineal and suprasellar tumors, tissue diagnosis and/or resection is not always necessary. Surgery is frequently indicated for other reasons, such as the presence of hydrocephalus at diagnosis, atypical/nondiagnostic radiographs, or due to nonspecific tumor markers. Unless otherwise indicated, tumor biopsy may be avoided in the following situations:

- Extremely high b-HCG combined with a very vascular suprasellar or pineal region tumor, which suggests NGGCT, most likely choriocarcinoma. The surgical risk is higher due to the vascularity, and for this reason, empiric adjuvant therapy may be advocated.
- Very high AFP with a heterogeneously enhancing suprasellar or pineal region tumor may suggest endodermal sinus tumor. Empiric therapy would be considered.
- Homogenously enhancing suprasellar or pineal region tumor with negative markers. Although controversial, some centers are willing to treat patients empirically based on the clinical picture and the radiographic findings consistent with a germinoma without histological confirmation or elevated tumor markers.[28]

17.11 Surgical Indications

Unlike many other pediatric CNS tumors, there is a limited role for complete resection in the treatment of most GCTs. Gross total resection is the treatment of choice for mature teratomas. However, the remainders of GCTs are treated with adjuvant therapy, with subsequent surgery performed if there is a histologic diagnostic uncertainty or if parts of the tumor do not respond to radiation therapy and/or chemotherapy.

The initial diagnosis of GCT can be confidently made without biopsy if there are characteristic clinical and radiographic findings combined with markedly elevated tumor markers. For example, pediatric patients presenting with enhancing pineal masses with markedly elevated AFP (endodermal sinus tumor) or b-HCG (choriocarcinoma) can often be treated with adjuvant therapy without tissue diagnosis.

However, if GCT is suspected and there are any noncharacteristic imaging findings or if tumor markers are only slightly elevated or in the normal range, a tumor biopsy is usually strongly considered.[8] If mature teratoma is diagnosed, gross total resection is often attempted. In the case of all other GCTs, adjuvant therapy is usually instituted without an attempt at resection.

In clinical practice, the common presence of hydrocephalus at the time of diagnosis often necessitates urgent ventricular drainage. Because most GCTs have an exposed surface within the third ventricle, endoscopic biopsy can often be readily performed at the time of ventricular access in the treatment of hydrocephalus in cases where the diagnosis cannot be made without histologic confirmation. When hydrocephalus is not present, tissue diagnosis can be made by stereotactic biopsy or craniotomy if necessary.

17.12 Surgical Technique

Hydrocephalus is often present at the time of diagnosis, providing an ideal route for access to GCTs. When biopsy is required, a combined endoscopic third ventriculostomy (ETV) and tumor biopsy is often the treatment of choice. When hydrocephalus is not present at diagnosis, tissue can be obtained by stereotactic biopsy, craniotomy, or endoscopically assisted craniotomy.

17.12.1 Endoscopic Biopsy/Endoscopic Third Ventriculostomy

- ETV and endoscopic biopsy (ENDOBX) can be performed during a single operation, either through a single burr hole (flexible endoscope) or through two separate burr holes (rigid endoscope).[30,31]
- ETV is usually performed prior to ENDOBX because bleeding from biopsy may obscure view for ETV.
- ETV success rate for treatment of hydrocephalus is high, approximately 68 to 89%.[10,30,31,32,33]

17.12.2 Stereotactic Biopsy

- More likely to be performed in a pineal region tumor than a suprasellar tumor because of surrounding vasculature.
- Frame or frameless biopsy.
- Need to carefully plan trajectory to avoid important vasculature.

17.12.3 Craniotomy

- Usually the initial approach of choice when a mature teratoma is strongly suspected or if hydrocephalus is not present at diagnosis.
- May be considered even when hydrocephalus is present at the time of diagnosis if the lesion is not accessible endoscopically or if the tumor is felt to be excessively vascular for an endoscopic biopsy.
- An endoscopically assisted craniotomy may be considered in certain situations in order to minimize exposure.[34]
- For pineal region tumors:
  - Midline infratentorial supracerebellar approach is the most commonly utilized.
  - Occipital transtentorial.
  - Transventricular.
  - Transcallosal.
- Suprasellar region tumors:
  - Pterional.
  - Subfrontal.

17.12.4 Ventricular Shunting

- Usually reserved for cases where ETV is either not technically possible or unsuccessful.

17.13 Postoperative Care

Postoperative care is similar to that rendered after typical ETV, endoscopic biopsy, or craniotomy.
- Steroids are often used on a limited basis before and after surgery.
- External ventricular drainage is often performed after ETV/biopsy. Proceed to clamping and drain removal depending on surgeon preference, the degree of bleeding after biopsy, and clinical status.
- Common neurologic sequelae include Parinaud's syndrome, convergence nystagmus, and other focal neurologic deficits related to hemorrhage.

17.14 Surgical Complications

17.14.1 Lack of Diagnosis

- A large multi-institutional study of 293 patients found endoscopic biopsy diagnostic 90% of the time.[32]

17.14.2 Sampling Error

- A large study showed that 27% of patients who underwent endoscopic biopsy eventually also had an open procedure. In this subset of patients, pathology was found to be discordant between endoscopic and open surgery 18% of the time. This discordant pathology only changed management 11% of the time.[32]

17.14.3 CSF Dissemination

- There is some concern that combined ETV plus endoscopic biopsy might lead to greater CSF dissemination of GCTs.
- Most studies show no increased risk of dissemination with endoscopic biopsy.[33,35]

17.14.4 Seizure

- Mayo clinic study showed that risk of seizure was higher in a transcallosal approach to lateral and third ventricle than with transcortical approach.[36]

17.14.5 Hemorrhage

- Cornell study of 86 patients showed 3.5% rate of hemorrhagic sequelae during endoscopic procedures for intraventricular tumors, with only 1 patient having relevant morbidity related to hemorrhage.[37]
- International study of endoscopic biopsy showed that there was always some bleeding, with 6% having severe hemorrhage.[32]

17.14.6 Death

- Rare, usually related to untreated hydrocephalus or severe bleeding.
- Only 1/59 patients with GCTs died within 30 days of surgery, according to the UK Pediatric CNS Tumor Registry.[38]
- Only 1/239 patients who underwent endoscopic biopsy died shortly after surgery.[32]

17.15 Radiation Therapy and Chemotherapy

The treatment for pediatric GCTs is dictated by the specific subtype of tumor and the extent of disease. The goal of treatment is to provide the best tumor control and cure rate while minimizing toxic long-term side effects. Treatment is therefore designed specifically to address the prognosis. Germinomas and mature teratomas have the best prognosis—the former managed by radiation with or without chemo and the latter managed by resection. The NGGCTs as a whole have a much worse prognosis. Historically, the standard treatment for all GCTs was craniospinal radiation, which was effective for pure germinomas, but produced unacceptable outcomes for patients with NGGCTs. In addition, the patients had significant morbidity from their treatment of the entire neuroaxis. Multiple studies have been conducted to reduce the dose of radiation, apply chemotherapy techniques, and reduce long-term side effect, while maintaining or improving long-term survival.

17.15.1 Germinomas

Germinomas are extremely sensitive to radiation. Empiric treatment, without biopsy, has been advocated by some investigators. However, biopsy is often performed when tumor markers are normal. Radiation therapy at doses of 50 Gy gives 85 to greater than 90% progression-free survival (PFS) rates, but has high long-term morbidity.[39] Chemotherapy alone has been attempted, and although many patients achieve a near-complete or complete response, most patients eventually relapse, and this method therefore has unacceptable PFS rates demonstrated at 84% 2-year survival.[12,40] Multiple studies have focused on reducing the dose and field of radiation combined with chemotherapy, and the results of these studies have led to the current treatment of choice—two to four cycles of chemotherapy (typically consisting of carboplatin and etoposide) and relatively low-dose radiation therapy of 24 to 36 Gy to the tumor site (s).[41,42] In addition, as the ventricular system is the primary area of relapse, typically 18 to 24 Gy is delivered to the whole ventricular field.[12]

17.15.2 NGGCTs

This group includes choriocarcinoma, endodermal sinus (yolk sac) tumors, embryonal carcinomas, and mixed GCTs (including mixed NGGCT elements with pure germinoma elements). Surgery is rarely needed for a tissue diagnosis in this group as tumor markers usually assist in making the diagnosis, although surgery may be indicated for hydrocephalus. Compared to germinomas, the NGGCTs are relatively resistant to radiation and have a worse prognosis. In the past, these tumors have been treated with craniospinal radiation and have had a 3-year survival rate of 20 to 45%.[12,39] Chemotherapy used prior to radiation has shown objective responses, including complete responses after two to four cycles of chemotherapy.[43,44] Chemotherapy without radiation has been attempted but 50% of patients treated by this method recurred, and at 65% 2-year survival, chemotherapy alone would not be considered acceptable for this group of patients.[40] Chemotherapy combined with radiation has been the focus of most research protocols to help improve the survival. Currently, the standard is chemotherapy (typically consisting of carboplatin, etoposide, and ifosfamide) followed by radiation therapy (45–54 Gy) to the tumor site (s). Whole ventricular field radiation of 30 Gy with or without craniospinal radiation is usually recommended. Institution of adjuvant therapy often reduces the size and vascularity of the tumor, thereby facilitating complete removal at the time of a second-look surgery, which may be indicated in the presence of residual or progressive disease after the completion of therapy.[41,42]

17.15.3 Teratomas

Surgical removal is the treatment of choice for mature teratoma. Chemotherapy and radiation are not typically recommended. Chemotherapy is employed in patients with immature teratomas; however, radiation therapy is controversial and likely has no role.[45] The best treatment for teratomas with malignant transformation is unclear.[12]

17.15.4 Relapse

Tumor recurrence occurs in 2 to 10% of patients with standard germinoma, and higher rates of relapse occur in NGGCT. Some recurrences are related to an incorrect initial diagnosis, to malignant transformation after therapy, or to simple local recurrence. Surgical biopsy and possible resection could be considered. If the patient has not yet received radiation, then salvage with focal or craniospinal radiation is recommended. Alternative chemotherapy agents have been reported with some success, such as cyclophosphamide, cisplatin, thiotepa, and others. High-dose chemotherapy with stem cell rescue has also been successful in some patients with or without additional focal radiation.[12,46,47]

17.16 Prognosis

The histologic subtype is the single most predictive factor of outcome.[42]

17.16.1 Germinomas

- Germinomas are highly curable with 10-year overall survival rates greater than 90% with biopsy followed by adjuvant therapy.[12]
- Studies have shown an excellent oncologic outcome with 40 to 50 Gy of radiation therapy to the whole ventricle or a larger field, but there is a high rate of complications including neuroendocrine deficiencies, growth retardation, and cognitive consequences.[42,48,49]
- Chemotherapy followed by reduced dose radiation therapy has produced 10-year PFS rates in the range of 75 to 93% with less complications than high-dose radiation therapy.[41,42]
- The degree of elevation of b-HCG has been controversial regarding a prognostic risk factor, but overall has not been shown to affect outcome.[50,51]

17.16.2 NGGCTs

- NGGCTs are relatively resistant to radiation therapy and chemotherapy and are associated with a less favorable outcome.[42,48,49]
- The addition of chemotherapy to radiation clearly improves the outcome of patients versus radiation alone.[52]
- A "sandwich" approach of chemotherapy, followed by radiation, followed by further chemotherapy, showed improved rates of 4-year survival of 74%.[44]
- Upfront chemotherapy can induce complete responses, but rates of 75% 6-year overall survival have been shown when used in combination with radiation.[53] Another study has shown a 5-year 79% event-free survival with the approach of chemotherapy followed by radiation.[54]
- Chemotherapy regimens must be chosen carefully, as some chemotherapy regimens have shown inferior results to others. The toxicities of each regimen must be considered, such as ototoxicity in particular when used in conjunction with radiation.[54]

17.17 Surgical Pearls

- Intracranial GCTs predominantly occur within the third ventricle, primarily in the pineal and suprasellar areas.
- While pineal and suprasellar region tumors in infants and children are often GCTs, there are many other tumor types that occur in these regions.
- GCTs have a propensity to be present along the entire neuraxis. If the clinical situation allows, obtain a brain and total spine MRI before performing surgery or initiating adjuvant therapy.
- If GCT is in the differential diagnosis, be sure to send serum tumor markers (AFP, b-HCG, PLAP) before making a decision to perform surgery. Also send CSF markers if they can be safely obtained. b-HCG can be minimally elevated even in germinomas.
- If tumor markers are highly suggestive of an NGGCT, such as choriocarcinoma (b-HCG) or endodermal sinus tumor (AFP), unless otherwise indicated, surgery may be avoided without a diagnostic biopsy or resection. Surgery is often performed for hydrocephalus, nondiagnostic radiographs or tumor markers, or residual disease after chemotherapy and/or radiation therapy.
- Mature teratoma is the only intracranial GCT for which complete, upfront resection is recommended. Germinoma is often biopsied, followed by radiation and chemotherapy. Other NGGCTs are often treated with upfront chemotherapy and radiation therapy, followed by resection of residual lesions if necessary.
- Obstructive hydrocephalus is often present at diagnosis and is the source of most of the common presenting symptoms (headache, vomiting, Parinaud's syndrome).
- Dilated ventricles at presentation provide a safe and effective route through which tissue diagnosis can be obtained endoscopically. Combined ETV and tumor biopsy, through either a single or dual burr hole approach, can effectively treat hydrocephalus and provide diagnostic tissue. Tiny biopsy specimens carry the risk of misdiagnosis due to sampling error.
- Germinomas biopsied followed by adjuvant therapy and completely resected mature teratomas carry an excellent prognosis. Other NGGCTs often carry a much poorer prognosis

17.18 Common Clinical Questions

1. What is the most common germ cell tumor of childhood?
2. For intracranial germ cell tumors, describe the most common general locations and the variations that occur based on gender.
3. Describe the World Health Organization's classification of germ cell tumors and tumor markers associated with the various tumors.
4. How do serum and/or CSF tumor marker levels impact surgical decision-making and expected prognosis?
5. What is the most common surgical approach to a child with obstructive hydrocephalus and a pineal region mass suspected to be germinoma? Describe the operative approach.

17.19 Answers to Common Clinical Questions

1. Sacrococcygeal teratomas account for close to 50% of all germ cell tumors prior to age 5. Intracranial germ cell tumors account for a small proportion of all germ cell tumors and occur with much less frequency than gonadal and other extragonadal locations (mediastinum, retroperitoneal, etc.).
2. Most intracranial germ cell tumors occur around the third ventricle. Males more commonly have tumors in the pineal region and females are more likely to have tumors in the suprasellar area.
3. The 2007 WHO classification of tumors divides intracranial germ cell tumors into germinomas and nongerminomatous germ cell tumors (NGGCTs). Pure germinomas tend to be negative for b-HCG and AFP. Syncytiotrophoblastic germinomas can frequently be positive for b-HCG. Endodermal sinus tumors (yolk sac tumors) typically secrete AFP. Choriocarcinomas typically secrete b-HCG. Mature teratomas are negative for b-HCG and AFP.
4. Patients with markedly elevated b-HCG and/or AFP likely have choriocarcinoma, endodermal sinus tumor, immature teratoma, or some other mixed GCT. These NGGCTs often carry a much worse prognosis than germinomas or teratomas, and they may benefit from chemotherapy or radiation therapy prior to attempted resection. Tumors that are negative for tumor markers are more likely to be germinoma, teratomas, or some other non-GCT. Upfront surgery is often performed in these tumors that are negative for tumor markers.
5. Children with obstructive hydrocephalus and a suspected pineal region germinoma are often treated with endoscopic third ventriculostomy and an endoscopic biopsy during the same operation. Use of a rigid endoscope usually requires two separate frontal burr holes in order to optimize the surgical angle for each stage of the procedure: ETV is performed through a burr hole near the coronal suture and tumor biopsy is performed through a more anterior frontal burr hole. Use of a flexible endoscope for ETV and biopsy can often be performed through a single burr hole.

References

[1] Lieuw K, Haas-Kogan D, Ablin A. Intracranial germ cell tumors. In: Gupta N, Banerjee A, Haas-Kogan D, eds. Pediatric CNS Tumors. Berlin: Springer-Verlag; 2004:107–121

[2] Frazier A, Amatruda J. Pediatric germ cell tumors. In: Orkin S, Fisher D, Look A, Lux S, Ginsburg D, Nathan D, eds. Oncology of Infancy and Childhood. Philadelphia, PA: Saunders Elsevier; 2009:911–961

[3] Altman RP, Randolph JG, Lilly JR. Sacrococcygeal teratoma: American Academy of Pediatrics Surgical Section Survey-1973. J Pediatr Surg. 1974; 9(3):389–398

[4] Isaacs H, Jr. Perinatal (fetal and neonatal) germ cell tumors. J Pediatr Surg. 2004; 39(7):1003–1013

[5] Bernstein L, Smith M, Liu L, Deapen D, Friedman D. Germ cell, trophoblastic and other gonadal neoplasms. In: SEER Cancer Statistics Review. Bethesda, MD: National Cancer Institute; 2007:125–137

[6] Ries L, Smith M, Gurney J, et al. Cancer incidence and survival among children and adolescents: United States SEER Program 1975–1995. In: National Cancer Institute SP, ed. Volume 99–4649. Bethesda, MD: NIH Publication, 1999:179

[7] Jennings MT, Gelman R, Hochberg F. Intracranial germ-cell tumors: natural history and pathogenesis. J Neurosurg. 1985; 63(2):155–167

[8] Echevarría ME, Fangusaro J, Goldman S. Pediatric central nervous system germ cell tumors: a review. Oncologist. 2008; 13(6):690–699

[9] Jellinger K. Primary intracranial germ cell tumours. Acta Neuropathol. 1973; 25(4):291–306

[10] Hayashi N, Murai H, Ishihara S, et al. Nationwide investigation of the current status of therapeutic neuroendoscopy for ventricular and paraventricular tumors in Japan. J Neurosurg. 2011; 115(6):1147–1157

[11] Matsutani M, Sano K, Takakura K, et al. Primary intracranial germ cell tumors: a clinical analysis of 153 histologically verified cases. J Neurosurg. 1997; 86(3):446–455

[12] Jubran RF, Finlay J. Central nervous system germ cell tumors: controversies in diagnosis and treatment. Oncology (Williston Park). 2005; 19(6):705–711, discussion 711–712, 715–717, 721

[13] Buetow SA. Epidemiology of testicular cancer. Epidemiol Rev. 1995; 17(2):433–449

[14] Louis D, Ohgaki H, Wiestler O, Cavenee WK. WHO classification of tumours of the central nervous system. In: Louis D, Ohgaki H, Wiestler O, Cavenee WK, eds. WHO Classification of Tumours of the Central Nervous System. Albany, NY: WHO Publication System; 2007:203

[15] Packer RJ, Cohen BH, Cooney K. Intracranial germ cell tumors. Oncologist. 2000; 5(4):312–320

[16] Sano K, Matsutani M, Seto T. So-called intracranial germ cell tumours: personal experiences and a theory of their pathogenesis. Neurol Res. 1989; 11(2):118–126

[17] Sano K. Pathogenesis of intracranial germ cell tumors reconsidered. J Neurosurg. 1999; 90(2):258–264

[18] Louis DN, Ohgaki H, Wiestler OD, et al. The 2007 WHO classification of tumours of the central nervous system. Acta Neuropathol. 2007; 114(2):97–109

[19] Parsa A, Pincus D, Feldstein N, Balmaceda C, Fetel M, Bruce J. Pineal region tumors. In: Keating R, Goodrich J, Packer R, eds. Tumors of the Pediatric Central Nervous System. New York, NY: Thieme, 2001:308–325

[20] Bjornsson J, Scheithauer BW, Okazaki H, Leech RW. Intracranial germ cell tumors: pathobiological and immunohistochemical aspects of 70 cases. J Neuropathol Exp Neurol. 1985; 44(1):32–46

[21] Okada Y, Nishikawa R, Matsutani M, Louis DN. Hypomethylated X chromosome gain and rare isochromosome 12p in diverse intracranial germ cell tumors. J Neuropathol Exp Neurol. 2002; 61(6):531–538

[22] Kamakura Y, Hasegawa M, Minamoto T, Yamashita J, Fujisawa H. C-kit gene mutation: common and widely distributed in intracranial germinomas. J Neurosurg. 2006; 104(3) Suppl: 173–180

[23] Iwato M, Tachibana O, Tohma Y, et al. Alterations of the INK4a/ARF locus in human intracranial germ cell tumors. Cancer Res. 2000; 60(8):2113–2115

[24] Zimmerman RA, Bilaniuk LT. Age-related incidence of pineal calcification detected by computed tomography. Radiology. 1982; 142(3):659–662

[25] Watanabe S, Aihara Y, Kikuno A, et al. A highly sensitive and specific chemiluminescent enzyme immunoassay for placental alkaline phosphatase in the cerebrospinal fluid of patients with intracranial germinomas. Pediatr Neurosurg. 2012; 48(3):141–145

[26] Miyanohara O, Takeshima H, Kaji M, et al. Diagnostic significance of soluble c-kit in the cerebrospinal fluid of patients with germ cell tumors. J Neurosurg. 2002; 97(1): 177–183

[27] Kawaguchi T, Kumabe T, Kanamori M, et al. Logarithmic decrease of serum alpha-fetoprotein or human chorionic gonadotropin in response to chemotherapy can distinguish a subgroup with better prognosis among highly malignant intracranial non-germinomatous germ cell tumors. J Neurooncol. 2011; 104(3):779–787

[28] Boop FA. Germ cell tumors. J Neurosurg Pediatr. 2010; 6(2): 123–, discussion 124

[29] Souweidane MM, Krieger MD, Weiner HL, Finlay JL. Surgical management of primary central nervous system germ cell tumors: proceedings from the Second International Symposium on Central Nervous System Germ Cell Tumors. J Neurosurg Pediatr. 2010; 6(2):125–130

[30] Ray P, Jallo GI, Kim RY, et al. Endoscopic third ventriculostomy for tumor-related hydrocephalus in a pediatric population. Neurosurg Focus. 2005; 19(6):E8

[31] O'Brien DF, Hayhurst C, Pizer B, Mallucci CL. Outcomes in patients undergoing single-trajectory endoscopic third ventriculostomy and endoscopic biopsy for midline tumors presenting with obstructive hydrocephalus. J Neurosurg. 2006; 105(3) Suppl:219–226

[32] Constantini S, Mohanty A, Zymberg S, et al. Safety and diagnostic accuracy of neuroendoscopic biopsies: an international multicenter study. J Neurosurg Pediatr. 2013; 11(6):704–709

[33] Shono T, Natori Y, Morioka T, et al. Results of a long-term follow-up after neuroendoscopic biopsy procedure and third ventriculostomy in patients with intracranial germinomas. J Neurosurg. 2007; 107(3) Suppl:193–198

[34] Uschold T, Abla AA, Fusco D, Bristol RE, Nakaji P. Supracerebellar infratentorial endoscopically controlled resection of pineal lesions: case series and operative technique. J Neurosurg Pediatr. 2011; 8(6):554–564

[35] Luther N, Stetler WR, Jr, Dunkel IJ, Christos PJ, Wellons JC, III, Souweidane MM. Subarachnoid dissemination of intraventricular tumors following simultaneous endoscopic biopsy and third ventriculostomy. J Neurosurg Pediatr. 2010; 5 (1):61–67

[36] Milligan BD, Meyer FB. Morbidity of transcallosal and transcortical approaches to lesions in and around the lateral and third ventricles: a single-institution experience. Neurosurgery. 2010; 67(6):1483–1496, discussion 1496

[37] Luther N, Cohen A, Souweidane MM. Hemorrhagic sequelae from intracranial neuroendoscopic procedures for intraventricular tumors. Neurosurg Focus. 2005; 19(1):E9

[38] O'Kane R, Mathew R, Kenny T, Stiller C, Chumas P. United Kingdom 30-day mortality rates after surgery for pediatric central nervous system tumors. J Neurosurg Pediatr. 2013; 12 (3):227–234

[39] Hoffman HJ, Otsubo H, Hendrick EB, et al. Intracranial germ-cell tumors in children. J Neurosurg. 1991; 74(4): 545–551

[40] Balmaceda C, Heller G, Rosenblum M, et al. Chemotherapy without irradiation–a novel approach for newly diagnosed CNS germ cell tumors: results of an international cooperative trial. The First International Central Nervous System Germ Cell Tumor Study. J Clin Oncol. 1996; 14(11): 2908–2915

[41] Matsutani M, Ushio Y, Abe H, et al. Japanese Pediatric Brain Tumor Study Group. Combined chemotherapy and radiation therapy for central nervous system germ cell tumors: preliminary results of a Phase II study of the Japanese Pediatric Brain Tumor Study Group. Neurosurg Focus. 1998; 5(1):e7

[42] Kanamori M, Kumabe T, Saito R, et al. Optimal treatment strategy for intracranial germ cell tumors: a single institution analysis. J Neurosurg Pediatr. 2009; 4(6):506–514

[43] Kellie SJ, Boyce H, Dunkel IJ, et al. Primary chemotherapy for intracranial nongerminomatous germ cell tumors: results of the second international CNS germ cell study group protocol. J Clin Oncol. 2004; 22(5):846–853

[44] Robertson PL, DaRosso RC, Allen JC. Improved prognosis of intracranial non-germinoma germ cell tumors with multimodality therapy. J Neurooncol. 1997; 32(1):71–80

[45] Garrè ML, El-Hossainy MO, Fondelli P, et al. Is chemotherapy effective therapy for intracranial immature teratoma? A case report. Cancer. 1996; 77(5):977–982

[46] Modak S, Gardner S, Dunkel IJ, et al. Thiotepa-based high-dose chemotherapy with autologous stem-cell rescue in patients with recurrent or progressive CNS germ cell tumors. J Clin Oncol. 2004; 22(10):1934–1943

[47] Malone K, Croke J, Malone C, Malone S. Successful salvage using combined radiation and ABMT for patients with recurrent CNS NGGCT following failed initial transplant. BMJ Case Rep. 2012; 2012:bcr2012006298

[48] Kersh CR, Constable WC, Eisert DR, et al. Primary central nervous system germ cell tumors. Effect of histologic confirmation on radiotherapy. Cancer. 1988; 61(11):2148–2152

[49] Shirato H, Nishio M, Sawamura Y, et al. Analysis of long-term treatment of intracranial germinoma. Int J Radiat Oncol Biol Phys. 1997; 37(3):511–515

[50] Ogino H, Shibamoto Y, Takanaka T, et al. CNS germinoma with elevated serum human chorionic gonadotropin level: clinical characteristics and treatment outcome. Int J Radiat Oncol Biol Phys. 2005; 62(3):803–808

[51] Sawamura Y, Ikeda J, Shirato H, Tada M, Abe H. Germ cell tumours of the central nervous system: treatment consideration based on 111 cases and their long-term clinical outcomes. Eur J Cancer. 1998; 34(1):104–110

[52] Itoyama Y, Kochi M, Kuratsu J, et al. Treatment of intracranial nongerminomatous malignant germ cell tumors producing alpha-fetoprotein. Neurosurgery. 1995; 36(3):459–464, discussion 464–466

[53] da Silva NS, Cappellano AM, Diez B, et al. Primary chemotherapy for intracranial germ cell tumors: results of the third international CNS germ cell tumor study. Pediatr Blood Cancer. 2010; 54(3):377–383

[54] Yoo KH, Lee SH, Lee J, et al. Improved outcome of central nervous system germ cell tumors: implications for the role of risk-adapted intensive chemotherapy. J Korean Med Sci. 2010; 25(3):458–465

18 Pineal Region Tumors

Scellig S.D. Stone, Alan R. Cohen

18.1 Introduction

Pineal region tumors account for less than 1% of central nervous system tumors in adults; however, this number is upward of 3% for pediatric brain tumors.[1] The prevalence is higher in Asian countries and males (~3:1 overall male:female ratio, ~12:1 for germ cell tumors [GCTs] specifically).

18.2 Anatomy and Physiology

The pineal gland sits within the pineal region, corresponding to the posterior incisural space (▶ Fig. 18.1).[2] The pineal region contains many critical neural and vascular structures, and a work-ing knowledge of this anatomy is of critical importance in order to successful navigate its confines surgically. The borders of the pineal region include:

- **Superior:** The splenium of the corpus callosum, hippocampal commissure, and posterior aspect of the tela choroidea.
- **Anterior:** The posterior aspect of the third ventricle including the habenular and posterior commissures, between which the pineal gland attaches, and the quadrigeminal plate.
- **Inferior:** The cerebellum, mainly vermis.
- **Lateral:** The pulvinar nucleus of the thalamus and the medial cerebral hemispheres.
- **Posterior:** The tentorial apex.

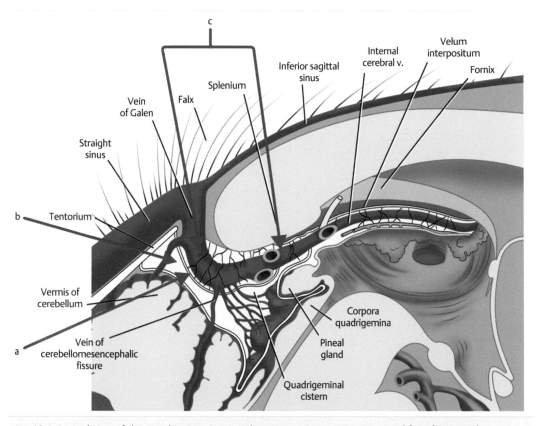

Fig. 18.1 Sagittal view of the pineal region. *Arrows* indicate approximate trajectories used for infratentorial supracerebellar **(a)** occipital transtentorial **(b)** and range of interhemispheric retrocallosal or transcallosal **(c)** surgical approaches.

Along with the gland, many critical vascular structures course through the pineal region, including:

- Arteries:
  - The posterior cerebral and superior cerebellar arteries.
  - The lateral and medial posterior choroidal arteries, the latter of which primarily supplies the pineal gland.
- Veins:
  - The vein of Galen.
  - The basal veins of Rosenthal.
  - The internal cerebral veins.
  - The internal occipital veins.
  - The vein of the cerebellomesencephalic fissure (also known as precentral cerebellar vein).

The pineal gland itself arises as a diencephalic diverticulum during embryogenesis.[3] It is mainly composed of pineocytes, melatonin-producing neurosecretory cells that are believed to regulate circadian rhythms, arranged in lobules among a fibrovascular and glial stroma. The gland typically develops radiographically visible calcifications by the second decade of life.[4]

18.3 Classification of Tumors

Pineal region tumors can be classified by identity and proportion using the following schema[1,5,6] (special note—published series generally include adults and the limited pediatric literature suggests some greater variability[7,8,9]):

- 60%—GCTs:
  - **Germinomas:** dysgerminoma, seminoma, atypical teratoma.
  - **Nongerminomatous GCTs** (NGGCTs):
    - Embryonal carcinoma.
    - Endodermal sinus tumor.
    - Choriocarcinoma.
    - Teratoma: only NGGCT either malignant or benign, more likely < age 3.
    - Mixed GCTs.
- 35%—neuroepithelial tumors:
  - **25%—pineal parenchymal tumors:**
    - Pineocytoma (WHO I) → astrocytic, neuronal or comb.
    - Differentiation more likely if > age 20.
    - Pineoblastoma (WHO IV) → pineocytic or retinoblastomatous differentiation more likely if < age 20.
    - Pineal parenchymal tumor of intermediate differentiation (WHO II, III).

- 10%—other neuroepithelial tumors:
  - Astrocytoma/glioblastoma.
  - Ependymoma.
  - Oligodendroglioma.
  - Choroid plexus papilloma/carcinoma.
  - Atypical teratoid rhabdoid tumor.
  - Papillary tumor of the pineal region (derived from subcommissural organ).
- 5%—other tumors:
  - Meningioma.
  - Hemangiopericytoma.
  - Lipoma.
  - Primary melanocytic tumors.
  - Metastases.
- Nonneoplastic lesions:
  - **Pineal cysts** (common incidental finding on autopsy or magnetic resonance imaging [MRI]).
  - **Arachnoid cyst.**
  - **Vascular malformations:**
    - Cavernous malformation.
    - Arteriovenous malformation.
    - Vein of Galen aneurysm.
  - **Dermoid/epidermoid cysts.**
  - **Infectious/inflammatory lesions** (abscess, tuberculoma, etc.).

18.4 Clinical Presentation

Pineal region tumors may present in several ways based on local mass-related and remote effects.

18.4.1 Local Mass-related Effects

- **Noncommunicating hydrocephalus** is the most common presentation:
  - Headache, vomiting, lethargy, memory disturbance, increasing head circumference, full/bulging fontanel, papilledema.
- **Parinaud's syndrome** due to quadrigeminal plate compression:
  - Supranuclear paralysis of conjugate upward gaze.
  - Light-near dissociation of accommodation (sluggish to light).
  - Paralysis of convergence.
- **Cerebellar dysfunction** due to cerebellar compression:
  - Ataxia, tremor.
- **Pineal apoplexy** manifesting as acute neurologic deterioration following hemorrhage:

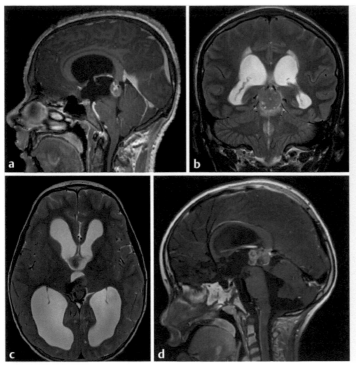

Fig. 18.2 MRI of (**a, b**) pineal region germinoma and (**c, d**) pineoblastoma. (**a**) Sagittal contrast-enhanced T1-weighted MRI demonstrating tandem pineal and suprasellar enhancing lesions. (**b**) Coronal T2-weighted image demonstrating lateral ventricular enlargement with transependymal flow, and displacement of the internal cerebral veins above and basal veins of Rosenthal laterally to the lesion. (**c**) Axial T2-weighted MRI demonstrating a mass in the posterior third ventricle/pineal region with associated hydrocephalus. The internal cerebral veins can be seen as flow voids draped over the posterior aspect of the lesion bilaterally. (**d**) Heterogeneously enhancing mass in the posterior third ventricle/pineal region.

- Headache, nausea, emesis, meningismus, visual disturbance, decreased level of consciousness.

18.4.2 Remote Effects

- Endocrinological disturbances:
  - Precocious puberty (luteinizing hormone–like effect of beta-human chorionic gonadotropin [beta-HCG] secretion).
  - Diabetes insipidus (DI; strong association with GCTs).
- *Radiculopathy/myelopathy* due to cerebrospinal fluid (CSF) seeding and drop metastases.
- *Symptoms of concomitant tumors*:
  - Retinoblastomas may occur in combination with pineoblastomas, referred to as "trilateral tumor."
  - Pineal region germinomas may present with a symptomatic suprasellar tandem lesion (DI, visual disturbance, hypopituitarism).

18.5 Investigations

18.5.1 Imaging

Contrast-enhanced craniospinal MRI is generally indicated to evaluate the lesion and look for evidence

of tandem or disseminated disease (▶ Fig. 18.2). Computed tomography (CT) may demonstrate characteristic patterns of calcification:

- Pineal parenchymal tumors may push or "explode" existing calcifications peripherally.
- Other tumors, such as germinomas, may "engulf" the calcified gland.

Calcification of the pineal gland prior to age 10 may suggest pathology; however, physiologic calcification has been reported at younger ages and thus should be interpreted with caution.[4] Choriocarcinoma has a tendency for hemorrhagic presentation.

18.5.2 Laboratory

GCT markers can narrow the diagnosis of pineal region tumors, although mixed GCTs may complicate interpretation.[10] Serum markers should be sent on all patients as they are nearly as sensitive as direct CSF sampling. In cases without obstructive hydrocephalus, CSF may be sampled by lumbar puncture for markers and cytology. Potentially useful markers include:

- Alpha-fetoprotein (AFP) → predominance suggests endodermal sinus (also known as "yolk sac") tumor

- Beta-HCG → predominance suggests choriocarcinoma.
- Placental alkaline phosphatase → predominance suggests germinoma.

Positive markers are diagnostic for malignant GCTs and obviate the need for a tissue diagnosis. Serial testing of markers can also provide a useful means of monitoring response to therapy and detecting occult metastases. In certain cases, it may also be useful to complete a full endocrine workup, including tests of pituitary function.

18.6 Management

A sellar/suprasellar lesion, midbrain compression, or obstructive hydrocephalus should prompt a formal ophthalmological evaluation. Emergent hydrocephalus may necessitate ventriculostomy placement for stabilization.

The presence of classic-appearing tandem or bifocal tumors in the pineal and suprasellar regions, without elevation of markers, is considered diagnostic for germinoma and generally negates the need for a tissue diagnosis. With classic appearance on imaging, upfront open resection should be considered for certain cases, such as meningioma, teratoma, and epidermoid. In all other scenarios, a tissue diagnosis is needed.

In the setting of hydrocephalus, endoscopic transventricular biopsy and CSF sampling for markers are preferred. Symptomatic obstructive hydrocephalus may be simultaneously treated by endoscopic third ventriculostomy (ETV), thus avoiding a shunt with subsequent potential for abdominal seeding of malignancy.

In the absence of hydrocephalus, stereotactic biopsy and/or cyst drainage is an option in experienced hands, with one large series of 370 patients indicating a diagnostic yield of 94%, morbidity of 8.1%, and mortality of 1.3%.[11] However, proximity with critical venous structures limits its use by many centers. Sampling error can also theoretically complicate any procedure involving minimal tissue sampling.

When less invasive tissue sampling is not applicable and a pathognomonic imaging/marker diagnosis is not made, open biopsy with CSF sampling should be considered.

18.7 Treatment and Outcomes

Overall treatment options include serial observation, surgical resection, focal and/or craniospinal radiation, and chemotherapy. These modalities are used in isolation or combination depending on the specific histopathologic diagnosis, and vary by institution. Typical treatments and outcomes for key tumors are summarized in ▶ Table 18.1.[5,6,12,13]

18.8 Endoscopic and Microsurgical Approaches

Although stereotactic biopsy is an option (see Management section), surgical treatment more commonly involves endoscopy or open microsurgery to achieve CSF diversion as needed, obtain a diagnosis, and resect the lesion when appropriate.

18.8.1 Anterior Neuroendoscopic

Endoscopic transventricular surgery, pioneered in the 1970s by Fukushima for the purpose of tumor biopsy, can permit sampling of CSF, treatment of hydrocephalus, and biopsy of pineal tumors.[14,15] Complete resection is precluded by the limited ability to achieve hemostasis, confined approach angles, and the small number and size of available instruments.

The patient is placed supine with a flexed neck. Generally, the nondominant hemisphere is transgressed. Planned entry points for tumor biopsy in the posterior third ventricle/pineal region are generally at or just medial to the midpupillary line, several centimeters anterior to the coronal suture, and can be refined using neuronavigation to visualize access to the lesion via straight passage through the foramen of Monro. In contrast, the optimal entry point for an ETV is more posterior, near the coronal suture. Rigid endoscopes generally provide the best optics and potentially most working ports for instrument flexibility; however, separate entry points may be required if both an ETV and tumor biopsy are performed. The use of a single burr hole somewhere between these optimal sites and angled scopes may resolve this issue (▶ Fig. 18.3).[16] Alternatively, a flexible endoscope can be used. Care must be taken to avoid retraction injury to the fornices. If needed, an ETV is

Table 18.1 Treatment strategies and outcomes for selected pineal region tumors

Tumor	Typical treatment strategy (*other options*)	Outcomes
GCTs		
Germinoma	Local radiation, craniospinal radiation + local boost, ± chemotherapy (*with lowered radiation dose*)	80–95% 5-y OS
Mature teratoma (congenital form)	Surgical resection	80–95% 5-y OS >90% mortality
Immature teratoma + malignant component	Surgical resection + local radiation, surgical resection alone (*+ craniospinal radiation + chemotherapy*) Surgical resection + craniospinal radiation (*+ local boost + chemotherapy*)	60–70% 5-y OS
Other malignant NGGCT	Craniospinal radiation + local boost ± surgical resection ± chemotherapy	25% 5-y OS
Pineal parenchymal tumors		
Pineocytoma	Initial observation, surgical resection (*+ local radiation or local radiation alone if < 3 cm*)	80–90% 5-y OS
Intermediate differentiation	Low grade: surgical resection (*+ chemotherapy ± radiation*) High grade: surgical resection + chemotherapy + radiation	75% 5-y OS 40% 5-y OS
Pineoblastoma	Craniospinal radiation + local boost + chemotherapy (*± surgical resection*)	10–20% 5-y OS, less if + CSF
Other notable tumors		
Low-grade glioma	Observation or individualized multimodality	75% 5-y OS
High-grade glioma	Radiation + chemotherapy (*± surgical resection*)	10% 5-y OS

Abbreviations: CSF, cerebrospinal fluid; GCTs, germ cell tumors; NGGCT, nongerminomatous germ cell tumor; OS, overall survival.

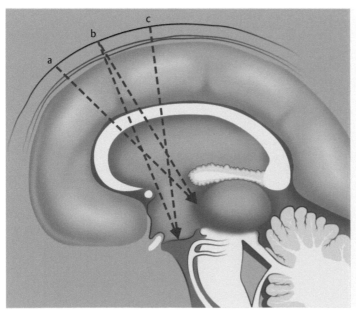

Fig. 18.3 Anterior neuroendoscopic trajectories as projected onto the midsagittal plane. The lateral position, typically at or just medial to the midpupillary line, is not depicted. **(a)** Optimal burr hole location for straight trajectory to biopsy posterior third ventricular lesion, **(b)** intervening entry point to permit both biopsy and third ventriculostomy, and **(c)** optimal burr hole location for third ventriculostomy.

generally performed prior to tumor biopsy because bleeding post biopsy can obscure visualization of anatomical landmarks. The success of endoscopic biopsy may be negatively affected by limited tissue sampling, although direct visualization of the lesion allows selective sampling from multiple regions. An external ventricular drain may be left in place when ETV function is uncertain or following excessive intraventricular hemorrhage.

18.8.2 Microsurgery

Although multiple options and variances exist, two main open approaches to the pineal region are most commonly used: the infratentorial supracerebellar and occipital transtentorial approaches (▶ Fig. 18.1).[15,17] A parietal posterior interhemispheric and other routes are also discussed briefly. The choice of approach is partially dictated by the extent of the lesion, its relationship to critical neurovascular structures in the pineal region, the goal(s) of surgery, and surgeon familiarity/comfort.

Infratentorial Supracerebellar

Pioneered by Krause and further refined/popularized by Stein in the early 1900s, this approach lends itself to small- to medium-sized lesions that are largely confined to the pineal region and below the vein of Galen.[18,19] Following the natural plane between the cerebellum and tentorium minimizes brain retraction (▶ Fig. 18.1).

Positioning

If performed using the sitting position, cerebellar retraction and venous pressure can be minimized, although downsides include the risk of venous embolism and surgeon discomfort. The prone position with neck flexion (or "Concorde" position) lessens the risk of venous embolism but necessitates cerebellar retraction in most cases. A modified lateral position can be employed to balance the pros and cons of these alternatives, although anatomic orientation may be less familiar.

Dissection

Through a midline skin incision, a bone flap is elevated extending just above the transverse sinus to the foramen magnum, with care taken to protect the torcular and transverse sinuses. The dura mater is opened with an inverse semicircular incision, based at the transverse sinuses, extending the full width of the craniotomy. Bridging veins from the midline superior cerebellar surface to the tentorium are sacrificed as needed; however, postoperative cerebellar venous congestion and swelling may occur if lateral veins are taken in excess. The precentral cerebellar vein and associated thick arachnoid membrane are typically taken and opened respectively, gaining exposure to the lesion (▶ Fig. 18.4).

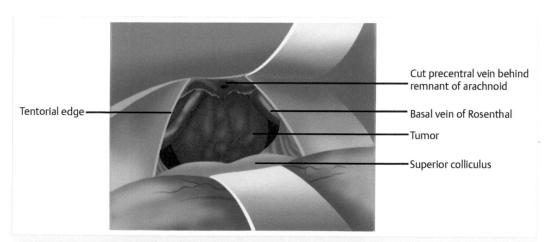

Tentorial edge

Cut precentral vein behind remnant of arachnoid

Basal vein of Rosenthal

Tumor

Superior colliculus

Fig. 18.4 View of a pineal region tumor after arachnoid opening from an infratentorial supracerebellar approach. Note the cerebellum retracted inferiorly.

Occipital Transtentorial

Initially described by Heppner in 1959 and later modified by Jamieson, this approach allows access to relatively large lesions extending beyond the pineal region and into the third ventricle and lesions in the region of the cerebellomesencephalic cistern (▶ Fig. 18.1).[20,21]

Positioning

The prone position with relatively neutral neck flexion allows a surgical trajectory perpendicular to the floor and generally provides the easiest orientation. Alternatively, a semi-lateral position may be used to allow gravity to retract the cerebral hemisphere.

Dissection

The skin incision can take the form of a three-sided flap designed to preserve scalp blood supply, or a paramedian incision with a superolaterally curved extension allowing lateral/inferior reflection of the scalp. A large bone flap is elevated extending just below and across the transverse and superior sagittal sinuses, respectively, allowing dural reflection across each. Bridging veins draining the occipital lobe into the superior sagittal sinus are generally safely anterior, but some entering the transverse sinus may partially obstruct access and warrant consideration of either limited sacrifice or a contralateral approach. An occipital ventriculostomy allows greater decompression of the ipsilateral occipital lobe and thus less chance of retraction injury. The tentorium is divided as needed from anterior to posterior, staying lateral to the straight and stopping short of the transverse sinuses (▶ Fig. 18.5). Further contralateral exposure can be gained by dividing the inferior sagittal sinus and incising the falx.

Posterior Interhemispheric Transcallosal and/or Retrocallosal

Originated by Dandy in the 1920s and later modified by others including McComb, this is primarily an option for lesions truly in the posterior third ventricle that push the internal cerebral veins posteriorly and inferiorly such that the lower angle associated with the above approaches would require excessive mobilization of the veins (▶ Fig. 18.1).[22,23]

Positioning

The patient may be placed prone with slight neck extension. Semi-prone positioning can be used to promote gravity retraction of the cerebral hemisphere, although orientation is more challenging. Preoperative assessment of bridging vein anatomy can help determine the optimal side of approach, with preference to the nondominant side if veins are not an issue.

Dissection

A coronally oriented straight skin incision across midline, or inverted U across midline and reflected inferolaterally, can be used to both maximize exposure and preserve scalp blood supply. A large bone flap over the vertex and extending across

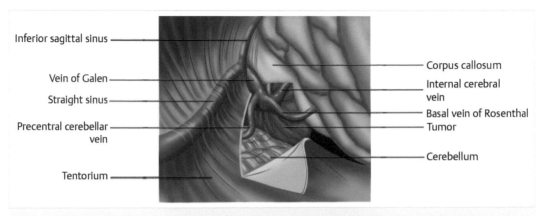

Fig. 18.5 View of pineal region tumor after dividing tentorium and opening arachnoid from a right occipital transtentorial approach.

midline allows greater flexibility to avoid bridging veins and alter trajectory. The dura is reflected over the superior sagittal sinus. After confirming trajectory and identifying/protecting the pericallosal arteries, a limited callosotomy or subsplenial approach is used to access the lesion.

Posterior Transcortical, Posterior Subtemporal, Paramedian Supracerebellar, Combined

These are rarely used due to the extent of brain transgressed, need for temporal lobe retraction, invasiveness, and/or limited exposure.[15,17] A transcortical approach is reserved for select cases with a very dilated lateral ventricle and is generally performed through a high parietal transcortical route in order to minimize injury to the visual pathways. For large lesions with significant anterior extension, a combined or staged approach using both a posterior pineal and an anterior route to the third ventricle may be needed.

18.9 Complications

The nature and expected frequency of complications related to surgical management of pineal tumors vary widely depending on the nature of individual lesions and the approach selected. Most modern series report permanent morbidity and mortality rates below 10%.[24]

Venous sinus injury during exposure can lead to air embolism, thus experienced anesthesia, blood product availability, a plan for management, and the use of end-tidal carbon dioxide and cardiac doppler monitors are recommended. Venous insufficiency and infarction can result from excessive interruption of cerebellar venous drainage, anterior occipital/posterior parietal/lateral occipital bridging veins. In the case of the cerebellum, this can lead to postoperative swelling with obstructive hydrocephalus or tonsillar herniation. Deep venous injury must be avoided and can lead to severe morbidity or mortality. Direct or indirect injury to brain regions from venous or arterial insufficiency, or retraction injury, can cause focal neurologic deficits such as cerebellar dysfunction, contralateral hemianopia due to visual cortex or optic radiation injury, contralateral hemiparesis, and contralateral sensory deficits including stereognosis. Retraction injury can be minimized through the use of temporary CSF drainage via lumbar drain or

ventriculostomy and/or hyperosmolar therapy. A corpus callosotomy of less than 2 cm in length is generally well tolerated; however, injury can rarely lead to disconnection syndromes. Excision of lesions closely abutting or involving the midbrain frequently results in at least transient extraocular movement abnormalities including impaired upgaze and convergence.

In the immediate postoperative period, intensive care unit monitoring is required with particular attention paid to signs of hemorrhage (particularly when an incomplete resection has been performed) and hydrocephalus. Should concern exist over the potential for seizures secondary to cortical injury, one may consider a prophylactic antiepileptic in the immediate postoperative period. A short course of peri- and postoperative steroids may be considered if considerable cerebral swelling is anticipated.

18.10 Common Clinical Questions

1. How do pineal region lesions typically present clinically?
2. Which pineal region lesions classically present with marked and relatively specific elevated serum and/or CSF AFP, and beta-HCG?
3. What features of a pineal region lesion may help a surgeon decide between using a supracerebellar infratentorial versus occipital transtentorial approach?
4. Name five pineal region tumors for which complete surgical resection is often the sole treatment.

18.11 Answers to Common Clinical Questions

1. Clinical features include: local mass-related effects (including symptoms of raised intracranial pressure due to hydrocephalus, Parinaud's syndrome due to quadrigeminal plate compression, cerebellar dysfunction due to compression, and less commonly pineal apoplexy following hemorrhage), remote effects (including endocrinological disturbances such as precocious puberty and DI, and radiculopathy/myelopathy due to CSF seeding), and symptoms of concomitant tumors (including ocular symptoms due to retinoblastoma or suprasellar lesions).

2. A marked and relatively specific elevation of AFP is classically seen with endodermal sinus tumors, and beta-HCG with choriocarcinoma.

3. The supracerebellar infratentorial approach lends itself to small- to medium-sized lesions that are largely confined to the pineal region and below the vein of Galen. The occipital transtentorial may be more appropriate for large lesions extending beyond the pineal region and into the third ventricle, or into cerebellomesencephalic cistern.

4. Complete surgical resection can be curative for many pineal region tumors. Examples include: meningioma, epidermoid, mature teratoma, pineocytoma, intermediately differentiated pineal parenchymal tumor with low-grade features, and low-grade glioma.

References

[1] Al-Hussaini M, Sultan I, Abuirmileh N, Jaradat I, Qaddoumi I. Pineal gland tumors: experience from the SEER database. J Neurooncol. 2009; 94(3):351–358

[2] Rhoton AL, Jr. Tentorial incisura. Neurosurgery. 2000; 47(3) Suppl:S131–S153

[3] Sadler TW. Langman's Medical Embryology. 9th ed. Philadelphia, PA: Lippincott Williams & Wilkins; 2004:534

[4] Barkovich AJ. Diagnostic Imaging Pediatric Neuroradiology. Salt Lake City, UT: Amirsys; 2007

[5] Louis DN. WHO Classification of Tumours of the Central Nervous System. 4th ed. Lyon: International Agency for Research on Cancer; 2007

[6] Perry A, Brat DJ. Practical Surgical Neuropathology: A Diagnostic Approach. Philadelphia, PA: Churchill Livingstone/ Elsevier; 2010

[7] Bailey S, Skinner R, Lucraft HH, Perry RH, Todd N, Pearson AD. Pineal tumours in the north of England 1968–93. Arch Dis Child. 1996; 75(3):181–185

[8] Edwards MS, Hudgins RJ, Wilson CB, Levin VA, Wara WM. Pineal region tumors in children. J Neurosurg. 1988; 68(5): 689–697

[9] Kang JK, Jeun SS, Hong YK, et al. Experience with pineal region tumors. Childs Nerv Syst. 1998; 14(1–2):63–68

[10] Bernstein M, Berger MS. Neuro-oncology: The Essentials. 2nd ed. New York, NY: Thieme; 2008

[11] Regis J, Bouillot P, Rouby-Volot F, Figarella-Branger D, Dufour H, Peragut JC. Pineal region tumors and the role of stereotactic biopsy: review of the mortality, morbidity, and diagnostic rates in 370 cases. Neurosurgery. 1996; 39(5): 907–912, discussion 912–914

[12] Villano JL, Propp JM, Porter KR, et al. Malignant pineal germ-cell tumors: an analysis of cases from three tumor registries. Neuro-oncol. 2008; 10(2):121–130

[13] Schild SE, Scheithauer BW, Haddock MG, et al. Histologically confirmed pineal tumors and other germ cell tumors of the brain. Cancer. 1996; 78(12):2564–2571

[14] Fukushima T, Ishijima B, Hirakawa K, Nakamura N, Sano K. Ventriculofiberscope: a new technique for endoscopic diagnosis and operation. Technical note. J Neurosurg. 1973; 38(2):251–256

[15] Little KM, Friedman AH, Fukushima T. Surgical approaches to pineal region tumors. J Neurooncol. 2001; 54(3):287–299

[16] Robinson S, Cohen AR. The role of neuroendoscopy in the treatment of pineal region tumors. Surg Neurol. 1997; 48(4): 360–365, discussion 365–367

[17] Yamamoto I. Pineal region tumor: surgical anatomy and approach. J Neurooncol. 2001; 54(3):263–275

[18] Bruce JN, Stein BM. The infratentorial supracerebellar approach. In: Apuzzo MLJ, ed. Surgery of the Third Ventricle. 2nd ed. Baltimore, MD: Williams & Wilkins; 1998:697–719

[19] Krause F. Chirurgie des Gehirns und Rückenmarks nach eigenen Erfahrungen. Berlin: Urban & Schwarzenberg; 1911

[20] Jamieson KG. Excision of pineal tumors. J Neurosurg. 1971; 35(5):550–553

[21] Heppner F. On operation technic in pinealoma [in German]. Zentralbl Neurochir. 1959; 19:219–224

[22] McComb JG, Levy ML, Apuzzo MLJ. The posterior interhemispheric retrocallosal and transcallosal approaches to the third ventricle region. In: Apuzzo MLJ, ed. Surgery of the Third Ventricle. 2nd ed. Baltimore, MD: Williams & Wilkins; 1998:743–777

[23] Dandy WE. An operation for the removal of pineal tumors. Surg Gynecol Obstet. 1921; 33:113–119

[24] Bruce JN. Pineal tumors. In: Winn HR, ed. Youmans Neurological Surgery. Vol 2. 6th ed. Philadelphia, PA: Elsevier Saunders; 2011:1359–1372

19 Intraventricular Tumors in Children

Bryan S. Lee, Vikram B. Chakravarthy, Nir Shimony, Violette M.R. Recinos

19.1 Introduction

Intraventricular tumors are rare primary central nervous system (CNS) neoplasms located within the ventricular system; these tumors occur more commonly in the pediatric population and make up 16% of all pediatric intracranial tumors.[1] Intraventricular tumors can be categorized into primary and secondary intraventricular tumors, depending on their origin. Primary tumors develop from within the ventricle, arising from the ependyma, subependymal glia of the ventricle, and choroid plexus, which include ependymoma, choroid plexus papilloma (CPP) and choroid plexus carcinoma (CPC), subependymal giant cell astrocytoma (SEGA), subependymoma, central neurocytoma, and intraventricular astrocytoma and meningioma.[2,3] Secondary tumors are also called paraventricular tumors that develop from the brain parenchyma, and bulge into the ventricle (greater than two thirds of the tumor volume by definition).[2] They include medulloblastoma, meningioma, astrocytoma, lymphoma, craniopharyngioma, and germ cell tumors. The most common intraventricular tumors in the pediatric population are ependymoma, CPP, and astrocytomas located in the lateral and frontal horns.[4] Other less common tumors include SEGA, oligodendroglioma, subependymoma, pilocytic astrocytoma in the cerebellum, neurocytoma, and CPC.[4] Pilocytic astrocytoma is considered the most common pediatric brain tumor, comprising 15% of pediatric brain tumors.[5] Pilocytic astrocytoma, however, is paraventricular in location and, therefore, comprises only a small fraction of all pediatric intraventricular tumors.[6]

- The incidence of pediatric cancer, including brain tumors, has increased over the last three decades.[7]
- Intraventricular tumors compose 0.8 to 1.6% of all pediatric CNS tumors. The majority of intraventricular tumors are benign.[4]
- Within the lateral ventricle, approximately 43% occur in the frontal horn and foramen of Monro, whereas 22% occur in the body and septum pellucidum, 20% in the atrium, 9% in the temporal horn, and 6% in the occipital horn.[3,8]
- Lateral ventricular tumors in younger children are most commonly CPPs and CPCs, where in the older pediatric group low-grade gliomas,

including ependymomas, pilocytic astrocytomas, and SEGAs, are more frequently found.[9]
- Genetic predisposition has been shown to be associated with intracranial tumors, and most of these congenital syndromes are transmitted as autosomal dominant traits within tumor suppressor genes.[4] Neurofibromatosis type I is associated with pilocytic astrocytoma, neurofibromatosis type II with ependymoma, tuberous sclerosis with SEGA, Turcot's syndrome with astrocytoma, Li–Fraumeni syndrome with malignant astrocytoma, and rhabdoid predisposition syndrome with CPC.[10]

19.2 Ependymoma

- Incidence and epidemiology: Ependymomas are circumscribed tumors that usually arise from the floor of the fourth ventricle, whereas in adults these tumors more commonly involve the spinal cord, and are commonly associated with calcification, hemorrhage, and cysts.[4] Ependymomas that occasionally grow out of the fourth ventricle through foramina of Luschka and Magendie to involve the cisterns are categorized as plastic ependymomas.[11] Ependymoma is a rare tumor with the incidence of 2.1 to 2.5 per 1 million children younger than 15 years of age; however, it is one of the most common intraventricular tumor in the pediatric population.[4,12]
- Prognosis: The time of diagnosis is known to determine the outcome in patients with ependymoma, likely secondary to lower rate of complete resection, no radiation therapy, and aggressive nature of the tumor itself.[13] The extent of resection is considered to be the most significant prognostic factor: 5-year overall survival (OS) for patients undergoing gross total resection is 66%, whereas it is 25% for subtotal resection.[14] Three-year progression-free survival rate for patients surgically treated overall was 26%.[15]
- Histopathology and neuroradiology: Most ependymomas are World Health Organization (WHO) grade II lesions and are well-delineated uniform cells with moderate cellularity and monomorphic round nuclei.[16] These cells exhibit perivascular pseudorosettes, also known as

Homer Wright rosettes, more commonly than true ependymal rosettes, also known as Flexner–Wintersteiner rosettes, and are typically GFAP positive (▶ Fig. 19.1). Ependymomas are well-demarcated lesions that are hypointense on T1-weighted magnetic resonance imaging (MRI) and hyperintense on T2-weighted MRI, with heterogeneous enhancement with gadolinium administration (▶ Fig. 19.2).[17]

19.3 Choroid Plexus Papilloma and Carcinoma

- Incidence and epidemiology: CPPs occur predominantly in the lateral ventricle in children, more specifically in the left atrium,

contrary to the fourth ventricular location in adults.[14,18] CPP tumors occur most frequently in pediatric patients younger than 3 years of age, and comprise approximately 0.5% of all intracranial tumors but almost 12% of all pediatric brain tumors for children younger than 2 years of age.[14]
- Prognosis: CPP treated surgically with complete resection is known to have 5-year survival rate of approximately 100%.[14] CPCs are frequently invasive with a relatively poor prognosis, with a 5-year OS rate of 40 to 50%.[18,19]
- Histopathology and neuroradiology: Histological hallmarks of CPP include single layer of cuboidal epithelial cells around a fibrovascular core, and positive staining for cytokeratin, GFAP, vimentin, and S100 (▶ Fig. 19.3). Whereas ependymomas

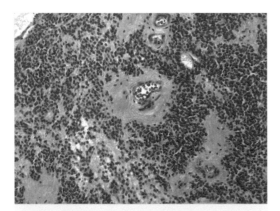

Fig. 19.1 Histopathology of ependymoma exhibiting perivascular pseudorosettes, also known as Homer Wright rosettes.

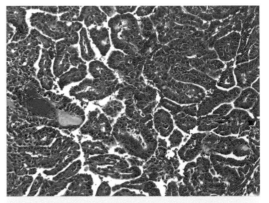

Fig. 19.3 Histopathology of CPP showing single layers of cuboidal epithelial cells around a fibrovascular core.

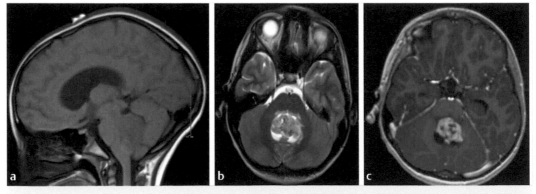

Fig. 19.2 MRI of ependymoma, demonstrating **(a)** a well-demarcated lesion hypo-/isointense on T1-weighted sagittal sequence and **(b)** hyperintense on T2-weighted axial sequence, **(c)** with heterogeneous enhancement with gadolinium on T1-weighted axial sequence.

are uniformly GFAP positive, CPPs are diffusely but not uniformly GFAP positive.[20] CPC is an aggressive neoplasm that is typically characterized by cellular anaplasia, nuclear pleomorphism, prominent mitoses, necrosis, and overall loss of differentiated papillary choroid structure.[20] CPCs retain cytokeratin positivity but less typically stain with S100.[21] CPP and CPC are both hypointense on T1-weighted sequence and hyperintense on T2-weighted sequence, with homogeneous enhancement with gadolinium administration (▶ Fig. 19.4 and ▶ Fig. 19.5).

19.4 Subependymoma

- Incidence and epidemiology: 82% of patients are older than 15 years of age, with majority being middle-aged and older males. Often found at autopsy in asymptomatic patients. Most are found to be smaller than 2 cm in size with symptomatic lesions measuring 3 to 5 cm in diameter. Patients commonly present with symptoms secondary to hydrocephalus, due to ventricular obstruction.[22]

- Prognosis: Benign lesions (WHO grade I) with low recurrence rate after gross total resection. Extraventricular extension is very rare.[23] Even with partial resection, postoperative adjuvant radiation or chemotherapy is not indicated due to a low risk for recurrence.

- Histopathology and neuroradiology: Subependymomas are typically found in the fourth ventricle and exhibit clusters of small nuclei in a dense fibrillary background of neuroglial fibers, often described as "islands of blue in a sea of pink"

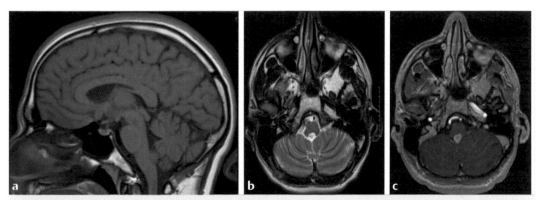

Fig. 19.4 MRI of CPP showing hypo-/isointense on **(a)** T1-weighted sagittal sequence and **(b)** hyperintense on T2-weighted axial sequence, **(c)** with homogeneous enhancement with gadolinium on T1-weighted axial sequence.

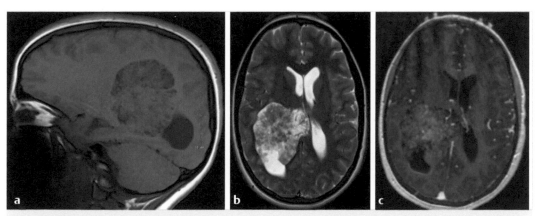

Fig. 19.5 MRI of CPC demonstrating **(a)** hypointensity on T1-weighted sagittal sequence and **(b)** hyperintensity on T2-weighted axial sequence, **(c)** with enhancement with gadolinium on T1-weighted axial sequence.

(► Fig. 19.6).[24,25] On MRI, they appear hypointense on T1-weighted sequence and hyperintense on T2-weighted sequence. Subependymoma in the lateral ventricles is the only intraventricular tumor that does not enhance with gadolinium administration on T1-weighted sequence.[24] Subependymoma in the fourth ventricle, however, can have heterogeneous contrast enhancement (► Fig. 19.7).[26] Calcification is present in 31% and cystic lesions are present in 18%.

19.5 Subependymal Giant Cell Astrocytoma

- Incidence and epidemiology: Most common neoplasm associated with tuberous sclerosis (20%), arising in the first two decades of life,

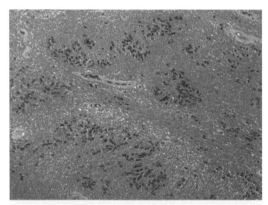

Fig. 19.6 Histopathology of subependymoma exhibiting clusters of small nuclei in a dense fibrillary background of neuroglial fibers.

typically presenting with seizures. SEGAs are slow-growing glioneuronal tumors, usually 2 to 3 cm at time of diagnosis, which eventually lead to ventricular obstructions.

- Prognosis: Benign (WHO grade I) tumors. Earlier diagnosis is associated with increased survival. Open-label, prospective clinical trial over 5 years demonstrated effectiveness of everolimus in preventing the growth of SEGA lesions with no significant toxicities or side effects. In this study, no patients progressed to requiring surgical intervention.[27]

- Histopathology and neuroradiology: SEGAs are located near the foramen of Monro. They are composed of relatively large cells that resemble gemistocytic astrocytes, but often have "ganglioid" nuclei with prominent nucleoli and elongated fibrillar processes.[28] Nuclear pleomorphism and mitoses may be present; however, they do not indicate anaplastic change. Immunohistochemistry demonstrates both glial- and neuronal-associated antigens.[28] On computed tomography (CT), SEGA appears iso- to hypodense with presence of calcifications. At times, they can be hyperdense, indicating presence of hemorrhage. On MRI, it demonstrates avidly contrast-enhancing mass in T1-weighted image, located at or near the foramen of Monro.[22]

19.6 Central Neurocytoma

- Incidence and epidemiology: Most commonly occur in older children and young adults, extremely rare in the pediatric age group,

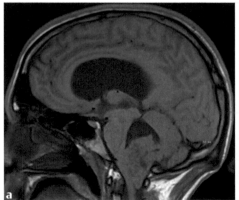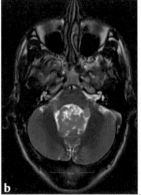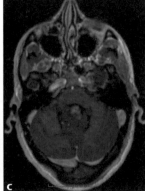

Fig. 19.7 MRI of subependymoma demonstrating (a) iso-/hypointensity on T1-weighted sagittal sequence and (b) iso-/hyperintensity on T2-weighted axial sequence, (c) with mild enhancement with gadolinium on T1-weighted axial sequence.

presenting with symptoms of elevated intracranial pressure. The median age in affected children is 16 years.[29] Constitute 0.25 to 0.5% of all intracranial tumors. Clinical presentation includes symptoms arising from elevated intracranial pressure, such as headaches, nausea/emesis, and visual deficits.

- Prognosis: Low-grade tumor (WHO II), good prognosis with surgical excision being the mainstay of treatment. Complete tumor removal leads to better tumor control and survival. There is little evidence of the use of adjuvant radiotherapy in children. However, after subtotal resections adjuvant radiotherapy can aid in local tumor control. Extraventricular extension is associated with poor prognosis. The atypical variant demonstrates increased Ki-67 activity leading to aggressive biologic behavior.[23]

- Histopathology and neuroradiology: Arising from the third or lateral ventricle in the region of the foramen of Monro with attachment to the septum pellucidum commonly. Composed of small, well-differentiated neurons with uniform round nuclei, fine chromatin, and occasional nucleoli in a loose neuropil-like background. Fixation artifact may demonstrate perinuclear clearing. Hematoxylin–eosin staining demonstrates immunoreactivity for synaptophysin and neuron-specific enolase. Atypical variant can present with microvascular proliferation, focal necrosis, and elevated mitotic activity.[28] On CT, calcifications are routinely found. On MRI, these tumors are T1 iso- to hypointense and T2 iso- to hyperintense, with mild to moderate heterogeneous contrast enhancement (▶ Fig. 19.8).[30]

19.7 Clinical Presentation

Clinical symptoms of intraventricular tumors are secondary to obstructive hydrocephalus from obstruction of cerebrospinal fluid (CSF) flow, or secondary to nonobstructive, communicating hydrocephalus from overproduction of CSF. Typical manifestations of hydrocephalus include headache, nausea, emesis, vision changes, papilledema, and altered mental status. In the younger age group, common signs and symptoms also include increased head circumference, irritability, and failure to thrive. More than half the pediatric patients younger than 2 years of age present with tense fontanelles, macrocrania, and diastasis of the cranial sutures.[14] Relatively uncommon features include seizures, memory loss due to mass effect on the fornix, and spontaneous hemorrhage.[8]

- The majority of tumors of the lateral and third ventricles are benign. Typically, clinical symptoms do not appear until the lesions enlarge to the size of a few centimeters causing mass effect on adjacent parenchyma.[31]

19.8 Surgical Approach and Techniques

Both primary and secondary intraventricular tumors can be removed via either standard open craniotomy or endoscopic approach. Traditionally, transcortical approach has been used, but more recently, transcallosal-interhemispheric approach is favored as it can provide direct access to the ventricles without passing through significant amounts of parenchyma.[32] Surgical approaches to

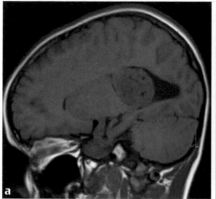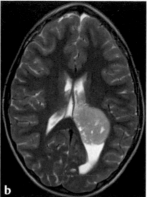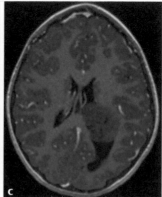

Fig. 19.8 MRI of central neurocytoma appearing **(a)** iso-/hypointense on T1-weighted sagittal sequence, **(b)** iso- to hyperintense on T2-weighted axial sequence, and **(c)** with mild heterogeneous gadolinium enhancement on T1-weighted axial sequence.

intraventricular tumors are summarized in the following (▸ Table 19.1).

- **Lateral ventricular tumors:** Anterior transsulcal approach, posterior transsulcal approach, posterior transcallosal approach, posterior temporal approach, and inferior temporal approach can be employed.
  - Anterior transsulcal (transsuperior frontal sulcus) approach is frequently used for tumors located in the anterior lateral ventricles and preferable for lesions with large, midline-draining cortical veins.[31]
  - Posterior transsulcal approach, in which craniotomy extends over the superior parietal lobule, is the preferred method to gain access to the atrium of the lateral ventricle. One should be careful not to injure the optic radiations in the lateral wall of the atrium.
  - Posterior transcallosal approach can provide easy access to the roof and medial portion of the atrium by splitting the splenium of the corpus callosum, but due to high risk of alexia, this approach should not be used in patients with homonymous hemianopsia contralateral to the dominant hemisphere.[31]
  - Posterior temporal approach provides access to the lateral part of the atrium, and as it exposes above the plane of the transverse sinus, care should be taken not to injure the vein of Labbé.
  - Inferior temporal approach is commonly used to gain access to tumors located in the temporal horns.
- **Anterior third ventricular tumors:** Transforaminal and interforniceal approach, lateral subfrontal approach, pterional approach, and endoscopic approach can be used.
  - Anterior transcallosal approach is the most frequently used as it provides several paths of dissection to open into the third ventricle without injuring the cortical tissue.[31] Lesions that are located anterior to the foramen of Monro and inferior to the third ventricle may not be easily accessible with this approach.[8]
  - Lateral subfrontal approach is useful for midline suprasellar and anterior third ventricular tumors.[8]
  - Pterional approach is used to gain access to suprasellar tumors that extend into the anterior third ventricle.[8]
  - Endoscopic approach is a suitable option for intraventricular tumors due to fluid-filled nature of the ventricles and the possibility of biopsy under direct visualization, and the ability to open obstruction via fenestration to restore normal CSF flow.[33] The risks and limitations of endoscopic approach include high bleeding risk due to no surrounding brain parenchyma to tamponade, the inability to remove tumors with high vascularity and fibrous consistency, and the possibility of the tumor being engulfed by adjacent neurovascular structures that cannot be mobilized.[2,31]
- **Posterior third ventricular tumors:** Transcallosal transvelum interpositum approach, infratentorial supracerebellar approach, and occipital transtentorial approach may be used.[31]
  - Transcallosal transvelum interpositum approach allows the choroidal dissection, removal, and reflection to gain visibility and to minimize contact with vessels.
  - Infratentorial supracerebellar approach is suitable for midline tumors in the pineal region as it avoids the need for retraction of the cerebral hemispheres.
  - Occipital transtentorial approach is useful for lesions with supra- or infratentorial components.[31]
- All surgical approaches are designed to minimize the disturbance of normal anatomy.
- The ideal surgical exposure involves creation of sufficient space for total resection if possible, visualization and identification of associated vessels, direct trajectory, and minimal brain retraction.[3,4,8,19]
- When approaching third ventricular tumors, the structures at most risk of injury include fornices and vessels within the velum interpositum, which include internal cerebral veins and the medial posterior choroidal arteries.[2]
- If tumor has cystic components, care should be taken during decompression not to allow the cystic components to escape into the ventricle or subarachnoid space and then cause aseptic meningitis. Tumors without cystic components should be internally decompressed to reduce tension in the surrounding structures.[31]

19.9 Postoperative Management and Complications

Postoperative care after surgical treatments of intraventricular tumors usually requires intensive care unit monitoring due to rather high rate of complications (up to 20%).[6] Patients are placed on

Table 19.1 Surgical approaches to intraventricular tumors[12,21,22,23,29,31,34]

Location	Approach	Benefits	Limits
Lateral ventricle			
Anterior lateral ventricles	Anterior transsulcal (transsuperior frontal sulcus)	Easy access to large tumors with midline-draining cortical veins	Difficult to expose contralateral lateral ventricle. Motor and sensory cortex at high risk of injury for tumors in midventricular location. High incidence of seizures
Midbody	Anterior transcallosal	Access to bilateral lateral ventricles. Avoidance of cortical incision. Decreased incidence of seizures	Risk of injuring bridging veins and causing venous hypertension. Risk of injuring basal ganglia and internal capsule
Atrium	Posterior transsulcal approach	Easy access to atrium with craniotomy that extends over superior parietal lobule	Risk of injuring optic radiations
	Posterior transcallosal approach	Easy access to roof and medial portion of atrium, trigone, and posterior body, reduced risk of damage to language area	Splitting of corpus callosum can result in alexia (avoid in patients with homonymous hemianopsia contralateral to dominant hemisphere), limited visualization of afferent vessels
	Posterior temporal approach	Easy access to lateral part of atrium	Risk of injuring vein of Labbé
Temporal horns	Inferior temporal approach	Easy access to temporal horns	Risk of injuring structures in temporal horn, including P2 artery, superior cerebellar artery, vein of Rosenthal, cranial nerve IV
Third ventricle			
Anterior third	Transforaminal, interforniceal	Several paths to open third ventricle without injuring cortex	Lesions anterior to foramen of Monro and inferior to third ventricle not accessible
	Lateral subfrontal	Easy access to midline suprasellar lesions	Injury of thin third ventricular floor
	Pterional	Easy access to suprasellar lesions that extend into anterior third ventricle	Poor visualization of ipsilateral third ventricular extension and contralateral opticocarotid and retrocarotid space
	Endoscopic	Minimally invasive, ability to biopsy, ability to fenestrate	High bleeding risk, inability to remove highly vascular and fibrous tumors, engulfing of tumors into adjacent neurovascular structures
Posterior third	Transcallosal transvelum interpositum	Choroidal dissection to gain visibility of vessels	Frequent distortion of anatomy
	Infratentorial supracerebellar	Easy access to midline structures in pineal region	Suboptimal for tumors extending laterally or supratentorially
	Occipital transtentorial	Easy access to tumors with supra- or infratentorial components with minimal retraction	Injury to internal cerebral vein and basal vein of Rosenthal

perioperative antibiotics for 24 hours and on high-dose steroids to be tapered off over 10 to 14 days. For patients with tumors resected via transcortical approach, antiepileptic medication is also used for seizure prophylaxis.[4] Complications include cerebral edema, intraventricular hemorrhage, subdural and epidural hematoma, and memory difficulties arising from forniceal injury.[34]

19.10 Common Clinical Questions

1. Where is the most common location of CPP in children and in adults?
2. What are histological hallmarks of ependymoma?
3. What is the only intraventricular tumor that does not enhance with contrast on MRI?
4. What are some commonly performed endoscopic procedures for intraventricular tumors?
5. What can result in significant blood loss when removing the intraventricular tumors?
6. What can prevent postoperative CSF obstruction and resultant symptoms of increased intracranial pressure, such as headaches and altered mental status?

19.11 Answers to Common Clinical Questions

1. CPP is most commonly located in lateral ventricle, more specifically left atrium, whereas it is fourth ventricle in adults.
2. Ependymoma is associated with perivascular pseudorosettes, also known as Homer Wright rosettes, more commonly than true ependymal rosettes, also known as Flexner–Wintersteiner rosettes.
3. Subependymoma in the lateral ventricles is the only intraventricular tumor that does not enhance with gadolinium administration on MRI.
4. Some commonly performed endoscopic procedures for intraventricular tumors include endoscopic septal fenestration, tumor biopsy with or without endoscopic third ventriculostomy (ETV), and endoscopic removal of tumors. Endoscopic management offers advantages, such as the ability to divert CSF via ETV or septal fenestration. Although endoscopic excision of solid intraventricular tumors remains challenging, tumor biopsy and cyst resection are commonly performed with high success rate.[35]

5. As most operative techniques result in creating exposure much smaller than the tumor itself, and as tumor gets removed in a piecemeal fashion, vascular supply to the tumor is not exposed early, resulting in possible large volume of blood loss.[35]
6. It is generally recommended to remove blood and air from within the ventricles. Moreover, placing cotton over the foramen of Monro during the early course of the surgery can also prevent pooling of blood into the third ventricle.

References

[1] Dolecek TA, Propp JM, Stroup NE, Kruchko C. CBTRUS statistical report: primary brain and central nervous system tumors diagnosed in the United States in 2005–2009. Neuro-oncol. 2013; 15(5):646–647

[2] Anderson RC, Walker ML. Neuroendoscopy. In: Albright AL, Pollack IF, Adelson PD, eds. Principles and Practice of Pediatric Neurosurgery. New York, NY: Thieme; 2008:131–144

[3] Santoro A, Salvati M, Frati A, Polli FM, Delfini R, Cantore G. Surgical approaches to tumours of the lateral ventricles in the dominant hemisphere. J Neurosurg Sci. 2002; 46(2):60–65, discussion 65

[4] Bettegowda C, Chen LC, Mehta VA, Jallo GI, Rutka JT. Supratentorial tumors in the pediatric population: multidisciplinary management. In: Quiñones-Hinojosa A, ed. Schmidek & Sweet Operative Neurosurgical Techniques. Philadelphia, PA: Elsevier; 2012:669–683

[5] Taylor MD, Sanford RA, Boop FA. Cerebellar pilocytic astrocytomas. In: Albright AL, Pollack IF, Adelson PD, eds. Principles and Practice of Pediatric Neurosurgery. New York, NY: Thieme; 2008:655–667

[6] Gökalp HZ, Yüceer N, Arasil E, et al. Tumours of the lateral ventricle. A retrospective review of 112 cases operated upon 1970–1997. Neurosurg Rev. 1998; 21(2–3):126–137

[7] Desmeules M, Mikkelsen T, Mao Y. Increasing incidence of primary malignant brain tumors: influence of diagnostic methods. J Natl Cancer Inst. 1992; 84(6):442–445

[8] Anderson RC, Ghatan S, Feldstein NA. Surgical approaches to tumors of the lateral ventricle. Neurosurg Clin N Am. 2003; 14(4):509–525

[9] Jelinek J, Smirniotopoulos JG, Parisi JE, Kanzer M. Lateral ventricular neoplasms of the brain: differential diagnosis based on clinical, CT, and MR findings. AJNR Am J Neuroradiol. 1990; 11(3):567–574

[10] Sévenet N, Sheridan E, Amram D, Schneider P, Handgretinger R, Delattre O. Constitutional mutations of the hSNF5/INI1 gene predispose to a variety of cancers. Am J Hum Genet. 1999; 65(5):1342–1348

[11] Courville CB, Broussalian SL. Plastic ependymomas of the lateral recess. Report of eight verified cases. J Neurosurg. 1961; 18:792–799

[12] Robinson LL. General principles of the epidemiology of childhood cancer. In: Pizzo PA, Poplack DG, eds. Principles and Practice of Pediatric Oncology. Philadelphia, PA: Lippincott; 1997:1–9

[13] Horn B, Heideman R, Geyer R, et al. A multi-institutional retrospective study of intracranial ependymoma in children:

identification of risk factors. J Pediatr Hematol Oncol. 1999; 21(3):203–211

[14] Souweidane MM. Brain tumors in the first two years of life. In: Albright AL, Pollack IF, Adelson PD, eds. Principles and Practice of Pediatric Neurosurgery. New York, NY: Thieme; 2008:489–510

[15] Geyer JR, Zeltzer PM, Boyett JM, et al. Survival of infants with primitive neuroectodermal tumors or malignant ependymomas of the CNS treated with eight drugs in 1 day: a report from the Childrens Cancer Group. J Clin Oncol. 1994; 12(8):1607–1615

[16] Weitman DM, Cogen PH. Infratentorial ependymoma. In: Keating RF, Goodrich JT, Packer RJ, eds. Tumors of the Pediatric Central Nervous System. New York, NY: Thieme; 2001:232–238

[17] Yuh EL, Barkovich AJ, Gupta N. Imaging of ependymomas: MRI and CT. Childs Nerv Syst. 2009; 25(10):1203–1213

[18] Ellenbogen RG, Winston KR, Kupsky WJ. Tumors of the choroid plexus in children. Neurosurgery. 1989; 25(3):327–335

[19] Berger C, Thiesse P, Lellouch-Tubiana A, Kalifa C, Pierre-Kahn A, Bouffet E. Choroid plexus carcinomas in childhood: clinical features and prognostic factors. Neurosurgery. 1998; 42(3):470–475

[20] Ellenbogen RG, Donovan DJ. Choroid plexus tumors. In: Keating RF, Goodrich JT, Packer RJ, eds. Tumors of the Pediatric Central Nervous System. New York, NY: Thieme; 2001:339–350

[21] Paulus W, Jänisch W. Clinicopathologic correlations in epithelial choroid plexus neoplasms: a study of 52 cases. Acta Neuropathol. 1990; 80(6):635–641

[22] Koeller KK, Sandberg GD, Armed Forces Institute of Pathology. From the archives of the AFIP. Cerebral intraventricular neoplasms: radiologic-pathologic correlation. Radiographics. 2002; 22(6):1473–1505

[23] Phi JH, Kim DG. Rare pediatric central neurocytomas. Neurosurg Clin N Am. 2015; 26(1):105–108

[24] Fishback JL. Neuropathology. In: Moore SP, Psarros TG, eds. The Definitive Neurological Surgery Board Review. Philadelphia, PA: Lippincott; 2005:108–133

[25] Gandolfi A, Brizzi RE, Tedeschi F, Paini P, Bassi P. Symptomatic subependymoma of the fourth ventricle. Case report. J Neurosurg. 1981; 55(5):841–844

[26] Chiechi MV, Smirniotopoulos JG, Jones RV. Intracranial subependymomas: CT and MR imaging features in 24 cases. AJR Am J Roentgenol. 1995; 165(5):1245–1250

[27] Franz DN, Agricola K, Mays M, et al. Everolimus for subependymal giant cell astrocytoma: 5-year final analysis. Ann Neurol. 2015; 78(6):929–938

[28] Gray F, Duyckaerts C, Girolami UD. Escourolle and Poirier's Manual of Basic Neuropathology. New York, NY: Oxford; 2014

[29] Rades D, Fehlauer F, Schild SE. Treatment of atypical neurocytomas. Cancer. 2004; 100(4):814–817

[30] Karthigeyan M, Gupta K, Salunke P. Pediatric central neurocytoma. J Child Neurol. 2017; 32(1):53–59

[31] Patel TR, Gould GC, Baehring JM, Piepmeier JM. Surgical approaches to lateral and third ventricular tumors. In: Quiñones-Hinojosa A, ed. Schmidek & Sweet Operative Neurosurgical Techniques. Philadelphia, PA: Elsevier; 2012:330–338

[32] Shucart WA, Stein BM. Transcallosal approach to the anterior ventricular system. Neurosurgery. 1978; 3(3):339–343

[33] Souweidane MM, Sandberg DI, Bilsky MH, Gutin PH. Endoscopic biopsy for tumors of the third ventricle. Pediatr Neurosurg. 2000; 33(3):132–137

[34] Apuzzo ML, Chikovani OK, Gott PS, et al. Transcallosal, interforncial approaches for lesions affecting the third ventricle: surgical considerations and consequences. Neurosurgery. 1982; 10(5):547–554

[35] Greenfield JP, Souweidane MM, Schwartz TH. Endoscopic approach to intraventricular brain tumors. In: Quiñones-Hinojosa A, ed. Schmidek & Sweet Operative Neurosurgical Techniques. Philadelphia, PA: Elsevier; 2012:351–356

20 Posterior Fossa Tumors

Christian A. Schneider, Nir Shimony, Karl F. Kothbauer

20.1 Introduction

Following accidents, the leading cause of death in children is cancer.[1] Tumors of the central nervous system (CNS) are the most common solid pediatric neoplasms.[2] Sixty percent of these tumors arise in the posterior fossa.[3] The symptoms of a posterior fossa tumor are more specific to its infratentorial localization than to its histological type. The most frequent complaints are symptoms related to hydrocephalus, followed by symptoms of brainstem, cerebellar, and cranial nerve (CN) dysfunction. Almost every patient with a newly diagnosed posterior fossa mass lesion must be rapidly evaluated and treated.[4] Because symptoms of irritability, vomiting, and headaches are such everyday complaints in a pediatricians' practice, the average symptomatic period to the diagnosis of a brain tumor is around 6 months, and 25% of all children have previously undergone gastrointestinal workup.[1] This explains why children with brain tumors are often seen in an emergency setting, when clinical decompensation is imminent. Especially acute obstructive hydrocephalus is feared and can lead to rapid clinical deterioration necessitating urgent cerebrospinal fluid (CSF) diversion surgery.[4]

Medulloblastoma (MB), pilocytic astrocytoma (PA), and ependymoma (EP) are the three most common tumors in the pediatric posterior fossa.[3] In all three, the extent of resection is the most important predictor of oncologic outcome (although for MB this statement is currently challenged[5]), meaning that the mere presence of a posterior fossa mass lesion usually implicates indication for surgery.[1] As a rule of thumb, tumor surgery should be performed as soon as possible but preferably in an elective setting, when the staff specialized in the management of these tumors is readily available. This includes neurosurgeon, neuroanesthetist, neuropathologist, neuromonitoring specialist, and neurosurgical scrub nurse.[4]

20.2 Neurosurgical Management of Pediatric Posterior Fossa Tumors

20.2.1 Diagnostic Evaluation

- Symptoms of increased intracranial pressure (ICP) or CN deficits usually lead to brain imaging before a neurosurgeon is involved. Obtaining a detailed history and a diligent neurological exam is self-evident.
- With the presence of a posterior fossa mass lesion, contrast-enhanced magnetic resonance imaging (MRI) of the head and the whole spine (to assess for drop metastases before postsurgical changes render the evaluation difficult) is mandatory.[4]
- There is no imaging modality that can determine the histology of a posterior fossa tumor with certainty, but experienced pediatric neuroradiologists are able to predict the histology in 90% of the cases.[1]
- A lumbar puncture is rarely needed preoperatively and can be even dangerous in the presence of a posterior fossa mass lesion. Diagnostic lumbar CSF is usually obtained in the postoperative period in tumors prone to spinal dissemination. A postoperative waiting period of 10 to 14 days is recommended to minimize the risk of false-positive lumbar CSF samples.[4,6]
- A formal ophthalmologic evaluation is useful when visual symptoms or oculomotor disturbances are present, to obtain a preoperative baseline examination. In case of dysfunction of the lower CNs with swallowing difficulty, facial weakness, hearing loss, or vestibular symptoms, ENT service should be consulted early.

20.2.2 Preoperative Management

- Admission and close observation of neurological status and vital signs in an intensive care setting are usually mandatory. Never discharge a patient with a newly diagnosed posterior fossa tumor! Especially in infants, circulatory response (bradycardia and hypertension) can be the only symptom of an acute deterioration. Close monitoring of head circumference and status of the fontanel in infants is part of that observation.

- Steroids are useful in the symptomatic patient and are generally administered on admission.
- Mannitol should be given in a surgical setting only or to buy time to an emergency surgical CSF diversion procedure, when acute hydrocephalic deterioration and herniation signs are present.
- Seizures rarely occur in posterior fossa tumors without leptomeningeal dissemination. The empiric administration of antiepileptic drugs in a seizure-free patient is not indicated.[4]
- Opiates and benzodiazepines are not contraindicated but can lead to severe respiratory depression in the presence of a significant posterior fossa mass lesion.
- Hydration and adequate administration of antiemetic drugs are important—especially in infants with frequent vomiting.
- Preoperative blood work must include a coagulation status and a type-and-screen evaluation.

20.3 Surgical Considerations

20.3.1 General

- The psychological impact on patients newly diagnosed with a brain tumor and their parents must be taken into account. Preoperative communication with the family is obviously of the utmost importance. In addition, updates from the operation theatre during surgery are always highly appreciated, especially during a long case. As a treating neurosurgeon, you will be following these patients for many years, meaning that establishing a relationship based on trust and communication at the beginning of treatment will make future management easier for all parties involved.
- Brain tumor resection can cause significant blood loss. This is especially concerning in infants with a small total blood volume. Anesthetist (availability of blood products), scrub nurse (preparation of patties, hemostatic materials, working bipolar coagulation forceps, and suction), and surgeon (meticulous hemostasis) should anticipate this and pay close attention to blood loss during the case (and

should also appreciate "hidden blood" in drainage bags, drapes, and pads).[1]

- Upon induction, the usual perioperative surgical antibiotic prophylaxis is administered (i.e., cefazolin 30 mg/kg). The authors recommend a single additional dose of steroids on induction (i.e., dexamethasone 8 mg). Occasionally, mannitol (0.5 g/kg) can be useful before opening the dura to help achieve a relaxed situation in the posterior fossa.[4]

Positioning

To access the posterior fossa, three options of patient positioning cover most of the surgeon's needs:

Prone and "Concorde" Position

After induction (supine), the head is fixed in a skull clamp (i.e., pediatric Mayfield, Sugita) and the patient flipped over onto the operating table, the latter padded with pressure distributing gel cushions and other positioning material. After adjusting the head and inclining it in the neck (for the "Concorde" position), the skull clamp is secured to the end of the table. Always leave a distance of two fingers width between chin and chest. The table is then adjusted in a reversed Trendelenburg fashion, until the operating field is horizontal. In children younger than 2 years, a horseshoe headrest is preferred to obviate the risk of complications related to pin fixation.[1]

Advantage: Standard midline approaches and paramedian approaches are covered. The risk of air embolism is low. The position for surgeon and assistant is comfortable and intuitive (face-to-face configuration of the microscope).

Disadvantage: The venous pressure is higher and the posterior fossa tighter compared to the sitting position.

Lateral Decubitus and "Park Bench" Position

The patient is positioned on his side with the head turned toward the floor. This position covers lateral approaches to the cerebellopontine angle and far lateral approaches to the ventral region of the brainstem.

Advantage: The cerebellar hemisphere follows gravity and "falls away" from the operating field. The risk of air embolism is low.

Disadvantage: The venous pressure is higher and the posterior fossa tighter compared to the sitting position.

Sitting Position

Some surgeons still prefer the sitting position under the aspect of a relaxed situation in the posterior fossa and a negative venous pressure, allowing for a fairly bloodless surgery. In pediatric neurosurgery, the sitting position is possible but mostly avoided.[1,7] Large osseous sinuses and an occipital sinus are often present, enhancing the risk of air embolism. In addition, rapid drainage of CSF can empty the ventricular system and lead to significant pneumocephalus and subdural hematomas.[1] If the sitting position is considered, preoperative echocardiography must exclude a patent foramen ovale being an absolute contraindication. Precordial Doppler sonography during the case is also mandatory, allowing for a fast reaction of the surgeon to air embolism (i.e., packing the operation field with wet compresses, waxing bony sinuses, performing hemostasis, and—ultimately—lowering the head of the patient).

Management of Hydrocephalus

- Obstructive triventricular hydrocephalus is reported in 80% of children with posterior fossa tumors and often is the factor responsible for symptoms and deterioration.[8,9]
- Thirty percent of these children will ultimately need a permanent CSF diversion after tumor resection.[10]
- Risk factors for a postresectional hydrocephalus requiring surgical treatment are[10,11]:
  - Age < 2 years.
  - Presence of transependymal edema.
  - Preresectional moderate or severe hydrocephalus.
  - Presence of cerebral metastases.
  - Diagnosis of MB, EP, or dorsal exophytic brainstem glioma.
- Some controversy exists about the best way to treat hydrocephalus secondary to posterior fossa tumors. The options are pre- or postoperative external ventricular drain (EVD), shunt, or endoscopic third ventriculostomy (ETV).
- ETV obviates the need for a shunt by creating an opening in the floor of the third ventricle, taking advantage of the much larger CSF resorption capacity of the external CSF spaces, bypassing a usually compressed aqueduct.
- Some evidence suggests that a preresectional ETV lowers the need for a postoperative shunt.[8,12] Opponents to this technique argue that in 70% of the cases hydrocephalus is sufficiently

treated by tumor removal, requiring neither ETV nor shunt, and that a prophylactic ETV puts the patients at risk of an additional intervention.

- Although only 30% of the patients will need CSF diversion after tumor removal, an EVD is often left behind during resection for safety reasons. The EVD is weaned during the following postoperative week. If EVD weaning is not successful, both options of ETV and shunt can be discussed again.
- The advantage of not having a permanent shunt in place, with all its downside of hardware failure, infection, and blockage, justifies in the authors' opinion the trial of a postresectional ETV, even if this could mean a prolongation of hospital stay in case shunting is ultimately needed.
- In the prone position, EVD positioning can be more difficult when choosing an occipital entry point. The use of a burr hole ultrasound probe is highly recommended to prevent catheter malpositioning and the need for several "attempts."
- Care must be taken to slowly release CSF from an EVD. Rapid changes in ICP can lead to circulatory reactions and, in the worst case, to perfusion issues of the retinas already at risk by the prone position. This problem can be addressed by immediately closing the EVD after placement to only drain CSF in the presence of a "tight posterior fossa."

Surgical Approaches to the Posterior Fossa

Midline Tumors

Many of the pediatric tumors in the posterior fossa are midline lesions arising from the brainstem or the roof of the fourth ventricle. Both intracranial approaches described in the following are covered with a midline suboccipital craniotomy. The inion is often palpable and the position of the transverse sinus is approximated by a line drawn from the inion to both auditory meatuses.[13] A straight midline incision is carried down to the bone along the midline avascular plane. The posterior arch of C1 and the spinous process of C2 are exposed to establish bony landmarks of the craniocervical junction. Care is taken not to injure the dura at this point because some patients present with a nonfused C1 arch, leaving a midline gap. Many surgeons routinely remove the C1 lamina, feeling that this helps normalizing CSF flow across the foramen magnum. Burr holes are then placed on either side just below the transverse sinus. Bilateral sharp dissection and the use of a Kerrison punch on the dorsal rim of the foramen magnum will create an entry point for the footplate of the craniotome to turn a bone flap up to the burr holes. When connecting both burr holes along the transverse sinus, care is taken not to injure an often-present occipital sinus in younger patients. In older children, a significant midline bony ridge can necessitate the use of a high-speed drill to complete the craniotomy. The bone flap is then elevated by cutting the occipital membrane at the foramen magnum. Meticulous hemostasis and padding of the craniotomy edges at this point prevents blood from entering the field after opening of the dura. The dura is incised in a **Y**-shaped fashion with the straight limb of the Y extending down across the plane of the foramen magnum. Bleeding is controlled with a step-by-step suturing of the dural edges or the application of hemoclips. The cerebellar hemispheres and the tonsils are immediately exposed; incision of the arachnoid with drainage of CSF usually leads to a relaxed situation in the operating field.[9,13]

Transvermian approach: After identification of the anatomical landmarks, the vermis is incised in its inferior part. The two halves of the vermis and the cerebellar tonsils are carefully retracted laterally, exposing the dorsal aspect of a fourth ventricular midline tumor. Both posterior inferior cerebellar arteries are usually seen and also displaced laterally. Planes around the tumor can be developed using cottonoids. In large tumors, central debulking with an ultrasound aspirator will allow for less traction when following the tumor–cerebellum interface later on. The noninvaded side of the cerebellar peduncle is first dissected exposing the floor of the fourth ventricle and the aqueduct. The transvermian approach allows for a better visualization of the rostral tumor aspects compared to the telovelar approach described in the following. However, it is limited in its lateral exposure, and the occurrence of cerebellar mutism is believed to be higher when the vermis is split and manipulated.[9,14,15]

Telovelar approach: The telovelar approach avoids splitting of the vermis and therefore tries to reduce the occurrence of cerebellar mutism. After a suboccipital posterior fossa craniotomy, the cerebellomedullary fissure is entered and the cerebellar tonsils are retracted laterally. On the floor of the fissure, the inferior medullary velum and the tela choroidea are encountered, the latter forming the caudal part of the roof of the fourth ventricle. After incising the tela choroidea, the fourth ventricle can be explored laterally to the foramina of Luschka on both sides. This allows the resection of midline tumors extending laterally. However, the rostral parts of a midline tumor are visualized less well by this approach.[9,13,14,15,16]

Transtentorial approach: Some midline tumors in the posterior fossa may extend high up to the quadrigeminal plate and the pineal region. In this localization, the working angle is suboptimal coming from a telovelar approach, and a transvermian approach would result in the destruction of the vermis with a consecutive high risk for cerebellar mutism. In this setting, a transtentorial approach can provide optimal visualization. A parasagittal craniotomy in the parietal region gives interhemispheric access to the superior aspect of the tentorium. The latter is incised and the most cranial part of the posterior fossa can be entered. The distance to the tumor, however, becomes considerably long and the use of intraoperative neuronavigation is almost mandatory. In addition, injury to the straight sinus may result in substantial bleeding deep down in the operation field, limiting the use of this surgical approach to experienced hands.[1]

Cerebellar Hemispheric Tumors

Accessing cerebellar hemispheric tumors is generally not as technically demanding. From a standard midline suboccipital craniotomy, as described, the tumor can be encountered by opening the cerebellar hemisphere along the folia at the point of the shortest distance of the tumor to the cerebellar surface.[9]

Lateral and Anterior Tumors

Retromastoid approach: This approach behind the sigmoid sinus covers most lateral tumors of the cerebellopontine angle. Again, the position of the transverse sinus is approximated by a line from the inion to the external auditory canal. The patient is positioned in a lateral decubitus fashion. From a curvilinear incision just medial to the mastoid, the bone is exposed. The sigmoid sinus is usually localized beneath the mastoid groove, and the connection of transverse and sigmoid sinus is found under the asterion. A single burr hole is placed inferiorly to the asterion and medially to the mastoid groove. A craniotomy flap is turned from the burr hole medially. If necessary, bone can be further removed with a drill or Kerrison punches to the anterior margin of the sigmoid sinus. The dura is opened in a **K**-shaped fashion and reflected with sutures. The cerebellum is then displaced downward with brain retractors over patties until drainage of CSF allows for a good visualization of the cerebellopontine angle. From this approach, the CNs from V to XII are accessible together with the tumors of that region.[13]

Far lateral approach: To access tumors ventral of the brainstem, the far lateral approach is used combining a lateral suboccipital craniotomy with the removal of the occipital condyle and the atlas down to the sulcus arteriosus. This approach is not straightforward even in experienced hands and will not be further discussed here.

Surgical Adjuncts

Intraoperative Neuromonitoring

- The use of somatosensory evoked potential, motor evoked potential, and brainstem auditory evoked potential monitoring has become routine in posterior fossa tumor surgery in most centers, especially for surgery in the cerebellopontine angle.[9]
- The impact of a best possible resection on oncologic outcome potentially compromises patient safety in regard to functional outcome. The use of intraoperative neuromonitoring should enable the surgeon to be safely as radical as possible. There is circumstantial evidence to this statement; class I evidence in randomized trials cannot be obtained for obvious ethical reasons.[17]
- The successful implementation of intraoperative neuromonitoring strongly depends on the teamwork of neurophysiologist (experience in acquisition and interpretation), anesthetist (using mainly intravenous anesthetic agents without paralytics), and surgeon (experience to tailor the procedure according to the monitoring feedback).[17]

Intraoperative Ultrasound

The use of intraoperative ultrasound is a reliable, fast, real-time, repeatable, and inexpensive adjunct to help the surgeon throughout the tumor resection. It is especially helpful in:
- Localizing the ventricles and guiding an EVD catheter during insertion.
- Localizing major vascular structures in the Doppler mode.
- Visualizing the tumor during approach and assessing for residual tumor after resection.
- Visualizing CSF pathways (i.e., flow through the aqueduct).
- Ruling out major hemorrhage into brain or ventricles.

Neuronavigation

- The use of intraoperative neuronavigation in posterior fossa tumor surgery is possible, although registering the patient's head in the prone or lateral position can be more demanding and the accuracy of the obtained registration must be carefully verified.
- Some surgeons feel that the use of neuronavigation in the posterior fossa does not give too much additional information, as the anatomical landmarks are quite straightforward. In the authors' view, however, neuronavigation is certainly useful when tailoring the craniotomy, especially its relations to the transverse and sigmoid sinus. Some evidence suggests that an exposed transverse sinus is more susceptible to air embolism, thrombosis, and hemorrhage, resulting in the recommendation to avoid carrying a suboccipital craniotomy on or over the transverse sinus.[18]

Intraoperative MRI

A growing number of centers are implementing intraoperative MRI (iMRI) as a surgical adjunct. Advocates of this technique argue that it influences intraoperative surgical decision-making in a significant amount of their patients, especially when a gross total resection is the surgical goal. It therefore might reduce the number of patients who need revision surgery for residual disease. The technique is safe for the pediatric population, although no prospective data exist whether the use of iMRI has a positive impact on oncologic outcome.[19,20]

Closure

Meticulous hemostasis before closure is naturally a general neurosurgical principle and is especially important in the posterior fossa, where hematoma formation next to the brainstem can have rapid devastating consequences. In addition, the occurrence of intraventricular hemorrhage often significantly extends hospitalization and certainly is not helpful when trying to avoid a shunt. The authors recommend a watertight dural closure, although there is no class I evidence available for that statement, regarding CSF leaks, infections, and the formation of pseudomeningoceles.[21,22,23] The choice of materials for dural augmentation (which is usually necessary) and dural sealant is at the discretion of the surgeon. The abundance of available products on the market is an indication of the fact that there is no perfect combination of product and technique. The authors recommend dural augmentation with allograft, sutured in a watertight fashion, and the application of some sealant (i.e., fleece bound or liquid fibrin glue). Then the bone flap is fixed with sutures or plates, and a meticulous multilayered closure of the muscles and especially the fascia and a running sutured skin closure are performed. Drains should be avoided whenever possible.

20.3.2 Postoperative Management

General

Extubation immediately after the procedure is usually possible and allows for a postoperative neurologic examination. Admission to the intensive care unit for at least overnight observation is mandatory with close assessment of neurological status and laboratory parameters.

Early MRI within 48 hours of surgery is routine for postoperative imaging in most centers. This has therapeutic consequences, as, in some tumors, revision surgery has to be considered in case of residual disease. The short interval to imaging is essential to differentiate between residual tumor and postsurgical changes.[1]

In case an EVD has been placed, CSF is routinely sent for cell count and bacteriology. When output volumes decrease, the drainage level is incrementally raised and the EVD eventually clamped. In an asymptomatic patient, the drain is then removed and the insertion site sutured. In case of symptoms, imaging and CSF diversion surgery must be discussed early.

Management of Complications

Hydrocephalus

See Management of Hydrocephalus.

Cerebellar Ataxia

Cerebellar ataxia is the most common complication of posterior fossa surgery. While the portion of the tumor invading one cerebellar peduncle can be resected aggressively, care should be taken to leave the other peduncle intact. Under this aspect, postoperative cerebellar ataxia usually resolves within weeks.[9] Steroids are routinely given in the attempt to accelerate clinical recovery.

Cerebellar Mutism

Cerebellar mutism (CM) is one of the feared complications after posterior fossa surgery. The literature on this syndrome is extensive but still the pathophysiology is poorly understood. CM is defined as a transient and delayed-onset (1–6 days postoperatively) mutism after a period of normal postoperative speech production. Clinical symptoms accompanying CM include: oropharyngeal apraxia, ataxia, hypokinesia, visual disturbances, and neurobehavioral symptoms (i.e., emotional lability).[24]

Proven risk factors for CM are: brainstem invasion, midline tumors, and MB histology. Possible risk factors comprise: preoperative language impairment, younger age, radical resection, incision of the vermis, and large tumor size.[24]

CM was believed to be a relatively benign complication, given its spontaneous remission and transient character. In more recent studies, however, formal neuropsychological evaluation of children with CM shows that affected patients are often left with significant neuropsychological impairment, including problems of attention, memory, processing speed, and verbal fluency, as well as behavioral deficits.[24,25,26]

Cranial Nerve Dysfunction

CN dysfunction is due to manipulation of either the nerves themselves or the brainstem at the level the CN nuclei. Nuclear CN impairment has a smaller chance of recovery.[9]

The spectrum seen after posterior fossa surgery includes abducens palsy, facial weakness, internuclear ophthalmoplegia, horizontal gaze palsy, swallowing difficulty, and vocal cord palsy.[9]

In tumors that arise from the brainstem or involve the lower CNs or the floor of the fourth ventricle, a delayed extubation with the presence of an ENT team to assess vocal cords and pharyngeal motility is recommended. In children affected by vocal cord paralysis or insensate pharynges, an early tracheostomy and gastrostomy should be discussed to prevent aspiration pneumonitis.[1]

Neurocognitive Defects

Apart of CM described earlier, posterior fossa tumors and their treatment (especially radiation therapy in infants) can result in significant impairment of the patient's neurocognitive functioning. Risk factors for postoperative neurocognitive deficits are the presence of preoperative deficits, severe hydrocephalus, invasion of the brainstem, and histological diagnosis of MB.[25]

Pseudomeningocele and CSF Leak

Even with the most meticulous closure techniques, postoperative pseudomeningocele formation and CSF leakage cannot completely be avoided. Evidently, a CSF leak significantly enhances the risk of wound infection and bacterial meningitis. Pseudomeningocele formation occurs in 25% and should first be conservatively managed and observed in the absence of a CSF leak.[9,23] In the presence of CSF leakage, however, a rapid surgical wound revision with insertion of a lumbar drain is needed to prevent infection. Recurrent CSF leaks or recurrent pseudomeningoceles can also be a symptom of hydrocephalus and will need CSF diversion surgery to control.[9]

Wound Infection and Bacterial Meningitis

Wound infections after posterior fossa surgery are especially feared, as they not only prolong hospitalization but also add significant morbidity to the procedure (i.e., postinfectious hydrocephalus). Wound infections must lead to rapid revision surgery, followed by empiric antibiotic treatment until cultures allow for a resistance-adapted antibiotic regime. The Infectious Diseases Service should always be consulted.

Aseptic Meningitis

The presence of blood in the subarachnoid space can lead to postoperative headaches, fever, irritability, photophobia, neck stiffness, and CSF pleocytosis, mimicking bacterial meningitis. The latter has to be excluded with CSF cultures. Aseptic meningitis can best be prevented with a meticulous hemostasis before closing. It usually responds well to low-dose steroid administration.[9]

20.4 Specific Pediatric Posterior Fossa Tumors

20.4.1 Overview

The "big three" tumors in the pediatric posterior fossa are: (1) medulloblastoma (MB), (2) pilocytic astrocytoma (PA), and (3) ependymoma (EP).[4] Less common are atypical teratoid/rhabdoid tumor (AT/RT), choroid plexus papilloma (CPP), and choroid plexus carcinoma (CPC). Occasionally encountered and not further discussed here are ganglioglioma, teratoma, hemangioblastoma, and dermoid/epidermoid cyst. All other tumor entities are very rare. Brainstem gliomas are covered elsewhere in this book.

20.4.2 Medulloblastoma

Epidemiology

MB is the most common malignant solid neoplasm of childhood and accounts for 25% of all pediatric brain tumors.[4,9] Eighty-five percent of all MBs arise from the cerebellar vermis, and a minority are found within the cerebellar hemispheres. Historically, MBs were considered to be PNETs (primitive neuroectodermal tumors) located in the posterior fossa—differentiating them from supratentorial PNETs. Current genetic fingerprinting, however, strongly suggests that supratentorial PNETs are genetically identical to other known tumor entities. Therefore, the term "PNET" disappeared in the current WHO classification.[27,28]

The median age at diagnosis is 7 years, with a slight predominance for Caucasian males. A series of predisposition syndromes are associated with the occurrence of MB, including Gorlin's syndrome, Turcot's syndrome, and Li–Fraumeni syndrome.[29]

Pathology

MBs are considered WHO grade 4 tumors.[28] Historically, histology appreciated four subtypes: (1) classic type, (2) desmoplastic/nodular type, (3) MB with extensive nodularity, and (4) large cell/anaplastic type.[30] Although there was some correlation of histological subtype and oncologic outcome, recent genotyping of MB tissue led to a novel stratification with a far better clinical

Table 20.1 Integrated medulloblastoma stratification in the context of clinical significance[28]

	Genetic profile	Histology	Prognosis
10%	MB, WNT-activated	Classic type	Low-risk tumor
		Large cell/anaplastic type (very rare)	Uncertain clinicopathological significance
30%	MB, SHH-activated, TP53-mutant	Classic type	Uncommon, high-risk tumor
		Large cell/anaplastic type	High-risk tumor; prevalent in children aged 7–17 y
		Desmoplastic/nodular type (very rare)	Uncertain clinicopathological significance
	MB, SHH-activated, TP53-wildtype	Classic type	Standard-risk tumor
		Large cell/anaplastic type	Uncertain clinicopathological significance
		Desmoplastic/nodular type (very rare)	Low-risk tumor in infants; prevalent in infants and adults
		Extensive nodularity	Low-risk tumor of infancy
25%	MB, non-WNT/non-SHH, group 3	Classic type	Standard-risk tumor
		Large cell/anaplastic type	High-risk tumor
35%	MB, non-WNT/non-SHH, group 4	Classic type	Standard-risk tumor
		Large cell/anaplastic type (rare)	Uncertain clinicopathological significance

Abbreviation: MB, medulloblastoma.

correlation. This novel stratification was adopted in the current WHO classification and is now listed in combination with the histologically defined subtypes.[28,31,32,33] ► Table 20.1 summarizes genetic profile, histology, and impact on prognosis. There is no doubt that genetic fingerprinting will become increasingly important in tumor stratification in general, and our knowledge on this topic is rapidly evolving.

Imaging

MB shows a wide variability on its MRI appearance. Typically, a T1-hypointense, T2-hyperintense, and patchy contrast-enhancing midline posterior fossa tumor corresponds to an MB. Calcifications and cyst formations are seen.[4] Leptomeningeal seeding is appreciated in one-third of the patients, usually along the spinal canal. The presence of spinal metastases on neuroimaging interestingly does not correlate with a positive CSF cytology and vice versa.[4]

Management

Patient survival and quality of life have significantly improved with the development of the current standard treatment regime of surgery, radiotherapy, and chemotherapy. However, this treatment leads to considerable morbidity, especially in infants younger than 3 years. Even if long-time survival is common nowadays, parents and patients have to face the fact that after craniospinal irradiation—to name one of the problems the percentage of individuals with academic degrees is significantly lower compared to the general population.[34]

In the very near future, however, treatment paradigms will dramatically change for MB patients. The implementation of genetic fingerprinting led to an abundance of new treatment protocols always in the context of multicenter trials. The traditional triad of surgery and radiochemotherapy obviously still has its place, especially in standard and high-risk situations. The identification of low-risk subgroups, however, will very soon lead to treatment de-escalation with an expected reduction of toxic side effects—without compromising oncologic survival. Moreover, potential drug targets are identified and evaluated—especially in SHH tumors.[35]

Surgery

Gross total resection is the goal of surgery in MB and the main predicting factor regarding oncologic outcome. Historically, residual tumor of more than 1.5 cm^2 (subtotal resection) was believed to justify revision surgery.[36] This statement is challenged in a recent trial.[5] It appears that there still is a role for best possible resection but not at too high a risk. Across all genetic subtypes of MB, there was no difference in overall survival (OS) when comparing subtotal (> 1.5 cm^2 residual) to near-total (< 1.5 cm^2 residual) to gross total (no residual) resection. However, there is a difference in progression-free survival comparing subtotal and near-total/gross total resection.[5] Apart from oncologic outcome, tumor removal obviously allows for tissue diagnostic and also treats accompanying hydrocephalus.

Radiation Therapy

MBs are reasonably radiosensitive and the implementation of craniospinal irradiation significantly prolonged survival, especially because these tumors are prone to seed along the neuraxis. Radiotherapy to the developing nervous system is mainly responsible for long-term neuropsychological sequelae, especially in children younger than 3 years. For that reason, every effort is made to avoid radiotherapy in these patients, or to postpone it until the age of 3 has been reached.[37] Acute side effects of radiotherapy comprise drowsiness, nausea, headache, lethargy, and fatigue. Long-term changes include cognitive impairment, growth abnormalities, hypopituitarism, hearing loss, moyamoya vasculopathy, and secondary neoplasms.[38]

Chemotherapy

Chemotherapy remains standard as an adjuvant treatment for MB patients. Treatment protocols, however, are rapidly changing and evolving, according to the novel MB stratification. A dedicated team of neuro-oncologists is indispensable to take the lead in the adjuvant treatment, as its complexity greatly increased with expanding knowledge about these tumors. This knowledge led to a number of trials with several treatment arms to especially reduce treatment toxicity. In addition to that, trial substances specifically targeting genetic pathway changes in MB subtypes are available and will hopefully soon lower side effects in standard treatment or offer salvage treatment for progressive disease.[35]

Follow-up

During treatment, MRI of brain and spine are recommended every 3 months for 18 months, followed by MRI of the brain every 6 months and MRI of the spine every 12 months, until the patient is in remission for 5 years. After that, annual MRI of brain and spine is performed.[39]

20.4.3 Pilocytic Astrocytoma

Epidemiology

PA is the most common pediatric cerebellar neoplasm and occurs at a mean age of 7 years.[4] There is no gender predilection, and these tumors are rarely diagnosed under 1 or over 40 years of age.[9] Fifty percent are seen within the cerebellar hemispheres, but PAs can be found in any location of the neuraxis—the optic pathway, thalamus, and hypothalamus being also common sites.[4]

Pathology

PAs are considered WHO grade 1 tumors.[28] They show a benign biological behavior with a slow growth, good macroscopic delineation, and high survival rates. Histologically, a biphasic pattern of loose glial and compacted piloid tissue is typical, the latter with abundant Rosenthal's fibers. On the immunohistochemical and molecular level, the demonstration of a high proliferative index does not correlate with a worse clinical course.[40] In cerebellar PAs, a single "signature" mutation leads to the activation of the MAPK pathway, an interesting future drug target.[41] While supratentorial and brainstem PAs have a strong association with neurofibromatosis type 1, cerebellar PAs do not show this feature and are mostly sporadic tumors.[4] In supratentorial and brainstem PAs, the status of the BRAF gene (mutation vs. fusion) has a big impact on biological behavior and BRAF evaluation is about to become routine in the diagnostic workup for these tumors.[42]

Imaging

Four patterns are typical morphologic imaging findings: (1) an enhancing mural nodule with a nonenhancing cyst, (2) an enhancing mural nodule with an intensely enhancing cyst, (3) a solid mass with no cystic component, and (4) a necrotic mass with a central nonenhancing zone.[43] Leptomeningeal dissemination is seen, but not incompatible with long-term survival.[44]

Management

Surgery

Complete resection of a PA is considered curative.[45] The resection of the mural nodule is crucial; the role of resection of the cyst wall is discussed controversially, as there seems to be no impact on survival. Subtotal resection leads to higher recurrence rates, but does not affect survival. Therefore, the risk of returning to the operating room for postoperative residual tumor must be carefully balanced against the option of serial MRI follow-up.[45] There is no role for upfront adjuvant radiation therapy or chemotherapy in PA. These options are reserved for recurrence or leptomeningeal spread.[4] When chemotherapy is considered, the knowledge of the BRAF status will allow for an individual prognosis: tumors with a BRAF fusion respond much better than tumors with a BRAF V600E mutation.[42]

Follow-up

When early postoperative imaging demonstrates gross total resection, MRI at 3 months is recommended, followed by annual MRI. In the case of residual tumor, imaging intervals should be tailored accordingly. As in other tumor entities, genetic fingerprinting led to a growing number of multicenter trials investigating optimal treatment for genetically different PAs.[42]

20.4.4 Ependymoma

Epidemiology

EP is the third most frequent brain tumor in the pediatric population and can be located throughout the CNS.[46] Seventy percent of all EPs occur in the posterior fossa—frequently in infants and young children—while older children and adults are more prone to supratentorial and spinal EPs. The mean age at the time of diagnosis is 4 years, but a quarter of all patients are younger than 3 years. Males are 1.4 times more likely to develop EP than females are.[9]

Pathology

The new WHO classification still differentiates subependymoma and myxopapillary EP (grade 1), classic (grade 2), and anaplastic EP (grade 3).[28] In addition, RELA fusion–positive EPs are newly listed. This mutation is reserved for supratentorial tumors and is quite consistently found.[47] Similar to MBs, supra- and infratentorial EPs are genetically different. The elucidation of that finding will most certainly have therapeutic implications in the future.

Histologically, EPs are glial neoplasms arising from ependymal cell layers adjacent to the ventricular system or the central spinal canal.[8] Histology

of EP is quite uniform, showing cells with oval or round nuclei, typically arranged in pseudorosettes around vessels. Similar to MB, there is no connection of histomorphologic features to the clinical course (within the same WHO grade).[46] For posterior fossa EPs, transcriptional profiling showed the existence of two large subgroups: posterior fossa A and B EPs (PFA and PFB). PFA patients are younger, have laterally located tumors with a balanced genome, and are much more likely to exhibit recurrence, metastasis at recurrence, and death, compared to PFB patients.[48]

Imaging

EPs in the posterior fossa are found either midline, arising from the roof or floor of the fourth ventricle (likely PFB EPs), or in the cerebellopontine angle (likely PFA EPs), encasing CNs and vascular structures, rendering resection extremely challenging. Typically, EPs appear hypointense in T1, hyperintense in T2, and hyperintense in FLAIR (fluid-attenuated inversion recovery) studies. Calcifications and intratumoral hemorrhages are common.[4] Leptomeningeal seeding does occur, mostly in the lumbosacral region, and 10% of the patients do have a positive CSF cytology at presentation.[4]

Management

Surgery

EP is a surgical disease. Complete surgical resection is the therapeutic goal and primary significant predictor of oncologic outcome. In fact, 5-year survival rate drops from 70 to 30% when residual tumor is appreciated on early postoperative MRI.[49] This circumstance warrants the strong consideration of second-look surgery to chase tumor remnants. The tendency to encase neurovascular structures, however, makes aggressive resection especially in the cerebellopontine angle a dangerous endeavor, and is connected with significant morbidity.[49] Recurrences should also be addressed surgically if possible, as they often occur at the primary tumor site.[49] Unfortunately, prognosis of recurrent EP is very poor, with a median survival time ranging from 8 to 24 months.[49]

Radiation Therapy

EPs are radiosensitive, making adjuvant radiation therapy mandatory in patients older than 3 years. About 45 to 56 Gy are administered to the tumor bed. In the absence of spinal dissemination in imaging or CSF cytology, craniospinal irradiation is not indicated, as it did not show to lower distant treatment failure rate.[49] Re-irradiation or radiosurgery can be considered in children with recurrent EP, although morbidity of re-irradiation is high.[50,51]

Chemotherapy

Currently, there is no established chemotherapy protocol in the treatment of EP. Bridging chemotherapy in infants is administered—usually cyclophosphamide and vincristine—to defer radiotherapy, but response rates are as low as 50%.[52]

Follow-up

The intervals of follow-up imaging largely depend on the achievement of a surgical gross total resection and should be chosen on an individual basis. The presence of residual tumor should warrant a closer follow-up, as relapses are frequent.

20.4.5 Atypical Teratoid/Rhabdoid Tumor

Epidemiology

AT/RT is a relatively new tumor entity, listed in the WHO classification since 2000.[28] AT/RTs form 1% of all pediatric brain tumors. A third occurs in the cerebellum or cerebellopontine angle. There is a 3:2 male predominance, and the median age of onset lies at 26 months. CSF dissemination is identified in 25% of the patients at the time of diagnosis. The prognosis is dismal, with an OS of 18 months without dissemination and 8 months with dissemination.[53]

Pathology

Using conventional histopathologic methods, AT/RTs show nests or sheets of rhabdoid cells, but also contain regions that are indistinguishable to MB. This circumstance led to the relatively late first description of AT/RTs in 1987. This also implies the possibility of sampling error in small biopsies.[4] Immunohistological staining for nuclear INI1 (absent in AT/RT and present in MB) and the identification of monosomy 22 help in placing the diagnosis.[54]

Imaging

There are no characteristic imaging features for AT/RT. The tumor shows similarities with MB, with an isointense T1 signal, heterogeneous T2 signal, and a patchy contrast enhancement.[4]

Management

Surgery

Similar to all tumors discussed, gross total resection of AT/RTs treats the consequences of a posterior fossa mass lesion, allows for tissue diagnosis, and is also believed to have a positive impact on oncologic outcome, although this effect is not as satisfying as with MBs or EPs.[55] The interface between cerebellum and AT/RTs can be ill-defined, and tumors found in the cerebellopontine angle often encase neurovascular structures, rendering resection difficult. Gross total resection is feasible in about 30% of the patients.[9]

Radiation Therapy

Postoperative radiation therapy is statistically effective. The gain in median OS, however, is only 10 months (OS 8.5 months without, 18.4 months with radiotherapy).[55] Many patients show evidence of disseminated disease at presentation, so usually craniospinal irradiation is administered. The known restrictions for the irradiation of children younger than 3 years apply, being of special importance in AT/RTs, as a large proportion of patients is younger than 3 years at the time of diagnosis.

Chemotherapy

Standard chemotherapy has not proven to be particularly effective in AT/RT. This led to the evaluation of high-dose alkylator-based chemotherapy with stem cell rescue.[56] The addition of intrathecal chemotherapy in recent studies increased OS at 2 years to 70%.[55] Novel approaches include the administration of a dendritic cell–based vaccination, reported as being successful in individual patients.[57]

Follow-up

Short survival times in patients diagnosed with AT/RT usually lead to symptom-based follow-up imaging.

20.4.6 Choroid Plexus Papilloma and Choroid Plexus Carcinoma

Epidemiology

Choroid plexus tumors are rare and comprise 0.5% of all pediatric CNS neoplasms.[4] They can occur in all age groups, but 70% of them are diagnosed before the age of 2 years. Male patients are affected more frequently with a ratio of 1.3:1.[58] Anatomically, they are distributed along the ventricular system, the choroid plexus as the tissue of origin given. In younger children, the lateral ventricles are affected more frequently, whereas in older children and adults choroid plexus tumors are localized rather in the fourth ventricle and the cerebellopontine angle.[58]

Pathology

According to the WHO, three classes of choroid plexus tumors are differentiated: CPP is assigned a WHO grade 1 and its anaplastic variant a grade 2. CPC receives a WHO grade 3.[28] Histologically, CPPs resemble normal choroid plexus tissue. CPP does not show necrosis, brain invasion, or mitotic figures, in contrast to CPC, where marked cytological atypia, nuclear pleomorphism, frequent mitoses, vascular proliferation, hemorrhage, and brain infiltration are seen.[59] Anaplastic CPPs present an intermediate degree of nuclear atypia and mitotic figures.[58] A number of genetic syndromes are known to predispose to CPP and CPC, like Li–Fraumeni syndrome, neurofibromatosis type 2, Aicardi's syndrome, Down's syndrome, and von Hippel–Lindau disease.[60] This led to the discovery of a range of chromosomal imbalances at the molecular level of these tumors.[60]

Imaging

Homogenous tumors with a "frondlike" appearance in close anatomical relation to the ventricular system and associated hydrocephalus are the typical imaging appearance of choroid plexus tumors. They appear isointense in T1 and heterogeneous in T2 sequences, with a marked contrast enhancement. Differentiation of CPP from CPC is not possible on imaging, although CPC is more prone to brain invasion and peritumoral edema than CPP. Calcifications are common.[58]

Management

Surgery

Again, the extent of surgical resection is a significant prognostic factor, especially in CPC.[4] The marked vascularity of these tumors is one of the surgical challenges. This even led to the implementation of preresectional chemotherapy to minimize blood loss.[61] Resection of a WHO grade 1 CPP is considered curative. Anaplastic CPPs are primarily managed surgically, and adjuvant treatment is discussed when dissemination or recurrence occurs.[59]

Radiation Therapy

Radiation therapy is indicated in CPCs and anaplastic CPPs with postoperative residual disease, recurrence, or dissemination.[58] As in all pediatric brain tumors, radiation therapy is deferred in children younger than 3 years whenever possible.

Chemotherapy

The combination of radiation therapy and chemotherapy is routinely administered in CPC.[62] With this treatment regime, OS at 2 years is 100% for CPP, 89% for anaplastic CPP, and 36% for CPC.[59] The use of preresectional chemotherapy in CPC—after biopsy to establish the diagnosis—has to be given strong consideration. Given the young age of the patients, upfront surgical resection can lead to the loss of several blood volumes. After chemotherapy, tumor tissue becomes fibrotic and less vascularized, allowing for a relatively bloodless removal.[61]

Follow-up

Follow-up intervals are dictated by the WHO grading of choroid plexus tumors. In CPP grade 1, annual MRI of the brain after early resection control is sufficient. In anaplastic CPP and CPC, close MRI observation of brain and spine is recommended.

20.5 Common Clinical Questions

1. Name the three most common tumors in the pediatric posterior fossa and the most important factor for a good oncologic outcome.
2. What are clinically important features of a posterior fossa mass lesion?
3. What are the main predicting factors for a persistent hydrocephalus after resection of a posterior fossa tumor?
4. What histological subtypes are differentiated in medulloblastoma and what is the reason for the proposal of a new genetic stratification?
5. What is the primary option when residual ependymoma is seen on postresectional early MRI?

6. What is an intriguing histological feature of pilocytic astrocytoma when correlated to clinical outcome?

20.6 Answers to Common Clinical Questions

1. The three most common tumors in the pediatric posterior fossa are: (1) medulloblastoma, (2) pilocytic astrocytoma, and (3) ependymoma. The achievement of a good resection is the most important factor for a good oncologic outcome in all three.
2. Special to posterior fossa mass lesions is their anatomical relation to vital structures in a confined space. Hydrocephalus due to blockage of CSF pathways can result in rapid clinical deterioration; invasion of brainstem or encasement of lower CNs can lead to significant morbidity.
3. Risk factors for a postresectional hydrocephalus comprise: (1) age < 2 years, (2) presence of transependymal edema, (3) preresectional moderate or severe hydrocephalus, (4) presence of cerebral metastases, and (5) histological diagnosis of medulloblastoma, ependymoma, or dorsal exophytic brainstem glioma.
4. Histologically, four types of medulloblastomas (MB) are differentiated: (1) classic MB, (2) desmoplastic/nodular-type MB, (3) MB with extensive nodularity, and (4) large cell anaplastic MB. The clinical prognosis, however, correlates better with the new molecular stratification.
5. The prognosis of ependymoma strongly depends on surgical gross total resection. In case of postoperative residual tumor, reoperation must be considered if resection of the remnant seems to be safely possible.
6. The presence of high mitotic activity, cellular atypia, and microvascular proliferation does not affect grading and clinical outcome of PA.

References

[1] Boop FA, Sanford RA, Taylor MD. Surgical management of pediatric posterior fossa tumors. In: Nanda A, ed. Principles of Posterior Fossa Surgery. New York, NY: Thieme; 2012

[2] Fleming AJ, Chi SN. Brain tumors in children. Curr Probl Pediatr Adolesc Health Care. 2012; 42(4):80–103

[3] Dolecek TA, Propp JM, Stroup NE, Kruchko C. CBTRUS statistical report: primary brain and central nervous system tumors diagnosed in the United States in 2005–2009. Neuro-oncol. 2012; 14 Suppl 5:v1–v49

[4] Weeks A, Fallah A, Rutka JT. Posterior fossa and brainstem tumors in children. In: Abdulrauf SI, Ellenbogen RG, Sekhar LN, eds. Principles of Neurological Surgery. Philadelphia, PA: Saunders/Elsevier; 2012

[5] Thompson EM, Hielscher T, Bouffet E, et al. Prognostic value of medulloblastoma extent of resection after accounting for molecular subgroup: a retrospective integrated clinical and molecular analysis. Lancet Oncol. 2016; 17(4):484–495

[6] Pang J, Banerjee A, Tihan T. The value of tandem CSF/MRI evaluation for predicting disseminated disease in childhood central nervous system neoplasms. J Neurooncol. 2008; 87 (1):97–102

[7] Harrison EA, Mackersie A, McEwan A, Facer E. The sitting position for neurosurgery in children: a review of 16 years' experience. Br J Anaesth. 2002; 88(1):12–17

[8] Due-Tønnessen BJ, Helseth E. Management of hydrocephalus in children with posterior fossa tumors: role of tumor surgery. Pediatr Neurosurg. 2007; 43(2):92–96

[9] Jung TY, Rutka JT. Posterior fossa tumors in the pediatric population: multidisciplinary management. In: Quiñones-Hinojosa A, Schmidek HH, eds. Schmidek & Sweet: Operative Neurosurgical Techniques: Indications, Methods, and Results. Vol 1. 6th ed. Philadelphia, PA: Elsevier/Saunders; 2012

[10] Riva-Cambrin J, Detsky AS, Lamberti-Pasculli M, et al. Predicting postresection hydrocephalus in pediatric patients with posterior fossa tumors. J Neurosurg Pediatr. 2009; 3(5):378–385

[11] Foreman P, McClugage S, III, Naftel R, et al. Validation and modification of a predictive model of postresection hydrocephalus in pediatric patients with posterior fossa tumors. J Neurosurg Pediatr. 2013; 12(3):220–226

[12] Bhatia R, Tahir M, Chandler CL. The management of hydrocephalus in children with posterior fossa tumours: the role of pre-resectional endoscopic third ventriculostomy. Pediatr Neurosurg. 2009; 45(3):186–191

[13] Baird LC, Javalkar V, Nanda A. Basic concepts in posterior fossa surgery. In: Nanda A, ed. Principles of Posterior Fossa Surgery. New York, NY: Thieme; 2012

[14] Rhoton AL, Jr. Cerebellum and fourth ventricle. Neurosurgery. 2000; 47(3) Suppl:S7–S27

[15] Tanriover N, Ulm AJ, Rhoton AL, Jr, Yasuda A. Comparison of the transvermian and telovelar approaches to the fourth ventricle. J Neurosurg. 2004; 101(3):484–498

[16] Mussi AC, Rhoton AL, Jr. Telovelar approach to the fourth ventricle: microsurgical anatomy. J Neurosurg. 2000; 92(5):812–823

[17] Macdonald DB, Skinner S, Shils J, Yingling C, American Society of Neurophysiological Monitoring. Intraoperative motor evoked potential monitoring - a position statement by the American Society of Neurophysiological Monitoring. Clin Neurophysiol. 2013; 124(12):2291–2316

[18] Gharabaghi A, Rosahl SK, Feigl GC, et al. Image-guided lateral suboccipital approach: part 2-impact on complication rates and operation times. Neurosurgery. 2008; 62(3) Suppl 1:24–29, discussion 29

[19] Yousaf J, Avula S, Abernethy LJ, Mallucci CL. Importance of intraoperative magnetic resonance imaging for pediatric brain tumor surgery. Surg Neurol Int. 2012; 3 Suppl 2:S65–S72

[20] Kubben PL, van Santbrink H, ter Laak-Poort M, et al. Implementation of a mobile 0.15-T intraoperative MR system in pediatric neuro-oncological surgery: feasibility and correlation with early postoperative high-field strength MRI. Childs Nerv Syst. 2012; 28(8):1171–1180

[21] Lam FC, Kasper E. Augmented autologous pericranium duraplasty in 100 posterior fossa surgeries–a retrospective case series. Neurosurgery. 2012; 71(2) Suppl Operative: ons302–ons307

[22] Barth M, Tuettenberg J, Thomé C, Weiss C, Vajkoczy P, Schmiedek P. Watertight dural closure: is it necessary? A prospective randomized trial in patients with supratentorial craniotomies. Neurosurgery. 2008; 63(4) Suppl 2:352–358, discussion 358

[23] Steinbok P, Singhal A, Mills J, Cochrane DD, Price AV. Cerebrospinal fluid (CSF) leak and pseudomeningocele formation after posterior fossa tumor resection in children: a retrospective analysis. Childs Nerv Syst. 2007; 23(2):171–174, discussion 175

[24] Pitsika M, Tsitouras V. Cerebellar mutism. J Neurosurg Pediatr. 2013; 12(6):604–614

[25] Di Rocco C, Chieffo D, Pettorini BL, Massimi L, Caldarelli M, Tamburrini G. Preoperative and postoperative neurological, neuropsychological and behavioral impairment in children with posterior cranial fossa astrocytomas and medulloblastomas: the role of the tumor and the impact of the surgical treatment. Childs Nerv Syst. 2010; 26(9):1173–1188

[26] Muzumdar D, Ventureyra EC. Treatment of posterior fossa tumors in children. Expert Rev Neurother. 2010; 10(4):525–546

[27] Sturm D, Orr BA, Toprak UH, et al. New brain tumor entities emerge from molecular classification of CNS-PNETs. Cell. 2016; 164(5):1060–1072

[28] Louis DN, Perry A, Reifenberger G, et al. The 2016 World Health Organization Classification of Tumors of the Central Nervous System: a summary. Acta Neuropathol. 2016; 131 (6):803–820

[29] Taylor MD, Mainprize TG, Rutka JT. Molecular insight into medulloblastoma and central nervous system primitive neuroectodermal tumor biology from hereditary syndromes: a review. Neurosurgery. 2000; 47(4):888–901

[30] Louis DN, Ohgaki H, Wiestler OD, et al. The 2007 WHO classification of tumours of the central nervous system. Acta Neuropathol. 2007; 114(2):97–109

[31] Northcott PA, Shih DJ, Peacock J, et al. Subgroup-specific structural variation across 1,000 medulloblastoma genomes. Nature. 2012; 488(7409):49–56

[32] Northcott PA, Korshunov A, Witt H, et al. Medulloblastoma comprises four distinct molecular variants. J Clin Oncol. 2011; 29(11):1408–1414

[33] Northcott PA, Korshunov A, Pfister SM, Taylor MD. The clinical implications of medulloblastoma subgroups. Nat Rev Neurol. 2012; 8(6):340–351

[34] Ris MD, Walsh K, Wallace D, et al. Intellectual and academic outcome following two chemotherapy regimens and radiotherapy for average-risk medulloblastoma: COG A9961. Pediatr Blood Cancer. 2013; 60(8):1350–1357

[35] Rudin CM, Hann CL, Laterra J, et al. Treatment of medulloblastoma with hedgehog pathway inhibitor GDC-0449. N Engl J Med. 2009; 361(12):1173–1178

[36] Zeltzer PM, Boyett JM, Finlay JL, et al. Metastasis stage, adjuvant treatment, and residual tumor are prognostic factors for medulloblastoma in children: conclusions from the Children's Cancer Group 921 randomized phase III study. J Clin Oncol. 1999; 17(3):832–845

[37] Dhall G, Grodman H, Ji L, et al. Outcome of children less than three years old at diagnosis with non-metastatic medulloblastoma treated with chemotherapy on the "Head Start" I and II protocols. Pediatr Blood Cancer. 2008; 50(6):1169–1175

[38] Gajjar A, Chintagumpala M, Ashley D, et al. Risk-adapted craniospinal radiotherapy followed by high-dose chemotherapy and stem-cell rescue in children with newly diagnosed medulloblastoma (St Jude Medulloblastoma-96): long-term results from a prospective, multicentre trial. Lancet Oncol. 2006; 7(10):813–820

[39] Gottardo NG, Gajjar A. Current therapy for medulloblastoma. Curr Treat Options Neurol. 2006; 8(4):319–334

[40] Tibbetts KM, Emnett RJ, Gao F, Perry A, Gutmann DH, Leonard JR. Histopathologic predictors of pilocytic astrocytoma event-free survival. Acta Neuropathol. 2009; 117(6):657–665

[41] Forshew T, Tatevossian RG, Lawson AR, et al. Activation of the ERK/MAPK pathway: a signature genetic defect in posterior fossa pilocytic astrocytomas. J Pathol. 2009; 218(2):172–181

[42] Sadighi Z, Slopis J. Pilocytic astrocytoma: a disease with evolving molecular heterogeneity. J Child Neurol. 2013; 28 (5):625–632

[43] Lee YY, Van Tassel P, Bruner JM, Moser RP, Share JC. Juvenile pilocytic astrocytomas: CT and MR characteristics. AJR Am J Roentgenol. 1989; 152(6):1263–1270

[44] Aryan HE, Meltzer HS, Lu DC, Ozgur BM, Levy ML, Bruce DA. Management of pilocytic astrocytoma with diffuse leptomeningeal spread: two cases and review of the literature. Childs Nerv Syst. 2005; 21(6):477–481

[45] Due-Tønnessen BJ, Helseth E, Scheie D, Skullerud K, Aamodt G, Lundar T. Long-term outcome after resection of benign cerebellar astrocytomas in children and young adults (0–19 years): report of 110 consecutive cases. Pediatr Neurosurg. 2002; 37(2):71–80

[46] Shu HK, Sall WF, Maity A, et al. Childhood intracranial ependymoma: twenty-year experience from a single institution. Cancer. 2007; 110(2):432–441

[47] Parker M, Mohankumar KM, Punchihewa C, et al. C11orf95-RELA fusions drive oncogenic NF-κB signalling in ependymoma. Nature. 2014; 506(7489):451–455

[48] Witt H, Mack SC, Ryzhova M, et al. Delineation of two clinically and molecularly distinct subgroups of posterior fossa ependymoma. Cancer Cell. 2011; 20(2):143–157

[49] Vinchon M, Leblond P, Noudel R, Dhellemmes P. Intracranial ependymomas in childhood: recurrence, reoperation, and outcome. Childs Nerv Syst. 2005; 21(3):221–226

[50] Merchant TE, Boop FA, Kun LE, Sanford RA. A retrospective study of surgery and reirradiation for recurrent ependymoma. Int J Radiat Oncol Biol Phys. 2008; 71(1):87–97

[51] Stafford SL, Pollock BE, Foote RL, Gorman DA, Nelson DF, Schomberg PJ. Stereotactic radiosurgery for recurrent ependymoma. Cancer. 2000; 88(4):870–875

[52] Grundy RG, Wilne SA, Weston CL, et al. Children's Cancer and Leukaemia Group (formerly UKCCSG) Brain Tumour Committee. Primary postoperative chemotherapy without radiotherapy for intracranial ependymoma in children: the UKCCSG/SIOP prospective study. Lancet Oncol. 2007; 8(8):696–705

[53] Athale UH, Duckworth J, Odame I, Barr R. Childhood atypical teratoid rhabdoid tumor of the central nervous system: a meta-analysis of observational studies. J Pediatr Hematol Oncol. 2009; 31(9):651–663

[54] Janson K, Nedzi LA, David O, et al. Predisposition to atypical teratoid/rhabdoid tumor due to an inherited INI1 mutation. Pediatr Blood Cancer. 2006; 47(3):279–284

[55] Chi SN, Zimmerman MA, Yao X, et al. Intensive multimodality treatment for children with newly diagnosed CNS atypical teratoid rhabdoid tumor. J Clin Oncol. 2009; 27(3):385–389

[56] Tekautz TM, Fuller CE, Blaney S, et al. Atypical teratoid/rhabdoid tumors (ATRT): improved survival in children 3 years of age and

older with radiation therapy and high-dose alkylator-based chemotherapy. J Clin Oncol. 2005; 23(7):1491–1499

[57] Ardon H, De Vleeschouwer S, Van Calenbergh F, et al. Adjuvant dendritic cell-based tumour vaccination for children with malignant brain tumours. Pediatr Blood Cancer. 2010; 54(4): 519–525

[58] Gupta N. Choroid plexus tumors in children. Neurosurg Clin N Am. 2003; 14(4):621–631

[59] Wrede B, Hasselblatt M, Peters O, et al. Atypical choroid plexus papilloma: clinical experience in the CPT-SIOP-2000 study. J Neurooncol. 2009; 95(3):383–392

[60] Rickert CH, Wiestler OD, Paulus W. Chromosomal imbalances in choroid plexus tumors. Am J Pathol. 2002; 160(3):1105–1113

[61] Schneider C, Kamaly-Asl I, Ramaswamy V, et al. Neoadjuvant chemotherapy reduces blood loss during the resection of pediatric choroid plexus carcinomas. J Neurosurg Pediatr. 2015; 16(2):126–133

[62] Wrede B, Liu P, Wolff JE. Chemotherapy improves the survival of patients with choroid plexus carcinoma: a meta-analysis of individual cases with choroid plexus tumors. J Neurooncol. 2007; 85(3):345–351

21 Brainstem Gliomas

Mari L. Groves, Rafael U. Cardenas, Nir Shimony, George I. Jallo

21.1 Introduction

Primary brainstem tumors encompass 10 to 20% of all central nervous system tumors in the pediatric population.[1] They most commonly present in childhood with a mean age of diagnosis of 7 to 9 years,[2,3] although they can occur at any age. There are 150 to 300 cases each year[4,5] in the United States. There is no gender predilection. In the adults, brain stem tumors are rarer, comprising only about 2% of all brain tumors,[6] and represent a greater diversity of pathology.[7] Approximately 80% of brainstem gliomas are diffuse intrinsic pontine gliomas (DIPGs) and carry a poor prognosis.[1] However, the remaining 15 to 20% of brainstem gliomas are low-grade astrocytomas, and these portend a more favorable course. Magnetic resonance imaging (MRI) provides the most precise information regarding the tumor epicenter and most likely diagnosis, which can then predict its biological behavior.[8] Choux and colleagues proposed a radiographic classification that defines brain tumors by four types: diffuse (type I), intrinsic focal (type II), exophytic focal (type III), and cervicomedullary (type IV)[9] (▶ Fig. 21.1).

- Type I tumors are diffuse brainstem gliomas and account for 75% of all brainstem tumors. Diffuse lesions are typically hypointense on T1-weighted sequences that are noncontrast enhancing and have some hyperintensity on T2-weighted images. These lesions are most commonly found within the pons and are malignant fibrillary astrocytomas (WHO grade III or IV).
- Type II lesions are focal, intrinsic tumors that can be cystic or solid. These lesions are most commonly low-grade gliomas (WHO I or II). T1-weighted images show variable contrast enhancement, but uniform enhancement can be characteristic of pilocytic astrocytomas.
- Type III lesions are defined as focal exophytic tumors that arise from the subependymal glial tissue of the fourth ventricle and grow both dorsal and laterally.
- Type IV lesions are cervicomedullary tumors with a presentation and behavior similar to intramedullary spinal cord gliomas. These lesions are typically low grade, noninfiltrative with growth that is confined by the white matter of the corticospinal tract and medial lemniscus.

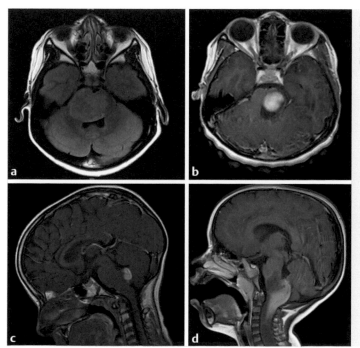

Fig. 21.1 Four types of brain tumors: **(a)** type I, diffuse; **(b)** type II, focal; **(c)** type III, dorsally exophytic; and **(d)** type IV, cervicomedullary.

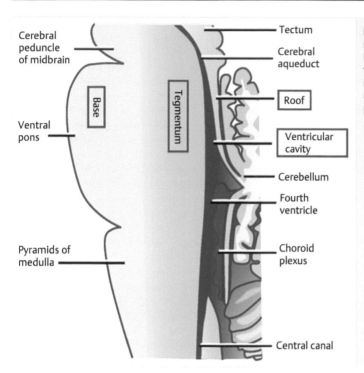

Cerebral peduncle of midbrain

Base

Tegmentum

Ventral pons

Pyramids of medulla

Tectum

Cerebral aqueduct

Roof

Ventricular cavity

Cerebellum

Fourth ventricle

Choroid plexus

Central canal

Fig. 21.2 Sagittal profile of the brainstem. There are four major parts of the brainstem that are contiguous throughout the medulla, pons, and midbrain: ventricular cavity, roof, tegmentum, and base. (Reproduced with permission from Alberstone et al.[10])

21.2 Anatomy

The brainstem, or mesencephalon, is composed of the midbrain, pons, and medulla. These are then broken into four areas: the ventricular cavity, roof, tegmentum, and base[10] (▶ Fig. 21.2).

- Ventricular cavity: extending from the rostral extent of the cerebral aqueduct of Sylvius to the obex and the beginning of the central canal of the spinal cord. Comprises the central canal as well as the fourth ventricle.
- Roof: overlying the ventricular cavity and comprised of the choroid plexus and tela choroidea of the fourth ventricle, the cerebellum, and the tectum.
- Tegmentum: ventral to the ventricular cavity and containing the cranial nerves (CNs) and their nuclei, major long ascending tracts, and the reticular formation.
- Base: comprised of the medullary pyramids, ventral pons, and crura cerebri of the midbrain. The major long descending tracts including the corticospinal, corticobulbar, and corticopontine tracts also traverse this space.

CN III through XII are located within the brainstem and are grouped into longitudinal columns. These columns carry their own functional distinction

with motor nuclei located medially and sensory nuclei located laterally. The medial columns are composed of somatic and visceral motor nuclei.[10]

- Column 1: immediately adjacent to midline and composed of neurons that innervate the striated muscles of the head and neck arising from embryonic myotomes.
  - Oculomotor nucleus (III): located in the midbrain at the level of the superior colliculus, just ventral to the cerebral aqueduct.
  - Trochlear nucleus (IV): located in the midbrain at the level of the inferior colliculus, just ventral to the cerebral aqueduct.
  - Abducens nucleus (VI): located in the pons, just ventral to the floor of the fourth ventricle.
  - Hypoglossal nucleus (XII): located in the medulla, just ventral to the floor of the fourth ventricle.
- Column 2: located lateral and ventral to column 1 and comprised of neurons that innervate the striated muscles of the head and neck derived from the branchial arches.
  - Motor nucleus of the trigeminal nerve (V): located in the pons.
  - Facial motor nucleus (VII): located in the pons.
  - Nucleus ambiguous (IX and X): located in the medulla.

- Nucleus of the spinal accessory nerve (XI): extends from the medulla into the cervical region of the spinal cord.
- Column 3: located immediately lateral to column 1: consists of nuclei of preganglionic parasympathetic neurons.
  - Edinger–Westphal nucleus (III): located in midbrain.
  - Superior and inferior salivatory nuclei (VII and IX, respectively): located in medulla.
  - Dorsal motor nucleus of the vagus (X): located in medulla.
- Lateral columns containing three sensory nuclei. Each sensory nucleus receives inputs from several different CN.
  - Trigeminal sensory nucleus, comprised of three distinct nuclei: the mesencephalic nucleus, main sensory nucleus, and the spinal trigeminal tract nucleus.
  - Vestibular and cochlear nuclei: extending from the rostral medulla into the pons.
  - Solitary nucleus: located in the medulla.

There are four long tracts, two ascending and two descending, that traverse the brainstem.
- The spinothalamic tract is the most lateral in the brainstem.
- The medial lemniscus, corticospinal, and corticobulbar tracts lie medially within the brainstem.
- The reticular formation extends from the higher cortical regions and the thalamus to the spinal cord and consists of the parvocellular zone and the magnocellular zone. These interneurons are responsible for motor, respiratory and cardiovascular control, sensory control, and consciousness.

21.3 Examination

Physical examination of patients with brainstem lesions includes a thorough neurological exam with special attention to CN function. Three important components should be ascertained during the workup: signs and symptoms related to the intra-axial component, signs and symptoms of hydrocephalus, and symptom onset. A complete clinical picture includes a thorough history and physical. A historical account may include old school pictures that may be helpful to track new cranial neuropathies, declining school performance, recurrent upper respiratory tract infections, or changes in voice.[11] More malignant lesions will present with rapidly presenting symptoms, whereas low-grade lesions present with a longer prodrome of months to years. They can impact multiple CN signs, ataxia, long tract signs, or cerebellar signs.[12] Interruption of corticospinal tract fibers will result in upper motor neuron syndromes including the loss of fine motor skills, spasticity, initial hyporeflexia followed by hyperreflexia, and up-going extensor plantar reflex.[12] The most common cranial neuropathies are CN VI and VII weakness.[13]

- Tectal lesions primarily compress the sylvian aqueduct causing obstructive hydrocephalus and oculomotor paresis.
- Midbrain lesions are typically low-grade gliomas.
- Focal pontine lesions have a poorer prognosis and present with facial paresis, hearing loss, or long tract findings.
- Focal medullary lesions present with lower CN deficits manifesting as vocal changes, swallowing difficulty, or pneumonias due to microaspirations.
- Tumors with a large dorsal exophytic component present with symptoms due to direct compression of the brainstem or with elevated intracranial pressure.
- Obstructive hydrocephalus manifests as headaches, ataxia, intractable vomiting, blurry vision secondary to papilledema, and torticollis.
- Cervicomedullary tumors may also present with medullary dysfunction as well as cervical cord dysfunction. This includes chronic neck pain, progressive cervical myelopathy with associated weakness, and spasticity.

21.4 Nonsurgical Management

Treatment options include:
- Radiation therapy/radiosurgery.
- Chemotherapy.
- Immunotherapy and other experimental therapies.

Nonsurgical management is the mainstay of therapy in more malignant lesions, such as diffuse pontine tumors. Patients with anaplastic astrocytoma or glioblastoma typically have poor prognosis and should be managed with palliative therapies. For patients who went biopsy and found to have mutation K27 M, prognosis is poor and the lesion should be treated as high grade glioma regardless to the tumor appearane in imaging. For these lesions, surgery has a very limited role and includes possible biopsy or cerebrospinal fluid (CSF) diversion since surgical resection carries significant morbidity with a low likelihood of altering therapy or outcomes. High-risk medical patients, or those with significant comorbidities, should be considered for nonoperative management.

- Diffuse glioma of midline structures (former DIPG): undergo standard conventional radiation therapy consisting of daily fractions given 5 days a week for up to 6 weeks with a total dose of approximately 54 Gy.[1,5,14,15]
- Radiation does not change overall survival, but there is a prolongation of progression-free survival.[16]
- Once tumor progression is noted in DIPG, patients will rapidly deteriorate. The median time between progression and death range from 1 to 4.5 months.[1]
- Historically, there is no clear survival benefit with chemotherapy as a stand-alone therapy or as an adjunct to radiotherapy for DIPG.[1]
- Using specific molecular targets as well as antiviral therapy may increase the utility of adjuvant chemotherapy in some tumor subtypes.

Low-grade lesions such as midbrain or tectal tumors may be observed, as the natural history of these lesions is quite indolent. These patients typically do well following treatment of the obstructive hydrocephalus.[17,18,19] Systematic surveillance should be implemented to assess for any worsening hydrocephalus or tumor growth. In cases of type II to IV lesions that are unresectable or partially resected, radiation and chemotherapy may be offered. These regimens are typically based on protocols developed for the treatment of supratentorial lesions. Tumor response was correlated with higher Karnofsky performance score, higher peripheral dose, smaller tumor volume, and longer symptom duration before radiation on univariate analysis and with Karnofsky performance score alone on multivariate analysis.

21.5 Surgical Indications

Surgery for brainstem tumors should be offered for focal lesions, if there is a questionable diagnosis, or if the biopsy results will alter treatment for a patient in a prospective clinical trial (▶ Fig. 21.3).

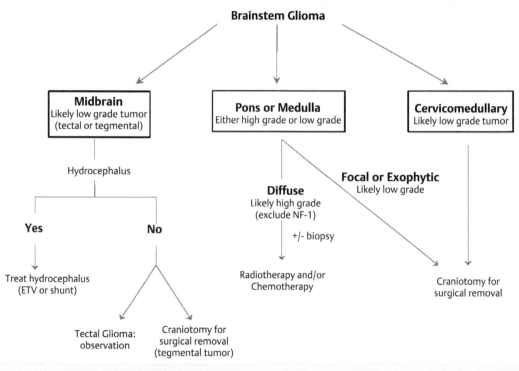

Fig. 21.3 Treatment paradigm for brainstem gliomas.

Surgical treatment should also take into consideration if there is concern for obstructive hydrocephalus. If there is obstruction at the level of the cerebral aqueduct, an endoscopic third ventriculostomy (ETV) may be considered. Patients who undergo an ETV have an 80 to 100% chance of remaining shunt-free with excellent control of the hydrocephalus.[1,19,20]

Appropriate candidates are identified based on the location and focality of the brainstem lesion. Surgical goals aim to resect as much tumor as possible while minimizing neurological sequelae. This is more amenable in focal tumors, as surgical morbidity is higher given the proximity to critical areas of the brainstem.[13] Brainstem biopsy may be indicated in more atypical type I tumors to provide a histopathological diagnosis as well as prognostic information and to guide therapeutic decision-making for more atypical lesions.[21]

21.6 Surgical Technique

Most operative approaches to brainstem tumors require a suboccipital, telovelar approach. For lesions that seem to be laterally situated, a suboccipital paramedian approach may be considered.

Preoperative considerations:
- Intraoperative monitoring is key for safe resection of brainstem lesions. This includes brainstem function monitoring of auditory evoked potential and somatosensory evoked potential. CN monitoring includes CN III, VI, VII, IX, X, and XII and should be set up to record direct motor stimulation from the floor of the fourth ventricle.
- Microsurgical equipment needed: an operating microscope, microsurgical dissectors, an ultrasonic surgical aspiratory device, and a retraction device.

Operative considerations:
- Anesthesiologists should expect neuromonitoring.
- The length of the endotracheal tube should be taken into consideration as the patients will be placed with neck flexion.
- Patients are placed in a prone position.
- Frazier burr hole may be prepared in the event CSF relaxation is needed.
- Internal debulking should be employed for all intrinsic brainstem tumors.
- The safest point of entry is typically where the intrinsic tumor is closest to the surface entry point. This should also be put in context of safe

entry zones in the floor of the fourth ventricle (▶ Fig. 21.4).
- Zone 1: Suprafacial triangle measures 16 mm in greatest distance. This region is superior to the facial colliculus and 5 mm lateral to the midline and away from the medial longitudinal fascicle. It will extend superiorly to below the trochlear nucleus.
- Zone 2: Infrafacial triangle measures < 9 mm and is located inferior to the facial colliculus and the abducens nucleus. The mediolateral borders include the medial longitudinal fascicle and the facial nucleus, respectively.
- Other sulci can provide a zone of safe entry: supracollicular sulcus, the infracollicular sulcus, the lateral mesencephalic sulcus, the median sulcus, the area acustica, the posterior intermediate sulcus, the posterior median fissure below the obex, and the posterior lateral sulcus.

21.7 Complications

Surgical complications include stroke, CN deficits, motor or sensory deficits, brainstem hemorrhage, CSF leak, pseudomeningocele formation, meningitis, or hydrocephalus. CN deficits include transient or permanent diplopia, facial palsy, dysphagia, vocal cord paralysis, or loss of cough or gag with the need for a tracheostomy or gastrostomy tube.
- Retraction injury may cause direct damage, edema, or infarction from compromise of the adjacent vessels, leading to facial sensory, motor, auditory, and speech deficits.
- Transient bradycardia and hypotension may be seen when working close to the nuclei of CN V and IX. When this occurs, cease manipulation of the surgical site until symptoms improve. Any attempt to proceed with surgery could lead to a cardiac event.
- Cerebellar mutism and pseudobulbar syndromes may result from excessive traction along the cerebellar hemispheres and transection of the vermis. Cerebellar mutism is a transient complication, and patients will experience a lack of speech output with intact speech comprehension. This may be associated with an oral pharyngeal apraxia.
- Splitting the cerebellar vermis may also cause equilibratory disturbances with truncal ataxia, staggering gait, oscillation of the head and trunk, and nystagmus on assuming an erect position.

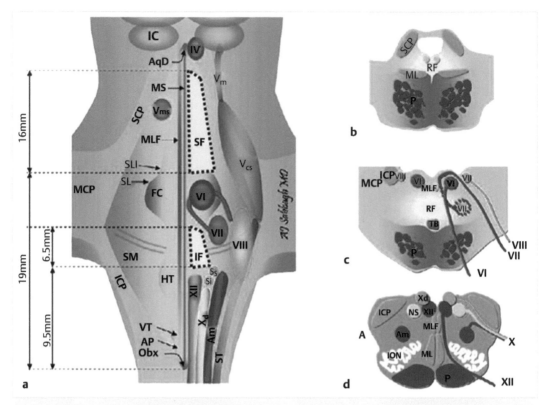

Fig. 21.4 Safe entry zones of the brainstem. Artist's rendering of the brainstem from a dorsal view **(a)** with illustrated safe entry zones and relevant nuclei and neural structures. The infrafacial and suprafacial triangles are highlighted as safe entry zones in the dorsal pons. Corresponding axial sections through the **(b)** upper, **(c)** mid, and **(d)** lower pons are illustrated. Am, nucleus ambiguus of CN IX and X with parasympathetics on its medial border; AP, area postrema; AqD, aqueduct of Sylvius; CTT, central tegmental tract; FC, facial colliculus; HT, hypoglossal triangle; IC, inferior colliculus; ICP, inferior cerebellar peduncle; IF, infrafacial triangle; ION, inferior olivary nucleus; MCP, middle cerebellar peduncle; ML, medial lemniscus; MLF, medial longitudinal fascicle; MS, median sulcus; N, nucleus; Obx, obex; P, pyramid; Pn TPF, pontine nuclei and transverse pontine fibers; SCP superior cerebellar peduncle; SF, suprafacial triangle; SL, sulcus limitans; SLI, sulcus limitans incisure; SM, striae medullares; Ss and Si, superior and inferior salivatory nuclei; ST, spinal trigeminal tract; STT, spinothalamic tract; TB, trapezoid body; Vcs, chief (sensory) nucleus of CN V; Vm, mesencephalic nucleus of CN V; Vms, motor (mastication) nucleus of CN V; VT, vagal triangle; Xd, dorsal vagal nucleus; IV, trochlear nucleus; VI, abducens nucleus; VII, facial nucleus and fiber tracks and nerve; VIII, vestibular nucleus and nerve; XII, hypoglossal nucleus and nerve. (Reproduced with permission from Sabbagh et a. [Fig. 58.4].[22])

- The posterior inferior cerebellar artery wraps around and underneath the cerebellar tonsils. It is susceptible to damage during the initial approach and tumor resection.
- Internal debulking is key as there is typically not a clear plane between the tumor and the brainstem. Attempts to create a plane will lead to damage of the surrounding brainstem as well as perpetuate retraction injury and lead to postoperative CN defects.
- Avoid excessive bipolar use along the brainstem. Most bleeding will stop with gentle pressure

and/or antifibrinolytic agents. Chasing bleeding vessels within the brainstem will result in additional CN defects.
- If intraoperative neuromonitoring changes occur from possibly ischemic changes, then raising the mean arterial pressure (MAP) to a high-normal range should be attempted as in a standard stroke protocol. This should be used in the context of adequate hemostasis.
- Dexamethasone should be used postoperatively to help address retraction injury edema.

- Prior to extubation, patients should be evaluated for adequate motor and respiratory drive. Lower pontine and medullary lesions may require intubation postoperatively until this can safely be assessed. If there has been compromise, patients may experience a gradual CO_2 retention and respiratory collapse due to an inadequate respiratory drive.

21.8 Postoperative Care

Early perioperative care should identify immediate CN deficits to ensure safe extubation and adequate respiratory drive. Patients who do not have an adequate respiratory drive should be considered for early tracheostomy to help facilitate early mobilization and rehabilitation. Patients with cerebellar mutism or oral pharyngeal dysphagia may not be safe for oral intake, and if there is concern for persistent aspiration, then a gastrostomy tube should be considered. Other CN abnormalities should be assessed. If the patient has incomplete eye closure, adequate corneal care as well as a potential lead weight may be considered. For more permanent facial weakness, a facial nerve transfer may be considered to help with facial reanimation. Surgery within the pons may result in transient or permanent diplopia. If this occurs, ophthalmologic treatment with special eyeglass prisms may be necessary.[23]

An MRI should be obtained to evaluate the extent of resection as well as any concerns within the surgical site. If an intraventricular drain was used during surgery, this should be weaned in a standard fashion. Perioperative steroids will also need to be weaned over a 1- to 2-week course.

21.9 Outcomes

The prognosis for patients with DIPG is extremely poor, with a prognosis similar to glioblastoma. DIPGs carry a 10% overall survival rate at 2 years, with a median survival time of < 1 year.[1,12,14,24] The median survival for pediatric patients is 18 months after diagnosis.[1,16]

Other focal brainstem tumors have a better prognosis. One series of focal tumors described a 4-year survival rate of 87.4% and a 4-year disease-free survival rate of 58.8%.[14] The most important prognostic factor was the extent of resection. Another series of low-grade brainstem tumors had a 5-year progression-free survival and overall survival rate of 57 and 89%, respectively.[25] In this series, pathology was an important prognostic factor

on survival, with pilocytic astrocytomas having a 1-year survival rate of 95 ± 5% versus fibrillary astrocytomas at 23 ± 11%.[26] For low-grade lesions, surgical re-resection may be considered for patients who have had growth within an area of recurrent tumor, or in patients whose initial surgery was halted due to changes in intraoperative monitoring or vital sign abnormalities.

Factors associated with poor outcome[12,26]:
- Diffuse glioma of midline structures (former DIPG).
- Age younger than 2 years.
- Presence of CN palsies, particularly abducens nerve palsy.
- Long tract signs on symptoms.
- Pontine location.
- Encasement of the basilar artery.
- Shorter duration of symptoms before diagnosis.

Factors associated with favorable outcomes[12,14]:
- Patients with neurofibromatosis.
- Older age.
- Longer duration of symptoms before diagnosis.

21.10 Surgical Pearls

- Internal debulking is key as there is typically not a clear plane between the tumor and the brainstem. Attempts to create a plane will lead to damage of the surrounding brainstem, as well as perpetuate retraction injury and lead to postoperative CN defects.
- Retraction injury may cause direct damage, edema, or infarction from compromise of the adjacent vessels, leading to facial sensory, motor, auditory, and speech deficits.
- Transient bradycardia and hypotension may be seen when working close to the nuclei of CN V and IX. When this occurs, cease manipulation of the surgical site until symptoms improve. Any attempt to proceed with surgery could lead to a cardiac event.
- Avoid excessive bipolar use along the brainstem. Most bleeding will stop with gentle pressure and/or antifibrinolytic agents. Chasing bleeding vessels within the brainstem will result in additional CN defects. If intraoperative neuromonitoring changes occur from possibly ischemic changes, then raising the MAP to a high-normal range should be attempted as in a standard stroke protocol. This should be used in the context of adequate hemostasis.
- Dexamethasone should be used postoperatively to help address retraction injury edema.

- Prior to extubation, patients should be evaluated for adequate motor and respiratory drive. Lower pontine and medullary lesions may require intubation postoperatively until this can safely be assessed. If there has been compromise, patients may experience a gradual CO_2 retention and respiratory collapse due to an inadequate respiratory drive.

21.11 Common Clinical Questions

1. How do brainstem gliomas commonly present?
2. What is the role of surgery for DIPGs?
3. What preoperative considerations must be made for patients with brainstem gliomas?
4. What is the clinical indication for a second surgical resection?

21.12 Answers to Common Clinical Questions

1. Three important components should be ascertained during the initial workup for a brainstem lesion: signs and symptoms related to the intra-axial component (paying special attention to CN dysfunction), signs and symptoms of hydrocephalus, and symptom onset. The more rapidly progressive lesions typically portend a poor prognosis.
2. For patients presenting with atypical DIPGs, a biopsy may be indicated for diagnosis and to help guide therapeutic strategies. The need for CSF diversion should also be assessed as these patients are at risk for obstructing the normal CSF outflow pathway.
3. Intraoperative neuromonitoring is key for avoiding complications. Patients should have appropriate brainstem reflexes and centers monitored. The endotracheal tube should be at the appropriate length to account for neck flexion. A Frazier burr hole should be prepared in the event that CSF relaxation is needed. Internal debulking should be employed for all intrinsic brainstem tumors to limit damage to the surrounding brainstem and minimize retraction edema.
4. For low-grade lesions, surgical re-resection may be considered for patients who have had growth within an area of recurrent tumor, or in patients whose initial surgery was halted due to changes in intraoperative monitoring or vital sign abnormalities.

References

[1] Hargrave D, Bartels U, Bouffet E. Diffuse brainstem glioma in children: critical review of clinical trials. Lancet Oncol. 2006; 7(3):241–248

[2] Littman P, Jarrett P, Bilaniuk LT, et al. Pediatric brain stem gliomas. Cancer. 1980; 45(11):2787–2792

[3] Berger MS, Edwards MS, LaMasters D, Davis RL, Wilson CB. Pediatric brain stem tumors: radiographic, pathological, and clinical correlations. Neurosurgery. 1983; 12(3):298–302

[4] Allen J. Brain stem glioma. Neurol Neurosurg. 1983; 4:2–7

[5] Walker DA, Punt JA, Sokal M. Clinical management of brain stem glioma. Arch Dis Child. 1999; 80(6):558–564

[6] White HH. Brain stem tumors occurring in adults. Neurology. 1963; 13:292–300

[7] Louis DN, Perry A, Reifenberger G, et al. The 2016 World Health Organization classification of tumors of the central nervous system: a summary. Acta Neuropathol. 2016;131:803–820

[8] McCrea HJ, Souweidane MM. Brainstem gliomas. In: Albright AL, Pollack IF, Adelson PD, eds. Principles and Practice of Pediatric Neurosurgery. 3rd ed. New York, NY: Thieme; 2015

[9] Choux M, Lena G, Do L. Brainstem tumors. In: Choux M, Di Rocco C, Hockley A, eds. Pediatric Neurosurgery. New York, NY: Churchill Livingstone; 2000:471–491

[10] Alberstone CD, Benzel EC, Najm IM, Steinmetz MP, eds. Brainstem. In: Anatomic Basis of Neurologic Diagnosis. New York, NY: Thieme; 2009

[11] Abbott R, Shiminski-Maher T, Epstein FJ. Intrinsic tumors of the medulla: predicting outcome after surgery. Pediatr Neurosurg. 1996; 25(1):41–44

[12] Kaplan AM, Albright AL, Zimmerman RA, et al. Brainstem gliomas in children. A Children's Cancer Group review of 119 cases. Pediatr Neurosurg. 1996; 24(4):185–192

[13] Behnke J, Christen HJ, Brück W, Markakis E. Intra-axial endophytic tumors in the pons and/or medulla oblongata. I. Symptoms, neuroradiological findings, and histopathology in 30 children. Childs Nerv Syst. 1997; 13(3):122–134

[14] Sandri A, Sardi N, Genitori L, et al. Diffuse and focal brain stem tumors in childhood: prognostic factors and surgical outcome. Experience in a single institution. Childs Nerv Syst. 2006; 22(9):1127–1135

[15] Bartels U, Hawkins C, Vézina G, Kun L, Souweidane M, Bouffet E. Proceedings of the diffuse intrinsic pontine glioma (DIPG) Toronto Think Tank: advancing basic and translational research and cooperation in DIPG. J Neurooncol. 2011; 105 (1):119–125

[16] Frazier JL, Lee J, Thomale UW, Noggle JC, Cohen KJ, Jallo GI. Treatment of diffuse intrinsic brainstem gliomas: failed approaches and future strategies. J Neurosurg Pediatr. 2009; 3(4):259–269

[17] Ternier J, Wray A, Puget S, Bodaert N, Zerah M, Sainte-Rose C. Tectal plate lesions in children. J Neurosurg. 2006; 104(6) Suppl:369–376

[18] Wellons JC, III, Tubbs RS, Banks JT, et al. Long-term control of hydrocephalus via endoscopic third ventriculostomy in children with tectal plate gliomas. Neurosurgery. 2002; 51 (1):63–67, discussion 67–68

[19] Javadpour M, Mallucci C. The role of neuroendoscopy in the management of tectal gliomas. Childs Nerv Syst. 2004; 20 (11–12):852–857

[20] Pollack IF, Hoffman HJ, Humphreys RP, Becker L. The long-term outcome after surgical treatment of dorsally exophytic brain-stem gliomas. J Neurosurg. 1993; 78(6):859–863

[21] Cartmill M, Punt J. Diffuse brain stem glioma. A review of stereotactic biopsies. Childs Nerv Syst. 1999; 15(5):235–237, discussion 238

[22] Sabbagh AJ, Albanyan AA, Al Yamany MA, Bunyan R, Abdelmoity AT, Soualmi LB. Brainstem glioma 1: pons. In: Nader R, Sabbagh AJ, eds. Neurosurgery Case Review: Questions and Answers. New York, NY: Thieme; 2009:198–202

[23] Jallo GI, Freed D, Roonprapunt C, Epstein F. Current management of brainstem gliomas. Ann Neurosurg. 2003; 3: 1–17

[24] Wagner S, Warmuth-Metz M, Emser A, et al. Treatment options in childhood pontine gliomas. J Neurooncol. 2006; 79 (3):281–287

[25] Fried I, Hawkins C, Scheinemann K, et al. Favorable outcome with conservative treatment for children with low grade brainstem tumors. Pediatr Blood Cancer. 2012; 58(4):556–560

[26] Fisher PG, Tihan T, Goldthwaite PT, et al. Outcome analysis of childhood low-grade astrocytomas. Pediatr Blood Cancer. 2008; 51(2):245–250

22 Intramedullary Spinal Cord Tumors

Karl F. Kothbauer

22.1 Introduction

Tumors arising from tissue elements within the spinal cord are a small subgroup of central nervous system (CNS) tumors in children. They are considered particularly threatening because of their localization in between densely packed fiber tracts that are all essential for motor control, movement coordination, and different modalities of sensation. Some of the first operations in adults were performed in the first decade of the 19th century by Eiselsberg in Vienna[1] and Elsberg in New York.[2] Later, Greenwood pioneered intramedullary surgery in the 1950s,[3,4,5] and subsequently, series in the modern era of microsurgery appeared,[6,7,8,9] also including series of children.[10]

22.2 Neurosurgical Management of Intramedullary Spinal Cord Tumors[11,12,13,14,15, 16,17,18,19]

22.2.1 Diagnostic Evaluation

Symptoms such as neck or back pain or neurologic dysfunction most often lead to spinal imaging before a pediatric neurosurgeon is consulted.[12] Obtaining a detailed history and a diligent neurological exam is essential.

Magnetic resonance imaging (MRI) of the entire spine is the imaging modality of choice.

Spinal tap for cerebrospinal fluid (CSF) analysis is not required for the diagnostic workup of the great majority of spinal cord tumors.

Interdisciplinary management and evaluation, particularly involving pediatric neurology and oncology, is essential not only for brain tumors but also for spinal cord tumors.

22.2.2 Preoperative Management

The preoperative workup can mostly be done in an outpatient setting.

Steroids can be useful for symptomatic patients and are administered upon hospital admission.

Preoperative blood work must include a coagulation status and a type-and-screen evaluation.

22.2.3 Surgical Considerations

General

The great majority of intramedullary tumors can be removed with elective surgery. However, as with brain tumors, the psychological impact on patients newly diagnosed with a spinal cord tumor and their parents must be taken very seriously.[20] Preoperative communication with the family is extremely important. Obtaining written consent from the parents should be done as early as possible to ensure sufficient time to consider the decision for surgery.

Phone calls from the operating room by the anesthesiologist to update the family on the progress of surgery were found to be extremely well received by all families.

Blood loss in spinal cord surgery in children is usually limited, but may be a factor for younger children and infants with a small total blood volume. The anesthesia team (availability of blood products), scrub nurse (preparation of Cottonoids, hemostatic materials, working bipolar coagulation forceps, and suction), and surgeon (meticulous hemostasis) should anticipate blood loss and pay close attention to blood loss during the surgery (including "hidden blood" in drainage bags, drapes, and Cottonoids).

At a minimum of 30 minutes before incision, perioperative surgical antibiotic prophylaxis is administered, usually cefazolin 30 mg/kg, together with a single dose of steroids on induction (i.e., dexamethasone 4–8 mg).

Positioning

All surgeries for removal of intramedullary spinal cord tumors are performed with the patient in prone position. A rigid head fixation (Sugita or Mayfield) is used for all cervical and upper thoracic exposures at least down to T5. For surgeries further caudally, a neutral head positioning in a soft headrest or a sideways position of the head can be used. However, care has to be taken to avoid too strong lateral rotation for long cases.

It is essential to use soft pads to avoid positional injuries to knees, hips, elbows, toe tips, etc. Soft gel rolls must be used in a body-parallel or transverse fashion to ensure relaxed position of the abdomen to minimize venous pressure.

Approach

A linear midline incision is used. The laminae are exposed in an anatomic layer, preserving the integrity of the musculature and the fascia using a monopolar cautery, utilizing the coagulation mode. It is imperative to gently pull the muscle layers laterally in toto but *not* forge between them as this will cause bleeding, poor wound healing, and pain. The exposed laminae are cut out laterally using a pediatric craniotome. Depending on the number of levels exposed in children, it may be possible to leave the cranial attachment intact and just pull the laminae aside and cover them with drapes. Otherwise, they are removed and preserved. After careful hemostasis, the wound surface is covered with large Cottonoids laterally from the skin to the dura. Then the dura is opened craniocaudally and tacked up laterally. Sometimes, the arachnoid can be opened separately and tacked sideways to expose the cord.

Surgical Adjuncts

Intraoperative Neuromonitoring

The use of motor evoked potential (MEP) and somatosensory evoked potential monitoring must be routine for spinal cord tumor surgery. Including anal sphincter MEPs and monitoring of bulbocavernosus reflex may be useful in cases involving the conus.[21,22]

The best possible extent of resection carries a significant risk of neurological injury. The use of intraoperative neuromonitoring enables the surgeon to be as radical as possible and still preserve long-term function.

The successful application of intraoperative neuromonitoring strongly depends on the teamwork of neurophysiologist (experience in acquisition and interpretation), anesthesiologist (using only intravenous anesthetic agents without muscle relaxants), and surgeon (experience to tailor the procedure according to the monitoring feedback).[22]

Intraoperative Ultrasound[23]

Intraoperative ultrasound is an easy-to-use imaging adjunct for spinal cord surgery. It is especially helpful in:
- Determining the craniocaudal extent of the solid tumor portion.
- Making sure the laminar exposure is sufficient.
- Visualizing cystic tumor component.

- Visualizing residual tumor which may not be apparent on the microscopic view.

Intraoperative Imaging

Intraoperative imaging other than ultrasound at this time is mainly limited to fluoroscopy to determine the correct level of the spinal exposure. It may well be that in the near future the extent of resection of intramedullary tumors will also be determined intraoperatively using intraoperative MRI.

Fluorescent dyes (5-ALA) are used for a variety of brain tumor resections, particularly glioblastoma. The use of 5-ALA fluorescence has also been reported in adult spinal cord tumors.[24]

Ultrasonic Aspirator

The ultrasound aspirator is an essential tool for all neurosurgical tumor resections and also has a key function in spinal cord tumor removal.[25] However, the use of intraoperative MEP monitoring has allowed identifying intraoperative events of significance for postoperative neurological dysfunction. One important result was the observation of intraoperative injury attributed to the use of the ultrasound aspirator (CUSA). This was interpreted such that the propagation of ultrasound in intact tissue reaches the surrounding spinal cord tissue and causes injury there. Since the CUSA continues to be essential for resection of tumors, its utilization was modified to remove tumor portions only after at least partially detaching them rather than going into the intact tumor volume with the CUSA for a primary internal debulking.

Microsurgical Laser

The microsurgical laser is an extremely useful tool for surgery on the spinal cord,[26] as it allows for incision into very soft and particularly very firm tumor tissue with great precision and an acceptable tissue depth penetration. Laser used in conjunction with the microsuction permits piecemeal resection similar to the use of bipolar and suction but without the bipolar's effect of the vasculature, or its electrical artifact prohibiting simultaneous monitoring.

22.2.4 Closure

Meticulous hemostasis of the resection cavity is mandatory. Based on experiences documented by intraoperative monitoring changes, the bipolar coagulation of small bleeding vessels in the wall of the resection cavity, particularly near the anterior spinal artery, must be avoided. Small bleeders can be controlled by Gelfoam, Avitene, or Floseal®, or simply by mild compression and irrigation. The dura must be closed using a running locked 4–0 suture. Braided or monofilic sutures can be used. It appears that braided sutures have less propensity for CSF leakage along the suture stitches, but no clear evidence for this exists. The dura can be covered with Surgicel. Routine use of additional hemostatic materials is not required and can be limited to specific circumstances.

Sometimes, epidural veins may bleed again once the dural tack-up is released for closure. These venous hemorrhages are usually well controlled by bipolar coagulation of the veins toward the lateral edges of the spinal canal. Bleeding from bony elements can be controlled with bone wax. The laminae that were removed at the beginning of surgery should be reinserted with fixation on both sides on every level. In younger children, small burr holes must be made in the laminae and the lateral stumps of the cut laminae. Fixation is made using size 1 Vicryl sutures. In older children, titanium microplates, normally used for craniotomy flaps, are optimal for this fixation. It is essential to ensure that the spinal canal is not narrowed by tilted or displaced laminae to avoid spinal cord compression.[27] The soft-tissue closure begins with not-too-tight 1 Vicryl resorbable sutures to adapt the paraspinal muscles. These sutures should include the spinous processes and/or the interspinous ligaments in order to reconstruct the functional integrity between muscles and the osseous elements. The aponeurotic fascial layer must then be sutured tightly, preferably with inverted suture technique. This is the realistically "watertight" layer which should be closed with extreme care to avoid CSF leakage. Subcutaneous 3–0 Vicryl sutures are applied in an inverted fashion. The skin should be closed using a running-locked suture technique as the final barrier for CSF leakage and with meticulous care to achieve skin adaptation.

As a rule, no wound drains are used in order to minimize CSF leakage and infection.

22.2.5 Postoperative Management

General

All patients are extubated in the operating room after surgery and then transferred to a pediatric intensive care unit for a duration of about 24 hours.

Vitals signs and pain score are documented every 30 minutes until about 5 hours postoperatively and hourly thereafter. Checkup of key neurological functions, particularly motor function, is assessed at the same time.

Pain results from a rather large back incision with a large wound surface and significant detachment of the spinal muscles. Pain therefore must be treated prophylactically and on an as-needed basis to ensure a low level of postoperative pain. Intrathecal injection of morphine at the end of surgery has been shown to be an extremely effective pain management for the first 24 hours.[28]

On the first postoperative day, MRI is routinely performed to assess the extent of tumor removal and the presence of spinal cord compression due to hemorrhage or displaced laminae.

Following imaging, the patient is transferred to a regular floor. Steroids are tapered over a 5-day period.

The patient is encouraged to move freely and receives assistance by physiotherapists for initial mobilization. Getting out of bed should be accomplished on day 1 or no later than day 2. Depending on the initial status and the progress of recovery, it may be possible to discharge the child home after about a week from the operation. If the neurological situation requires inpatient neurorehabilitation, this should be organized in a timely fashion. Most of the time, the plan will be outlined already before surgery, to minimize delays due to waiting times and insurance approvals.

Management of Complications

Postoperative Neurologic Deficits

Postoperative paralysis is possible after spinal cord surgery. Its interpretation depends on the intraoperative findings of MEP and D-wave monitoring. If the neurophysiologic data predict a temporary motor deficit (loss of MEPs with preservation of D-wave), a paraparesis is the expected postoperative status and does not require further treatment other than careful examination to detect a trend toward improvement and initial supportive physiotherapy. Should neuromonitoring indicate intact motor control (MEPs present at the closing baseline) and the patient exhibits para- or monoparesis, then immediate MRI reimaging or even immediate revision of the surgical site must be considered. MEP monitoring is 100% sensitive to postoperative motor deficits[29] and therefore a late surgical problem such as hematoma or spinal cord swelling within the dural sac must be considered. Both require timely revision.

A certain degree of postoperative sensory dysfunction must be considered as normal after spinal cord tumor resection.

Bladder Management

A Foley catheter is inserted after induction of anesthesia for intraoperative fluid management and bladder emptying. Usually, the catheter is removed on the second or third postoperative day. It may take a few days for bladder emptying to normalize. Both long-term incontinence and overflow bladder are rare after spinal cord tumor removal, unless the tumor directly involved the conus medullaris.

Pseudomeningocele and CSF leakage

Even in the best of surgical hands, the "watertight" dural closure is not a complete assurance that CSF will not seep into the epidural space and the wound—hence, the importance of a meticulous multilayer closure! Thus, a degree of CSF accumulation in the tissue or between layers is often seen on postoperative MRI scans, and sometimes, accumulation is also visible and/or palpable under the skin. Most of the time, this will subside without intervention. In such large "pseudomeningoceles," some action may be necessary, and the first measure is prescribing acetazolamide (250 mg every 12 hours), which reduces the production of CSF by about 50%.[30] Clinical experience exists as to the efficacy of this treatment.

Nevertheless, CSF under the skin is a manageable problem. CSF leakage through the incision may be a sign of poor wound closure or of incipient infection, or in rare cases an indicator for hydrocephalus. CSF leakage must prompt bloodwork to assess the presence of infection, a spinal tap with release of at least 20 mL of CSF to divert pressure and obtain CSF analysis. In some cases, the skin may be resutured and the leak stopped with a few single stitches. In the absence of infection and of further leakage, the patient may be observed as an inpatient and after a few days the leakage may resolve. If it does not, and/or if infection is present, a wound revision to irrigate and completely reclose is necessary. At that time, it is most often useful to insert a temporary lumbar CSF drain and keep the patient on strict bedrest to assist wound healing. Drainage should be pressure-controlled at ear level and limited to a maximum average of 20 to 25 mL/hour.

Spinal Deformity

Kyphosis or scoliosis may occur after spinal cord tumor surgery.[31,32] Sometimes, particularly in cystic tumors, scoliosis is part of the presenting clinical syndrome, and may progress following the compromise to spinal stability by the operation. In children and young adults in particular, it is desirable to avoid large stabilization surgery as the growth of the spine may be significantly impaired by stabilization. Stabilization may even be a cause for progressive deformity if it interferes with normal growth! Nevertheless, if kyphosis with subsequent spinal canal narrowing and spinal cord compression occurs, corrective surgery may nonetheless be required. It is an important principle to provide posterior decompression first, if a front-back approach is necessary, as an anterior correction without prior posterior decompression carries a significant risk for surgical compression and paraplegia.

Wound Infection and Bacterial Meningitis

Wound infections after spinal cord surgery appear to be very rare. If they occur, they may be associated with CSF leakage and the same principles apply as stated earlier. If overt wound infection with dehiscence and purulent secretion is clinically seen, urgent, i.e., same-day, wound revision using extensive irrigation and debridement is indicated. If this occurs, only a limited number of resorbable sutures should be used for closure and the skin is best closed with deep 0 braided sutures using the Donati technique. In this situation, a wound drain with minimal or no suction cannot be avoided. A separate lumbar CSF drain may be needed as well. After obtaining microbiology samples, empiric antibiotics should be started, and antibiotic regimen improved as cultures and sensitivity testing become available.

22.3 Specific Types of Intramedullary Spinal Cord Tumors

22.3.1 Overview

The distribution of tumor types in the pediatric population significantly differs from the adult. In children, the prevailing tumor type is pilocytic astrocytoma,[10,19] while in adults ependymomas are most frequent. Gangliogliomas occur as well as other rare tumor types such as hemangioblastomas.[33]

Malignant tumors such as glioblastoma are very rare and usually manifest with rapid neurologic deterioration.[34] Dissemination of tumors from other locations, such as medulloblastomas, may be found. Intermediate-type tumors graded WHO 3 have been reported[35] and are believed to require adjuvant treatment including chemotherapy and, depending on the patient's age, also radiation.

22.3.2 Pilocytic Astrocytoma

Epidemiology

They comprise more than half of all intramedullary tumors in childhood.[12,19,36]

Imaging

Pilocytic astrocytomas are more frequently centrally located but may have eccentric extensions. Cystic components are frequent and these tumors typically show enhancement with gadolinium. Differential diagnosis vis-à-vis ependymomas can be difficult based on MRI alone.

Management

Most complete surgical resection with the preservation of neurologic function is the cornerstone of treatment.[14,18,36,37,38] There is ample evidence and experience about the rationale for surgical resection early on[39,40] as well as the optimal outcome achieved by gross total resection,[19] albeit small remnants of tumor appear not to affect this outcome.[14]

Surgery

Gross total resection must be attempted and is often possible. However, the surgical strategy should put priority on the preservation of neurologic function, particularly the ability to walk. Therefore, the last remnants of a tumor need not be chased, as small residual appears not to significantly impact survival.[14] If a large residual remains at a time when neuromonitoring indicates that no further injury can be tolerated, it is quite possible to switch to a two-stage resection.

The particulars of pilocytic astrocytoma resection are defined by its frequent appearance of having a tumor capsule and thus a well-visible demarcation to the surrounding normal tissue. This may mimic the appearance of ependymoma. However, pilocytic astrocytomas also have areas of diffuse margins to the spinal cord just like a diffuse astrocytoma would have. And this dual appearance must be considered in order to avoid a resection attempt which may cause injury to the normal cord, as one gets "into a wrong layer" when dissecting a capsulelike surface further into a diffuse margin area. The laser is useful to detach tumor tissue and the CUSA to remove such detached tumor bulk. Neuromonitoring with MEPs should constantly be used to always know the functional integrity of the motor pathways. Cysts should be opened early on to achieve decompression in the event of swelling upon dural incision.

Radiation Therapy

There is no rationale to treat pediatric patients with low-grade spinal cord astrocytomas (diffuse of pilocytic) with radiation therapy. The downside of additional cord injury, growth arrest of the affected parts of the spine, or even asymmetric growth may be negative consequences. However, if unusual tumor types are found with WHO 3 or even 4,[35] radiotherapy may well be necessary to prolong survival.

Chemotherapy

The use of chemotherapy based on temozolomide has been tried anecdotally but is not an established treatment for pilocytic astrocytomas. Progression-free survival of 5 years has been observed in patients with growth of residual disease. Higher grade tumors may require chemotherapy with either temozolomide or other regimens.[41]

Follow-up

The MRI scan on postoperative day 1 serves as a quality control for surgery. After 3 months, a baseline MRI should be obtained to assess the presence or absence of residual tumor, cystic formations, scarring, and cord atrophy. If there is no residual tumor, yearly follow-up MRIs are indicated. There is no evidence as to the overall duration of follow-up. It may or may not be acceptable to cease yearly MRIs after a decade.

If residual tumor is found, a first follow-up scan is scheduled for 6 months, and if the residual is stable, yearly scans thereafter are planned.

22.3.3 Ganglioglioma

Epidemiology

These are the third most common intramedullary tumor in childhood comprising 12% of pediatric intramedullary tumors.[19]

Imaging

Gangliogliomas appear to form large tumors, often with considerable cystic components. They are more irregular in texture and configuration than pilocytic astrocytomas, and certainly more so than ependymomas. They also tend to form nodules of solid tumor and cystic components.

Management

Surgery

Complete resection is attempted with very similar aspects as those for pilocytic astrocytomas.

The other aspects are the same as in pilocytic astrocytoma.

22.3.4 Ependymoma

Epidemiology

It is the second most common tumor type in children.[19]

Pathology

Ependymomas are glial neoplasms arising from ependymal cell layers adjacent to the ventricular system or the central spinal canal. Histology of ependymoma is quite uniform, showing cells with oval or round nuclei, typically arranged in pseudorosettes around vessels. Classic ependymoma is grade 2 in the WHO scheme. Subependymomas are rare variants which are classified as WHO 1 as are the conus-cauda variant, the myxopapillary ependymoma.[17]

Imaging

Ependymomas typically are central tumors. They often develop "polar" cyst with some hemorrhagic component. They most often homogenously enhance with gadolinium administration.

Management

Surgery

The complete resection is most important in this subgroup, as they may be considered cured when removed completely. The resection most often is possible along a cleavage plane which surrounds the entire tumor. Only in the anterior wall the tumor vessels arise usually from the anterior spinal artery and must be carefully dissected away from the tumor to avoid vascular injury and subsequent ischemia. It is imperative to avoid bipolar coagulation of these vessels, particularly too close to the anterior spinal artery. It has been clearly shown in the analysis of monitoring data that injury occurred at the time of vessel obliteration. Alternatively, mild compression usually stops bleeding, and if it does not, new hemostatic materials such as Floseal® will.

Subependymomas[42] appear to be sometimes septated with stretches of normal tissue between tumor strands. This may be difficult to detect but important to avoid injury.

Radiation Therapy

Radiation is avoided in all spinal cord ependymomas. However, recently a survival benefit was demonstrated in myxopapillary ependymoma[43] patients who underwent surgery plus radiation versus those who only underwent surgery. However, the downside of radiation treatment to the growing spine must still be carefully weighed against this probably small benefit.

Chemotherapy

No effective chemotherapy is available for spinal cord ependymomas.

Follow-up

The intervals of follow-up imaging largely depend on the achievement of a surgical gross total resection and should be chosen on an individual basis. The presence of residual tumor should warrant a closer follow-up, as relapses are possible.

22.3.5 Diffuse Astrocytoma and Mixed Gliomas

Epidemiology

Usually these astrocytoma variants figure in the "other" category of publications.[19] Therefore, their true incidence is difficult to know. Nevertheless, diffuse astrocytomas and gliomas with oligodendroglias components do occur.

Imaging

These rare tumors may have the diffuse, nonenhancing characteristics their cousins in the brain have. However, tumors of mixed histological composition may be heterogeneous and thus appear with nodules, cysts, and asymmetric cord enlargements, very similar to the appearance of pilocytic tumors.

Management
Surgery

Complete resection with consideration of the aspects put forth earlier on pilocytic astrocytomas is the preferred surgical goal.

Radiation Therapy

In low-grade tumors, no adjuvant treatment is warranted.

Chemotherapy

In low-grade tumors, no adjuvant treatment is warranted.

Follow-up

The follow-up can be the same as for pilocytic astrocytomas.

22.3.6 Hemangioblastoma
Epidemiology

Hemangioblastomas are the typical spinal cord tumors of patients affected by the autosomal dominant von Hippel–Lindau disease. These patients often have multiple spinal cord hemangioblastomas, which may grow unpredictably, form cysts and significant spinal cord edema, and thus may require multiple surgeries over the years.[44]

Imaging

Hemangioblastomas typically have intense vascularization, which is shown well both on gadolinium-enhanced and on T2 images. They typically but not in every case develop adjacent cysts and frequently cause intense cord edema, presumably as a precursor to cyst formation. This is the tumor type that can be conclusively diagnosed on imaging alone. Very rarely, for instance in a high cervical or craniocervical localization, it may be indicated to perform a preoperative angiogram. Partial embolization of feeding arteries may be possible at that time, rendering the surgical resection somewhat easier by reducing the intense blood flow through these tumors.

Management
Surgery

Only complete surgical resection is possible for hemangioblastomas. They are very well delineated and can be meticulously removed from the cord with minimal damage. The presence of cysts may make the exposure easier. Large tumors must be approached with great care as the thin capsule may easily permit hemorrhage, which may be uncontrollable until the entire tumor is removed and the feeding arteries obliterated. Under no circumstances must the draining vein or veins be coagulated first, as this would result in intense swelling and hemorrhage and subsequent cord damage.

Hemangioblastomas cannot be partially removed as bleeding would stop only after the entire lesion is gone. Still the use of neuromonitoring is helpful to reassure the surgeon of intact pathways and to indicate whether spinal cord edema reaches a threatening intensity. If this is the case, the dura must not be closed primarily after tumor removal. It may be necessary to insert a longitudinal dural extension graft to prevent a type of "compartment syndrome" of the cord within the dural sac.

Radiation Therapy

No adjuvant treatment is warranted.

Chemotherapy

No adjuvant treatment is warranted.

Follow-up

Once resected, hemangioblastomas with documented complete removal can be considered cured and do not require yearly follow-up.

However, in patients with von Hippel–Lindau disease, lifelong follow-up with yearly imaging is strictly required to ensure early detection of newly arising or progressive tumors.

22.3.7 High-grade Glial Tumors

Epidemiology

High-grade tumors, particularly glioblastomas of the spinal cord, are rare but they do occur.[34,45]

Pathology

Glioblastomas are a rare exception. They have the same tissue characteristics as glioblastomas in the brain. Anaplastic astrocytoma has been described and frequently follows the diffuse astrocytoma pattern with added features of vascular proliferation and increased cellularity. Mixed astrocytomas with anaplastic features have been rarely seen. The grade 3 ganglioglioma is a rare type which also has received some attention.[35]

Imaging

The appearance of malignant tumors on MRI is heterogeneous. Diffuse anaplastic astrocytomas can appear as diffuse, even nonenhancing extensions of the cord. Contrast enhancement, nodules, and cystic components can all occur. Most likely, these tumors are eccentric in the cord, may extent through the pia to the cord surface, and cause significant adjacent edema.

Surgery

The extent of resection should be strictly limited to what is functionally permissible based on neuromonitoring in order to absolutely avoid a significant motor deficit.[34] In malignant tumors, such dysfunction is more likely to be present already before surgery. Surgery is essential to establish the histologic diagnosis, which determines the choice of adjuvant treatment and follow-up.

Adjuvant Therapy

Radiation Therapy

Radiation therapy can be indicated even in children older than 3 years to improve progression-free survival. To minimize the impact of radiation on the growth of the spine, proton beam radiation may be considered to avoid a large dose absorption into the vertebral bodies and the facet joints.

Chemotherapy

For glioblastomas, the standard treatment plan for cerebral glioblastomas would be used[46] in the same way as for those occurring in the brain. Other treatments have been tried with some success.[35,41]

22.4 Summary

Neurological and oncologic outcome must be clearly distinguished.

The neurologic result of spinal cord tumor resection depends on a number of factors. The one documented factor independently contributing to the postoperative outcome, usually the motor outcome and more specifically the ability to walk, is the preoperative baseline. The better the motor status before surgery, the more likely the postoperative motor function will be satisfactory as well.[39,40] This is well understood with a concept of ongoing structural damage to the motor pathways, which may reach a critical level only at which clinical dysfunction begins to appear. At this stage, the compensatory mechanisms may already be close to being exhausted and thus the ability of the spinal cord to tolerate the inevitable trauma of surgery limited.

The approach into the cord practically always is through the posterior part, thus injuring the sensory pathways. Therefore, almost always some degree of sensory dysfunction is present after surgery.[18] Usually, this does not result in a significant degree of long-term morbidity as compensation occurs and is supported by neurorehabilitation.

The motor outcome of spinal cord surgery in children is remarkably favorable.[10,11,12,14,19,36,38,47] Paraplegia is and should be an extreme exception.

The oncologic outcome is determined by the type and grade of the histological diagnosis on one side and the extent of resection on the other.[13,14,19,36] The progression-free survival is clearly longer with gross total resection than subtotal resection. The work of Constantini et al has shown that small tumor residuals as determined on postoperative MRI scans do not change this outcome unless the resection is less than about 85%, below which progression will occur frequently and early.[14] Clearly, high-grade tumors have an unfavorable prognosis as compared to low-grade tumors.[34]

22.5 Common Clinical Questions

1. Name the most common tumor in the spinal cord in children.
2. What is the typical presentation of a low-grade astrocytoma in the thoracic cord in children?

3. What is the treatment of choice for intramedullary spinal cord hemangioblastoma?
4. What is the role of adjuvant treatment for intramedullary astrocytomas WHO 3?
5. What is the best technique for small vessel bleeder hemostasis after spinal cord tumor resection?

22.6 Answers to Common Clinical Questions

1. Pilocytic astrocytoma.
2. Nocturnal back pain.
3. Complete surgical resection alone.
4. Most complete surgical resection followed by chemotherapy and radiation treatment (for children older than 3 years).
5. Irrigation, mild compression, Avitene. Avoid bipolar coagulation.

References

[1] Eiselsberg Av, Ranzi E. Über die chirurgische Behandlung der Hirn- und Rückenmarkstumoren. Arch Klin Chir. 1913; 102(2):309–468

[2] Elsberg CA, Beer E. The operability of intramedullary tumors of the spinal cord. A report of two operations with remarks upon the extrusion of intraspinal tumors. Am J Med Sci. 1911; 142:636–647

[3] Greenwood J, Jr. Total removal of intramedullary tumors. J Neurosurg. 1954; 11(6):616–621

[4] Greenwood J. Intramedullary tumors of spinal cord. A follow-up study after total surgical removal. J Neurosurg. 1963; 20:665–668

[5] Greenwood J, Jr. Surgical removal of intramedullary tumors. J Neurosurg. 1967; 26(2):276–282

[6] Malis LI. Intramedullary spinal cord tumors. Clin Neurosurg. 1978; 25:512–539

[7] Stein BM. Surgery of intramedullary spinal cord tumors. Clin Neurosurg. 1979; 26:529–542

[8] Fischer G, Mansuy L. Total removal of intramedullary ependymomas: follow-up study of 16 cases. Surg Neurol. 1980; 14(4):243–249

[9] Guidetti B, Mercuri S, Vagnozzi R. Long-term results of the surgical treatment of 129 intramedullary spinal gliomas. J Neurosurg. 1981; 54(3):323–330

[10] Epstein F, Epstein N. Surgical treatment of spinal cord astrocytomas of childhood. A series of 19 patients. J Neurosurg. 1982; 57(5):685–689

[11] Epstein F. Spinal cord astrocytomas in childhood. In: Homburger F, ed. Progress in Experimental Tumor Research. Vol 30. Basel: S. Karger; 1987:135–153

[12] Epstein FJ, Farmer J-P. Pediatric spinal cord tumor surgery. Neurosurg Clin N Am. 1990; 1(3):569–590

[13] Constantini S, Houten J, Miller DC, et al. Intramedullary spinal cord tumors in children under the age of 3 years. J Neurosurg. 1996; 85(6):1036–1043

[14] Constantini S, Miller DC, Allen JC, Rorke LB, Freed D, Epstein FJ. Radical excision of intramedullary spinal cord tumors: surgical morbidity and long-term follow-up evaluation in 164 children and young adults. J Neurosurg. 2000; 93(2) Suppl:183–193

[15] Jallo GI, Kothbauer KF, Epstein FJ. Intrinsic spinal cord tumor resection. Neurosurgery. 2001; 49(5):1124–1128

[16] Brotchi J. Intrinsic spinal cord tumor resection. Neurosurgery. 2002; 50(5):1059–1063

[17] Bagley CA, Kothbauer KF, Wilson S, Bookland MJ, Epstein FJ, Jallo GI. Resection of myxopapillary ependymomas in children. J Neurosurg. 2007; 106(4) Suppl:261–267

[18] McGirt MJ, Chaichana KL, Atiba A, Attenello F, Woodworth GF, Jallo GI. Neurological outcome after resection of intramedullary spinal cord tumors in children. Childs Nerv Syst. 2008; 24(1):93–97

[19] Ahmed R, Menezes AH, Awe OO, Torner JC. Long-term disease and neurological outcomes in patients with pediatric intramedullary spinal cord tumors. J Neurosurg Pediatr. 2014; 13(6):600–612

[20] Shiminski-Maher T, Woodman C, Keene N. Childhood Brain & Spinal Cord Tumors: A Guide for Families, Friends and Caregivers. 2nd ed: Bellingham, WA: Childhood Cancer Guides; 2014

[21] Kothbauer KF. Intraoperative neurophysiologic monitoring for intramedullary spinal-cord tumor surgery. Neurophysiol Clin. 2007; 37(6):407–414

[22] Sala F, Kothbauer K. Intraoperative neurophysiological monitoring during surgery for intramedullary spinal cord tumors. In: Nuwer M, ed. Intraoperative Monitoring of Neural Function. Vol. 8. Amsterdam: Elsevier; 2008:632–650

[23] Epstein FJ, Farmer J-P, Schneider SJ. Intraoperative ultrasonography: an important surgical adjunct for intramedullary tumors. J Neurosurg. 1991; 74(5):729–733

[24] Millesi M, Kiesel B, Woehrer A, et al. Analysis of 5-aminolevulinic acid-induced fluorescence in 55 different spinal tumors. Neurosurg Focus. 2014; 36(2):E11

[25] Fasano VA, Zeme S, Frego L, Gunetti R. Ultrasonic aspiration in the surgical treatment of intracranial tumors. J Neurosurg Sci. 1981; 25(1):35–40

[26] Jallo GI, Kothbauer KF, Epstein FJ. Contact laser microsurgery. Childs Nerv Syst. 2002; 18(6)(–)(7):333–336

[27] Abbott R, Feldstein N, Wisoff JH, Epstein FJ. Osteoplastic laminotomy in children. Pediatr Neurosurg. 1992; 18(3):153–156

[28] Poblete B, Konrad C, Kothbauer KF. Intrathecal morphine analgesia after cervical and thoracic spinal cord tumor surgery. J Neurosurg Spine. 2014; 21(6):899–904

[29] Kothbauer KF, Deletis V, Epstein FJ. Motor-evoked potential monitoring for intramedullary spinal cord tumor surgery: correlation of clinical and neurophysiological data in a series of 100 consecutive procedures. Neurosurg Focus. 1998; 4(5):e1

[30] Rubin RC, Henderson ES, Ommaya AK, Walker MD, Rall DP. The production of cerebrospinal fluid in man and its modification by acetazolamide. J Neurosurg. 1966; 25(4):430–436

[31] McGirt MJ, Chaichana KL, Attenello F, et al. Spinal deformity after resection of cervical intramedullary spinal cord tumors in children. Childs Nerv Syst. 2008; 24(6):735–739

[32] Yao K, Kothbauer KF, Bitan F, Constantini S, Epstein FJ, Jallo GI. Spinal deformity and intramedullary tumor surgery. Childs Nerv Syst. 2000; 16:530

[33] Deutsch H, Shrivistava R, Epstein F, Jallo GI. Pediatric intramedullary spinal cavernous malformations. Spine. 2001; 26(18):E427–E431

[34] McGirt MJ, Goldstein IM, Chaichana KL, Tobias ME, Kothbauer KF, Jallo GI. Extent of surgical resection of malignant

astrocytomas of the spinal cord: outcome analysis of 35 patients. Neurosurgery. 2008; 63(1):55–60, discussion 60–61

[35] Schneider C, Vosbeck J, Grotzer MA, Boltshauser E, Kothbauer KF. Anaplastic ganglioglioma: a very rare intramedullary spinal cord tumor. Pediatr Neurosurg. 2012; 48(1):42–47

[36] Scheinemann K, Bartels U, Huang A, et al. Survival and functional outcome of childhood spinal cord low-grade gliomas. Clinical article. J Neurosurg Pediatr. 2009; 4(3):254–261

[37] Jallo GI, Danish S, Velasquez L, Epstein F. Intramedullary low-grade astrocytomas: long-term outcome following radical surgery. J Neurooncol. 2001; 53(1):61–66

[38] McGirt MJ, Chaichana KL, Atiba A, Attenello F, Yao KC, Jallo GI. Resection of intramedullary spinal cord tumors in children: assessment of long-term motor and sensory deficits. J Neurosurg Pediatr. 2008; 1(1):63–67

[39] Morota N, Deletis V, Constantini S, Kofler M, Cohen H, Epstein FJ. The role of motor evoked potentials during surgery for intramedullary spinal cord tumors. Neurosurgery. 1997; 41(6): 1327–1336

[40] Woodworth GF, Chaichana KL, McGirt MJ, et al. Predictors of ambulatory function after surgical resection of intramedullary spinal cord tumors. Neurosurgery. 2007; 61 (1):99–105, discussion 105–106

[41] Allen JC, Aviner S, Yates AJ, et al. Children's Cancer Group. Treatment of high-grade spinal cord astrocytoma of childhood with "8-in-1" chemotherapy and radiotherapy: a pilot study of CCG-945. J Neurosurg. 1998; 88(2):215–220

[42] Jallo GI, Zagzag D, Epstein F. Intramedullary subependymoma of the spinal cord. Neurosurgery. 1996; 38(2):251–257

[43] Feldman WB, Clark AJ, Safaee M, Ames CP, Parsa AT. Tumor control after surgery for spinal myxopapillary ependymomas: distinct outcomes in adults versus children: a systematic review. J Neurosurg Spine. 2013; 19 (4):471–476

[44] Roonprapunt C, Silvera VM, Setton A, Freed D, Epstein FJ, Jallo GI. Surgical management of isolated hemangioblastomas of the spinal cord. Neurosurgery. 2001; 49(2):321–327, discussion 327–328

[45] Cohen AR, Wisoff JH, Allen JC, Epstein F. Malignant astrocytomas of the spinal cord. J Neurosurg. 1989; 70(1): 50–54

[46] Stupp R, Mason WP, van den Bent MJ, et al. European Organisation for Research and Treatment of Cancer Brain Tumor and Radiotherapy Groups, National Cancer Institute of Canada Clinical Trials Group. Radiotherapy plus concomitant and adjuvant temozolomide for glioblastoma. N Engl J Med. 2005; 352(10):987–996

[47] Nadkarni TD, Rekate HL. Pediatric intramedullary spinal cord tumors. Critical review of the literature. Childs Nerv Syst. 1999; 15(1):17–28

23 Tumors of the Spinal Column

Dominic N.P. Thompson, Nir Shimony

23.1 Introduction

In pediatric practice, spinal tumors are less frequent than intracranial tumors and also much less common than in adult practice. Approximately one-third of spinal tumors in childhood are extradural, the remainder being intramedullary or intradural but extramedullary.

The term **spinal column tumors** is used here to encompass those tumors that arise in the extradural space and the paraspinal regions as well as from the bony and cartilaginous elements of the spine. A variety of tumor types, both benign and malignant, may be encountered in these locations, although both the age of the patient and the anatomical site of origin will aid in refining the differential diagnosis in individual cases.

The management of spinal column tumors is guided by:
• Biology of the tumor.
• Neurological status of the patient.
• Spinal deformity or instability.

Tumors of extradural origin are more likely to be malignant than intradural tumors. Spinal column tumors may be part of a more systemic malignant disease and, in such cases, surgery alone is unlikely to be curative; it is therefore important that these cases be managed by a multidisciplinary neuro-oncology team to ensure that the timing, objectives, and extent of surgery are agreed and appropriate.

Severe neurological deterioration mandating emergency intervention is rare in pediatric spinal column tumors, and thus, there is usually time to permit appropriate investigations and planning of intervention.

Vertebral collapse with deformity or instability will mean that spinal stabilization will have to be considered as part of the surgical strategy. Even if there is no evidence of deformity or instability at the outset, late postsurgical deformity is a significant risk following laminectomy or laminoplasty, particularly in a growing child, and these risks need to be factored into the clinical decision-making process.[1]

23.2 Clinical Presentation

23.2.1 Pain

Spinal pain is present in up to two-thirds of cases of spinal tumor at the time of diagnosis. The pain is frequently poorly localized and may have been present for many months. Constant pain or pain of increasing intensity, pain that wakes the child at night, or pain that is associated with radicular spread or sensory impairment is of particular significance and warrants prompt investigation.[2,3]

23.2.2 Weakness

Along with pain, weakness is one of the commonest findings in children with spinal tumor. In the infant, weakness can be easily overlooked until the late stages of spinal cord compression. In an older child, a limp, fatigability, a tendency to trip, or falls may be the manifestations of lower limb weakness. Examination findings are typically those of upper motor neurone type with hyperreflexia.

23.2.3 Mass

Extension of a spinal or paraspinal mass into the adjacent soft tissue can result in a palpable mass in a thin child. A soft-tissue mass in association with a bone tumor is suggestive of malignancy.

23.2.4 Spinal Deformity

Scoliosis is present in approximately one-quarter of cases. Rapid curve progression or atypical or left-sided curves should prompt the search for an underlying spinal lesion or spinal cord anomaly. Torticollis may herald the presence of a tumor involving the upper cervical spine or craniovertebral junction.

23.2.5 Sphincter Disturbance

This is an unusual presenting symptom in childhood but one that is easily overlooked as it may not have been recognized by the parent or child.

Findings include an enlarged bladder, incomplete bladder emptying, a history of urinary infection, or frank incontinence. Disturbance of rectal continence is less common and, when it occurs, is a later sign; neurogenic sphincter disturbance almost always affects the bladder first.

23.3 Investigations

Numerous modalities are available to investigate spinal tumors; investigations are chosen with the following in mind:
• Refining the differential diagnosis.
• Evaluating the site and extent of the lesion, and its effect on the neuraxis (spinal cord and nerve roots).
• Evaluating the extent of bone involvement.
• Assessment of spinal deformity.
• Determination of instability.

The most commonly required investigations are the following.

23.3.1 Spinal MRI

The whole spine should be imaged with and without contrast. Magnetic resonance imaging (MRI) provides the best modality to assess the effect of the lesion on the neuraxis.[4]

23.3.2 Spinal CT

High-resolution computed tomography (CT) scan (using bone window algorithm) of the involved area is used where detailed bony information is required, for example, in assessing extent of bone involvement or suitability for instrumental fixation. CT-guided biopsy of the lesion will be useful in cases of suspected malignancy.

23.3.3 Plain X-rays

Plain X-rays are unlikely to provide additional diagnostic information, although they often have a role in assessing spinal deformity or in cases of suspected instability, for example, flexion/extension X-rays in cervical lesions.

23.3.4 Additional Investigations

There are certain investigations there are specific to the workup of certain tumor types (▶ Table 23.1).

Table 23.1 Additional investigations that may be used in the evaluation of particular tumor types

Investigation	Tumor type
Urinary catecholamines	Neuroblastoma (diagnosis)
MiBG scan	Neuroblastoma (staging)
Bone marrow aspirate	Neuroblastoma, lymphoma, Ewing's sarcoma (staging)
Radioisotope scan	Osteoid osteoma
Skeletal survey	Histiocytosis, malignant bone tumors (staging)
CT chest/abdomen	Malignant bone tumors (osteosarcoma, Ewing's sarcoma)
Spinal angiography	Hemangioma of bone, aneurysmal bone cyst

Abbreviations: CT, computed tomography; MiBG, metaiodobenzylguanidine.

23.4 Tumor Types

A wide range of tumor types can involve the spinal column either primarily or secondarily as a result of extension from adjacent tissues. Some of the more common benign and malignant tumors of the spinal column encountered in pediatric neurosurgical practice are shown in Box 23.1.

Box 23.1 Spinal column tumor types in children

• Malignant:
  - Neuroblastoma.
  - Osteogenic sarcoma.
  - Ewing's sarcoma (peripheral PNET).
  - Chordoma.
  - Lymphoma.
  - Metastases.
• Benign:
  - Hemangioma of bone.
  - Aneurysmal bone cyst.
  - Osteoid osteoma/osteoblastoma.
  - Histiocytosis.

23.4.1 Malignant

Malignant tumors of the spinal column present with spinal pain (this may have a radicular component), painful scoliosis, gait disturbance, or limb weakness. Bladder (or rarely bowel) incontinence is seen in lumbosacral malignancies when the conus or cauda equina are involved, although it is an unusual presenting feature in tumors higher in the spinal column. Systemic features such as weight loss and night sweats may be present particularly in lymphoma and Ewing's sarcoma (EWS).

Malignant tumors of the spinal column require multidisciplinary approach. Accurate pathological diagnosis can be difficult but is an essential prerequisite to treatment. CT-guided biopsy or open biopsy will usually be required in the first instance, although, in cases presenting with spinal compression, tumor tissue will be obtained at the time of the decompression procedure. Because of the propensity for hematogenous spread, staging investigations including CT chest, ultrasound abdomen, and bone marrow aspiration are required.

Surgery should be considered as an adjunctive therapy in the management of malignant tumors of the spinal column. Neoadjuvant and adjuvant chemotherapy have improved the prognosis for many malignant tumors largely due to their ability to shrink tumors, reduce vascularity, and thus optimize the chances of gross total resection.

Neuroblastoma

Spinal neuroblastoma (NB) is predominantly a tumor of infancy and younger children. The histogenesis of NB is uncertain, although these tumors are thought to originate in neural crest–derived peripheral nerve progenitors. Spinal NB commonly occurs along the sympathetic chain (and adrenal gland) and so is typically centered on the paravertebral region with secondary extension through the intervertebral foramina into the intraspinal compartment. The cells of origin are involved in catecholamine secretion, and this feature is exploited in diagnosis and workup, as metabolites from the catecholamine synthesis pathway are excreted via the kidney and can be detected in the urine. The metabolic activity of these tumors is also utilized in staging the disease; the radionuclide MiBG (metaiodobenzylguanidine) is taken up by NB and will permit identification of metastatic disease. Some of these tumors show a phenomenon of maturation toward more favorable pathology either on treatment or spontaneously, and so a spectrum of tumors ranging from malignant to benign is recognized in pediatric patients (neuroblastoma, ganglioneuroblastomas, ganglioneuroma; ▶ Fig. 23.1a).

The mainstay of treatment for NB is chemotherapy. Surgical decompression is reserved for cases presenting with severe deficit or rapidly evolving neurology; however, there is a high rate of post-surgical spinal deformity.

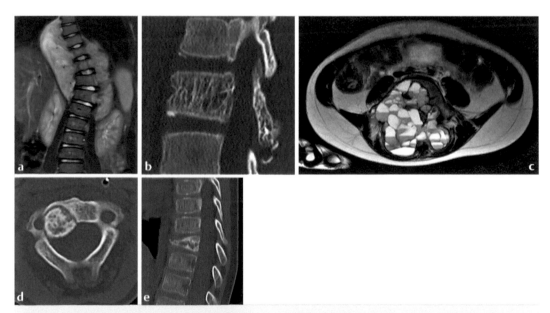

Fig. 23.1 Radiological appearances of spinal column tumors. (a) Paravertebral ganglioneuroma. (b) Hemangioma of bone. (c) Aneurysmal bone cyst. (d) Osteoid osteoma. (e) LCH (vertebra plana).

Osteogenic Sarcoma

Osteogenic sarcoma (OS) is the most common primary bone neoplasm in children and typically presents around the time of puberty. However, spinal involvement (either as primary lesion or site of metastasis) is seen in only 5% of cases.[5] Imaging reveals bone destruction, with a soft-tissue mass demonstrating variable degrees of mineralization. Tissue diagnosis is established by open or CT-guided biopsy. Neoadjuvant chemotherapy is used to reduce tumor volume, followed by maximal surgical resection of the involved field. Five-year survival for all OS is approximately 18%; spinal involvement portends a worse prognosis.

Ewing's Sarcoma (Peripheral PNET)

Also a tumor of the teenage years, 10% of cases of EWS involve the spine; however, in contrast with OS, there is a predilection for the lumbosacral region.[5] Histologically, these small round blue cell tumors are considered part of the primitive neuroectodermal tumor (PNET) spectrum. Metastatic spread is present in up to half of cases at the time of presentation.[2] On MRI, EWS appears as an area of lytic bone destruction with an associated mass lesion. As with OS, accurate tissue diagnosis is essential. Neoadjuvant chemotherapy is the initial treatment of choice, followed by wide local resection usually with instrumented fixation; radiation therapy is then used for postsurgical residual disease. Five-year survival is approximately 40%.

Lymphoma

Lymphoma involving the spine is rare and usually occurs late in the disease. Most lymphomas that involve the spine in childhood are B-cell lymphomas of the non-Hodgkin type and tend to occur in the adolescent age group. Spinal lymphoma characteristically spreads along nerve roots and through the intervertebral foramina. Pathological fractures are present in up to one-quarter of patients. Chemotherapy is the mainstay of treatment; surgery is reserved for cases of spinal disease refractory to primary treatment or for clinical symptoms or signs of spinal cord compression.

Chordoma

It is a rare tumor of notochordal origin with a predilection for the craniovertebral junction and the sacrum (together, these two sites comprise over two-thirds of cases). Subtypes include classical, chondroid, and dedifferentiated; the latter has a more aggressive natural history. Immunohistochemical techniques are often required to distinguish chordoma from chondrosarcoma that has a more favorable prognosis. Gross total en bloc resection provides the best long-term survival; however, this is usually only feasible for small volume, localized tumors (< 30 mL). Chordoma is only moderately radiosensitive; however, proton beam therapy has increased the dose of radiotherapy that can be safely delivered to residual or recurrent tumors. There is a high rate of local recurrence, and 5-year survival is approximately 60%.

23.4.2 Benign

Within the spectrum of benign spinal tumors, there are those that can be considered benign with favorable natural history (e.g., Langerhans cell histiocytosis [LCH] and osteoid osteoma) and those that are benign but locally aggressive (e.g., aneurysmal bone cyst [ABC], giant cell tumor of bone).[6,7]

Hemangioma

Hemangioma of bone is commonly an entirely benign, incidental MRI finding appearing as a discrete area of high T2 signal within the vertebral body. No treatment or follow-up is indicated. On occasion, however, spinal hemangioma can present as a locally infiltrative lesion with extension into the paraspinal tissues and spinal canal, resulting in spinal compression. On CT scan, these lesions have a characteristic pattern of vertical trabeculation (▶ Fig. 23.1b). These are highly vascular tumors, and where surgical intervention is required (usually due to pain or radiculomyelopathy), preoperative angiography and embolization should be considered. Following embolization, radical surgical excision with spinal reconstruction can be achieved. Successful treatment has also been described using vertebroplasty or direct ethanol injection. Focal radiotherapy may be required in cases of residual or recurrent disease.[8]

Aneurysmal Bone Cyst

This is a benign but locally aggressive lesion, and can occur in isolation or in conjunction with another pathology such as fibrous dysplasia or giant cell tumor of bone. ABCs commonly originate in the posterior elements but extension to the vertebral body is frequent. They characteristically consist of well-demarcated cysts, frequently containing chocolate-colored fluid due to old blood products, surrounded by a thin wall of reactive bone that tends to expand the vertebra and produces a "soap bubble" appearance on CT or MRI (▶ Fig. 23.1c). Despite the name, they are not particularly vascular at surgery (in contrast with hemangioma). Pain is the commonest presentation. Treatment options vary according to site and mode of presentation. The radiological features are usually diagnostic, and preliminary biopsy is rarely necessary. Where there is evidence of spinal compression, either en bloc resection or extensive curettage with grafting should be performed. Gross total resection should be the goal of therapy; instrumented spinal fixation will be required in most cases.[9] Postsurgical surveillance is required as there is a significant risk of local recurrence, particularly in partially resected lesions.[10] Transarterial selective embolization has hitherto been used as an adjunct to surgery; however, recent evidence suggests that this modality should be considered as a primary definitive treatment for ABC in the absence of instability or neurological compromise.[11] In children, due to the potentially hazardous late effects, radiotherapy is generally reserved for instances where primary treatment has failed.[12]

Osteoid Osteoma/Osteoblastoma

The distinction between these two entities is essentially a matter of size; pathological appearances are indistinguishable. Small lesions < 1.5 cm are termed osteoid osteoma, while the larger version is referred to as osteoblastoma. Clinical presentation is with local spinal pain that typically responds to nonsteroidal anti-inflammatory drugs. Neurological deficits are more commonly seen with osteoblastoma; also, osteoblastoma tends to have a higher rate of recurrence. Radiologically, there is often a central nidus of dense bone, frequently with sclerosis of the surrounding bone, resulting in a lucent halo around the lesion (this finding is more consistent in osteoid osteoma)[13] (▶ Fig. 23.1d). These appear as "hot spots" on radionuclide scanning. Complete surgical resection is the principal treatment. Radiotherapy is reserved for recurrence.

23.4.3 Langerhans Cell Histiocytosis

Langerhans cells are dendritic cells that are part of the immune system. LCH may occur as an isolated bone lesion (unifocal LCH), previously termed eosinophilic granuloma, or with multiple bony lesions (multifocal unisystem LCH). A more malignant form with widespread extraosseous tissue involvement is recognized (multifocal multisystem LCH). In children, 80% of cases are unifocal and the spine is involved in up to 25% of cases. The classical spinal appearance of LCH is vertebra plana (▶ Fig. 23.1e). There is often an associated soft lesion; although spinal cord compression is rare, pain rather than neurological compromise is the most common presentation.[14] Needle biopsy may be required for diagnosis. Treatment is indicated for multifocal lesions or extension into the spinal canal. Treatment consists of steroids, bisphosphonates, and chemotherapy, with a bracing regime to control spinal deformity. The role of surgery is limited to rare instances of spinal compression or cases of progressive spinal deformity.

23.4.4 Giant Cell Tumor of Bone

It is an extremely rare tumor in pediatric practice. These are locally aggressive tumors that require en bloc complete resection in order to attain long-term disease control.

23.4.5 Anatomical Site of Origin

Spinal column tumors show a predilection for certain patterns of growth and this can be of help in refining the differential diagnosis (▶ Fig. 23.2). This should be considered a rough guide and there will of course be exceptions.

23.4.6 Age

It is also important to consider the age of the child as many tumors have a propensity to occur at particular times in childhood (▶ Fig. 23.3).

23.5 Treatment Considerations

In children with vertebral column tumors, management strategies are formulated according to:
- Grade and stage of the tumor.
- The role of surgery in relation to other oncological modalities.
- The need to preserve of neurological function.
- The perceived effect of the tumor or surgical treatment on spinal stability and deformity.

For some malignant tumors, neoadjuvant treatment with chemotherapy or radiotherapy can optimize

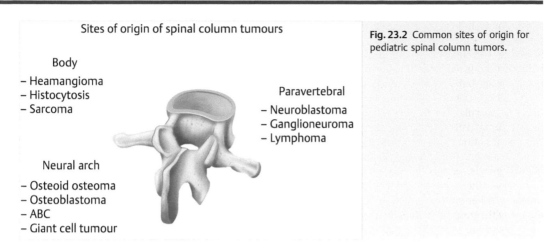

Sites of origin of spinal column tumours

Body
– Heamangioma
– Histocytosis
– Sarcoma

Paravertebral
– Neuroblastoma
– Ganglioneuroma
– Lymphoma

Neural arch
– Osteoid osteoma
– Osteoblastoma
– ABC
– Giant cell tumour

Fig. 23.2 Common sites of origin for pediatric spinal column tumors.

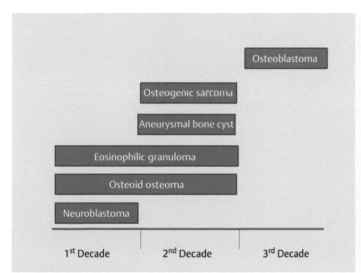

Fig. 23.3 Spinal column tumors according to age at presentation.

Osteoblastoma

Osteogenic sarcoma

Aneurysmal bone cyst

Eosinophilic granuloma

Osteoid osteoma

Neuroblastoma

1st Decade   2nd Decade   3rd Decade

the chances of successful surgical resection. Additionally, embolization can significantly reduce the vascularity of tumors such as hemangioma, thus reducing operative risk and facilitating radical surgical resection (▶ Table 23.2).

23.5.1 Surgical Planning

Once surgery is required, detailed multimodality imaging is essential to preoperative planning. Types of tumor resection include the following.

En Bloc Resection

For primary malignant tumors of bone, a complete oncological resection preserving all tumor margins should be pursued where possible. These are, however, complex surgeries requiring extensive exposures and reconstructive instrumentation. While most experience is in adults, these techniques can be applied to selected pediatric cases.

Determining the extent of resection, the surgical approach and the implications for spinal reconstruction can be aided by the use of a reproducible and validated approach to tumor staging such as the Weinstein-Boriani-Biagini (WBB) system.[15] Using this method, the vertebra is divided into radial segments and a series of concentric zones from intradural to extraspinal. This system is then used to define the most appropriate technique of en bloc resection. Broadly speaking, the following three types of resection are described.

Table 23.2 Treatment strategies for spinal column tumors in children

Tumor	Primary treatment	Additional treatment
Malignant		
Neuroblastoma	Neoadjuvant chemotherapy	Surgery[a]
Osteosarcoma	Neoadjuvant chemotherapy	Radical surgery
Ewing's sarcoma	Neoadjuvant chemotherapy + radiotherapy	Radical surgery
Lymphoma	Chemotherapy + radiotherapy	Surgery[a]
Chordoma	Radical surgery	Proton beam radiotherapy
Benign		
Hemangioma	Embolization/surgery	Radiotherapy
Aneurysmal bone cyst	Embolization/surgery	Radiotherapy
Osteoblastoma/osteoid osteoma	Surgery	None
Histiocytosis	Chemotherapy	Surgery (stabilization)

Note: For the child presenting with symptoms or signs of spinal cord compression, an initial emergency decompression may be required. These strategies are based on a known diagnosis and absence of clinical spinal cord compression.
[a]The role of surgery in these instances is for significant residual disease following first-line therapy.

Vertebrectomy

En bloc excision of the vertebral body and posterior elements, this is achieved either via separate anterior and posterior approaches or via a single posterior approach.

Sagittal Resection

For tumors that are lateralized to the vertebral bodies or posterior elements, a segmental resection may be performed comprising part of the vertebral body and any involved ipsilateral pedicle or hemilamina.

Posterior Arch Resection

An en bloc removal of the entire lamina and spinous process in circumstances where the pedicles are not involved.

23.5.2 Intralesional Resection

Most benign lesions are amenable to less extensive surgery and can be satisfactorily treated by an intralesional approach using piecemeal resection or curettage.

23.6 Complications and Their Prevention

Spinal tumor surgery, particularly major tumor resections, carry significant risks, many of which can be anticipated, and measures can be taken to minimize them.

23.6.1 Neurological

The spinal cord may be compromised at the time of presentation due to direct compression from the lesion or vertebral collapse, and remains vulnerable during tumor surgery. Perioperative steroid treatment is commenced prior to surgery. Intraoperative neurophysiological monitoring (motor evoked potentials, somatosensory evoked potentials) is generally recommended for all but the most minor of cases.

23.6.2 Vascular

Major blood loss should be anticipated; crossmatched blood and clotting factors are ordered preoperatively. Preoperative embolization should be considered in particular circumstances such as spinal hemangioma.

23.6.3 Deformity

The integrity of the spinal column may be compromised by tumor involvement or by surgical intervention. In many cases, spinal instrumentation will need to be performed concomitantly with the tumor resection; young age does not preclude the use of spinal instrumentation.

If there is no deformity at the time of presentation, then these patients can be followed with serial spinal X-rays to monitor for the emergence of delayed deformity. A customized spinal brace may reduce the rate of postsurgical deformity in children considered at increased risk.

23.7 Surgical Pearls

- Spinal pain is the commonest presenting symptom of spinal column tumors. *Red flag* symptoms include pain that is constant, nocturnal pain, pain with a radicular distribution, and pain associated with abnormal neurological examination.
- The spectrum of spinal column neoplasms in children is different compared with adults. The age of the patient and position of the tumor within the vertebra are valuable in refining the differential diagnosis.
- A soft-tissue mass associated with a bone tumor is suggestive of malignancy.
- Malignant spinal column tumors are rarely treated with surgery alone; these tumors require a coordinated multidisciplinary neuro-oncology approach.
- The potential for spinal deformity should be incorporated into neurosurgical management plan. Risk factors for progressive spinal deformity include: young age, scoliosis at the time of presentation, involvement of vertebral body and posterior elements, and multiple level laminectomies.
- Infection, particularly tuberculosis, can masquerade as a spinal column tumor. Consider ethnic background, history of foreign travel, and presence of systemic symptoms.

23.8 Common Clinical Questions

1. Which spinal column tumors typically occur in the posterior neural arch?
2. Can tumor resection be combined with spinal reconstruction?
3. What factors influence the neurosurgical management in an 18-month-old child found to have a paraspinal tumor with intraspinal extension?

23.9 Answers to Common Clinical Questions

1. Osteoid osteoma, osteoblastoma, ABC, and giant cell tumors of bone typically arise in

or primarily involve the posterior neural arch.
2. Spinal reconstruction, using strut grafting or instrumental fixation, can be used at the time of initial tumor resection. Typically, this is the case for malignant tumors requiring en bloc resections or where there is significant deformity at the time of presentation.
3. The commonest spinal column tumor in this age group with this pattern of growth is NB. Diagnosis can be made on the basis of urinary catecholamines or biopsy. The primary treatment modality in this instance will be chemotherapy. Even with intraspinal extension, immediate commencement of steroids and chemotherapy can result in rapid tumor regression without the need for neurosurgical intervention. Surgical decompression is reserved for cases presenting with clear neurological deficit or as second-line treatment for residual disease persisting after chemotherapy.

References

[1] Joaquim AF, Cheng I, Patel AA. Postoperative spinal deformity after treatment of intracanal spine lesions. Spine J. 2012; 12 (11):1067–1074

[2] Sciubba DM, Hsieh P, McLoughlin GS, Jallo GI. Pediatric tumors involving the spinal column. Neurosurg Clin N Am. 2008; 19(1):81–92

[3] Garg S, Dormans JP. Tumors and tumor-like conditions of the spine in children. J Am Acad Orthop Surg. 2005; 13(6):372–381

[4] Bloomer CW, Ackerman A, Bhatia RG. Imaging for spine tumors and new applications. Top Magn Reson Imaging. 2006; 17(2):69–87

[5] Kim HJ, McLawhorn AS, Goldstein MJ, Boland PJ. Malignant osseous tumors of the pediatric spine. J Am Acad Orthop Surg. 2012; 20(10):646–656

[6] Harrop JS, Schmidt MH, Boriani S, Shaffrey CI. Aggressive "benign" primary spine neoplasms: osteoblastoma, aneurysmal bone cyst, and giant cell tumor. Spine. 2009; 34 (22) Suppl:S39–S47

[7] Enneking WF, Spanier SS, Goodman MA. A system for the surgical staging of musculoskeletal sarcoma. 1980. Clin Orthop Relat Res. 2003(415):4–18

[8] Acosta FL, Jr, Sanai N, Chi JH, et al. Comprehensive management of symptomatic and aggressive vertebral hemangiomas. Neurosurg Clin N Am. 2008; 19(1):17–29

[9] Zenonos G, Jamil O, Governale LS, Jernigan S, Hedequist D, Proctor MR. Surgical treatment for primary spinal aneurysmal bone cysts: experience from Children's Hospital Boston. J Neurosurg Pediatr. 2012; 9(3):305–315

[10] Novais EN, Rose PS, Yaszemski MJ, Sim FH. Aneurysmal bone cyst of the cervical spine in children. J Bone Joint Surg Am. 2011; 93(16):1534–1543

[11] Amendola L, Simonetti L, Simoes CE, Bandiera S, De Iure F, Boriani S. Aneurysmal bone cyst of the mobile spine: the

therapeutic role of embolization. Eur Spine J. 2013; 22(3): 533–541

[12] Burch S, Hu S, Berven S. Aneurysmal bone cysts of the spine. Neurosurg Clin N Am. 2008; 19(1):41–47

[13] Zileli M, Cagli S, Basdemir G, Ersahin Y. Osteoid osteomas and osteoblastomas of the spine. Neurosurg Focus. 2003; 15(5):E5

[14] Peng X-S, Pan T, Chen L-Y, Huang G, Wang J. Langerhans' cell histiocytosis of the spine in children with soft tissue extension and chemotherapy. Int Orthop. 2009; 33(3):731–736

[15] Boriani S, Weinstein JN, Biagini R. Primary bone tumors of the spine. Terminology and surgical staging. Spine. 1997; 22 (9):1036–1044

Section V

Cerebrovascular Disorders

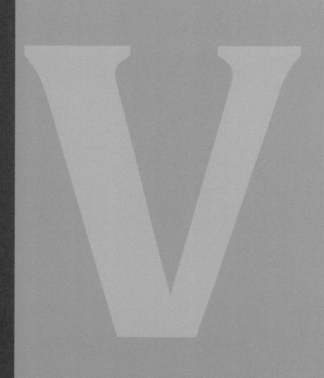

24 Aneurysms

Edward R. Smith

24.1 Introduction and Anatomy

Aneurysms are one of the most common vascular anomalies of the central nervous system, but are far less common in children than in adults. These structurally abnormal areas of arterial wall can cause bleeding, compression of adjacent structures, and concomitant loss of neurologic function. The epidemiology, pathophysiology, presentation, and treatment of pediatric intracranial aneurysms have features distinct from those in adult patients.

24.2 Epidemiology and Pathophysiology

It is estimated that the general prevalence of unruptured, asymptomatic intracranial aneurysm (across all ages) is 3.2% and only 0.5 to 4.6% of these are present in children.[1,2,3,4,5,6] Ruptured aneurysms in the pediatric population are also rare, with 0.6% of all aneurysmal subarachnoid hemorrhage (SAH) comprised of patients younger than 19 years.[3,6,7] Given a total of approximately 18,300 SAH cases annually, this means that there are only about 100 aneurysmal SAH cases each year in children.[8,9] Intracranial aneurysms are more common in males than females (especially in prepubertal children) at 2.7:1, with a shift to a female preponderance (similar to adults) at 3:1 to 5:1 in the postpubertal population.[6,10,11,12]

Location and size of aneurysms in children differ as compared to adults. Children are more likely to harbor aneurysms in the posterior circulation (25% in children vs. 8% in adults) and less likely to have anterior cerebral artery aneurysms (5–10% in children vs. 34% in adults), but roughly the same for internal carotid artery and middle cerebral artery lesions.[3,6,7,11,13] Children are less likely than adults to have multiple aneurysms, and two to four times more likely to have giant (> 2.5 cm) aneurysms than adults.[5,6,10,13]

The etiology of aneurysms in the pediatric population shifts with increasing age. Younger children, particularly younger than 5 years, have the majority of dissecting, fusiform aneurysms, while older children have a majority of saccular aneurysms.[6,10,13] Familial aneurysms are very rare, accounting for 5 to 20% of all reported cases in children and young adults, but less than 5% of prepubertal cases.[14,15] The causes of pediatric intracranial aneurysm are summarized in Box 24.1.

24.3 Presentation and Evaluation

Most aneurysms are asymptomatic and often are never detected. There are no formal screening guidelines for children with affected family members, nor for most genetic disorders (see preceding paragraph).[19] Generally, only family members of sibling pairs or three first-degree relatives who harbor known intracranial aneurysms are recommended for screening, usually with magnetic resonance imaging (MRI)/magnetic resonance angiography (MRA).[14,15,16,19]

For those that are found with symptoms, Box 24.2 and Box 24.3 outline the common presentations. In one series, over half of pediatric aneurysm patients presented with SAH, 33% presented with mass effect symptoms, and 11% were found after trauma.[6] Children with SAH from aneurysm often present with a low Hunt–Hess grade relative to adults, usually 1 to 3.[6,10,20,21]

Evaluation of a patient with a suspected SAH from an aneurysm includes history, neurologic and physical examination, and radiographic studies to define the anatomy of the lesion. Up to 90% of all nontraumatic SAH in children will result from a structural lesion.[22] These patients should be screened with computed tomography (CT) scan, and if a vascular lesion is suspected, a CT arteriogram (CTA) can be a means of identifying the presence of an aneurysm.[19] While lacking the detail of a catheter-based arteriogram, CTA affords the treating physician an immediate image outlining key anatomy of a lesion, information of critical importance in the setting of an acutely ill child. Patterns of SAH in pediatric aneurysm CT studies are summarized in the Box 24.4 (▶ Fig. 24.1).

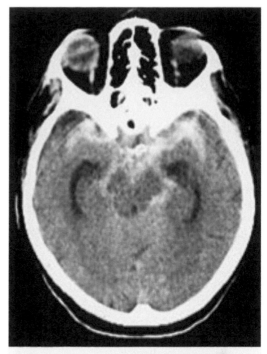

Fig. 24.1 Imaging appearance of aneurysmal subarachnoid hemorrhage on axial noncontrast head CT. Note early ventricular dilatation in temporal horns.

MRI is also useful in the diagnosis and delineation of the three-dimensional anatomy of an aneurysm, particularly with MRA. Overall, MRI/MRA was able to identify the source of SAH correctly in 66% of cases.[22] In contrast, catheter-based digital subtraction angiography (DSA)—the "gold standard" of imaging in aneurysm—was able to identify lesional pathology in 97% of patients, versus 80% of the time without DSA.[23] Angiography generally includes bilateral injection of both the internal

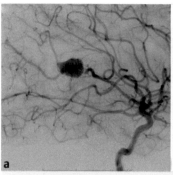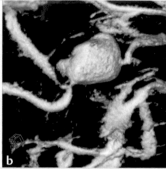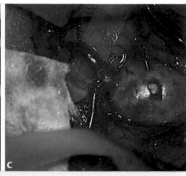

Fig. 24.2 **(a)** Appearance of aneurysm on conventional digital subtraction angiography (DSA), with distal middle cerebral dissecting lesion. **(b)** The same lesion visualized with three-dimensional reconstructions from the arteriogram. **(c)** An intraoperative photograph, as preparation is being made for a distal bypass and concomitant trapping of the aneurysm.

and external carotid arteries and the vertebral arteries in order to visualize all of the vessels. Three-dimensional angiography with computer-generated reconstruction is increasingly employed to depict lesional anatomy (▶ Fig. 24.2). With catheter angiography, a recent analysis of 241 consecutive pediatric patients revealed a 0% complication rate during the procedure and a 0.4% postprocedural complication rate. Evaluation should look for:
- Lesion size, orientation, and location.
- Neck anatomy.
- Daughter blisters.
- Other aneurysms (especially important with infectious lesions).

If the aneurysm is fusiform, the segment of vessel involved, delineation of normal borders, and involvement of perforators are important.

Standard preoperative laboratory studies (complete blood count, clotting times [prothrombin time/partial prothrombin time], type and cross [T&C] for blood bank, and a chemistry panel [Chem 7]) should be considered as pretreatment studies for aneurysms.

24.4 Treatment and Surgical Indications

The decision to treat or observe a given aneurysm can be complex and is best made by a multidisciplinary team including neurosurgeons, endovascular specialists, and neurologists. If treatment is planned, success is predicated on removing the lesion from circulation while preserving normal blood flow to the brain. This can be achieved by

open surgery, endovascular techniques, or a combination of approaches (Box 24.5).

> **Box 24.5 Treatment approaches for pediatric intracranial aneurysm**
>
> - Surgical:
>   - Clipping (obliteration of lesion).
>   - Clip reconstruction (rebuild arterial wall/lumen).
>   - Trapping of lesion (+/– revascularization with bypass).
> - Endovascular:
>   - Embolization (coil/glue).
>   - Stenting (+/– embolization).
>   - Parent artery occlusion.

The advent of endovascular therapy has revolutionized the treatment of pediatric aneurysms, providing options unavailable to earlier generations of physicians. The relatively noninvasive nature of the approach is particularly attractive in children. It is important to note that there is a great deal of evolution of this field, limiting long-term outcome data. Consequently, it is important, when possible, to have cases reviewed at institutions that offer both endovascular and open techniques in order to provide a balanced approach to formulating care plans.[17,24]

The rarity of pediatric aneurysms precludes firm guidelines for treatment indications.[19] In general, aneurysms that have ruptured or that demonstrate enlargement over time, or symptomatic lesions should be considered for treatment. Depending on location and patient status, it may be reasonable to treat aneurysms greater than 3 mm in size, particularly given the long expected lifespan of children. Mycotic aneurysms sometimes will regress with effective antibiotic therapy, obviating the need for other interventions. In addition, flow-related aneurysms located proximal to a lesion such as an arteriovenous malformation (AVM) may regress following definitive treatment of the primary lesion (such as resection of the AVM), demonstrating another scenario when direct aneurysm treatment might not be required.[25,26]

While debatable, lesions 2 mm or smaller in size and those located outside the subarachnoid space are sometimes followed. Much controversy—on both sides—surrounds the large study of unruptured aneurysms published in 1998, but it is important to recognize that these were predominantly adult patients, with questionable relation to the pediatric population, given the differences in lifespan, aneurysm etiology, and risk factors.[1,7]

24.5 Surgical Technique

The variability of aneurysm size, location, and presentation makes each case unique. There is an obvious difference between a critically ill child with an unexpected hemorrhage and an asymptomatic lesion. However, there are general principles able to be applied to all surgical cases.[27] Approaches should be selected to maximize access to the lesion, avoid eloquent neurologic cortex (if possible), and afford the surgeon visualization of proximal vessels to achieve temporary clip placement if needed. Placement of a ventriculostomy (EVD) or lumbar drain can sometimes help with brain relaxation or control of hydrocephalus, but it is critical to recognize that overdrainage of cerebrospinal fluid (CSF) can result in hemorrhage from sudden shifts in aneurysmal transmural pressure. Appropriate patient preparation, with large-bore intravenous access, arterial line monitoring, and other adjuncts, such as a bladder catheter, is important. Controlling blood pressure and administration of medications for antibiotic (with an EVD) or antiepileptic control need to be considered. If trapping is an option, the availability of a bypass graft (scalp artery, radial artery, etc.) with access needs to be planned in advance.

24.5.1 Preoperative Preparation

Communication with nursing and anesthesia before the case will streamline care. In general, equipment should include an operating microscope, multiple suctions, a craniotome, bipolar

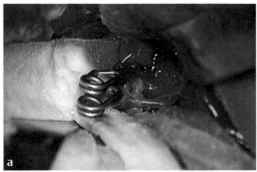
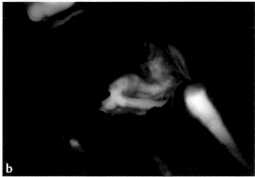

Fig. 24.3 Intraoperative image of aneurysm clipping with **(a)** Conventional microscope, and **(b)** Indocyanine green (ICG) dye image. Note ICG image demonstrates patency of parent vessel (below clips) with complete obliteration of aneurysm (no filling with dye).

electrocautery (nonstick, if available), aneurysm clips, and a retraction system. The anesthesia team should prepare with multiple large-bore intravenous catheters and attempt to have blood products in the operating room. It is good practice to have the microscope draped and clips selected prior to opening the incision, in order to be prepared for emergencies. Availability of intraoperative angiography and/or indocyanine green (ICG) on the microscope to confirm real-time aneurysm obliteration with parent vessel patency is helpful (▶ Fig. 24.3). Agents to manage temporary clipping, such as barbiturates or propofol, and hypothermia and vasoactive medications are important. Adenosine can be used to briefly reduce blood flow in order to better visualize the anatomy of an unexpected rupture.

24.5.2 Operative Approach

Blood pressure shifts should be minimized, particularly during pinning (sometimes local anesthetic injection prior to pin placement can help to blunt blood pressure changes). Frameless stereotaxy can aid in operative planning, ensuring a wide opening with full access to the aneurysm and good visualization. Control of proximal vessels is key, potentially including the carotid artery in the neck. During the craniotomy, care should be taken to avoid tearing the dura and subjacent vessels. Ultrasound can help with localization using real-time imaging. Once open, a clear strategy should be outlined prior to attacking the lesion.

Critical to aneurysm surgery is avoiding intraoperative rupture. If SAH has already occurred, gentle clot removal with sharp dissection when possible can reduce risk of unexpected rupture. Preparing a site for proximal control with temporary clip application is a good strategy. Once ready to clip, careful inspection of surrounding anatomy can help to ensure obliteration of the aneurysm without inadvertent occlusion of small perforators. Evaluation of parent vessel patency and aneurysm occlusion can be performed with intraoperative Doppler, ICG administration, and/or catheter angiography.

24.6 Complications

- Bleeding from intraoperative rupture is the most immediate complication of surgery, and risks are magnified in smaller children, who have little reserve. The loss of one-quarter of blood volume can induce shock, and there may be rapid decompensation in children, which mandates careful monitoring and replacement of blood products by the operative team.
- Stroke may occur from perforator/parent vessel occlusion or emboli/dissection caused by injury to the arterial tree during manipulation (reported at 6–8%).[10,17]
- Hydrocephalus can result from blood in the subarachnoid space or ventricles (reported at 14%).[10]
- Vasospasm can occur following SAH (reported in 21% of pediatric cases).[10]
- Cerebral salt wasting (CSW) is an often underrecognized consequence of SAH and should be considered in the posthemorrhage period if major fluid or sodium shifts are observed.

Overall, surgical morbidity and mortality vary widely dependent on age, aneurysm type, and presentation. Recent series describe average mortality rates of 1 to 3% and morbidity rates of 8 to 14%.[17,28]

24.7 Postoperative Care and Follow-up

Immediate postoperative care centers on confirming that the aneurysm has been fully obliterated (with imaging) and maintaining hemodynamic stability with good blood pressure control (keeping the patient normotensive to sometimes slightly hypertensive, in order to avoid vasospasm). In general, most patients will spend a period of time in the intensive care unit and then often mobilize to the wards. In addition to immediate operative complications, there are problems specific to SAH, including hydrocephalus, vasospasm, and CSW. For patients with SAH, the first week or so after ictus is the key period for developing these conditions. Frequent neurologic examinations should be supplemented with imaging (such as CT/MRI for hydrocephalus and CTA/MRA/transcranial Doppler/angiography for vasospasm). Some patients may benefit from so-called triple-H therapy—hypertension, hypervolemia, and hemodilution—in order to reduce the risk of vasospasm (only after aneurysm treatment).[31,32] The use of calcium channel–blocking agents, such as nimodipine, is unclear in children.

Follow-up will frequently consist of an office visit about 1 month postoperatively, then annually thereafter. In addition to the perioperative angiogram to confirm obliteration of the aneurysm, an MRI/MRA at 6 months may be helpful as a baseline study, to be compared to subsequent annual MRI/MRA. Imaging is performed annually for 5 years, if feasible, with some centers suggesting lifetime imaging every 3 to 5 years thereafter.[31] An angiogram (DSA) is often performed at 1 year postoperatively to confirm durable cure.

24.8 Outcomes

There is a wide range of reported outcomes for pediatric aneurysms, with "good" posttreatment outcomes ranging from 13 to 95% and treatment-related mortality ranging from 3 to 100%.[32] Shunting will be required for 14% of patients with hydrocephalus after SAH.[10] Overall, from a clinical perspective, of patients who survive treatment, 91% (with a mean of 25 years of follow-up) go on to enjoy independent living, with high rates of university graduation and employment.[12] Radiographically, one study reviewed a group of 59 patients with aneurysms who were treated when they were children and had an average of 34 years of follow-up.[33] In this series, 41% developed recurrent or de novo aneurysms after treatment. The annual rate of hemorrhage was 0.4%, with four deaths. The only identified risk factor adding to recurrent or de novo aneurysm development was smoking.[33] These data, while obviously limited in part by the absence of current imaging technologies and surgical techniques at the time of patient treatment, nonetheless underscore the need for continued follow-up in pediatric intracranial aneurysm patients.

24.9 Surgical Pearls

- Ensure all equipment is prepared before starting the case: draped microscope, clip selection, multiple suctions, blood in the room.
- Communication with anesthesia and nursing is critical to provide best care, including planned clipping times and intraoperative rupture.
- Minimizing blood pressure shifts (such as using deep local anesthesia for pinning) and CSF shifts (limiting CSF drainage to a few milliliters at a time) can reduce the risk of re-rupture.
- It is good practice to periodically zoom out and inspect the surface of the brain for unexpected bleeding or swelling. Misplaced retractors or compression of veins can cause problems if unrecognized.
- Sharp dissection and gentle retraction are important to avoid tearing the aneurysm dome.
- Proximal control is critical, including consideration of the neck if anterior circulation aneurysms are being treated.
- Intraoperative imaging tools (ICG, angiography) can improve the accuracy of clip placement and parent/perforator vessel preservation.

24.10 Common Clinical Questions

1. What are some modifiable risk factors that contribute to aneurysm formation in children?
2. If an aneurysm is found in a child, what are the screening recommendations for siblings and other relatives?
3. Where are the most common locations of traumatic aneurysms?
4. What steps are helpful in the immediate management of a child presenting with a hemorrhage from an aneurysm?

24.11 Answers to Common Clinical Questions

1. While adult intracranial aneurysms are often associated with modifiable risk factors—

including hypertension, obesity, high cholesterol, diabetes, and alcohol and drug abuse—the only shared major risk seems to be smoking. It makes sense for children to control all the other risk factors as well, but smoking appears to have a major contribution, particularly to the development of recurrent or growing residual aneurysms.[6,33]

2. There are no fixed screening recommendations for family members of children found to harbor intracranial aneurysms. While the risk of acquired aneurysms (posttraumatic, postinfectious, postsurgical, etc.) in related family members is not genetic, the evidence for or against screening relatives of children with spontaneous aneurysms is limited. Current data suggest increased risk with a sibling pair or three first-degree relatives with known aneurysms.[14,15,16]

3. Traumatic intracranial aneurysms can occur after trauma or surgery. They are most commonly found in the anterior circulation, especially around the cavernous sinus and pericallosal artery.[16,30]

4. The following steps are warranted for the child who presents with an intracranial hemorrhage. It is important to note that severity of presentation can vary greatly and thus treatment has to be individually tailored. If a child presents with an SAH without a clear etiology on initial evaluation, aneurysm (and AVM) should be considered and a CT angiogram (CTA) may be helpful in the acute setting to identify the presence of a lesion. (If no clear lesion is found, repeat imaging in 4–6 weeks with MRI/MRA should be performed to evaluate the hemorrhage cavity after the clot has cleared.)

- Access: large-bore intravenous (at least two), arterial line, bladder catheter (airway intubation if unable to protect airway), and nasogastric tube if intubated.
- Blood pressure control (labetalol or Nipride) with goal of normotension for age.
- Intracranial pressure control—external ventricular drain if hydrocephalus (Note: avoid overdrainage of CSF to prevent re-rupture, often no more than 5 mL at a time), Head of bed (HOB) elevated.
- Antiepileptic medication if concern for seizure.

References

[1] Vlak MH, Algra A, Brandenburg R, Rinkel GJ. Prevalence of unruptured intracranial aneurysms, with emphasis on sex, age, comorbidity, country, and time period: a systematic review and meta-analysis. Lancet Neurol. 2011; 10(7):626–636

[2] Sedzimir CB, Robinson J. Intracranial hemorrhage in children and adolescents. J Neurosurg. 1973; 38(3):269–281

[3] Locksley HB, Sahs AL, Knowler L. Report on the cooperative study of intracranial aneurysms and subarachnoid hemorrhage. Section II. General survey of cases in the central registry and characteristics of the sample population. J Neurosurg. 1966; 24(5):922–932

[4] Roche JL, Choux M, Czorny A, et al. Intracranial arterial aneurysm in children. A cooperative study. Apropos of 43 cases [in French]. Neurochirurgie. 1988; 34(4):243–251

[5] Gerosa M, Licata C, Fiore DL, Iraci G. Intracranial aneurysms of childhood. Childs Brain. 1980; 6(6):295–302

[6] Gemmete JJ, Toma AK, Davagnanam I, Robertson F, Brew S. Pediatric cerebral aneurysms. Neuroimaging Clin N Am. 2013; 23(4):771–779

[7] International Study of Unruptured Intracranial Aneurysms Investigators. Unruptured intracranial aneurysms–risk of rupture and risks of surgical intervention. N Engl J Med. 1998; 339(24):1725–1733

[8] Roger VL, Go AS, Lloyd-Jones DM, et al. American Heart Association Statistics Committee and Stroke Statistics Subcommittee. Executive summary: heart disease and stroke statistics-2012 update: a report from the American Heart Association. Circulation. 2012; 125(1):188–197

[9] Go AS, Mozaffarian D, Roger VL, et al. American Heart Association Statistics Committee and Stroke Statistics Subcommittee. Heart disease and stroke statistics–2013 update: a report from the American Heart Association. Circulation. 2013; 127(1):e6–e245

[10] Garg K, Singh PK, Sharma BS, et al. Pediatric intracranial aneurysms–our experience and review of literature. Childs Nerv Syst. 2014; 30(5):873–883

[11] Lasjaunias P, Wuppalapati S, Alvarez H, Rodesch G, Ozanne A. Intracranial aneurysms in children aged under 15 years: review of 59 consecutive children with 75 aneurysms. Childs Nerv Syst. 2005; 21(6):437–450

[12] Koroknay-Pál P, Lehto H, Niemelä M, Kivisaari R, Hernesniemi J. Long-term outcome of 114 children with cerebral aneurysms. J Neurosurg Pediatr. 2012; 9(6):636–645

[13] Allison JW, Davis PC, Sato Y, et al. Intracranial aneurysms in infants and children. Pediatr Radiol. 1998; 28(4):223–229

[14] Broderick JP, Sauerbeck LR, Foroud T, et al. The Familial Intracranial Aneurysm (FIA) study protocol. BMC Med Genet. 2005; 6:17

[15] Brown RD, Jr, Huston J, Hornung R, et al. Screening for brain aneurysm in the Familial Intracranial Aneurysm study: frequency and predictors of lesion detection. J Neurosurg. 2008; 108(6):1132–1138

[16] Aeron G, Abruzzo TA, Jones BV. Clinical and imaging features of intracranial arterial aneurysms in the pediatric population. Radiographics. 2012; 32(3):667–681

[17] Hetts SW, Narvid J, Sanai N, et al. Intracranial aneurysms in childhood: 27-year single-institution experience. AJNR Am J Neuroradiol. 2009; 30(7):1315–1324

[18] Dunn IF, Woodworth GF, Siddiqui AH, et al. Traumatic pericallosal artery aneurysm: a rare complication of transcallosal surgery. Case report. J Neurosurg. 2007; 106(2) Suppl:153–157

[19] Roach ES, Golomb MR, Adams R, et al. American Heart Association Stroke Council, Council on Cardiovascular Disease in the Young. Management of stroke in infants and children: a scientific statement from a Special Writing Group of the American Heart Association Stroke Council and the Council on Cardiovascular Disease in the Young. Stroke. 2008; 39(9):2644–2691

[20] Hunt WE, Hess RM. Surgical risk as related to time of intervention in the repair of intracranial aneurysms. J Neurosurg. 1968; 28(1):14–20

[21] Hunt WE, Kosnik EJ. Timing and perioperative care in intracranial aneurysm surgery. Clin Neurosurg. 1974; 21: 79–89

[22] Beslow LA, Jordan LC. Pediatric stroke: the importance of cerebral arteriopathy and vascular malformations. Childs Nerv Syst. 2010; 26(10):1263–1273

[23] Al-Jarallah A, Al-Rifai MT, Riela AR, Roach ES. Nontraumatic brain hemorrhage in children: etiology and presentation. J Child Neurol. 2000; 15(5):284–289

[24] terBrugge KG. Neurointerventional procedures in the pediatric age group. Childs Nerv Syst. 1999; 15(11–12):751–754

[25] Hayashi S, Arimoto T, Itakura T, Fujii T, Nishiguchi T, Komai N. The association of intracranial aneurysms and arteriovenous malformation of the brain. Case report. J Neurosurg. 1981; 55(6):971–975

[26] Watanabe H, Nakamura H, Matsuo Y, et al. Spontaneous regression of cerebral arterio-venous malformation following major artery thrombosis proximal to dominant feeders: a case report [in Japanese]. No Shinkei Geka. 1995; 23(4):371–376

[27] Sanai N, Auguste KI, Lawton MT. Microsurgical management of pediatric intracranial aneurysms. Childs Nerv Syst. 2010; 26(10):1319–1327

[28] Kakarla UK, Beres EJ, Ponce FA, et al. Microsurgical treatment of pediatric intracranial aneurysms: long-term angiographic and clinical outcomes. Neurosurgery. 2010; 67(2):237–249, discussion 250

[29] Origitano TC, Wascher TM, Reichman OH, Anderson DE. Sustained increased cerebral blood flow with prophylactic hypertensive hypervolemic hemodilution ("triple-H" therapy) after subarachnoid hemorrhage. Neurosurgery. 1990; 27(5):729–739, discussion 739–740

[30] Nahed BV, Ferreira M, Naunheim MR, Kahle KT, Proctor MR, Smith ER. Intracranial vasospasm with subsequent stroke after traumatic subarachnoid hemorrhage in a 22-month-old child. J Neurosurg Pediatr. 2009; 3(4):311–315

[31] Tonn J, Hoffmann O, Hofmann E, Schlake HP, Sörensen N, Roosen K. "De novo" formation of intracranial aneurysms: who is at risk? Neuroradiology. 1999; 41(9):674–679

[32] Huang J, McGirt MJ, Gailloud P, Tamargo RJ. Intracranial aneurysms in the pediatric population: case series and literature review. Surg Neurol. 2005; 63(5):424–432, discussion 432–433

[33] Koroknay-Pál P, Niemelä M, Lehto H, et al. De novo and recurrent aneurysms in pediatric patients with cerebral aneurysms. Stroke. 2013; 44(5):1436–1439

25 Arteriovenous Malformations

Edward R. Smith

25.1 Introduction and Anatomy

Arteriovenous malformations (AVMs) are relatively common intracranial developmental vascular anomalies consisting of direct arterial-to-venous connections without intervening capillaries. There is no functional neural tissue within the confines of the lesion.[1] Malformations can range from simple single-channel arteriovenous fistulas to a complex tangled nidus connecting enlarged feeding arteries to draining veins (including vein of Galen malformations, reviewed as a distinct entity in another chapter of this book). AVMs have the capacity to grow, particularly in children, likely through a combination of hemodynamic changes (mechanical stretch and enlargement of vessels) and vasculogenesis (developing new vessels in response to elaboration of vascular growth factors and ischemic drive). Enlargement of an AVM seems to alter the adjacent brain. Functional magnetic resonance imaging (MRI) data have suggested that the presence of an AVM in an eloquent area of the brain may be associated with "migration" of the function to adjoining cortex or to the homolog on the contralateral hemisphere.[2,3] This migration or displacement of functional neuronal tissue has important implications for surgical planning.

While most AVMs are thought to be isolated developmental lesions, there are known genetic conditions predisposing individuals to multiple AVMs. Mutations in RASA-1 (a GTPase activating protein) are associated with problems in vessel development, including familial high-flow arteriovenous lesions and/or cutaneous capillary malformations in a small number of families.[4] Hereditary hemorrhagic telangiectasia (HHT) is a genetic condition that predisposes affected individuals to AVMs throughout the body. Thirty-five percent of multiple intracranial AVMs associated with HHT were in children, while the mean age at presentation for HHT is 35 years.[5]

Aneurysms are also found in conjunction with many AVMs. In approximately 7 to 25% of cases of cerebral AVM, there is an associated arterial aneurysm on a feeding pedicle. The prevailing hypothesis is that these aneurysms are flow-related and are most commonly seen in high-flow lesions. These flow-related aneurysms can spontaneously regress following the reduction in blood flow after treatment of the AVM.[6,7]

25.2 Epidemiology and Pathophysiology

AVM is the most common symptomatic high-flow intracranial vascular abnormality in adults and children.[8] The overall frequency of detection for AVMs—including asymptomatic lesions found at autopsy—was 1.4% (46 among 3,200 brain tumor cases).[9] Looking only at those lesions detected because of symptoms, the annual incidence was reported as 1.1 per 100,000.[10] Of those that are symptomatic, about 20% will manifest before 15 years of age.[11] Children comprise 12 to 18% of all AVMs from major centers, and the overall prevalence in children is about 0.02% of the pediatric population.[12,13,14,15] Most AVMs present in adulthood, with a mean age of presentation of approximately 30 to 40 years. AVMs are equally distributed between males and females in the pediatric population.

Neurological signs and symptoms commonly relate to intracranial or subarachnoid hemorrhage from a vessel in the malformation or from a coexistent arterial aneurysm. Symptoms may also relate to cerebral ischemia that is due to diversion of blood to the AVM from the normal cerebral circulation ("steal") or secondary to stagnation causing increased venous pressure secondary to the AVM. Enlarged anomalous vessels may compress or distort adjacent cerebral tissue or cause obstructive hydrocephalus by interfering with the normal circulation or cerebrospinal fluid. Communicating hydrocephalus can result from earlier hemorrhage or venous hypertension.

25.3 Presentation and Evaluation

Hemorrhage and seizure are the most common presenting symptoms for pediatric AVM, but findings may also include headache, focal neurologic deficits, and cognitive decline.[16,17,18,19] Children with AVM are more likely to present with intracranial hemorrhage than adults: 80 to 85% in some pediatric series.[13,20] For children known to have an AVM, the annual risk of hemorrhage has been estimated at 2 to 4%.[21,22] Hemorrhagic events from an AVM in childhood have been associated with a 25% mortality rate.[23] In contrast to earlier reports suggesting that smaller AVMs may have a higher risk of bleeding, more recent data have shown that size is not a major determinant in the risk for hemorrhage.[24,25] A spontaneous intraparenchymal hemorrhage in a child should raise concerns for the presence of an AVM or tumor. Rebleeding rates have been reported to be approximately 6% within the first 6 months.

Evaluation of a patient with an AVM includes history, neurologic and physical examination, and radiographic studies to define the anatomy of the lesion.[26] Most patients present with a new neurological deficit: unusually severe headache ("worst headache of my life") or seizure. These patients should be screened with computed tomography (CT) scan, and if a vascular lesion is suspected, a CT arteriogram (CTA) can be a means of identifying the presence of an AVM. While lacking the detail of a catheter-based arteriogram, CTA affords the treating physician an immediate image outlining key anatomy of a lesion, information of critical importance in the setting of an acutely ill child.

MRI is also useful in the diagnosis and delineation of the three-dimensional anatomy of an AVM. MRI better localizes parenchymal structures relative to the AVM, even if there is a high suspicion of AVM based on the CT or CTA findings and angiography is planned. Chronic ischemic changes, presumably a result of "steal" phenomenon or venous hypertension, may be identified on MRI as bright signal of the surrounding brain on FLAIR (fluid-attenuated inversion recovery) or T2 images (▶ Fig. 25.1).

Catheter-based digital subtraction angiography (DSA) is the "gold standard" of imaging in AVM, establishing the nature and extent of the lesion to its blood supply and its venous drainage.[27] Angiography generally includes bilateral injection of both the internal and external carotid arteries and the vertebral arteries in order to visualize all of the vessels supplying the AVM (▶ Fig. 25.2). Three-dimensional angiography with computer-generated reconstruction is increasingly employed to depict lesional anatomy. It is important to underscore that 15% of cerebral AVMs receive some

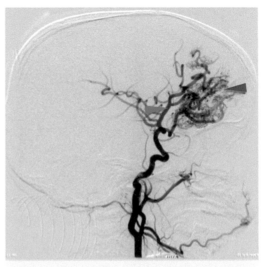

Fig. 25.2 Appearance of AVM on catheter digital subtraction angiography (DSA). Lateral right internal carotid artery injection demonstrates high-flow right frontal AVM. Note markedly dilated feeding artery (*green arrowhead*) and cluster of dysplastic vessels comprising the nidus (*red arrowhead*).

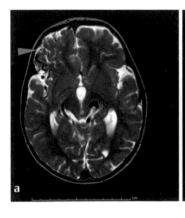 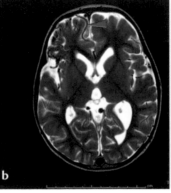

Fig. 25.1 Imaging appearance of AVM on MRI. Axial T2 images show typical flow voids in right frontal lobe (*green arrowhead*) and prominent arterial feeder from anterior cerebral artery (*red arrowhead*).

blood supply from ipsilateral or contralateral meningeal arteries.[28] With catheter angiography, a recent analysis of 241 consecutive pediatric patients revealed a 0% complication rate during the procedure and a 0.4% postprocedural complication rate. Evaluation should look for:

- High-flow versus low-flow lesions.
- Outflow stenoses.
- Varices in subarachnoid or ventricular spaces.
- Number and location of feeding vessels.[29]

Standard preoperative laboratory studies (complete blood count, clotting times (prothrombin time/partial prothrombin time), type and cross [T&C] for blood bank, and a chemistry panel [Chem 7]) should be considered as pretreatment studies for AVM.

25.4 Treatment and Surgical Indications

Treatment is predicated on obliteration of the lesion, which can be achieved by surgery, radiation, embolization, or a combination of therapies. Multimodality therapy of AVM has been advocated by several investigators.[20,30,31,32] Neurointerventionalists, radiation oncologists, and neurosurgeons work together to determine the best strategy for a particular patient. Using a multimodality approach, angiographic obliteration rates of 92.9% have been reported. The choice to operate is based on several factors: (1) eloquence of cortical location (speech, motor function, and sensation), (2) pattern of venous drainage, (3) size, (4) associated aneurysms, (5) recent hemorrhage, (6) clinical deterioration, and (7) risk of complication from other modalities of therapy (such as radiation injury to the developing brain).[31,33] Several of these factors are combined in the Spetzler–Martin[34] grade (▶ Table 25.1) that incorporates eloquence of location, pattern of venous drainage, and size and is considered predictive of outcome from surgical management. (While a revised, simplified version of the Spetzler–Martin system has been proposed, most institutions continue with the original classification.[35]) Regarding surgical indications, in general, if a lesion is surgically accessible with minimal morbidity, it is reasonable to consider resection, given expected lifespan of children and morbidity of hemorrhage, as outlined in the American Heart Association guidelines.[36]

Table 25.1 Spetzler–Martin AVM grading scale

Size	
0–3 cm	1
> 3–6 cm	2
> 6 cm	3
Location	
Noneloquent	0
Eloquent	1
Deep venous drainage	
Not present	0
Present	1

25.4.1 Radiation

Conventional fractionated radiation is not helpful in the majority of AVMs; however, stereotactic radiosurgery offers cure rates of up to 90% in lesions smaller than 3 cm in size. This approach is beneficial for surgically inaccessible lesions or in patients who are high-risk surgical candidates. Shortcomings of this approach include a delay of up to 3 years for lesion obliteration and exposure to radiation in children. Radiation has increased risk in younger populations, making its application less appealing in those children younger than 3 years.

The long delay between treatment and lesion obliteration in radiosurgery for AVMs means that the child is at risk of the complication of bleeding during this interval. Patients with small (less than 3-cm diameter), deep-seated lesions (in the basal ganglia, internal capsule, and thalamus) are the best candidates for radiosurgery. A study of 42 children with lesions in these locations documented a 62% angiographic cure rate within 2 years.[37] However, radiosurgery in these sites have shown a higher risk of rebleeding when compared to AVMs treated in other areas of the brain.[38] Young children have risk of radiation-induced damage, including injury to the surrounding developing brain and potential for development of secondary malignancies. These risks limit radiation use to older children in most cases.

25.4.2 Embolization

Although not traditionally used as a stand-alone treatment for AVMs other than in rare cases with a small nidus and a small number of feeding pedicles, there is a growing literature on the use of newer embolization agents (Onyx) for definitive treatment of brain AVM in adults. However, the situation in children is more complex, and embolization is rarely used as a stand-alone modality, as the recurrence rate is higher and lesion immaturity may preclude complete visualization angiographically. Regardless, embolization is a significant aid in the treatment of AVMs, reducing their blood supply and facilitating operative approaches (usually < 72 hours before surgery). Embolization also has a role in targeted treatment of nonoperative lesions, by occluding areas at risk of hemorrhage such as aneurysms or high-risk varices (those that are intraventricular).

25.5 Surgical Technique

The variability of AVM size, location, and vascular pedicles makes each case unique. However, there are general principles able to be applied to all AVM surgical cases. Approaches should be selected to maximize access to the lesion, avoid eloquent neurologic cortex (if possible), and afford the surgeon visualization of feeding and draining vessels to permit proximal control of blood flow.

25.5.1 Preoperative Preparation

Communication with nursing and anesthesia before the case will streamline care. In general, equipment should include an operating microscope, multiple suctions, a craniotome, bipolar electrocautery (nonstick, if available), AVM/aneurysm clips, and a retraction system. The anesthesia team should prepare with multiple large-bore intravenous catheters and attempt to have blood products in the operating room. It is good practice to have the microscope draped and clips selected prior to opening the incision, in order to be prepared for emergencies.

Operative approach: Frameless stereotaxy can aid in operative planning, ensuring a wide opening with full access to AVM vessels and good visualization. Ultrasound can help with localization using real-time imaging. During the craniotomy, care should be taken to avoid tearing the dura and subjacent vessels. Once open, a clear strategy should be outlined prior to attacking the lesion. Progression from feeding arteries to draining veins is critical, as is avoidance of entering the nidus if possible (▶ Fig. 25.3). Repeated inspection of the surgical field is helpful to ensure that no compression of draining veins exists. Detailed examination of the operative bed after completion is key to avoiding inadvertent residual lesion, as is perioperative imaging if possible.

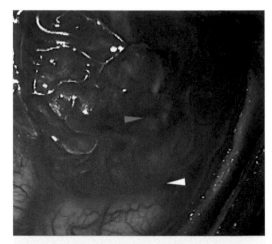

Fig. 25.3 Intraoperative image of AVM. Intraoperative photograph demonstrates appearance of AVM on the surface of the brain. Note the dilated, abnormal vessels extending up to the sulcal border (*white arrowhead*). This lesion had been treated with preoperative embolization, and the intra-arterial embolic agent is black (Onyx) and can be seen occluding a feeder at the anterior margin of the lesion (*green arrowhead*).

25.6 Complications

• Bleeding is the most immediate complication of surgery, and risks are magnified in smaller children, who have little reserve. The loss of one-quarter of blood volume can induce shock and there may be rapid decompensation in children, which mandates careful monitoring and replacement of blood products by the operative team.

• Normal perfusion pressure breakthrough is a phenomenon that is thought to occur after resection of high-flow AVMs in which the blood previously transmitted through the AVM is redirected to smaller, normal vasculature after the AVM has been removed, with subsequent inability of the vessels to handle the increased flow. This can result in brain swelling, increased intracranial pressure, seizure, neurologic dysfunction, or hemorrhage. The problem may be minimized by staged preoperative embolization and rigorous blood pressure control postoperatively.

• Neurologic deficit can occur following AVM resection, although specific rates are hard to derive, given the wide variability in AVM size and location.

Overall, there is low postoperative morbidity in low-grade (I–III) Spetzler–Martin lesions (ranging from 0 to 12%), along with a high rate of complete obliteration (up to 100%), suggesting that surgical resection of these lesions is warranted, especially when performed in experienced centers.[20,31,39,40]

25.7 Postoperative Care and Follow-up

Immediate postoperative care centers on hemodynamic stability with good blood pressure control (keeping the patient normotensive to sometimes slightly hypotensive, in order to avoid reperfusion hemorrhage). In general, most patients will spend a period of time in the intensive care unit and then often mobilize to the wards. Follow-up will frequently consist of an office visit about 1 month postoperatively and then annually thereafter. In addition to the perioperative angiogram to confirm obliteration of the AVM, an MRI/magnetic resonance angiography (MRA) at 6 months may be helpful as a baseline study, to be compared to subsequent annual MRI/MRA. Imaging is performed annually for 5 years, if feasible. An angiogram (DSA) is often performed at 1 year postoperatively to confirm durable cure.

25.8 Outcomes

In pediatric patients with grade I to III Spetzler–Martin AVMs treated by resection,[40] good recovery was achieved in 90% and deaths occurred at a rate of 5%. Radiographic obliteration rates were 89%. These data strongly support resection as a primary treatment for patients with Spetzler–Martin grade I or II AVM. The low postoperative morbidity in children with these lesions (ranging from 0 to 12%), along with a high rate of complete obliteration (up to 100%), suggests that delayed control, inherent to radiosurgery, might not be warranted.[20,31,39,40]

For comparison, a similar group of patients treated with radiosurgery alone had a reported 80% efficacy of lesion obliteration at 36 months, with 4 out of 53 patients having recurrent hemorrhage posttreatment.[41] One large pediatric AVM study included 40 patients and confirmed radiographic obliteration of the AVM nidus in 35% of the patients.[42] The cumulative posttreatment hemorrhage rate was 3.2% per patient per year in the first year and 4.3% per patient per year over the first 3 years.[42] These rates of obliteration, which are notably lower than that reported in the adult population, were potentially complicated by a slightly larger than average size of treated AVM in the study group. In contrast, when a group of 53 pediatric patients was stratified by AVM size (< 3, 3–10, and > 10 mL), in the smallest and middle group, obliteration rates of 80 and 64.7% were reported.[41]

25.9 Surgical Pearls

- Always obliterate feeding arteries before occluding or dividing draining veins, as hemorrhage can result if outflow is interrupted while blood is still entering the AVM.
- Avoid entering the body of the nidus, trying instead to work circumferentially around the lesion. If bleeding occurs, it is important to note that AVM vessels often do not coagulate well due to their dysplastic nature. Consequently, it is usually better to cover the area with a small square of Gelfoam and compress gently rather than to dive into the nidus with bipolar electrocautery.
- It is good practice to periodically zoom out and inspect the surface of the brain for unexpected bleeding or swelling. Misplaced retractors or compression of draining veins can cause problems if unrecognized.
- Careful examination of the resection cavity at the completion of the surgery is important to reduce the risk of missing residual nidus.
- If possible, perioperative imaging (particularly with DSA) can help ensure complete resection and minimize the possibility of postoperative hemorrhage from residual AVM.

25.10 Common Clinical Questions

1. What are the outcomes associated with the different Spetzler–Martin grades?
2. What sort of outcomes can be expected for more complex, large AVMs treated with multimodality therapies?
3. What considerations should be reviewed in the setting of a patient diagnosed with an AVM who is pregnant?
4. What steps are helpful in the immediate management of a child presenting with a hemorrhage from an AVM?

25.11 Answers to Common Clinical Questions

1. For patients treated operatively, outcomes can be predicted by the Spetzler–Martin grade. Grade I had 0% deficits, grade II had 5% deficits, grade III had 16% deficits, grade IV had 27% deficits, and grade V had 31% deficits.[34] Looking specifically at children, a more recent report describes an 89% radiographic obliteration rate and 5% morbidity and 5% mortality rate for grade I to III lesions.[40]

2. The efficacy of multimodality treatment of large, complex lesions is supported by a group of 53 children at a 3-year follow-up in whom a 58% cure rate was noted for AVMs greater than 6 cm in diameter.[43]

3. Treatment of a known AVM should be undertaken prior to pregnancy, whenever possible. There are rare situations of documented intracranial AVM in a pregnancy. Either the AVM was not addressed prior to gestation or neurological sequelae led to its discovery. Data in this small group of patients are inconclusive, particularly with regard to the rate of hemorrhage during the pregnancy.[44,45,46,47,48,49,50] MRI is safe for initial evaluation of the anatomy of the lesion.[51] No specific recommendations can be made if the AVM is diagnosed during pregnancy, because individual risk–benefit relationships need to be assessed. If the mother has an untreated or partially treated AVM, caesarean section should be considered.[40,48,50,52]

4. The following steps are warranted for the child who presents with an intracranial hemorrhage. It is important to note that severity of presentation can vary greatly and thus treatment has to be individually tailored. If a child presents with an intraparenchymal hemorrhage without a clear etiology on initial evaluation, AVM should be considered and a CT angiogram (CTA) may be helpful in the acute setting to identify the presence of dilated vessels or nidus. (If no clear lesion is found, repeat imaging in 4–6 weeks with MRI should be performed to evaluate the hemorrhage cavity after the clot has cleared.)
   - Access: Large-bore intravenous (at least two), arterial line, bladder catheter (airway intubation if unable to protect airway), and nasogastric tube if intubated.
   - Blood pressure control (labetalol or Nipride) with goal of normotension for age.
   - Intracranial pressure control—external ventricular drain if hydrocephalus (Note: avoid overdrainage of CSF to prevent re-rupture, often no more than 5 mL at a time), head of bed (HOB) elevated.
   - Antiepileptic medication if concern for seizure.

References

[1] Friedlander RM. Clinical practice. Arteriovenous malformations of the brain. N Engl J Med. 2007; 356(26): 2704–2712

[2] Mine S, Hirai S, Yamakami I, Ono J, Yamaura A, Nakajima Y. Location of primary somatosensory area in cerebral arteriovenous malformation involving sensorimotor area [in Japanese]. No To Shinkei. 1999; 51(4):331–337

[3] Vates GE, Lawton MT, Wilson CB, et al. Magnetic source imaging demonstrates altered cortical distribution of function in patients with arteriovenous malformations. Neurosurgery. 2002; 51(3):614–623, discussion 623–627

[4] Thiex R, Mulliken JB, Revencu N, et al. A novel association between RASA1 mutations and spinal arteriovenous anomalies. AJNR Am J Neuroradiol. 2010; 31(4):775–779

[5] Lasjaunias P. Vascular Diseases in Neonates, Infants and Children. Berlin: Springer Verlag; 1997

[6] Hayashi S, Arimoto T, Itakura T, Fujii T, Nishiguchi T, Komai N. The association of intracranial aneurysms and arteriovenous malformation of the brain. Case report. J Neurosurg. 1981; 55 (6):971–975

[7] Watanabe H, Nakamura H, Matsuo Y, et al. Spontaneous regression of cerebral arterio-venous malformation following major artery thrombosis proximal to dominant feeders: a case report [in Japanese]. No Shinkei Geka. 1995; 23(4):371–376

[8] Gonzalez LF, Bristol RE, Porter RW, Spetzler RF. De novo presentation of an arteriovenous malformation. Case report and review of the literature. J Neurosurg. 2005; 102(4):726–729

[9] Olivecrona H, Riives J. Arteriovenous aneurysms of the brain, their diagnosis and treatment. Arch Neurol Psychiatry. 1948; 59(5):567–602

[10] Jessurun GA, Kamphuis DJ, van der Zande FH, Nossent JC. Cerebral arteriovenous malformations in The Netherlands Antilles. High prevalence of hereditary hemorrhagic telangiectasia-related single and multiple cerebral arteriovenous malformations. Clin Neurol Neurosurg. 1993; 95(3):193–198

[11] Di Rocco C, Tamburrini G, Rollo M. Cerebral arteriovenous malformations in children. Acta Neurochir (Wien). 2000; 142 (2):145–156, discussion 156–158

[12] Celli P, Ferrante L, Palma L, Cavedon G. Cerebral arteriovenous malformations in children. Clinical features and outcome of treatment in children and in adults. Surg Neurol. 1984; 22(1):43–49

[13] Kahl W, Kessel G, Schwarz M, Voth D. Arterio-venous malformations in childhood: clinical presentation, results after operative treatment and long-term follow-up. Neurosurg Rev. 1989; 12(2):165–171

[14] Kader A, Goodrich JT, Sonstein WJ, Stein BM, Carmel PW, Michelsen WJ. Recurrent cerebral arteriovenous malformations after negative postoperative angiograms. J Neurosurg. 1996; 85(1):14–18

[15] D'Aliberti G, Talamonti G, Versari PP, et al. Comparison of pediatric and adult cerebral arteriovenous malformations. J Neurosurg Sci. 1997; 41(4):331–336

[16] Graf CJ, Perret GE, Torner JC. Bleeding from cerebral arteriovenous malformations as part of their natural history. J Neurosurg. 1983; 58(3):331–337

[17] Heros RC, Korosue K, Diebold PM. Surgical excision of cerebral arteriovenous malformations: late results. Neurosurgery. 1990; 26(4):570–577, discussion 577–578

[18] Jomin M, Lesoin F, Lozes G. Prognosis for arteriovenous malformations of the brain in adults based on 150 cases. Surg Neurol. 1985; 23(4):362–366

[19] Itoyama Y, Uemura S, Ushio Y, et al. Natural course of unoperated intracranial arteriovenous malformations: study of 50 cases. J Neurosurg. 1989; 71(6):805–809

[20] Humphreys RP, Hoffman HJ, Drake JM, Rutka JT. Choices in the 1990s for the management of pediatric cerebral arteriovenous malformations. Pediatr Neurosurg. 1996; 25 (6):277–285

[21] Brown RD, Jr, Wiebers DO, Forbes G, et al. The natural history of unruptured intracranial arteriovenous malformations. J Neurosurg. 1988; 68(3):352–357

[22] Ondra SL, Troupp H, George ED, Schwab K. The natural history of symptomatic arteriovenous malformations of the brain: a 24-year follow-up assessment. J Neurosurg. 1990; 73 (3):387–391

[23] Altschuler E, Lunsford LD, Kondziolka D, et al. Radiobiologic models for radiosurgery. Neurosurg Clin N Am. 1992; 3(1): 61–77

[24] Norris JS, Valiante TA, Wallace MC, et al. A simple relationship between radiological arteriovenous malformation hemodynamics and clinical presentation: a prospective, blinded analysis of 31 cases. J Neurosurg. 1999; 90(4):673–679

[25] Stefani MA, Porter PJ, terBrugge KG, Montanera W, Willinsky RA, Wallace MC. Angioarchitectural factors present in brain arteriovenous malformations associated with hemorrhagic presentation. Stroke. 2002; 33(4):920–924

[26] Ogilvy CS, Stieg PE, Awad I, et al. Stroke Council, American Stroke Association. Recommendations for the management of intracranial arteriovenous malformations: a statement for healthcare professionals from a special writing group of the Stroke Council, American Stroke Association. Circulation. 2001; 103(21):2644–2657

[27] Pott M, Huber M, Assheuer J, Bewermeyer H. Comparison of MRI, CT and angiography in cerebral arteriovenous malformations. Bildgebung. 1992; 59(2):98–102

[28] Newton TH, Cronqvist S. Involvement of dural arteries in intracranial arteriovenous malformations. Radiology. 1969; 93(5):1071–1078

[29] Ellis MJ, Armstrong D, Vachhrajani S, et al. Angioarchitectural features associated with hemorrhagic presentation in pediatric cerebral arteriovenous malformations. J Neurointerv Surg. 2012:2011–010198

[30] Ter Brugge K, Lasjaunias P, Chiu M, Flodmark O, Chuang S, Burrows P. Pediatric surgical neuroangiography. A multicentre approach. Acta Radiol Suppl. 1986; 369:692–693

[31] Hoh BL, Chapman PH, Loeffler JS, Carter BS, Ogilvy CS. Results of multimodality treatment for 141 patients with brain arteriovenous malformations and seizures: factors associated with seizure incidence and seizure outcomes. Neurosurgery. 2002; 51(2):303–309, discussion 309–311

[32] Lee BB, Do YS, Yakes W, Kim DI, Mattassi R, Hyon WS. Management of arteriovenous malformations: a multidisciplinary approach. J Vasc Surg. 2004; 39(3):590–600

[33] Fisher WS, III. Therapy of AVMs: a decision analysis. Clin Neurosurg. 1995; 42:294–312

[34] Spetzler RF, Martin NA. A proposed grading system for arteriovenous malformations. J Neurosurg. 1986; 65(4):476–483

[35] Spetzler RF, Ponce FA. A 3-tier classification of cerebral arteriovenous malformations. Clinical article. J Neurosurg. 2011; 114(3):842–849

[36] Roach ES, Golomb MR, Adams R, et al. American Heart Association Stroke Council, Council on Cardiovascular Disease in the Young. Management of stroke in infants and children: a scientific statement from a Special Writing Group of the American Heart Association Stroke Council and the Council on Cardiovascular Disease in the Young. Stroke. 2008; 39(9):2644–2691

[37] Andrade-Souza YM, Zadeh G, Scora D, Tsao MN, Schwartz ML. Radiosurgery for basal ganglia, internal capsule, and thalamus arteriovenous malformation: clinical outcome. Neurosurgery. 2005; 56(1):56–63, discussion 63–64

[38] Pollock BE, Gorman DA, Brown PD. Radiosurgery for arteriovenous malformations of the basal ganglia, thalamus, and brainstem. J Neurosurg. 2004; 100(2):210–214

[39] Morgan MK, Rochford AM, Tsahtsarlis A, Little N, Faulder KC. Surgical risks associated with the management of Grade I and II brain arteriovenous malformations. Neurosurgery. 2004; 54(4):832–837, discussion 837–839

[40] Kiriş T, Sencer A, Sahinbaş M, Sencer S, Imer M, Izgi N. Surgical results in pediatric Spetzler-Martin grades I-III intracranial arteriovenous malformations. Childs Nerv Syst. 2005; 21(1):69–74, discussion 75–76

[41] Levy EI, Niranjan A, Thompson TP, et al. Radiosurgery for childhood intracranial arteriovenous malformations. Neurosurgery. 2000; 47(4):834–841, discussion 841–842

[42] Smyth MD, Sneed PK, Ciricillo SF, et al. Stereotactic radiosurgery for pediatric intracranial arteriovenous malformations: the University of California at San Francisco experience. J Neurosurg. 2002; 97(1):48–55

[43] Chang SD, Marcellus ML, Marks MP, Levy RP, Do HM, Steinberg GK. Multimodality treatment of giant intracranial arteriovenous malformations. Neurosurgery. 2003; 53(1):1–11, discussion 11–13

[44] Horton JC, Chambers WA, Lyons SL, Adams RD, Kjellberg RN. Pregnancy and the risk of hemorrhage from cerebral arteriovenous malformations. Neurosurgery. 1990; 27(6): 867–871, discussion 871–872

[45] Lanzino G, Jensen ME, Cappelletto B, Kassell NF. Arteriovenous malformations that rupture during pregnancy: a management dilemma. Acta Neurochir (Wien). 1994; 126(2–4):102–106

[46] Karlsson B, Lindquist C, Johansson A, Steiner L. Annual risk for the first hemorrhage from untreated cerebral arteriovenous malformations. Minim Invasive Neurosurg. 1997; 40(2):40–46

[47] Yih PS, Cheong KF. Anaesthesia for caesarean section in a patient with an intracranial arteriovenous malformation. Anaesth Intensive Care. 1999; 27(1):66–68

[48] Trivedi RA, Kirkpatrick PJ. Arteriovenous malformations of the cerebral circulation that rupture in pregnancy. J Obstet Gynaecol. 2003; 23(5):484–489

[49] Piotin M, Mounayer C, Spelle L, Moret J. Cerebral arteriovenous malformations and pregnancy: management of a dilemma [in French]. J Neuroradiol. 2004; 31(5):376–378

[50] English LA, Mulvey DC. Ruptured arteriovenous malformation and subarachnoid hemorrhage during emergent cesarean delivery: a case report. AANA J. 2004; 72(6):423–426

[51] Shojaku H, Seto H, Kakishita M, Yokoyama M, Ito J. Use of MR angiography in a pregnant patient with thalamic AVM. Radiat Med. 1996; 14(3):159–161

[52] Terao M, Kubota M, Tamakawa S, Kawada K, Ogawa H. Anesthesia for cesarean section in a patient with intracranial A-V malformation [in Japanese]. Masui. 1995; 44(12):1700–1702

26 Pediatric Cavernous Malformations

Rajiv R. Iyer, Mari L. Groves, Nir Shimony, George I. Jallo

26.1 Introduction/ Epidemiology

Cavernous malformations (CMs), also referred to as cavernous angiomas, or cavernomas, occur throughout the central nervous system (CNS) and are angiographically occult vascular lesions made up of closely packed thin-walled sinusoidal vessels without interspersed neural tissue. The majority of CMs are supratentorial, but infratentorial and intraspinal lesions are also known to occur.[1,2] In the pediatric population, CMs can cause significant morbidity manifesting in the form of headaches or seizures, as well as acute hemorrhage causing more severe neurological decline. CMs have been reported to occur in 0.4 to 0.5% of the general population and are more common in adults, while approximately 25% occur in the pediatric age group.[3,4,5,6] There is no clear gender predilection associated. The majority of CMs in the pediatric population are solitary and sporadic. However, those with multiple CMs, or in patients with a positive family history, a high index of suspicion should be maintained for an inherited form of this disorder.[7] Familial forms of this disorder demonstrate autosomal dominant inheritance and are caused by genetic mutations in the *CCM1*, *CCM2*, and *CCM3* genes on chromosomes 7q, 7p, and 3q, respectively.[8,9,10,11,12] In patients found to have an intraspinal CM, there is thought to be an increased risk of harboring other CMs within the neuraxis, warranting radiographic screening.[13] Risk factors for the development of CMs are not well understood, but may include prior radiation therapy or the presence of venous anomalies.[14,15,16,17,18]

26.2 Pathology

Macroscopically, CMs are well-circumscribed, lobulated lesions separated from neural parenchyma that have a "mulberrylike," purplish appearance due to the presence of partial thrombosis and a low rate of blood flow through the vascular channels within (▶ Fig. 26.1a). The immediately surrounding brain or spinal cord parenchyma may be gliotic due to chronic inflammation and often contains hemosiderin staining from prior hemorrhage. Histologically, CMs consist of densely packed sinusoidal vessels lined by a thin layer of endothelium embedded in a collagenlike stroma. The tight junction barrier of this endothelium, however, has increased permeability due in part to a lack of astrocyte foot processes.[19] The blood vessels of CMs are also devoid of smooth muscle, pericytes, and other properties of mature endothelium, and typically demonstrate hyalinization (▶ Fig. 26.1b). For these reasons, there is thought to be recurrent red blood cell extravasation and resultant microhemorrhages of different ages. Varying degrees of calcification may also be present.

26.3 Diagnostic Imaging

In contrast with CNS vascular lesions such as arteriovenous malformations, arteriovenous fistulas, and aneurysms, CMs are typically undetectable on cerebral angiography and are thus classified as angiographically occult.[20,21] These lesions are frequently asymptomatic and have been increasingly detected in an incidental manner with the

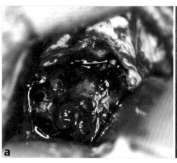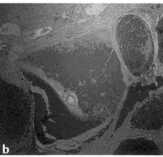

Fig. 26.1 (a) Gross appearance of cavernous malformation demonstrating "mulberrylike" appearance caused by concurrent thrombosis and low blood flow through the lesion. (b) Photomicrograph of a CM demonstrating closely interspersed sinusoidal channels and red blood cell extravasation.

widespread use of magnetic resonance imaging (MRI).[22] In the acute setting, computed tomography (CT) imaging serves a use in detecting acute hemorrhage and large lesions; however, MRI remains the most sensitive study for the detection of CMs.[23,24] In fact, early studies demonstrated that CT imaging detected only approximately 36% of CMs that were evident on MRI.[7] Zabramski and colleagues in 1994 described a classification system for CMs based on their imaging characteristics. Type I lesions are characterized by subacute hemorrhage as evidenced by hyperintensity on T1-weighted imaging and a quick transformation from a hyper- to hypointense lesion on T2-weighted MRI. Type II lesions demonstrate concurrent hemorrhage and thrombosis, correlating with the underlying pattern of repeating hemorrhage and clotting over time. These lesions feature a reticulated pattern of high and low signal intensity at their core, surrounded by a hypointense rim on T2-weighted imaging that corresponds to circumferential hemosiderin deposition, with a classic "popcornlike" appearance on MRI (▶ Fig. 26.2). Type III lesions contain chronic hemosiderin deposition, while type IV CMs are punctate and easier to detect with gradient echo (GRE) sequences, and histopathologically may be considered capillary telangiectasias.[25] Compared to T2-weighted fast spin-echo sequences, T2-weighted GRE sequences are better at detecting chronic hemosiderin deposition and deoxyhemoglobin. Especially relevant for familial cases of CMs, susceptibility-weighted imaging has been thought to have an even higher sensitivity than T2-weighted imaging for detection of small CMs.[26] CMs typically demonstrate minimal, if any, enhancement following administration of gadolinium. An association exists between CMs and the coexistence of a developmental venous anomaly (DVA). This association has been reported to be approximately 20%, and in the majority of hemorrhagic cases leading to the diagnosis of a DVA on imaging, an associated CM was present at the location of hemorrhage.[18,27]

26.4 Clinical Presentation

26.4.1 Intracranial CMs

Similar to the adult population, the majority of CMs in the pediatric population are supratentorial in location, while approximately 20% are infratentorial.[28,29] The average age at presentation has been reported to be around 10 years, although they can arise at any point from neonatal stages, throughout adolescence and into adulthood.[28,29,30,31,32] Supratentorial CMs generally occur in the cortical regions and subcortical white matter, but in other rare circumstances are found in deeper locations such as the basal ganglia, hypothalamus, ventricular system, optic chiasm, pineal region, and others.[28,33]

In young children without a family history, asymptomatic identification of CMs is generally uncommon. When symptoms do arise, they are attributable to hemorrhage. This can be subdivided into chronic microhemorrhages that cause surrounding parenchymal edema and irritation over time, and large intralesional or intraparenchymal hemorrhages that cause acute neurological deficits or deterioration. For many children with supratentorial CMs, their primary presentation is with seizures.[28,31,34] In other patients, medical attention is sought due to headaches or neurological deficit. Repeated hemorrhages in certain patients can cause progressive CM growth and associated mass effect; these individuals may present from signs of

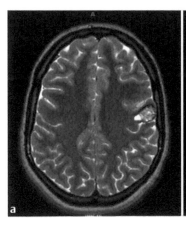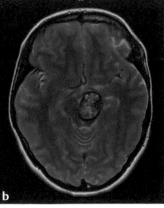

Fig. 26.2 (a) T2-weighted magnetic resonance image (MRI) demonstrating left frontal precentral gyrus CM exhibiting a reticulated core of hypo- and hyperintensity and a T2-hypointense surrounding rim. (b) T2-weighted MRI demonstrating left midbrain and cerebral peduncle CM in a 14-year-old girl who presented with pupillary dilation.

elevated intracranial pressure or focal neurological deficit.

Infratentorial CMs consist primarily of brainstem and cerebellar lesions. Patients with brainstem CMs may exhibit a myriad of signs and symptoms including cranial nerve deficits, sensory disturbances, hemiparesis, altered level of consciousness, and hydrocephalus.[35] Acute or progressive headaches that localize to the occipital region, cerebellar dysfunction, and, less commonly, cranial nerve palsies or acute neurological decline are some of the clinical signs and symptoms associated specifically with cerebellar CMs.[36,37] In the pediatric population, due to the relatively high incidence of posterior fossa tumors, lesion characteristics such as an associated venous anomaly or the presence of blood of different ages should lead the clinician to maintain a higher index of suspicion for CMs. However, given the high incidence in children of primary brain tumors in the posterior fossa, a differential diagnosis must be maintained.

26.4.2 Intraspinal CMs

Intraspinal CMs comprise about 5% or less of all pediatric CMs affecting the neuraxis.[29] These lesions can be classified as intramedullary, intradural extramedullary, and extradural, with intramedullary CMs being the predominant subtype. Given the rarity of these lesions, the literature describing their typical presentation and guiding their clinical management is limited to scattered case reports and small case series.[38,39,40,41,42,43] Although rare, intraspinal CMs can lead to significant morbidity given the high density of functionally critical neural tissue that lies adjacent. Commonly, patients will present with neck or back pain, sensory disturbances such as paresthesias or frank numbness, and motor weakness, myelopathy, and bowel or bladder dysfunction. Any constellation of these symptoms in a child should raise the suspicion of an intramedullary lesion such as a CM. Importantly, patients with intraspinal CMs should undergo pan-neuraxis imaging to rule out the presence of other such lesions, as there is a higher prevalence of coexisting CMs in these patients.[39,44]

26.5 Natural History

Several studies have attempted to elucidate the natural history of CMs in the adult population in order to help clinicians define their hemorrhagic risk and to guide clinical management following diagnosis. Rates of hemorrhage are typically defined as either events per lesion-year or events per person-year, and have been reported to be between 0.7 and 22.9%.[25,45,46,47,48,49,50] Unfortunately, these studies are heterogeneous with respect to the amount of familial CM cases as well as the number of truly asymptomatic patients they contain. One consensus feature of these studies, however, is that prior CM hemorrhage itself confers risk for subsequent hemorrhage.

In the pediatric population, there are substantially less data shedding light on the natural history of CMs. In 2012, Al-Holou and colleagues evaluated over 14,000 patients under the age of 25 years who underwent MRI of the brain and found 164 CMs in 92 patients, 42% of whom were asymptomatic. At follow-up, the authors discovered a hemorrhage rate of 1.6% per patient-year and 0.9% per lesion-year in the group of patients with incidentally discovered CMs. Similar to reports in the adult population, for those patients who at some point presented with acute neurological symptoms, the hemorrhage rate was higher at 8% per patient-year. Importantly, factors associated with a higher hemorrhagic rate included an infratentorial location, consistent with previous reports, as well as the presence of a DVA.[51,52]

More recently, Gross and colleagues evaluated a cohort of 167 pediatric patients (younger than 21 years) with CMs, 26% of whose lesions were incidentally discovered. Overall annual hemorrhage rate was determined to be 3.3% per lesion-year, and 1.2% in subgroup analysis of solitary, incidental CMs. Overall hemorrhage rate was determined to be 11.3% for previously hemorrhagic lesions. Importantly, of 11 untreated hemorrhagic CMs with greater than 5-year follow-up, temporal relation to prior hemorrhage played a role in subsequent hemorrhage risk: annual hemorrhage rates were 18% within 3 years of prior CM hemorrhage, decreasing to 4.8 and 3.3% at 3 and 5 years of respective follow-up. This temporal clustering of CM hemorrhages has been previously reported.[53] Overall, multivariate analysis of their cohort yielded risk factors for CM hemorrhage that included prior hemorrhage, associated DVAs, and a brainstem location.[31]

26.6 Surgical Indications, Techniques, and Outcomes

Pediatric patients with neuraxis CMs represent a heterogeneous group with varying age, presentation, and number of lesions. Given these variables, treatment options must be tailored for each patient and each clinical scenario encountered. As the natural history of CMs in the pediatric population becomes better defined, surgical indications also become elucidated. In asymptomatic patients with incidentally discovered CMs, and especially those with higher-risk, deep-seated lesions, expectant observation is appropriate with serial imaging over time to monitor lesion growth or clinically silent hemorrhage.[54,55] For symptomatic patients, surgical excision is the mainstay of treatment, as children have a longer time course to develop progression of clinical symptoms from lesion growth or repeated hemorrhage over time. Like other clinical decisions in the pediatric population, the risks and benefits of action and inaction must be weighed for those patients with CMs. Generally, in children, an aggressive treatment strategy involving surgical excision is undertaken when lesions are safely accessible, symptomatic, or demonstrate evidence of current or prior hemorrhage.[32] This is especially true for easily accessible supratentorial lesions in noneloquent regions. For deep-seated lesions, such as thalamic or brainstem CMs, or those in eloquent cortex, management is more controversial and surgical morbidity must be weighed against the benefit of resection. A pattern of repeated hemorrhage or progressive neurological deficit due to mass effect may indicate surgical intervention for such CMs.[56,57] For brainstem CMs, exophytic lesions and those that come to the pial surface are more appropriate for surgical intervention, as these features minimize the chance of harm to normal neural tissue. Appropriate surgical planning must include a thorough knowledge of the vital structures in the vicinity of the lesion, including white matter tracts that are intolerant to retraction, brainstem nuclei, perforating vessels, and draining veins. Morbidity in these cases may result from incomplete CM resection and hematoma formation.[56]

In those patients who present with a neurological deficit due to an acutely hemorrhagic CM, acute decline due to elevated intracranial pressure and mass effect may warrant immediate intervention. Typically, however, these lesions are managed initially with supportive therapy and rehabilitation following the initial hemorrhagic event. Weeks later, after swelling and edema have subsided, excision can be performed to prevent further morbidity due to repeat hemorrhages that have been shown to temporally cluster after the initial event.[53]

Surgical intervention is often employed for children who present with medically refractory seizures due to supratentorial CMs. It is important that seizure semiology localizes to the lesion, which in some cases may require EEG (electroencephalographic) monitoring. In patients with multiple CMs, it is especially important to discern which lesion may be symptomatic prior to surgery. For those who undergo surgery for CM-induced epilepsy, improved seizure control postoperatively can generally be expected. In some cases, continued medical therapy is required to prevent seizures postoperatively, while, in others, doses can be weaned.[33,58] Some studies have suggested that excision of surrounding hemosiderin-stained neural parenchyma may improve seizure control postoperatively.[59,60] Others, however, suggest that good seizure control can result without the need for such extensive resections.[33,61] Therefore, when undertaking CM resection for medically refractory epilepsy, more extensive surgery may decrease the likelihood of postoperative seizures, but caution should be used in lesions that are adjacent to or within functionally relevant areas so as to not cause iatrogenic deficits due to resection of nonlesional tissue.[28]

Surgical excision often utilizes the safest and most direct approach to the target lesion with the intent of leaving functional cortex and other deeper, vital structures unharmed. Under close neurophysiological monitoring, resection of the CM is often best accomplished by circumferentially dissecting the lesion away from adjacent neural parenchyma. Generally, entering the CM during resection is inadvisable, as it can lead to difficult-to-control bleeding and may risk incomplete resection. However, in some cases of deep cortical lesions and brainstem CMs, dissection along the periphery of the lesion is not possible without causing retraction injury to functionally critical surrounding structures and may thus warrant piecemeal resection and internal debulking. Typically, if a DVA is encountered, this is preserved. Meticulous hemostasis is critical following CM resection and careful inspection of the resection cavity helps avoid remnant lesion, which can lead to lesion recurrence or repeat hemorrhage.

Surgery is often well tolerated in children with CMs. Several series over the recent decades describe the international experience with CMs in the pediatric population.[28,29,32,33,55,62] Overall mortality rates are very low and are commonly 0%. The majority of reports consist primarily of supratentorial CMs with outcomes often reported as good or excellent. Cerebellar CMs in the pediatric population have also been shown to have excellent surgical outcomes with low morbidity and mortality.[37] Not surprisingly, deep-seated CMs, including brainstem CMs, demonstrate a higher rate of postoperative morbidity. These rates have been reported to be approximately 12 to 30%.[35,56] In many cases of brainstem CMs, transient neurological deficits are seen postoperatively, which tend to improve over time. However, permanent neurological injury is also possible. Overall, brainstem CM surgery in the pediatric population is well tolerated, and the higher rate of morbidity for these lesions emphasizes the importance of choosing appropriate surgical candidates after weighing the risks and benefits of intervention, as well as the safest surgical approach for lesion resection.[63,64]

Intramedullary CMs are rare in children but are often managed surgically due to the risk of intramedullary hemorrhage and progressive myelopathy over time. With simple laminectomy and intradural exploration, these lesions can be resected under electrophysiological guidance with maintenance of preoperative function and possible neurological improvement over time.[39]

26.7 Radiosurgery

The role of radiosurgery is a highly debated topic in the management of CMs. There are little data supporting its use as a first-line therapy in the pediatric population. Various reports suggest a decrease in hemorrhage rates following radiosurgery, but it has been suggested that these studies demonstrate an unusually high pretreatment hemorrhage rate.[35] Within 2 to 3 years of radiosurgery, rates of hemorrhage are reported to be between 8.8 and 32%. However, after this time period, hemorrhage rates appear to drop to 1.1 to 4.5%. Rates of morbidity including neurological deficit following radiosurgery have been reported to be between 13 and 26%.[65,66,67,68] Overall, it remains to be determined whether hemorrhage rates following radiosurgery differ significantly from the natural history of these lesions in the pediatric population. For children, first-line therapy should be surgery for symptomatic lesions, while the role of radiosurgery as opposed to observation alone for inaccessible lesions or poor surgical candidates requires further elucidation.

26.8 Common Clinical Questions

1. In what locations do CMs occur in the pediatric population and what are some risk factors associated with hemorrhage?

2. What are the common presenting symptoms for children with CMs?
3. What is the recommended treatment strategy for symptomatic supratentorial and infratentorial CMs?

26.9 Answers to Common Clinical Questions

1. In children, the most common location for CMs is in the supratentorial compartment. As many as 80% of lesions are found in the cerebrum. Other areas where one may find these lesions are in the infratentorial compartment, which can be subdivided into cerebellar CMs and brainstem CMs. Intraspinal CMs are rare but, when encountered, are typically intramedullary in location. Suggested risk factors for hemorrhage include prior hemorrhage, an infratentorial location, and the presence of a DVA.

2. The most common presenting symptom for CMs in children is seizures. Other symptoms depend on lesion location and the temporal acuity of hemorrhage. With chronic, repeated hemorrhages, seizures and headaches are possible, and if hemorrhage is acute, symptoms from elevated intracranial pressure or mass effect can occur, including focal neurological deficits. Cerebellar dysfunction, cranial nerve palsies, and hydrocephalus are possible with infratentorial lesions. Intraspinal lesions can present with motor weakness, sensory disturbances, or chronic myelopathy due to hemosiderin irritation and gliosis surrounding the lesion.

3. Observation with serial imaging is often employed for asymptomatic lesions found in children. Overall, however, an aggressive treatment approach is used in children with CMs to prevent morbidity later in life. Surgical treatment is the therapeutic mainstay for symptomatic lesions that are surgically accessible and demonstrate evidence of current or prior hemorrhage. Resection of the hemosiderin rim for cases of medically refractory epilepsy can help decrease the likelihood of postoperative seizures, but this method should be limited to noneloquent cortical areas. Symptomatic cerebellar lesions can be surgically removed with good results. Brainstem lesions that are exophytic or lie in close proximity to a pial surface are better suited for surgical intervention. Repeated

hemorrhages and progressive neurological deficit are reasons to consider surgical intervention for brainstem CMs.

References

[1] Lena G, Ternier J, Paz-Paredes A, Scavarda D. Central nervous system cavernomas in children [in French]. Neurochirurgie. 2007; 53(2–3, Pt 2):223–237

[2] McCormick WF, Hardman JM, Boulter TR. Vascular malformations ("angiomas") of the brain, with special reference to those occurring in the posterior fossa. J Neurosurg. 1968; 28(3):241–251

[3] Del Curling O, Jr, Kelly DL, Jr, Elster AD, Craven TE. An analysis of the natural history of cavernous angiomas. J Neurosurg. 1991; 75(5):702–708

[4] Herter T, Brandt M, Szüwart U. Cavernous hemangiomas in children. Childs Nerv Syst. 1988; 4(3):123–127

[5] Maraire JN, Awad IA. Intracranial cavernous malformations: lesion behavior and management strategies. Neurosurgery. 1995; 37(4):591–605

[6] Otten P, Pizzolato GP, Rilliet B, Berney J. 131 cases of cavernous angioma (cavernomas) of the CNS, discovered by retrospective analysis of 24,535 autopsies [in French]. Neurochirurgie. 1989; 35(2):82–83, 128–131

[7] Rigamonti D, Hadley MN, Drayer BP, et al. Cerebral cavernous malformations. Incidence and familial occurrence. N Engl J Med. 1988; 319(6):343–347

[8] Bergametti F, Denier C, Labauge P, et al. Société Française de Neurochirurgie. Mutations within the programmed cell death 10 gene cause cerebral cavernous malformations. Am J Hum Genet. 2005; 76(1):42–51

[9] Gault J, Sain S, Hu LJ, Awad IA. Spectrum of genotype and clinical manifestations in cerebral cavernous malformations. Neurosurgery. 2006; 59(6):1278–1284, discussion 1284–1285

[10] Laberge-le Couteulx S, Jung HH, Labauge P, et al. Truncating mutations in CCM1, encoding KRIT1, cause hereditary cavernous angiomas. Nat Genet. 1999; 23(2):189–193

[11] Liquori CL, Berg MJ, Siegel AM, et al. Mutations in a gene encoding a novel protein containing a phosphotyrosine-binding domain cause type 2 cerebral cavernous malformations. Am J Hum Genet. 2003; 73(6):1459–1464

[12] Sahoo T, Johnson EW, Thomas JW, et al. Mutations in the gene encoding KRIT1, a Krev-1/rap1a binding protein, cause cerebral cavernous malformations (CCM1). Hum Mol Genet. 1999; 8(12):2325–2333

[13] Vishteh AG, Zabramski JM, Spetzler RF. Patients with spinal cord cavernous malformations are at an increased risk for multiple neuraxis cavernous malformations. Neurosurgery. 1999; 45(1):30–32, discussion 33

[14] Baumgartner JE, Ater JL, Ha CS, et al. Pathologically proven cavernous angiomas of the brain following radiation therapy for pediatric brain tumors. Pediatr Neurosurg. 2003; 39(4):201–207

[15] Duhem R, Vinchon M, Leblond P, Soto-Ares G, Dhellemmes P. Cavernous malformations after cerebral irradiation during childhood: report of nine cases. Childs Nerv Syst. 2005; 21(10):922–925

[16] Heckl S, Aschoff A, Kunze S. Radiation-induced cavernous hemangiomas of the brain: a late effect predominantly in children. Cancer. 2002; 94(12):3285–3291

[17] Larson JJ, Ball WS, Bove KE, Crone KR, Tew JM, Jr. Formation of intracerebral cavernous malformations after radiation treatment for central nervous system neoplasia in children. J Neurosurg. 1998; 88(1):51–56

[18] Rigamonti D, Spetzler RF. The association of venous and cavernous malformations. Report of four cases and discussion of the pathophysiological, diagnostic, and therapeutic implications. Acta Neurochir (Wien). 1988; 92(1–4):100–105

[19] Clatterbuck RE, Eberhart CG, Crain BJ, Rigamonti D. Ultrastructural and immunocytochemical evidence that an incompetent blood-brain barrier is related to the pathophysiology of cavernous malformations. J Neurol Neurosurg Psychiatry. 2001; 71(2):188–192

[20] Rigamonti D, Drayer BP, Johnson PC, Hadley MN, Zabramski J, Spetzler RF. The MRI appearance of cavernous malformations (angiomas). J Neurosurg. 1987; 67(4):518–524

[21] Tomlinson FH, Houser OW, Scheithauer BW, Sundt TM, Jr, Okazaki H, Parisi JE. Angiographically occult vascular malformations: a correlative study of features on magnetic resonance imaging and histological examination. Neurosurgery. 1994; 34(5):792–799, discussion 799–800

[22] Labauge P, Brunereau L, Laberge S, Houtteville JP. Prospective follow-up of 33 asymptomatic patients with familial cerebral cavernous malformations. Neurology. 2001; 57(10):1825–1828

[23] Gomori JM, Grossman RI, Goldberg HI, Hackney DB, Zimmerman RA, Bilaniuk LT. Occult cerebral vascular malformations: high-field MR imaging. Radiology. 1986; 158(3):707–713

[24] Lemme-Plaghos L, Kucharczyk W, Brant-Zawadzki M, et al. MRI of angiographically occult vascular malformations. AJR Am J Roentgenol. 1986; 146(6):1223–1228

[25] Zabramski JM, Wascher TM, Spetzler RF, et al. The natural history of familial cavernous malformations: results of an ongoing study. J Neurosurg. 1994; 80(3):422–432

[26] de Souza JM, Domingues RC, Cruz LC, Jr, Domingues FS, Iasbeck T, Gasparetto EL. Susceptibility-weighted imaging for the evaluation of patients with familial cerebral cavernous malformations: a comparison with t2-weighted fast spin-echo and gradient-echo sequences. AJNR Am J Neuroradiol. 2008; 29(1):154–158

[27] Töpper R, Jürgens E, Reul J, Thron A. Clinical significance of intracranial developmental venous anomalies. J Neurol Neurosurg Psychiatry. 1999; 67(2):234–238

[28] Acciarri N, Galassi E, Giulioni M, et al. Cavernous malformations of the central nervous system in the pediatric age group. Pediatr Neurosurg. 2009; 45(2):81–104

[29] Mazza C, Scienza R, Beltramello A, Da Pian R. Cerebral cavernous malformations (cavernomas) in the pediatric age-group. Childs Nerv Syst. 1991; 7(3):139–146

[30] Bergeson PS, Rekate HL, Tack ED. Cerebral cavernous angiomas in the newborn. Clin Pediatr (Phila). 1992; 31(7):435–437

[31] Gross BA, Du R, Orbach DB, Scott RM, Smith ER. The natural history of cerebral cavernous malformations in children. J Neurosurg Pediatr. 2015:1–6

[32] Scott RM, Barnes P, Kupsky W, Adelman LS. Cavernous angiomas of the central nervous system in children. J Neurosurg. 1992; 76(1):38–46

[33] Mottolese C, Hermier M, Stan H, et al. Central nervous system cavernomas in the pediatric age group. Neurosurg Rev. 2001; 24(2–3):55–71, discussion 72–73

[34] Bilginer B, Narin F, Hanalioglu S, Oguz KK, Soylemezoglu F, Akalan N. Cavernous malformations of the central nervous system (CNS) in children: clinico-radiological features and management outcomes of 36 cases. Childs Nerv Syst. 2014; 30(8):1355–1366

[35] Porter RW, Detwiler PW, Spetzler RF, et al. Cavernous malformations of the brainstem: experience with 100 patients. J Neurosurg. 1999; 90(1):50–58

[36] Amato MC, Madureira JF, Oliveira RS. Intracranial cavernous malformation in children: a single-centered experience with 30 consecutive cases. Arq Neuropsiquiatr. 2013; 71(4):220–228

[37] Knerlich-Lukoschus F, Steinbok P, Dunham C, Cochrane DD. Cerebellar cavernous malformation in pediatric patients: defining clinical, neuroimaging, and therapeutic characteristics. J Neurosurg Pediatr. 2015; 16(3):256–266

[38] Ardeshiri A, Özkan N, Chen B, et al. A retrospective and consecutive analysis of the epidemiology and management of spinal cavernomas over the last 20 years in a single center. Neurosurg Rev. 2016; 39(2):269–276, discussion 276

[39] Deutsch H, Shrivistava R, Epstein F, Jallo GI. Pediatric intramedullary spinal cavernous malformations. Spine. 2001; 26(18):E427–E431

[40] Lopate G, Black JT, Grubb RL, Jr. Cavernous hemangioma of the spinal cord: report of 2 unusual cases. Neurology. 1990; 40(11):1791–1793

[41] McCormick PC, Michelsen WJ, Post KD, Carmel PW, Stein BM. Cavernous malformations of the spinal cord. Neurosurgery. 1988; 23(4):459–463

[42] Tong X, Deng X, Li H, Fu Z, Xu Y. Clinical presentation and surgical outcome of intramedullary spinal cord cavernous malformations. J Neurosurg Spine. 2012; 16(3):308–314

[43] Tu YK, Liu HM, Chen SJ, Lin SM. Intramedullary cavernous haemangiomas: clinical features, imaging diagnosis, surgical resection and outcome. J Clin Neurosci. 1999; 6(3):212–216

[44] Cohen-Gadol AA, Jacob JT, Edwards DA, Krauss WE. Coexistence of intracranial and spinal cavernous malformations: a study of prevalence and natural history. J Neurosurg. 2006; 104(3):376–381

[45] Aiba T, Tanaka R, Koike T, Kameyama S, Takeda N, Komata T. Natural history of intracranial cavernous malformations. J Neurosurg. 1995; 83(1):56–59

[46] Kondziolka D, Lunsford LD, Kestle JR. The natural history of cerebral cavernous malformations. J Neurosurg. 1995; 83(5):820–824

[47] Kupersmith MJ, Kalish H, Epstein F, et al. Natural history of brainstem cavernous malformations. Neurosurgery. 2001; 48(1):47–53, discussion 53–54

[48] Moriarity JL, Wetzel M, Clatterbuck RE, et al. The natural history of cavernous malformations: a prospective study of 68 patients. Neurosurgery. 1999; 44(6):1166–1171, discussion 1172–1173

[49] Porter PJ, Willinsky RA, Harper W, Wallace MC. Cerebral cavernous malformations: natural history and prognosis after clinical deterioration with or without hemorrhage. J Neurosurg. 1997; 87(2):190–197

[50] Robinson JR, Awad IA, Little JR. Natural history of the cavernous angioma. J Neurosurg. 1991; 75(5):709–714

[51] Al-Holou WN, O'Lynnger TM, Pandey AS, et al. Natural history and imaging prevalence of cavernous malformations in children and young adults. J Neurosurg Pediatr. 2012; 9(2):198–205

[52] Li D, Hao SY, Tang J, et al. Clinical course of untreated pediatric brainstem cavernous malformations: hemorrhage risk and functional recovery. J Neurosurg Pediatr. 2014; 13(5):471–483

[53] Barker FG, II, Amin-Hanjani S, Butler WE, et al. Temporal clustering of hemorrhages from untreated cavernous malformations of the central nervous system. Neurosurgery. 2001; 49(1):15–24, discussion 24–25

[54] Fortuna A, Ferrante L, Mastronardi L, Acqui M, d'Addetta R. Cerebral cavernous angioma in children. Childs Nerv Syst. 1989; 5(4):201–207

[55] Giulioni M, Acciarri N, Padovani R, Frank F, Galassi E, Gaist G. Surgical management of cavernous angiomas in children. Surg Neurol. 1994; 42(3):194–199

[56] Bertalanffy H, Gilsbach JM, Eggert HR, Seeger W. Microsurgery of deep-seated cavernous angiomas: report of 26 cases. Acta Neurochir (Wien). 1991; 108(3–4):91–99

[57] Steinberg GK, Chang SD, Gewirtz RJ, Lopez JR. Microsurgical resection of brainstem, thalamic, and basal ganglia angiographically occult vascular malformations. Neurosurgery. 2000; 46(2):260–270, discussion 270–271

[58] Acciarri N, Giulioni M, Padovani R, Galassi E, Gaist G. Surgical management of cerebral cavernous angiomas causing epilepsy. J Neurosurg Sci. 1995; 39(1):13–20

[59] Baumann CR, Schuknecht B, Lo Russo G, et al. Seizure outcome after resection of cavernous malformations is better when surrounding hemosiderin-stained brain also is removed. Epilepsia. 2006; 47(3):563–566

[60] Wang X, Tao Z, You C, Li Q, Liu Y. Extended resection of hemosiderin fringe is better for seizure outcome: a study in patients with cavernous malformation associated with refractory epilepsy. Neurol India. 2013; 61(3):288–292

[61] Cohen DS, Zubay GP, Goodman RR. Seizure outcome after lesionectomy for cavernous malformations. J Neurosurg. 1995; 83(2):237–242

[62] Di Rocco C, Iannelli A, Tamburrini G. Cavernomas of the central nervous system in children. A report of 22 cases. Acta Neurochir (Wien). 1996; 138(11):1267–1274, discussion 1273–1274

[63] Braga BP, Costa LB, Jr, Lemos S, Vilela MD. Cavernous malformations of the brainstem in infants. Report of two cases and review of the literature. J Neurosurg. 2006; 104(6) Suppl:429–433

[64] Di Rocco C, Iannelli A, Tamburrini G. Cavernous angiomas of the brain stem in children. Pediatr Neurosurg. 1997; 27(2):92–99

[65] Amin-Hanjani S, Ogilvy CS, Candia GJ, Lyons S, Chapman PH. Stereotactic radiosurgery for cavernous malformations: Kjellberg's experience with proton beam therapy in 98 cases at the Harvard Cyclotron. Neurosurgery. 1998; 42(6):1229–1236, discussion 1236–1238

[66] Chang SD, Levy RP, Adler JR, Jr, Martin DP, Krakovitz PR, Steinberg GK. Stereotactic radiosurgery of angiographically occult vascular malformations: 14-year experience. Neurosurgery. 1998; 43(2):213–220, discussion 220–221

[67] Kondziolka D, Lunsford LD, Flickinger JC, Kestle JR. Reduction of hemorrhage risk after stereotactic radiosurgery for cavernous malformations. J Neurosurg. 1995; 83(5):825–831

[68] Lunsford LD, Khan AA, Niranjan A, Kano H, Flickinger JC, Kondziolka D. Stereotactic radiosurgery for symptomatic solitary cerebral cavernous malformations considered high risk for resection. J Neurosurg. 2010; 113(1):23–29

Section VI

Developmental and Congenital Cranial Disorders

VI

27 Chiari Malformations

Karl F. Kothbauer

27.1 Introduction

What is today called Chiari I malformation was originally described in 1891.[1] It is a developmental anomaly of the hindbrain. Herniation of the cerebellar tonsils through the foramen magnum into the cervical spinal canal is its primary feature.

Four types of Chiari malformation are described[2]:

1. Chiari I (also known as cerebellar ectopia) is defined as the caudal displacement of the cerebellar tonsils below the level of the foramen magnum with obliteration of the cisterna.
2. Chiari II (also known as Arnold–Chiari malformation)[3] is a more severe and extensive hindbrain anomaly with caudal displacement of brainstem, cerebellar tonsils, vermis, posterior inferior cerebellar arteries (PICAs), and the fourth ventricle. It often includes a cervicomedullary kink and cranially directed cranial nerve roots. Brainstem dysfunction is a typical finding. Chiari II occurs with myelomeningocele and hydrocephalus, and frequently is associated with syringomyelia.[4]
3. Chiari III consists of herniation of the posterior fossa contents into an occipitocervical encephalomeningocele. It also includes a cervical spina bifida. Chiari III is the severest form of the Chiari complex[5] and is considered incompatible with survival.
4. Chiari IV is the rarest and mildest form. It is characterized by cerebellar hypoplasia, but no herniation.[5]

Sometimes a transitional form of Chiari I malformation with morphological signs of brainstem dysplasia but without spina bifida is referred to as Chiari 1.5.[5] This transitional form is regarded as Chiari I malformation in the present context.

Syringomyelia (also known as hydromyelia), the formation of a longitudinal cavity within the spinal cord, is present in about 50 to 70% of the patients with Chiari I malformation[6,7] and in up to 95% of patients with Chiari II.[4,8,9]

Many attempts to explain the syrinx formation have been made. Gardner and Angel postulated a delayed and incomplete embryonic closing of the central canal with an (at least potentially) open communication from the fourth ventricle into the central canal of the spinal cord. In his hydrodynamic theory, he suggested that the extension of the syrinx cavity is caused by a "water hammer" effect, i.e., a pulsatile transmission of the cerebrospinal fluid (CSF) from the fourth ventricle into the central canal.[10]

Later, Williams modified this theory to the "craniospinal pressure dissociation hypothesis,"[11] where the craniospinal pressure differences due to venous pulsations, rather than Gardner arterial pulse waves, were put forward as the primary mechanism responsible for the syrinx formation.

In 1994, Oldfield et al[12] used dynamic magnetic resonance imaging (MRI) to study the pulsatile movement of the CSF in the posterior fossa and the cervical spinal canal before and after decompressive surgery. This newer concept suggests that the obstruction at the foramen magnum caused by crowding of the tonsils results in a block of the CSF flow during systole. This causes a systolic wave in the spinal CSF that acts on the surface of the spinal cord. This results in progression of syringomyelia by repeated compression of the cord, probably by mechanical disruption of the cord tissue with every pressure wave, and by forcing fluid into the cord from the outside in. It has been suggested that the pulsatile pressure waves force CSF into the cord through the perivascular and interstitial spaces. In addition, the syrinx fluid is propelled longitudinally within the syrinx during each cardiac cycle. This together may be responsible for the origin and persistence of syringomyelia. Armonda et al[13] showed the changes in pulsatile CSF flow before and after posterior fossa decompression.

Based on these pathophysiological concepts, a full array of surgical strategies has been advocated in the treatment of Chiari I malformation and syringomyelia. The common denominator of all these strategies is posterior craniovertebral decompression. There is little controversy about this principle. However, the details of the procedure, its extent and invasiveness, and the technique of dural closure are subject to considerable debate.

27.2 Anatomy

As a group of developmental disorders, Chiari malformations are characterized by an abnormal anatomy of the structures of the craniocervical junction. Usually, this involves only the intradural structures, but it may also be associated with a degree of abnormality of the osteoarticular apparatus of the craniocervical junction.

Intradural anatomy. The normal location of the cerebellar tonsils and the presence and size of the cisterna magna are the primary anatomical structures changed in Chiari. The cerebellar tonsils are dislocated caudally into the cervical spinal canal to a varying degree. Usually, displacement of at least a few millimeters (> 3 mm) below the level of the foramen magnum is required to call the finding "Chiari." Absence or very small size of the cisterna magna appears more physiologically relevant. Descent of the tonsils below the level of the C2 vertebral arch is not infrequent.

Anatomical changes in Chiari II malformation are more extensive, with more structures to be caudally dislocated, such as the vermis and the lower brainstem. In addition, a medullary kink may be present and the caudal cranial nerves may have an upward course.

Chiari II is more often associated with bony abnormalities than Chiari I. These abnormalities include primarily an elevation of the dens with a ventral indentation of the brainstem. Occipitalization of the atlas, a bifid posterior atlas arch, and an occipital bony keel with far ventral indentation may occur.

27.3 Clinical Findings

Not infrequently in the era of MRI, Chiari I malformation is an incidental finding, discovered, for instance, in the course of evaluation after trauma. A correlation between general symptoms such as headache and the presence of Chiari must be carefully evaluated.

The variety of presenting symptoms of Chiari I malformation is shown in Box 27.1 and does include headaches. Clinical findings upon examination are equally diverse, as they include potential dysfunction of all systems located in and traversing the craniocervical junction (Box 27.2). Characteristically, if neurological dysfunction is found, three syndromes are defined in Chiari malformation.[14]

1. Foramen magnum syndrome (20%): headaches in about one-third of patients, ataxia, corticospinal and sensory deficits, cerebellar signs, and lower cranial nerve dysfunction, such as swallowing difficulties or nasal speech.

2. Central cord syndrome (60%): characteristically associated with syringomyelia. Dissociated sensory loss, lower motor neuron syndrome with muscle atrophy, and pyramidal signs.

3. Cerebellar syndrome (10%): ataxia, nystagmus, dysarthria.

Box 27.1 Symptoms of Chiari I malformation

- Pain
- Headache
- Neck pain
- Shoulder pain
- Arm pain
- Facial pain
- Diplopia
- Numbness
- Weakness
- Tinnitus
- Nasal speech
- Dizziness
- Hearing loss
- Hiccup

Box 27.2 Clinical findings of Chiari I malformation

- Hyperreflexia
- Nystagmus
- Gait disturbance
- Hand muscle atrophy
- Cape sensory loss
- Ataxia
- Oculomotor disturbance
- Lower cranial nerve dysfunction
- Babinski's sign

27.4 Diagnostic Evaluation

Imaging with MRI is the hallmark of modern diagnosis in this condition. All other imaging modalities may be required here and there under certain conditions, but not regularly. MRI shows all necessary anatomical changes which constitute the diagnosis of Chiari malformations and those that are required to make therapeutic decisions, as well

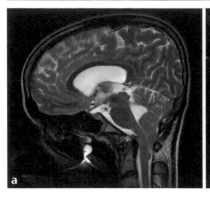
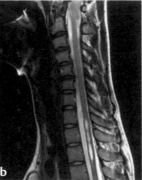

Fig. 27.1 Significant caudal displacement of the **(a)** cerebellar tonsils and **(b)** cervicothoracic syringomyelia in a 16-year-old girl with Chiari I malformation who presented with bilateral fifth nerve palsy.

as those that are needed for surgical planning. This includes particularly syringomyelia (▶ Fig. 27.1).

Computed tomography (CT) may sometimes be necessary to assess the bone situation at the craniovertebral junction. The MRI findings for Chiari malformation are defined in the anatomical description. The specific findings on imaging for Chiari II malformation are listed in Box 27.3.[2]

Box 27.3 Anatomic imaging findings in Chiari II malformation

- Bend deformity of medulla
- Tectal fusion (tectal beaking)
- Enlarged interthalamic adhesion
- Elongation of medulla
- Low attachment of tentorium
- Steep sinus rectus
- Hydrocephalus
- Syringomyelia
- Trapped fourth ventricle
- Cerebellomedullary compression
- Agenesis of corpus callosum
- Microgyria
- Platybasia

27.5 Nonsurgical Management

There is no nonsurgical treatment for this condition. The decision whether or not to perform surgery depends on the symptoms, the extent of the anatomical abnormality, and, in particular, the presence of significant structural damage such as syringomyelia.

The natural history of untreated Chiari I malformation is not well known, but in a larger series of observed cases a relatively benign evolution is suggested.[15]

27.6 Surgical Indications

The decision for or against surgery must be strictly viewed from the best interest of the patient. Symptoms such as pain that can be reasonably associated with the pathology should warrant surgery. "Reasonably associated" may not be so easily defined, but neck pain and shoulder pain (due to indentation of cervical nerve roots or compression of the spinal trigeminal nerve complex) fall in this category. Neurological dysfunction as in one of the three syndromes will constitute a surgical indication. In asymptomatic patients, the presence of structural tissue damage in the form of syringomyelia, even if (yet) asymptomatic, is considered an indication for surgery. Certainly, a previously observed patient with newly developed syrinx or symptoms would also qualify for surgery.

Chiari II malformations are much less frequently significant for craniocervical crowding, but if they are, maybe due to cyst formation or bony narrowing, decompression may be indicated as well. Since most patients with Chiari II are patients with spina bifida, and the majority of them still have shunted hydrocephalus, it is imperative to ensure proper shunt function or patent third ventriculostomy prior to posterior decompression.

27.7 Surgical Technique

Penfield and Coburn first performed a posterior fossa decompression in the late 1930s (their first patient died in the first night after surgery).[16]

In 1941, Adams et al[17] suggested to treat Chiari malformation with a decompression of the cervical spinal cord and the cerebellum. Gustafson and Oldberg already suggested that syringomyelia might respond to unblocking of the craniospinal CSF pathways,[18] even before Gardner and Angel.[10]

Surgery for Chiari malformation is closely intertwined with surgical treatment of the frequently associated syringomyelia.

The "correct" way to treat Chiari malformations is one of the most disputed issues in pediatric neurosurgery. The common ground is that a posterior fossa decompression should be made. Some suggest that this craniectomy must be of considerable size[19]; some even combine this with some form of cranioplasty.[20]

This author prefers small craniectomies, aimed at significantly enlarging the foramen magnum. Some authors advocate that the craniectomy alone may be sufficient,[21] while some argue that the dura must be opened.[22] Some try to only open the dura, but not the arachnoid.[23] Interestingly, while there appear to be a large number of centers where it is custom practice to microsurgically shrink the cerebellar tonsils upward, there are comparatively few reports about this practice.[22,24,25,26]

Closure of the dura again is disputed. In the older literature, the dura was just left open.[27] Today, mostly the dura is closed with some form of graft. Autografts from the fascia lata, pericranium, or the nuchal ligament were proposed.[20,28] Most report dural closure with an artificial dural substitute,[12,28,29] which is also the preference of this author. The use of fascia lata requires a second incision at the thigh, which is uncomfortable, and all autografts carry a significant risk of strong scar tissue formation, which may in fact obliterate the CSF spaces at the craniovertebral junction rather than keep them open.

Many of these technical questions are handled according to the experience and reflected choice of the individual surgeon rather than being based on a scientific consensus or even scientific evidence.

Since different choices of surgical technique nonetheless mostly lead to comparable and favorable surgical results and all appear to have a more or less low complication rate, it may also be argued that individual patients with individual circumstances and anatomical context may benefit from individual surgical technique choices.

Syringomyelia associated with Chiari malformation is treated only with craniovertebral decompression. Contrary to prior practice, myelotomy and placement of a syringosubarachnoid drainage are considered only in cases with persistent or progressive syrinx after primary posterior craniovertebral decompression.[30]

27.8 Complications

Complications after craniovertebral decompression are rare but do occur, and their prevention requires adherence to meticulous surgical technique and proper postoperative monitoring. The first patient reported to have undergone decompressive surgery died from respiratory depression in the first night after surgery.[16]

Postoperative respiratory problems may occur also in modern neurosurgical practice and thus require proper monitoring at an intensive care unit (ICU) overnight after surgery. Wound-healing difficulties, CSF leakage, or subcutaneous collection may occur. This must be avoided by employing meticulous surgical technique with duroplasty, watertight muscle and fascial closure using size 1 absorbable sutures, subcutaneous sutures, and a running locked skin suture with meticulous adaptation of the skin edges. Even a seemingly minor skin scab after less-than-optimal suture may result in CSF leakage and a host of subsequent problems including revision, infection, intracranial hypotension, and an unhappy family.

Neurological dysfunction after craniovertebral decompression is very infrequent. Vascular damage to the PICA has been implied and may play a role, but usually the PICA is well visible and damage to it or excessive manipulation which may result in local vasospasm must be avoided. This author has once experienced the development of significant swelling of the protruding cerebellar tonsils, which was reflected in significant changes in intraoperative motor evoked potential (MEP) monitoring. MEP loss indicated a severe unilateral damage to the corticospinal system. This was addressed by rapid decompressive resection of the cerebellar tonsils until CSF drainage and gained space by resection provided sufficient decompression. A hemiparesis was seen postoperatively, which fortunately, and in accordance with the neurophysiological profile, was only transient.[31] The routine use of intraoperative monitoring for avoidance of neurological complications is debated[32] but not generally accepted.

Surgical decompression for Chiari II malformation is less frequently indicated. If it is performed, the anatomy of the venous sinuses in the posterior fossa must be appreciated. As the posterior fossa is small and the sinus rectus steep, the torcula may be quite close to the foramen magnum, and particularly in younger children an occipital sinus may

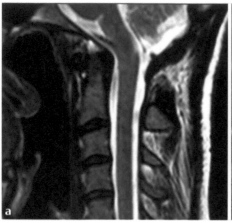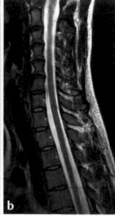

Fig. 27.2 MRI 10 years after surgery in the same patient who has fully recovered in 3 months after surgery with normalization of the **(a)** posterior fossa and no evidence for **(b)** syringomyelia.

be present, both of which pose a risk for serious hemorrhage if opened.

27.9 Postoperative Care

Patients must be monitoring in an ICU setting overnight after surgery. Postoperative pain management must be aggressive using acetaminophen, NSAID, and opioids to largely suppress immediate pain from the rather large incision, which involves—painfully—the neck muscles. Respiratory and circulatory monitoring is essential, even though in this day and age respiratory depression may indeed be a rare occurrence.

An MRI scan is recommended on postoperative day 1 to document adequate decompression, rule out hematoma, and provide an early comparison of a syrinx to postoperative syrinx size as well as a baseline for later assessment of syrinx evolution.

The patient must be mobilized out of bed on postoperative day 1, and remains hospitalized for a few days. External support with collars is unnecessary and should not be considered; rather, rapid normalization of neck movement in spite of initial pain should be encouraged. Skin sutures must be removed after 2 weeks, to ensure healing without CSF leakage. Patients should remain on light activities after discharge. A postoperative surgical visit should be scheduled after 4 to 6 weeks, following which full activities can be resumed. MRI follow-up is unnecessary if no syrinx was present. In the presence of syrinx, a first follow-up is recommended 3 to 6 months postoperative. Later MRI follow-up depends on the evolution of a syrinx.

27.10 Outcomes

Decompression of Chiari I malformation is usually effective in alleviating pain but not as much in reversing already present neurologic dysfunction.[6]

Cerebellar symptoms apparently also respond well to decompression.[2] The results from decompression in Chiari II patients appear to be less favorable, a finding attributed to the underlying developmental anomaly not treatable with mechanical decompression alone. In Chiari II patients, the underlying disability strongly defines the clinical situation and this may be less due to Chiari and more due to paraplegia. Syringomyelia must be followed and the expectation is that a syrinx will decrease in size or nearly obliterate (▶ Fig. 27.2).

27.11 Surgical Pearls

- Bony decompression aims at enlargement of the foramen magnum.
- Lateral decompression at the foramen magnum is essential.
- Removal of the posterior arch of the atlas must be as wide laterally as the foramen magnum decompression.
- Dural opening should be **Y**-shaped.
- The pia of the cerebellar tonsils is microsurgically shrunk by carefully applying bipolar coagulation, which is very effective in "pulling" the dislocated tissue upward.
- Arachnoid strands become visible and may be stretched upon shrinking of the tonsils and must

be carefully divided to avoid ripping on the pia of the brainstem or vessels that may be attached in them.

- The dura is closed with an inverted triangular piece of artificial dural graft which fits well into the **Y**-shaped opening. Dural closure should be with a running locked suture, as watertight as possible.
- The muscular and fascial layers are tightly sutured with individual size 1 resorbable sutures. The fascial layer sutures are optimally watertight when inverted and placed very close. The skin should be closed with a watertight running locked monofilic suture of size 3–0 or, in smaller children, 4–0.

27.12 Common Clinical Questions

1. Describe the primary pathology of Chiari I malformation.
2. What are the most frequent signs and symptoms of Chiari II malformation?
3. What would be a plausible indication for surgery in a patient with an incidental finding of Chiari I malformation?
4. Why is an artificial dural graft preferable to an autograft such as fascia lata or pericranium?
5. What is the treatment of syringomyelia associated with Chiari malformation?
6. What is the co-prevalence of Chiari II malformation and spina bifida?

27.13 Answers to Common Clinical Questions

1. Displacement of the cerebellar tonsils below the level of the foramen magnum and obliteration of the cisterna magna.
2. Pain (Headache, Neck- and shoulder pain), foramen syndrome, central cord syndrome, cerebellar syndrome.
3. Presence of syringomyelia.
4. Because autografts tend to shrink with healing and scar formation.
5. Craniovertebral decompression.
6. Chiari II only occurs in patients with spina bifida.

References

[1] Chiari H. Ueber Veränderungen des Kleinhirns infolge von Hydrocephalie des Grosshirns. Dtsch Med Wochenschr. 1891; 17:1172–1175

[2] Greenberg MS. Handbook of Neurosurgery. Vol. 1. 5th ed. New York, NY: Thieme; 2001

[3] Arnold J. Myelocyste, Transposition von Gewebskeimen und Sympodie. Beitr Pathol Anat. 1894; 16:1–28

[4] McLone DG, Knepper PA. The cause of Chiari II malformation: a unified theory. Pediatr Neurosci. 1989; 15(1):1–12

[5] Iskandar BJ, Oakes WJ. Chiari malformations. In: Albright AL, Pollack IF, Adelson PD, eds. Principles and Practice of Pediatric Neurosurgery. 1st ed. New York, NY: Thieme; 1999:165–187

[6] Dyste GN, Menezes AH, VanGilder JC. Symptomatic Chiari malformations. An analysis of presentation, management, and long-term outcome. J Neurosurg. 1989; 71(2):159–168

[7] Krieger MD, McComb JG, Levy ML. Toward a simpler surgical management of Chiari I malformation in a pediatric population. Pediatr Neurosurg. 1999; 30(3):113–121

[8] Cahan LD, Bentson JR. Considerations in the diagnosis and treatment of syringomyelia and the Chiari malformation. J Neurosurg. 1982; 57(1):24–31

[9] Aubin ML, Vignaud J, Jardin C, Bar D. Computed tomography in 75 clinical cases of syringomyelia. AJNR Am J Neuroradiol. 1981; 2(3):199–204

[10] Gardner WJ, Angel J. The mechanism of syringomyelia and its surgical correction. Clin Neurosurg. 1958; 6:131–140

[11] Williams B. The distending force in the production of "communicating syringomyelia". Lancet. 1969; 2(7613):189–193

[12] Oldfield EH, Muraszko K, Shawker TH, Patronas NJ. Pathophysiology of syringomyelia associated with Chiari I malformation of the cerebellar tonsils. Implications for diagnosis and treatment. J Neurosurg. 1994; 80(1): 3–15

[13] Armonda RA, Citrin CM, Foley KT, Ellenbogen RG. Quantitative cine-mode magnetic resonance imaging of Chiari I malformations: an analysis of cerebrospinal fluid dynamics. Neurosurgery. 1994; 35(2):214–223, discussion 223–224

[14] Paul KS, Lye RH, Strang FA, Dutton J. Arnold-Chiari malformation. Review of 71 cases. J Neurosurg. 1983; 58(2): 183–187

[15] Strahle J, Muraszko KM, Kapurch J, Bapuraj JR, Garton HJ, Maher CO. Natural history of Chiari malformation Type I following decision for conservative treatment. J Neurosurg Pediatr. 2011; 8(2):214–221

[16] Penfield W, Coburn DF. Arnold-Chiari malformation and its operative treatment. Arch Neurol Psychiatry. 1939; 42(5): 872–876

[17] Adams RD, Schatzki R, Scoville WB. The Arnold Chiari malformation. N Engl J Med. 1941; 225(4):125–131

[18] Gustafson WA, Oldberg E. Neurologic significance of platybasia. Arch Neurol Psychiatry. 1939; 42(5):872–876

[19] Milhorat TH, Chou MW, Trinidad EM, et al. Chiari I malformation redefined: clinical and radiographic findings for 364 symptomatic patients. Neurosurgery. 1999; 44(5): 1005–1017

[20] Sakamoto H, Nishikawa M, Hakuba A, et al. Expansive suboccipital cranioplasty for the treatment of syringomyelia

associated with Chiari malformation. Acta Neurochir (Wien). 1999; 141(9):949–960, discussion 960–961

[21] Yundt KD, Park TS, Tantuwaya VS, Kaufman BA. Posterior fossa decompression without duraplasty in infants and young children for treatment of Chiari malformation and achondroplasia. Pediatr Neurosurg. 1996; 25(5):221–226

[22] Batzdorf U. Chiari malformation and syringomyelia. In: Appuzzo MLJ, ed. Brain Surgery. Vol. 2. 1st ed. New York, NY: Churchill Livingstone; 1993:1985–2201

[23] Hida K, Iwasaki Y, Koyanagi I, Sawamura Y, Abe H. Surgical indication and results of foramen magnum decompression versus syringosubarachnoid shunting for syringomyelia associated with Chiari I malformation. Neurosurgery. 1995; 37(4):673–678, discussion 678–679

[24] Fischer EG. Posterior fossa decompression for Chiari I deformity, including resection of the cerebellar tonsils. Childs Nerv Syst. 1995; 11(11):625–629

[25] Won DJ, Nambiar U, Muszynski CA, Epstein FJ. Coagulation of herniated cerebellar tonsils for cerebrospinal fluid pathway restoration. Pediatr Neurosurg. 1997; 27(5):272–275

[26] Depreitere B, Van Calenbergh F, van Loon J, Goffin J, Plets C. Posterior fossa decompression in syringomyelia associated

with a Chiari malformation: a retrospective analysis of 22 patients. Clin Neurol Neurosurg. 2000; 102(2):91–96

[27] Williams B. A blast against grafts–on the closing and grafting of the posterior fossa dura. Br J Neurosurg. 1994; 8(3):275–278

[28] Feldstein NA, Choudhri TF. Management of Chiari I malformations with holocord syringohydromyelia. Pediatr Neurosurg. 1999; 31(3):143–149

[29] Weinberg JS, Freed DL, Sadock J, Handler M, Wisoff JH, Epstein FJ. Headache and Chiari I malformation in the pediatric population. Pediatr Neurosurg. 1998; 29(1):14–18

[30] Alzate JC, Kothbauer KF, Jallo GI, Epstein FJ. Treatment of Chiari I malformation in patients with and without syringomyelia: a consecutive series of 66 cases. Neurosurg Focus. 2001; 11(1):E3

[31] Kothbauer KF, Deletis V, Epstein FJ. Motor-evoked potential monitoring for intramedullary spinal cord tumor surgery: correlation of clinical and neurophysiological data in a series of 100 consecutive procedures. Neurosurg Focus. 1998; 4(5):e1

[32] Sala F, Squintani G, Tramontano V, Coppola A, Gerosa M. Intraoperative neurophysiological monitoring during surgery for Chiari malformations. Neurol Sci. 2011; 32 Suppl 3:S317–S319

28 Encephaloceles

Elizabeth J. Le, Rafael U. Cardenas, Mari L. Groves

28.1 Introduction

An *encephalocele* is a protrusion of cerebral tissue, leptomeninges, and cerebrospinal fluid (CSF) through calvarial and dural defects beyond the confines of the skull, while a *cephalocele* refers to the herniation of any combination of these components.[1] Encephaloceles may be rare neurodevelopmental lesions present at birth (primary) or acquired due to traumatic, postsurgical, inflammatory, or neoplastic causes (secondary).[2]

28.2 Classification

While several classification schemes have been proposed in the past, current encephalocele classification is based on the anatomic location of the skull defect (▶ Fig. 28.1). These lesions are initially divided into *anterior* and *posterior* groups. Within the anterior division, encephaloceles may be *sincipital* (extending between the frontal or facial bones) or *basal* (protruding inferiorly through the skull base). Posterior encephaloceles may be *occipital*, *occipitocervical*, *temporal*, or *parietal*.[3] Further subclassification may be performed through assessment of detailed computed tomography (CT) or magnetic resonance imaging (MRI) for the precise location of the lesion and its anatomic contents.

28.3 Pathogenesis

Although the pathogenesis underlying the development of encephaloceles is not fully understood, these lesions are thought to develop from an error in neural development occurring after primary and secondary neurulation with incomplete ectodermal dysjunction. During primary neurulation, which occurs between the third and fourth gestational weeks, the future brain and majority of the spinal cord form through a progression of embryonic folding and midline fusion. Abnormalities arising during the initial closure of the neural tube, at the rostral (cranial) neuropore, may result in disorders such as anencephaly, in which the involved neural tissue is exposed and disorganized. After primary neurulation, differentiation of the ectoderm (future epidermis) and neuroepithelium (future brain and spinal cord) takes place. Because encephaloceles typically contain well-developed neural and mesenchymal tissues encompassed by normal skin, their development must ensue after primary neurulation.[4] The characteristic protrusion of neural tissue is thought to arise during mesodermal differentiation. Mesoderm, which forms the meninges and skull, normally migrates between the ectoderm and neuroepithelial layers. However, scarring and subsequent adhesion of these ectodermal layers may prevent mesodermal intercalation. During the

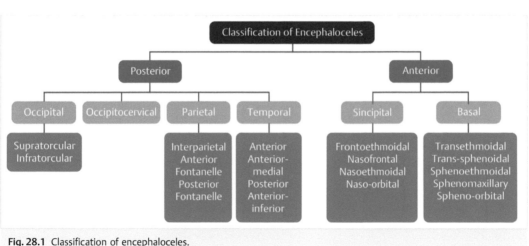

Fig. 28.1 Classification of encephaloceles.

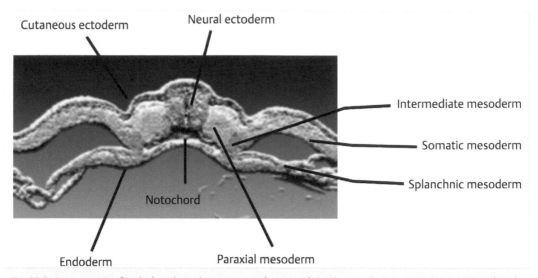

Fig. 28.2 Cross section of a chick embryo demonstrating features of the three embryonic germ layers. (Reproduced with permission from Albright AL, Pollack IF, Adelson PD. Principles and Practice of Pediatric Neurosurgery. 3rd ed. New York, NY: Thieme; 2015, Fig. 2.3.B.)

rapid growth of the telencephalon, even a small region of mesenchymal insufficiency or weakness may allow for herniation of cerebral tissue extracranially[5] (▶ Fig. 28.2).

Both environmental and genetic factors may promote the development of primary encephaloceles. For instance, the development of the posterior variety has been associated with low maternal fibrate levels, vitamin A usage, and exposure to sodium arsenate, while the risk of developing anterior encephaloceles has been correlated with exposure to fungal molds and pesticides.[6,7] Other external causes of encephaloceles, such as warfarin exposure and amniotic band syndrome, may present with other associated findings.

28.3.1 Warfarin Syndrome

Low birth weight, mental retardation, hydrocephaly, seizures, nasal hypoplasia, bone stippling, limb shortening, and optic atrophy.

28.3.2 Amniotic Band Syndrome

Tissue bands, ring constrictions and amputations of digits or limbs, distal syndactyly, microcephaly, irregular or asymmetric encephaloceles, microphthalmia, bizarre orofacial clefts.

Though the vast majority of congenital encephaloceles are sporadic, there are rare cases of lesions with genetic etiologies. While the molecular pathogenesis underlying encephaloceles development remains largely unknown, encephaloceles may be found as a component of certain rare autosomal recessive syndromes (▶ Table 28.1).[8,9,10,11,12,13]

28.4 Epidemiology

The overall incidence of encephalocele is unknown as the majority of congenital encephaloceles lead to spontaneous abortion. Furthermore, epidemiologic data collection is difficult in developing nations, where a significant number of these lesions are found. Similarly, the true incidence of secondary encephaloceles is also unknown. For primary encephaloceles, the frequency varies according to type and geographic location. The overall incidence is reported as 0.8 to 3.0 per 10,000 live births, which accounts for approximately 10 to 20% of all cases of craniospinal dysraphism. Occipital encephaloceles account for 85% of all encephaloceles and occur at a rate of 0.8 to 4.0 per 10,000 live births in North America, Europe, and northern Asia, while sincipital encephaloceles are significantly less frequent in these geographic locations. Conversely, sincipital encephaloceles are the most common type in Southeast Asia, areas of Russia, and central Africa, where they may be found in 1 in 5,000 live births, while occipital encephaloceles occur at a lower rate. In most series

Table 28.1 Congenital syndromes associated with encephaloceles

Syndrome	Description	Features
Walker–Warburg syndrome	The most severe congenital muscular dystrophy, which affects development of muscles, brain, and eyes Caused by mutations of one of several genes that produce proteins that glycosylate α-dystroglycan	Hypotonia, muscle weakness/atrophy, lissencephaly, hydrocephalus, cerebellar and brainstem abnormalities, microphthalmia, buphthalmos, corneal opacities, cataracts, optic nerve abnormalities, retinal dysplasia, *occipital encephaloceles*
Meckel's syndrome	Characterized by polycystic kidneys, encephaloceles, and polydactyly, as well as a variety of neural tube, facial, cardiac, bone, and genitourinary system abnormalities Caused by mutations in at least one of eight genes that produce proteins involved in cilia structure and function	Polycystic kidneys, polydactyly, *occipital encephaloceles*, hepatic fibrosis, holoprosencephaly, microphthalmia, retinal dysplasia, orofacial clefts, ambiguous external genitalia, other neural tube defects, cardiac anomalies
Knobloch's syndrome	Characterized by severe vision problems and a skull defect Caused by mutations in the *COL18A1* gene that produces proteins that form collagen XVIII	High myopia, vitreoretinal degeneration, retinal detachment, macular degeneration, normal intelligence, *occipital encephaloceles*
Roberts' syndrome	Characterized by limb and facial abnormalities as well as intellectual impairment Caused by mutations in the *ESCO2* gene, which makes a protein involved in chromatid adhesion during cell division	Hypomelia, phocomelia, abnormal/missing digits, joint contractures, orofacial clefts, micrognathia, ear abnormalities, hypertelorism, down-slanting palpebral fissures, beaked nose, microcephaly, *frontal encephaloceles*, heart, kidney, genital abnormalities
Von Voss–Cherstvoy syndrome	May represent a group of syndromes with radial and hematologic abnormalities Unknown pathogenesis	Phocomelia of upper limbs, variable brain abnormalities, urogenital anomalies, thrombocytopenia, *occipital encephaloceles*
Frontonasal dysplasia	Abnormal development of head and face prenatally Mutations in the *ALX1* or *ALX3* genes (autosomal dominant inheritance with *ALX4* mutation) which make homeobox proteins	Ocular hypertelorism, broad nose, no nasal tip, orofacial clefts, *frontal encephaloceles*, widow's peak hairline, corpus callosal abnormalities, intellectual disability

of congenital encephaloceles, the basal variety is very rare in Western countries and represents only 5% of all cases.[14,15,16]

28.5 Clinical Findings and Diagnosis

Encephaloceles may be diagnosed during the prenatal period through routine fetal ultrasound or MRI, which may also provide detailed characterization regarding the location and type of lesion. Amniocentesis may reveal normal to elevated α-fetoprotein and acetylcholinesterase levels depending on epithelialization of the encephalocele.

This information may aid in prenatal counseling regarding prognosis, as well as planning of delivery, postnatal surgery, and management. A vaginal delivery may be possible with relatively small lesions, but larger encephaloceles may necessitate a C-section.[17,18,19]

Although encephaloceles are usually obvious at birth, subtle herniations may require a high level of suspicion for detection, particularly in the setting of other congenital abnormalities. MRI is utilized to identify such occult lesions. During the postnatal period, MRI is also used to classify encephaloceles, demonstrate the extent of neural herniation, predict the amount of functional cerebral tissue within the sac, evaluate for the presence and degree of hydrocephalus, and determine the presence of other abnormalities of the craniocervical axis. Magnetic resonance angiography/venography (MRA/MRV) may be performed to assess for the presence of neurovascular structures within the herniation sac and characterize the relationship of the encephaloceles to the surrounding vasculature. Further information may be obtained from volumetric (three-dimensional) CT imaging, which can aid in craniofacial reconstruction planning.[20,21]

28.6 Surgical Management

While encephaloceles vary widely in location and outcomes, the basic principles of management are constant:
- Removal of the herniation sac.
- Preservation of functional neurovascular elements.
- Prevention of CSF leakage through careful closure of meninges and nondysplastic skin.
- Correction of cosmetic deformity.

Ongoing advances in neurosurgical technique, cranial imaging, surgical equipment, and minimally invasive approaches have made encephalocele repair safer and more accessible.[2,22,23]

28.7 Posterior Encephaloceles

28.7.1 Clinical Findings

Posterior encephaloceles include lesions arising in the occipital, occipitocervical, parietal, and temporal regions. Herniation of cerebral tissue in each location results in a variety of clinical findings.

Occipital Encephaloceles

Occipital encephaloceles typically occur in the midline within the area between the lambda and foramen magnum and may be supratorcular or infratorcular, relative to their relationship with the confluence of the sinuses. These lesions are nearly always fully covered with skin and vary in appearance, size, and content, ranging from small outpouchings containing only CSF and nonfunctional gliotic tissue to large herniations sacs that may include portions of functional cortex, brainstem, and cerebellum involving the entire occiput. Furthermore, the remaining intracranial contents tend to move posterocaudally, resulting in the frontal lobes being partially displaced into the middle fossa and the posterior temporal lobes shifted into the posterior fossa. Herniation of cerebral contents posteriorly also results in displacement of the torcula, transverse sinuses, and tentorium as well as brainstem distortion and kinking (▶ Fig. 28.3).

Clinical presentation varies depending on the size and contents of the encephalocele. Normal respirations and neurologic function may be observed in patients with only a small amount of cerebral herniation, while cranial nerve deficits, poor sucking and feeding, spasticity, blindness, and developmental delay may be associated with larger masses.

In 15 to 20% of patients with occipital encephaloceles, other central nervous system anomalies or neural tube defects may be found, such as cortical

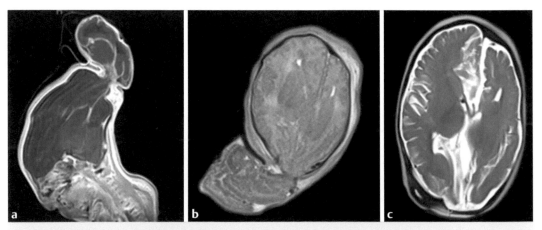

Fig. 28.3 (a) T1 contrast-enhanced sagittal MRI demonstrates large occipital encephalocele with prominent vessels within the defect. (b) T2 FLAIR (fluid-attenuated inversion recovery) axial MRI shows the extent of brain tissue contained within the herniated sac. (c) T2 HASTE (half-Fourier acquisition single-shot turbo spin echo) axial MRI shows adequate resection of the defect and reconstruction.

dysplasia, thalamic fusion, callosal agenesis or dysplasia, dysgenesis of the cecum and vermis, posterior fossa cysts, an absent, rudimentary or inverted cerebellum (ventral displacement of the cerebellar hemispheres around the anterolateral aspect of the brainstem), a small posterior fossa, and hydromyelia. In addition, hydrocephalus is present in 16 to 65% of cases. Hydrocephalus is important to identify as it significantly affects prognosis and outcome for these patients (▶ Fig. 28.4). Occipital encephaloceles are also associated with cranial abnormalities such as microcephaly, microphthalmia, facial clefts, skull base deformity, and sloping forehead due to caudal displacement of the frontal, temporal, and occipital lobes. Other systemic anomalies in the cardiac, renal, limb, and genital areas also frequently accompany occipital encephaloceles and indicate a global dysfunction of development.

Occipitocervical Encephaloceles

Occipitocervical encephaloceles include both a cranial and cervical spinal defect. Again, clinical presentation varies depending on the size and contents of the encephalocele. However, hydrocephalus is often a significant component of the clinical presentation, with focal neurologic findings being a less prominent feature. Associated congenital anomalies may be found in 50% of children, similar to those found with occipital encephaloceles.[24]

Parietal Encephaloceles

Parietal encephaloceles extend through defects between the lambda and bregma. These lesions also vary in configuration, from large lesions to small subscalp lesions consisting only of dura, fibrous tissue, and dysplastic brain tissue (atretic parietal cephaloceles), which are thought to be an involuted true encephaloceles.[25] These lesions are often accompanied by a variety of abnormalities including Chiari II malformations, diencephalic cysts, vermis agenesis, midline porencephaly, agenesis of the corpus callosum, holoprosencephaly, communication with the lateral ventricles, and Dandy–Walker cysts. In comparison to patients with occipital lesions, parietal encephaloceles are associated with a highly unfavorable prognosis. The poor functional outcomes are mainly due to the associated cerebral malformations, which are often more frequent and severe than those found with the more common types of encephaloceles.

Temporal Encephaloceles

Temporal encephaloceles arise at the pterion or asterion and are often apparent during early infancy, though some lesions may be an occult cause of temporal lobe seizures.[26] The clinical presentation may vary based on the particular location of the herniation.
- *Anterior temporal* defects occur within the sphenoid wing, resulting in herniation of brain tissue into the posterior orbital area, causing unilateral pulsating exophthalmos.
- *Anterior medial* defects occur in the anterior wall of middle fossa and sphenoid sinus, often found incidentally or due to CSF rhinorrhea (▶ Fig. 28.5).
- *Posterior temporal* defects project through the tegmen tympani and extend into the tympanic antrum or epitympanic recess. These lesions

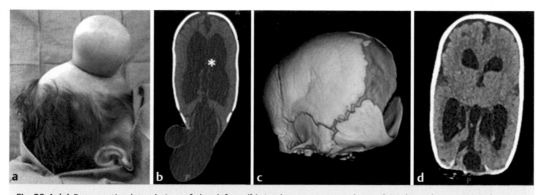

Fig. 28.4 (a) Preoperative lateral view of the defect. **(b)** Axial non-contrast-enhanced CT shows large occipital meningoencephalocele. Note the presence of significant ventricular dilatation (star). **(c)** 3D CT reconstruction demonstrates large posterior calvarial bone defect. **(d)** Axial non-contrast-enhanced CT shows adequate reconstruction of the defect with decrease in ventricular size after shunt insertion (shunt catheter not shown).

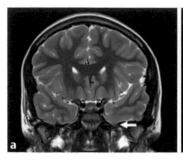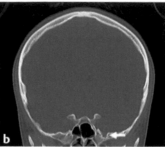

Fig. 28.5 (a) Preoperative T2 coronal MRI demonstrating a focal bony defect in the greater wing of the sphenoid with protrusion of temporal cortex and CSF. **(b)** Bony defect is again demonstrated in a coronal non-contrast-enhanced CT.

present with rhinorrhea, otorrhea, or CSF within the middle ear, resulting in decreased hearing or meningitis.

- *Anterior-inferior temporal* defects herniate through the anterior floor of the infratemporal fossa and most commonly present with simple or complex partial seizures.

28.7.2 Surgical Management

For any encephalocele, the timing of surgery should be based on the integrity of the skin overlying the lesion, presence of other systemic anomalies, and overall prognosis. When the skin overlying the lesion is intact, surgery may be performed electively. In the meantime, a thorough evaluation by a pediatrician and geneticist should be performed as well as complete examination of the cranial vault and cervical spine with MRI and possibly volumetric CT in order to aid in surgical planning.

The outcomes of encephalocele repair are particularly reliant upon the proficiency of the surgical team with treatment of such lesions as well as pediatric patients in general. Given the rarity of these anomalies, particularly in North America, neurosurgeons or plastic surgeons may encounter only a few cases during their career. Most would encourage such patients to be referred to craniofacial centers with expertise in treating encephaloceles. Similarly, experienced pediatric neuroanesthesiologists who can meticulously maintain normothermia and adequate blood volume in these patients are integral members of the surgical team in order to limit the risk of morbidity and mortality.

For occipital and occipitocervical lesions, the patient is positioned prone on a padded horseshoe headrest overlying two well-padded chest rolls with thorough cushioning of the face and pressure

points of the body, including the forehead, maxillary eminences, chest, iliac crests, and knees. Extreme care should be taken to prevent pressure on the eyes. The neck may be flexed as needed for adequate exposure, particularly in cases of occipitocervical lesions. The encephalocele sac should be secured to prevent inadvertent movement that may cause torsion of the contents. The occipital and upper cervical regions are then sterilely prepared and draped. A horizontal or vertical (for cervical or low-lying occipital encephaloceles) elliptical skin incision extending circumferentially around the lesion is made. Utilizing monopolar cautery at a low setting, a dissection plane is created between the skin and abnormal epithelium to the pericranium. Violation of the galea should be avoided in order to prevent significant blood loss from the highly vascular scalp. This dissection should extend from normal skin and skull to the skull defect and neck of the herniation sac. With cervical lesions, the normal cervical spine levels caudal to the defect should be exposed with a limited laminectomy. Subsequently, the plane between the dura and the bone defect should be carefully delineated. At this time, decompression of the sac may be accomplished by CSF drainage and the contents of the herniation sac may be explored. Both gliotic tissue and abnormal neural elements should be amputated, though any normal neurovascular structures should be meticulously preserved. A specimen may be sent for culture. If possible, the dura may be closed primarily, or with a dural graft (pericranium or collagen-based dural substitutes) in order to achieve a watertight closure. Frequently, the skull defect is small enough that no graft is necessary. In some larger defects, closure may be performed in a delayed fashion once calvarial development is sufficient to perform a split-thickness graft. If the defect is large and early repair is necessary, an autologous graft may be harvested from a rib or normal calvarial region. Other materials, such as methyl methacrylate, hydroxyapatite bone cement, and demineralized bone matrix may also be utilized.[27,28,29] In patients with large amounts of herniated functional neural tissue and vascular structures, "expansion cranioplasties" have been described to aid in preservation of cerebral material. In young infants capable of regenerating new calvarial bone at the donor site, outward-expanding barrel stave osteotomies are performed and the skin opening is extended to adjacent parietal regions with subsequent harvesting of full-thickness craniotomy fitting the shape of the skull defect. The donor site contains osteogenic dura that will ossify and create new bone within 2 to 6 months.[30] In addition, a variety of strategies have been described to expand the intracranial cavity in order to accommodate the herniated neural elements. One method involves the use of tantalum mesh to expand the cranium and incorporate the herniated brain tissue into the cranial cavity. Daily digital compression of the tantalum mesh is then used to slowly invaginate the residual encephalocele into the compliant cranial cavity, obliterating it over a course of 3 to 4 months.[31] A similar approach is the ventricular volume reduction technique, which involves first closing the encephalocele with a dural patch graft, which then allows the intraventricular pulse pressure to produce a hydrocephalic state. The herniated neural elements are then transposed into the enlarged intracranial cavity during ventriculoperitoneal shunting.[32] After repair of the calvarial defect or closure of dura, if cranioplasty is deferred, redundant skin is resected and the skin edges are approximated in order to achieve a tension-free, cosmetic closure.

Parietal encephaloceles may be repaired similarly to those of the occipital region. For temporal encephaloceles, the location and size of the defect dictates the approach. For encephaloceles of the middle fossa, both the transmastoid approach and middle cranial fossa approach, as well as a combination of both, have been used for repair. Larger lesions may be approached more effectively through the middle fossa, while those impinging on the ossicular chain may be better suited from a combined procedure.[33] Anterior temporal lesions may be repaired through a standard pterional craniotomy, while posterior encephaloceles may be addressed with a subtemporal craniotomy.[3] The same principles regarding surgical management of the herniation sac and closure apply regardless of the approach.

Postoperatively, it is of utmost importance to monitor for hydrocephalus in order to avoid CSF leakage, which tends to occur more frequently with posterior encephaloceles. The wound should undergo frequent examination for evidence of leakage of CSF or the development of pseudomeningocele. Head circumference should be measured daily, while ventricular size should be monitored with serial ultrasounds. A ventriculoperitoneal shunt should be inserted if hydrocephalus becomes clinically significant in order to prevent CSF leakage and wound compromise.

28.7.3 Outcome

For all children with encephaloceles, approximately 40% can be expected to have a normal neurologic and functional outcome, while 60% can be expected to be significantly mentally and physically impaired. Historically, children with posterior encephaloceles were thought to have worse functional outcomes than those with anterior lesions, with less than half of patients able to live independently and function in society. Over time, independent factors associated with neurologic status have been determined, including the presence of hydrocephalus, other brain abnormalities, seizure disorders, and functional brain tissue within the herniation sac.[34] In fact, recent series of children with treated encephaloceles demonstrated that the location of the lesion was not a significant predictor of outcome, while hydrocephalus and associated intracranial anomalies were predictive of developmental delay.[35] Thus, children with occipital encephaloceles may seem to exhibit worse physical, emotional, cognitive, and overall health outcomes due to the fact that hydrocephalus and seizure disorders occur more frequently in children with occipital encephaloceles compared to those with anterior encephaloceles. The treatment of hydrocephalus and seizure disorders can improve the long-term outcome of these patients.[36]

28.8 Anterior Encephaloceles

Anterior encephaloceles may be either sincipital or basal lesions.

28.8.1 Sincipital Encephaloceles

Sincipital encephaloceles are located within the region of the foramen cecum, anterior to the cribriform plate, and often present as a forehead or nasal/

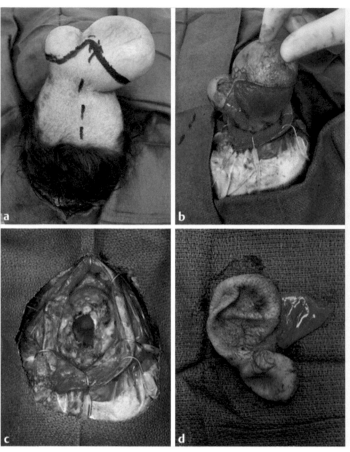

Fig. 28.6 (a) Preoperative image demonstrating a frontoethmoidal (sincipital) encephalocele. (b) Intra-operative photo demonstrating repair of the dural defect using a dural substitute graft following excision of the herniated glial tissue. (c) Sagittal T2-weighted MRI and (d) Axial T2-weighted MRI demonstrating the frontoethmoidal encephalocele.

nasional mass (▶ Fig. 28.6). Further subclassification occurs according to the location of the bone defect as well the course of the encephalocele sac.

- *Frontoethmoidal (interfrontal)* encephaloceles are relatively uncommon and produce a midline forehead mass between the nasion and bregma. They may be found in conjunction with large lipomas of the subcutaneous tissues of the forehead and corpus callosum.
- *Nasofrontal* encephaloceles extend through a midline defect in the junction between the frontal nasal bones. When small, they appear as a small protuberance at the nasion, while displacement of the nasal bones inferiorly and the medial walls laterally occurs when they are large. Furthermore, obstruction may result with extension to the nasal passages.
- *Nasoethmoidal* encephaloceles occur at the level of the foramen cecum with extension of the herniation sac anteroinferiorly as it passes between the nasal bones and nasal cartilage.

- *Naso-orbital* encephaloceles extend through the frontal ethmoidal junction inferolaterally and into the nasion and orbit at the level of the middle third of the frontal process of the maxilla. As a result, globe displacement, telecanthus, and nasolacrimal duct dysfunction causing epiphora and dacryocystitis may occur. Severity of ocular deformity may range from decreased global motility to anophthalmia.

Depending on the subtype, sincipital encephaloceles may present at birth as a visible mass causing marked craniofacial abnormality or they may not be detected until childhood or adulthood. While nasoethmoidal lesions may be occult, all other sincipital encephaloceles present at birth as a facial swelling that enlarges with crying or Valsalva's maneuver. Furthermore, sincipital encephaloceles are frequently accompanied by widening of the nasion due to displacement of the medial orbital walls (telecanthus), increased interpupillary distance (hypertelorism), cleft lip and palate, craniosynostosis, orbital dystopia, unilateral microphthalmos or anophthalmos, and epiphora.

Sincipital encephaloceles should be differentiated from other growths that may also originate in the naso-orbital or nasofrontal region, such as dermoid cysts or teratomas with or without a dermal sinus tract. Encephaloceles tend to be eccentric, pulsatile, and enlarge with crying, while other masses typically occur in the midline, lack pulsation, and are unaffected by crying. Similarly, nasoethmoidal encephaloceles, often detected in late childhood or adulthood, may need to be distinguished from nasal polyps. Encephaloceles occur more frequently in children and tend to be located in the midline, medial to the middle concha and attached firmly to the medial surface of the septum. They may cause nasal bridge widening and display a positive Furstenberg's sign, pulsation, and enlargement with jugular venous compression. Nasal polyps, however, are rare in the pediatric patients and tend to present as pedunculated masses arising from the turbinates rather than the midline. They are not associated with nasal bridge widening and have a negative Furstenberg's sign.[3,37,38]

28.8.2 Basal Encephaloceles

Basal encephaloceles present as mucosal-covered masses protruding through the posterior aspect of the anterior cranial fossa floor in the region of the cribriform plate and planum sphenoidale. These lesions may extend into the ethmoid sinus and nasal cavity or through the sphenoethmoid junction or sphenoid sinus and into the epipharynx. Because they are in close proximity to the suprasellar cisterns, they may contain important neural structures such as the hypothalamus, pituitary gland and stalk, optic chiasm, and vessels of the anterior circle of Willis. Additionally, these lesions may be occult and only detected during workup for other neurologic deficits. Further subclassification occurs based on the location of the herniated encephalocele sac.

- *Transethmoidal* encephaloceles occur through a defect within the cribriform plate that extends through the ethmoid sinuses into the anterior aspect of the nasal cavity.
- *Transsphenoidal* encephaloceles extend into the epipharynx or sphenoid sinus.
- *Sphenoethmoidal* encephaloceles occur in the posterior aspect of the junction between the cribriform plate and sphenoid bone, extending into the posterior nasal cavity.

- *Sphenomaxillary* encephaloceles extend into the maxillary sinus.
- *Spheno-orbital* encephaloceles herniate into the orbit via the superior orbital fissure and present with proptosis and exophthalmos. Other symptoms may include progressive visual loss, microphthalmos, coloboma, hydrophthalmos, anophthalmos, and microcornea. Other masses, such as teratomas, may also occur in this area, but encephaloceles can be distinguished by the presence of nasal obstruction, CSF rhinorrhea, and repeated bouts of meningitis.

While posterior encephaloceles are often associated with multiple systemic anomalies, the associated abnormalities of anterior encephaloceles tend to be limited to the cranial region.[2,39]

28.8.3 Surgical Management

Similar to their posterior counterparts, anterior encephaloceles are often covered by skin and, in the absence of CSF leakage or airway obstruction, these lesions may be treated electively. Again, a thorough evaluation by a pediatrician and geneticist should be performed as well as complete examination of the cranial vault with MRI and volumetric CT in order to aid in surgical planning.

Both the neurologic and cosmetic outcomes of anterior encephalocele repair are particularly reliant upon the proficiency of the surgical team with treatment of such lesions as well as pediatric patients in general. Treatment of anterior encephaloceles entails consideration of significant aesthetic and naso-orbital factors, such as correction of telecanthus, maintenance of the horizontal ocular axis, correction of hypertelorism, preservation of patent nasolacrimal ducts, and reconstruction of nasal abnormalities, and many would advocate that such patients be referred to craniofacial centers with expertise in treating complex craniofacial abnormalities. Surgery often occurs through a collaboration of services. While the neurosurgical team proceeds with encephalocele resection and dural closure, the plastic surgery team takes charge of cranial and craniofacial defect repair, ocular and nasal reconstruction, and dermal closure.

Anterior encephalocele repair should be performed during early infancy in order to prevent progressive craniofacial deformity due to an enlarging, pulsatile herniation sac. Surgery may be performed in a single operation or staged fashion. Single operations tend to be the procedure of choice. Similar to correction of single-suture syn-ostosis in early infancy, early single operations to repair anterior encephaloceles rely upon subsequent neurological and craniofacial development to form the cranium for optimal aesthetic results. Staged procedures occurring in later infancy and childhood provide the benefit of avoiding significant blood loss in an infant, interference with anterior facial development, and telecanthus recurrence after early reconstruction.

Both intracranial and extracranial approaches have been described for anterior encephalocele treatment. Intracranial approaches had been favored as safer due to the ability to expose dural defects and their contents as well as achieve a watertight closure free of contamination within the nasal cavity. The craniotomy utilized for an intracranial approach can range from a large bifrontal craniotomy to a small nasional craniotomy, with the less invasive procedures being favored in appropriate cases. However, as surgical instruments and techniques improve, minimally invasive endoscopic approaches continue to increase in feasibility, safety, and popularity. As with posterior encephaloceles, the main goals of surgery are correction of the deformity, prevention of CSF leakage, and preservation of functional neurovascular elements.

28.8.4 Sincipital and Basal Encephaloceles—Intracranial Approach

Prior to positioning, a lumbar drain may be placed if a complex dural repair is anticipated, in the setting of a large or relatively posterior defect, to aid in brain relaxation, and to minimize retraction on the developing brain. The patient is then positioned supine with the head on a padded horseshoe headrest. Thorough cushioning of the pressure points of the body should be performed. The encephalocele sac should be secured to prevent inadvertent movement that may cause torsion of the contents. The surgical field should then be sterilely prepared and draped. Next, a bicoronal incision is performed with meticulous hemostasis with preservation of a large, vascularized pericranial flap, which is reflected anteriorly. A bifrontal craniotomy may then be performed just superior to the floor of the anterior cranial fossa. For lesions located within the ethmoid or planum sphenoidale, such access will be sufficient, though extension laterally through a pterional craniotomy or temporally through a subtemporal craniotomy

may be required for lesions protruding into the orbit or infratemporal fossa. Alternatively, a smaller nasional craniotomy may be performed below the bregma when appropriate for some sincipital encephaloceles by removing a small rectangular piece of bone extending from eyebrow level to the tip of the nasal bone. The dura and base of the encephalocele are subsequently mobilized with inspection of its contents. If the contents do not require preservation, ligation of gliotic and nonfunctional tissue may be performed with care taken to resect the herniated mass flush with the floor of the anterior cranial fossa. With the nasional craniotomy, transection of nonfunctional tissue is performed parallel to the cribriform plate with subsequent removal of herniated matter from the orbits, maxillary, and nasal cavities. For basal encephaloceles, volume reduction of the sac may be more difficult as vital structures, such as the hypothalamus, anterior cerebral arteries, optic nerves, and optic chiasm, have a propensity to herniate in this location. Every attempt should be made to relocate vital structures into the cranial cavity. When possible, the dura is repaired primarily. The vascularized pericranial flap or collagen-based dural substitutes may be used to achieve a watertight closure when necessary. If needed, the vascularized pericranial flap may also be used to obliterate dead space and separate empty cavities from the intracranial cavity. The skull base, nasal, facial, and orbital deformities may be reconstructed using autologous bone graft from the infant's calvaria or a split-thickness graft in an older child.[3,40]

Following treatment of the encephalocele, facial anomalies should be addressed. The nasolacrimal ducts should be evaluated and preserved. If they appear obstructed, cannulation or dacryocystorhinostomy should be considered in order to prevent the development of dacryocystitis. Orbital appearance may be corrected through medial canthopexy to align the horizontal ocular axis and orbital translocation to reduce hypertelorism. Contouring of the frontal and nasal bones may be performed in order to create a normal nasofrontal angle. Following craniofacial repair, the skin edges of the bicoronal incision are approximated in order to achieve a tension-free, cosmetic closure.[2,3]

28.8.5 Endoscopic Repair—Extracranial Approach

Historically, intracranial approaches have been the preferred method for treating anterior encephaloceles, particularly those of the basal variety due to a tendency toward incomplete resection and postoperative CSF leaks with endoscopic approaches. Though traditional open craniotomy approaches allow for improved visualization and require less technical expertise, disadvantages include possible cosmetic deformity, disruption of bony growth centers in children, and increased morbidity. As surgical techniques and instruments have evolved, safety, efficacy, and versatility of endoscopic approaches have improved dramatically. Recent series have demonstrated success rates of 88 to 100%, complication rates of 12 to 23%, and failure rates of 15% for encephalocele repair using endoscopic approaches, which is comparable to that of transcranial approaches.[41,42,43] It is now generally accepted that minimally invasive approaches may effectively treat sincipital and basal encephaloceles in the absence of significant craniofacial deformity while avoiding a large coronal incision and craniotomy.[44] Factors that may limit use of an endoscopic approach include anatomic locations with limited access (lateral frontal region), chronic sinusitis, prior endoscopic sinus surgery, and unavailability of nasal tissue for repair.[41]

In preparation for an endoscopic approach, detailed preoperative imaging, frameless stereotaxis, and adequate endoscopic equipment (optics, irrigation, instruments, and cautery) are essential. The anterior skull base is typically accessed through an endonasal approach through one or a combination of four corridors, transnasal, transsphenoidal, transethmoidal, and transmaxillary, based on the location of the encephalocele. Once accessed, the defect must be circumferentially visualized with reduction of the herniation sac until it is flush with the skull base. At the defect site, the skull base should then be circumferentially demucosalized. The mucosal graft should be flush with the skull base and no overlap should occur between the in situ skull base mucosa and mucosal graft. Any overlap may result in mucocele development. Grafting may be performed using underlay, overlay, or combination of techniques with a variety of potential graft materials including septal mucoperiosteum, temporalis fascia, DuraGen, cadaveric fascia, free mucosal graft, or vascularized pedicled mucosal flap. Nasal packing is then placed in both nares to minimize postoperative nasal bleeding and to bolster the closure. It is typically removed within the first 24 hours postoperatively. Postoperative antibiotic use is controversial. Some advocate for antibiotics while nasal packing is in place for 24 hours or during the first 72 hours after surgery.[45] Preoperative lumbar drain placement is also a nonuniform practice as multiple series have shown a general decrease in use over time with no significant impact on morbidity or postoperative CSF leakage.[41,45]

Regardless of the approach, careful monitoring and prevention of postoperative CSF leak should be performed. The wound should undergo frequent examination for evidence of leakage of CSF or the development of pseudomeningocele. Head circumference should be measured daily, while ventricular size should be monitored with serial ultrasounds. A ventriculoperitoneal shunt should be inserted if hydrocephalus becomes clinically significant in order to prevent CSF leakage and wound compromise. Potential postoperative morbidities include dacryocystitis, wound infection, CSF leak, visual abnormalities, and anosmia.

28.8.6 Outcome

Historically, children with anterior encephaloceles were thought to have better predicted outcomes than children with posterior lesions. However, this is more likely due to the fact that hydrocephalus and seizure disorders are less frequently associated with sincipital and basal encephaloceles than occipital and parietal lesions. Furthermore, functional and neurologic outcomes for all children with encephaloceles tend to worsen in the presence of associated cranial, neuroanatomic, and systemic abnormalities. Cognitive function inversely correlates with the type and amount of functional cerebral tissue within the herniation sac. For patients with anteriorly located encephaloceles, prognosis tends to be excellent, with the exception of basal encephaloceles with herniation of vital structures. The majority of patients with nasofrontal encephaloceles tend to have normal or nearly normal intelligence and ultimately do well following repair of their congenital deformity.[34,35]

28.9 Surgical Pearls

- Ensure adequate preoperative evaluation—all medical abnormalities should be corrected prior to surgical treatment in order to minimize postoperative morbidity and mortality.
- Ensure adequate exposure—for anterior encephaloceles, the craniotomy should be placed low enough that the herniation sac can be adequately accessed and completely resected.

- Ensure complete resection—inadequate exposure and resection may lead to a persistent facial mass in anterior encephalocele surgery.
- Ensure monitoring for hydrocephalus—failure to identify hydrocephalus may lead to postoperative CSF leak, wound dehiscence, and infection.

28.10 Common Clinical Questions

1. What is the prognosis of patients with encephaloceles?
2. What are potential complications of anterior encephalocele repair?

28.11 Answers to Common Clinical Questions

1. For all children with encephaloceles, approximately 40% can be expected to have a normal neurologic and functional outcome, while 60% can be expected to be significantly mentally and physically impaired. Historically, children with anterior encephaloceles were thought to have better predicted outcomes than children with posterior lesions. However, this is more likely due to the fact that hydrocephalus and seizure disorders are less frequently associated with sincipital and basal encephaloceles than occipital and parietal lesions. Furthermore, functional and neurologic outcomes for all children with encephaloceles tend to worsen in the presence of associated cranial, neuroanatomic, and systemic abnormalities. Cognitive function inversely correlates with the type and amount of functional cerebral tissue within the herniation sac.
2. Potential complications include dacryocystitis, wound infection, CSF leak, visual abnormalities, and anosmia.

References

[1] Woodworth BA, Schlosser RJ, Faust RA, Bolger WE. Evolutions in the management of congenital intranasal skull base defects. Arch Otolaryngol Head Neck Surg. 2004; 130(11): 1283–1288

[2] Youmans JR, Winn HR. Youmans Neurological Surgery. 6th ed. Philadelphia, PA: Saunders/Elsevier; 2011

[3] Albright AL, Pollack IF, Adelson PD, Principles and Practice of Pediatric Neurosurgery. New York, NY: Thieme; 2008

[4] Copp AJ. Neurulation in the cranial region—normal and abnormal. J Anat. 2005; 207(5):623–635

[5] Gluckman TJ, George TM, McLone DG. Postneurulation rapid brain growth represents a critical time for encephalocele formation: a chick model. Pediatr Neurosurg. 1996; 25(3): 130–136

[6] Makelarski JA, Romitti PA, Rocheleau CM, et al. National Birth Defects Prevention Study. Maternal periconceptional occupational pesticide exposure and neural tube defects. Birth Defects Res A Clin Mol Teratol. 2014; 100(11):877–886

[7] Gaffield W, Keeler RF. Induction of terata in hamsters by solanidane alkaloids derived from Solanum tuberosum. Chem Res Toxicol. 1996; 9(2):426–433

[8] Salonen R, Paavola P. Meckel syndrome. J Med Genet. 1998; 35(6):497–501

[9] Seaver LH, Joffe L, Spark RP, Smith BL, Hoyme HE. Congenital scalp defects and vitreoretinal degeneration: redefining the Knobloch syndrome. Am J Med Genet. 1993; 46(2):203–208

[10] Vajsar J, Schachter H. Walker-Warburg syndrome. Orphanet J Rare Dis. 2006; 1:29

[11] Dorsett D. Roles of the sister chromatid cohesion apparatus in gene expression, development, and human syndromes. Chromosoma. 2007; 116(1):1–13

[12] Lubinsky MS, Kahler SG, Speer IE, Hoyme HE, Kirillova IA, Lurie IW. von Voss-Cherstvoy syndrome: a variable perinatally lethal syndrome of multiple congenital anomalies. Am J Med Genet. 1994; 52(3):272–278

[13] Allam KA, Wan DC, Kawamoto HK, Bradley JP, Sedano HO, Saied S. The spectrum of median craniofacial dysplasia. Plast Reconstr Surg. 2011; 127(2):812–821

[14] Suwanwela C. Geographical distribution of fronto-ethmoidal encephalomeningocele. Br J Prev Soc Med. 1972; 26(3):193–198

[15] Bhandari S, Sayami JT, K C RR, Banjara MR. Prevalence of congenital defects including selected neural tube defects in Nepal: results from a health survey. BMC Pediatr. 2015; 15: 133

[16] Sargiotto C, Bidondo MP, Liascovich R, Barbero P, Groisman B. Descriptive study on neural tube defects in Argentina. Birth Defects Res A Clin Mol Teratol. 2015; 103(6):509–516

[17] Miller E, Ben-Sira L, Constantini S, Beni-Adani L. Impact of prenatal magnetic resonance imaging on postnatal neurosurgical treatment. J Neurosurg. 2006; 105(3) Suppl: 203–209

[18] Kasprian GJ, Paldino MJ, Mehollin-Ray AR, et al. Prenatal imaging of occipital encephaloceles. Fetal Diagn Ther. 2015; 37(3):241–248

[19] Ahmed A, Noureldin R, Gendy M, Sakr S, Abdel Naby M. Antenatal sonographic appearance of a large orbital encephalocele: a case report and differential diagnosis of orbital cystic mass. J Clin Ultrasound. 2013; 41(5):327–331

[20] Tirumandas M, Sharma A, Gbenimacho I, et al. Nasal encephaloceles: a review of etiology, pathophysiology, clinical presentations, diagnosis, treatment, and complications. Childs Nerv Syst. 2013; 29(5):739–744

[21] Mahapatra AK. Giant encephalocele: a study of 14 patients. Pediatr Neurosurg. 2011; 47(6):406–411

[22] Holm C, Thu M, Hans A, et al. Extracranial correction of frontoethmoidal meningoencephaloceles: feasibility and outcome in 52 consecutive cases. Plast Reconstr Surg. 2008; 121(6):386e–395e

[23] Alexiou GA, Sfakianos G, Prodromou N. Diagnosis and management of cephaloceles. J Craniofac Surg. 2010; 21(5): 1581–1582

[24] Kotil K, Kilinc B, Bilge T. Diagnosis and management of large occipitocervical cephaloceles: a 10-year experience. Pediatr Neurosurg. 2008; 44(3):193–198

[25] Wong SL, Law HL, Tan S. Atretic cephalocele - an uncommon cause of cystic scalp mass. Malays J Med Sci. 2010; 17(3):61–63

[26] Morone PJ, Sweeney AD, Carlson ML, et al. Temporal lobe encephaloceles: a potentially curable cause of seizures. Otol Neurotol. 2015; 36(8):1439–1442

[27] Blum KS, Schneider SJ, Rosenthal AD. Methyl methacrylate cranioplasty in children: long-term results. Pediatr Neurosurg. 1997; 26(1):33–35

[28] Steinbok P. Repair of a congenital cranial defect in a newborn with autologous calvarial bone. Childs Nerv Syst. 2000; 16 (4):247–249, discussion 250

[29] Moss SD, Joganic E, Manwaring KH, Beals SP. Transplanted demineralized bone graft in cranial reconstructive surgery. Pediatr Neurosurg. 1995; 23(4):199–204, discussion 204–205

[30] Mohanty A, Biswas A, Reddy M, Kolluri S. Expansile cranioplasty for massive occipital encephalocele. Childs Nerv Syst. 2006; 22(9):1170–1176

[31] Gallo AE, Jr. Repair of giant occipital encephaloceles with microcephaly secondary to massive brain herniation. Childs Nerv Syst. 1992; 8(4):229–230

[32] Oi S, Saito M, Tamaki N, Matsumoto S. Ventricular volume reduction technique–a new surgical concept for the intracranial transposition of encephalocele. Neurosurgery. 1994; 34(3):443–447, discussion 448

[33] Gonen L, Handzel O, Shimony N, Fliss DM, Margalit N. Surgical management of spontaneous cerebrospinal fluid leakage through temporal bone defects–case series and review of the literature. Neurosurg Rev. 2016; 39(1):141–150, discussion 150

[34] Kiymaz N, Yilmaz N, Demir I, Keskin S. Prognostic factors in patients with occipital encephalocele. Pediatr Neurosurg. 2010; 46(1):6–11

[35] Lo BW, Kulkarni AV, Rutka JT, et al. Clinical predictors of developmental outcome in patients with cephaloceles. J Neurosurg Pediatr. 2008; 2(4):254–257

[36] Bui CJ, Tubbs RS, Shannon CN, et al. Institutional experience with cranial vault encephaloceles. J Neurosurg. 2007; 107(1) Suppl:22–25

[37] Adil E, Robson C, Perez-Atayde A, et al. Congenital nasal neuroglial heterotopia and encephaloceles: An update on current evaluation and management. Laryngoscope. 2016; 126(9):2161–2167

[38] Davis CH, Jr, Alexander E, Jr. Congenital nasofrontal encephalomeningoceles and teratomas; review of seven cases. J Neurosurg. 1959; 16(4):365–377

[39] David DJ, Sheffield L, Simpson D, White J. Fronto-ethmoidal meningoencephaloceles: morphology and treatment. Br J Plast Surg. 1984; 37(3):271–284

[40] Roux FE, Lauwers F, Oucheng N, Say B, Joly B, Gollogly J. Treatment of frontoethmoidal meningoencephalocele in Cambodia: a low-cost procedure for developing countries. J Neurosurg. 2007; 107(1) Suppl:11–21

[41] Rawal RB, Sreenath SB, Ebert CS, Jr, et al. Endoscopic sinonasal meningoencephalocele repair: a 13-year experience with stratification by defect and reconstruction type. Otolaryngol Head Neck Surg. 2015; 152(2):361–368

[42] Castelnuovo P, Bignami M, Pistochini A, Battaglia P, Locatelli D, Dallan I. Endoscopic endonasal management of encephaloceles in children: an eight-year experience. Int J Pediatr Otorhinolaryngol. 2009; 73(8):1132–1136

[43] Tabaee A, Anand VK, Cappabianca P, Stamm A, Esposito F, Schwartz TH. Endoscopic management of spontaneous meningoencephalocele of the lateral sphenoid sinus. J Neurosurg. 2010; 112(5):1070–1077

[44] Nyquist GG, Anand VK, Mehra S, Kacker A, Schwartz TH. Endoscopic endonasal repair of anterior skull base non-traumatic cerebrospinal fluid leaks, meningoceles, and encephaloceles. J Neurosurg. 2010; 113(5):961–966

[45] Bedrosian JC, Anand VK, Schwartz TH. The endoscopic endonasal approach to repair of iatrogenic and noniatrogenic cerebrospinal fluid leaks and encephaloceles of the anterior cranial fossa. World Neurosurg. 2014; 82(6) Suppl:S86–S94

29 Congenital Arachnoid Cysts

Gianpiero Tamburrini

29.1 Introduction

Congenital arachnoid cysts (ACs) are also called leptomeningeal cysts. This term excludes secondary "arachnoid" cysts (i.e., posttraumatic, postinfectious, etc.), lined with diseased or inflammatory arachnoidal membranes, and glioependymal cysts, lined with glial tissue and epithelial cells. True arachnoid cysta tend to involve more frequently the supratentorial compartment, sylvian fissure cysts representing the most common location.[1,2] Controversial issues do actually still exist concerning both the indications to surgical treatment and the type of surgery, the role of endoscopy having reached an increasingly relevant role in this context.[3,4,5]

29.2 Pathogenesis

True ACs are developmental lesions that arise from the splitting or duplication of the arachnoid membrane (thus they are in fact intra-arachnoid cysts).

The etiology of these lesions has long been the subject of debate.

- The most accepted theory is that they develop from a minor aberration in the development of the arachnoid mater from around week 15 of gestation onward, when the cerebrospinal fluid (CSF) is generated to gradually replace the extracellular ground substance between the external and the internal arachnoid membrane (endomeninx).[1] The malformative hypothesis is supported by the common location of ACs at the level of normal arachnoid cisterns, their occasional occurrence in siblings, the presence of accompanying anomalies of the venous architecture (i.e., the absence of the sylvian vein), and the association with other congenital anomalies (agenesis of the corpus callosum and Marfan's syndrome).
- Specific problems in the definition of the pathogenesis concern intraventricular ACs. For some authors, they represent a kind of "internal" meningocele; for others, they derive from the arachnoid layer and are transported along with the vascular mesenchyme when they invaginate through the choroidal fissure.[1,6]

29.3 Epidemiology

Congenital ACs have been reported to account for roughly 1% of atraumatic intracranial mass lesions. This relatively old figure is the result of a correlation between data obtained from the clinical experience in the era before computed tomography (CT)/magnetic resonance imaging (MRI) (0.7–2% of space-occupying lesions) and those obtained from autopsy observations (0.1–0.5% of incidental autoptic findings)[7]; relatively recent MR studies in healthy participants suggest that this rate is higher, approximating 1.5 to 2.0%.[8] Intracranial ACs are nearly always sporadic and single. They occur two or three times more often in males than in females and three to four times more often on the left side of the brain than on the right. The bilateral occurrence of more or less symmetrical cysts has been reported, although rarely, in normal as well as in neurologically impaired children. In the latter instance, especially in patients with bitemporal cysts, the differential diagnosis should be made with lesions resulting from perinatal hypoxia or metabolic diseases.

According to the information provided by large mixed series (i.e., including both children and adults), 6 to 90% of patients belong to the pediatric age group; it is recognized that the largest proportion of infantile cases occur during the first 2 years of life.[9]

The most common location for ACs is within the middle cranial fossa, 30 to 50% of lesions being found there. Another 10% occur over the cerebral convexity, 9 to 15% in the suprasellar region, 5 to 10% in the quadrigeminal plate cistern, 10% in the cerebellopontine angle (CPA), and 10% in the midline posterior fossa.[1,2] The anatomical classification and topographic distribution of the different types of ACs are summarized in ► Table 29.1.

29.4 Sylvian Fissure Cysts

29.4.1 Epidemiology

Sylvian fissure cysts alone account for about half of adult and one-third of pediatric cases. Their most accepted classification is the one of Galassi and

Table 29.1 Anatomical classification and topographical distribution of intracranial arachnoid cysts

Location	Percentage distribution
Supratentorial	
• Sylvian fissure	30–50
• Sellar region	9–15
• Cerebral convexity	4–15
• Interhemispheric fissure	5–8
• Quadrigeminal plate	5–10
Infratentorial	
• Median	9–17
• Cerebellar hemisphere	5–11
• Cerebellopontine angle	4–10
• Retroclival	0.5–3

colleagues who divided sylvian fissure cysts into three types, depending on their size and apparent communication (metrizamide CT study) with the normal CSF spaces[10] (▶ Fig. 29.1).

29.4.2 Clinical Manifestations

Sylvian fissure cysts may manifest clinically at any age, but they become symptomatic more frequently in children and adolescents than in adults, and in most series, infants and toddlers account for about a quarter of the cases.
- The diagnosis is frequently incidental.
- In symptomatic patients, the symptoms are often nonspecific, headache being the most common complaint.

Controversies exist concerning the management of asymptomatic children and children with aspecific clinical symptoms. Preventive surgery has been proposed with the objective of reducing the risk of spontaneous/posttraumatic cyst rupture, with consequent subdural hematomas, hygromas, and intracystic bleedings. From a review of the most recent literature, this risk is overall approximately 4.3% (relatively low), with the most frequent occurrences being the one of subdural hematomas (overall risk of 3.5%) and subdural hygromas (overall risk of 2.4%); intracystic bleedings have been only rarely reported.[11,12,13] The only risk factor almost uniformly considered for cyst rupture is a history of head injury, with 80 to 90% of the reported cases being posttraumatic.[11,12,13]
- Cyst rupture might mean spontaneous resolution of the cyst.[14,15]
- When symptomatic, rupture of the cyst in the subdural space is usually related to mild and gradually occurring clinical manifestations, so leaving the time for an adequate management; acute clinical symptoms are the object of sporadic reports, mostly in adult patients.[16,17]
- Surgical treatment itself has a related risk of postoperative subdural hygroma/hematoma, which is similar to the one reported for spontaneous/posttraumatic cases.[18]
- Surgery might not be able to prevent the rupture of the cyst. From a recent endoscopic series of 40 patients, 10% had a subdural hematoma/hygroma in the follow-up, in spite of the MR evidence of a reduction of the cyst volume in 50% of them.[19]

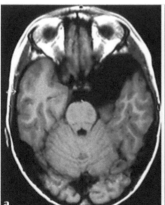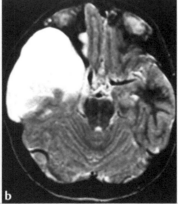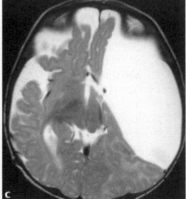

Fig. 29.1 MR example images of arachnoid cysts of the sylvian fissure. **(a)** Type I: the cyst is confined to the temporal pole. **(b)** Type II: the cyst extends to the middle third of the sylvian fissure. **(c)** Type III: the cyst extends to the whole temporal fossa and presents suprasylvian extension.

Among focal signs, mild proptosis and contralateral motor weakness may be noted in advanced cases.

- Seizures and signs of increased intracranial pressure (IICP) represent the clinical onset in about 20 to 35% of patients. When signs of IICP appear acutely, they are usually the consequence of an abrupt increase in the cyst volume, because of subdural or intracystic bleeding.[1,18]
- Mental impairment is found in only 10% of the cases; however, developmental delay and behavioral abnormalities are common in children with large lesions and are nearly constant and severe in patients with bilateral cysts.[20,21,22,23,24]

29.4.3 Radiological Findings

A localized bulging of the skull and/or asymmetrical macrocrania are characteristic features in half of the patients. CT in these cases reveals an outward bulging and thinning of the temporal squama and anterior displacement of the lesser and greater wings of the sphenoid bone. Cysts appear as well-defined lesions between the dura and the distorted brain, with the same density of CSF and without contrast enhancement. Cerebral ventricles are usually of normal size or minimally dilated.[6,10] MRI shows lesions to have hypointensity on T1-weighted and hyperintensity on T2-weighted images. Scanning of the vascular structures is useful in order to define the arteries and veins in relation to the cyst wall. Cine-flow sequences have been employed in the last 15 years as substitutes for metrizamide CT in order to define the presence or absence of communication between the cysts and the subarachnoid spaces.[25,26,27] This may be particularly important in asymptomatic patients, just as in patients with nonspecific clinical symptoms. In this context, further information that might indicate the need for surgery may be provided by ICP monitoring.[7,28,29,30] Perfusion MRI sequences and SPECT (single-photon emission computed tomography) studies have also been proposed; the latter may help to evaluate brain perfusion around the cyst walls.[31,32,33,34,35]

29.4.4 Surgical Management

There are essentially three surgical options, even in combination:

- Cyst marsupialization through open craniotomy.
- Endoscopic cyst marsupialization.
- Cyst shunting.

Open cyst marsupialization is considered the preferable surgical procedure. Successful open fenestration rates vary from 75 to 100%; moreover, a substantial reduction in the earlier morbidity rates has been reported in recent series and surgical mortality has been reduced to almost nil. Two issues concerning open surgery should be pointed out.

Total excision of the AC membranes is no longer considered worthwhile; large windows in a bipolar fashion are sufficient to allow CSF pulsations through the cyst cavity and reduce the risk of harming the adjacent cortex. A more focal cyst opening might also prevent CSF escape into the subdural space and the development of postoperative subdural hygromas.[36]

All vessels either traversing the cyst cavity or lying in the cyst membrane represent the normal vasculature and are therefore to be preserved.[3]

Pure endoscopic cyst marsupialization has been proposed as an alternative to open fenestration in recent years and has rapidly gained favor among physicians.[19,4] Endoscopy has also been used to assist open surgery in order to reduce the extension of the surgical approach. Alternating results of pure endoscopic techniques have been reported, with success rates ranging between 45 and 100%.[36]

Cyst diversions are obviously safer, but are accompanied by a high incidence of additional surgical procedures (around 30%) and the stigma of lifelong shunt dependency.[31,3]

29.5 Sellar Region Cysts

Sellar region cysts represent the second most common among supratentorial intracranial ACs. Affected males slightly outnumber females, with a male-to-female ratio of about 1.5:1. The cysts can be subdivided in two groups:

- Suprasellar cysts that develop above the diaphragma sellae.
- Intrasellar cysts that are found within the sellar cavity.

The latter are far less common than the former and are exceptional in children.

The term sellar region cysts includes neither the "empty sella" syndrome, nor intrasellar and/or suprasellar arachnoid diverticula. Metrizamide CT or cine-MRI studies are helpful in the differential diagnosis, showing neither contrast entering nor relevant CSF flow inside true cysts.[5]

It is largely accepted that sellar and suprasellar ACs can be considered a consequence of a lobulation of the prechiasmatic and interpeduncular arachnoid complex, physiologically composed of two distinct arachnoid sheets named as the diencephalic membrane and the mesencephalic membrane.

Intrasellar ACs are asymptomatic in about half of the cases. Headache is the most frequent complaint in symptomatic patients, and endocrinological disturbances are frequently associated. Suprasellar cysts have been reported to be symptomatic in more than 90% of cases. Most suprasellar cysts cause obstructive hydrocephalus since a superior part of the cyst wall protrudes into the third ventricle and thus obstructs the foramen or foramina of Monro. Obstructive hydrocephalus is the most common cause of the initial signs and is reported in nearly 90% of the patients. Ventriculomegaly may also be asymmetrical. Cases without any ventricular dilatation are very rare. Visual field defect and/or decreased visual acuity may occur due to compression of the chiasm. Endocrine function may be affected due to deflection of the stalk, protrusion of the cyst wall into the third ventricle, and very close proximity of the cyst to the hypothalamic–pituitary area. Growth hormone and corticotrophin production are the most frequently compromised hormonal activities Delayed menarche in women may also be noted.[5,37,38]

Suprasellar ACs have been shown to compromise neurocognitive function and psychological profiles in the pediatric age group. A typical manifestation of a suprasellar cyst is the "bobble-headed doll" syndrome, characterized by slow, rhythmic movements of the head in an anteroposterior direction; it has been reported in approximately 10% of children with suprasellar cysts.[5]

During prenatal life, in the neonatal period, and in infancy, echoencephalography is a useful diagnostic tool, allowing the evolution of this kind of lesion to be followed during the first months of life. An MRI examination should be performed whenever technically feasible. There are three characteristic diagnostic MRI features regarding suprasellar cysts: (1) vertical deflection of the optic chiasm/tracts, (2) upward displacement of the anterior mesencephalon and mammillary bodies, and (3) effacement of the ventral surface of the upper brainstem (e.g., pons). MRI studies are also important for the differential diagnosis between suprasellar ACs and other possible cystic lesions of the sellar region (i.e., Rathke's cleft cyst, cystic craniopharyngiomas, epidermoid cysts, etc.) (▶ Fig. 29.2).[5,37,38]

The rapid advances in endoscopic technologies have significantly changed the management of sellar region cysts. The endoscopic transnasal approach is ideally suited for pure intrasellar cysts and has substituted the traditional microsurgical approach to these lesions. Suprasellar cysts have been managed by only opening the cyst roof (endoscopic transventricular ventriculocystostomy) compared with opening both the cyst roof and the cyst floor (ventriculocystocisternostomy); the latter technique is actually considered safe and, if compared with ventriculocystostomy, is associated with a lower recurrence rate (5–10% vs. 25–40%). In fact, chronic mesencephalic compression by the cyst may lead to secondary aqueductal occlusion. In this scenario, apical membrane fenestration alone, although allowing for adequate cyst decompression, may not result in extraventricular

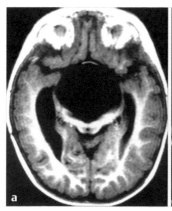
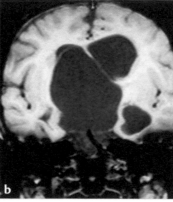

Fig. 29.2 Suprasellar arachnoid cyst. **(a)** Axial T1 MR image showing the extension of the cyst inside the third ventricle and the posterior displacement of the cerebral peduncles. **(b)** Coronal T1 image showing the extension of the cyst from the interpeduncular cistern to the right lateral ventricle.

CSF flow. The basal membrane fenestration, on the other hand, serves the purpose of allowing trapped fluid to pass into the basal cisterns and bypass the occluded aqueduct altogether. Shunting procedures have been practically abandoned. Although relatively safe, they are associated with a surprisingly high percentage of reoperations. Microsurgical excision, fenestration, or marsupialization has to be reserved for patients in whom the endoscopic management has failed or for patients with main extraventricular extension of the cyst walls (i.e., suprasellar ACs involving the medial aspect of the temporal lobe).[5,38]

It is important to remember that whatever the surgical treatment, endocrinological problems, if present, rarely resolve, with medical substitution therapy being required in most cases; similarly neurocognitive disturbances, when present, do not tend to improve with surgery. Visual symptoms and symptoms of intracranial hypertension, on the other hand, improve remarkably after surgery. Flow-sensitive MRI is needed to confirm a pulsation artifact in the follow-up period in order to confirm the presence of stable communication between the cyst and the CSF spaces.[5]

29.6 Cerebral Convexity Cysts

They are relatively uncommon (4–15% of all intracranial ACs); females are more frequently affected than males. We distinguish between two main varieties:

- Hemispherical cysts, huge fluid collections extending over most or all of the surface of one cerebral hemisphere.
- Focal cysts, small lesions generally involving the cerebral convexity.

Hemispheric cysts have been considered to be extreme extensions of sylvian fissure cysts, differing because of a compressed rather than an enlarged sylvian fissure and the absence of temporal lobe aplasia. They are most commonly discovered in infants presenting with macrocrania, bulging anterior fontanel, and cranial asymmetry. CT and MRI allow the differential diagnosis with chronic subdural fluid collections (subdural hygroma and hematoma) in most cases.[39]

Localized bulging of the skull usually suggests a focal cyst. In children, typically, neurological signs are lacking, whereas adults frequently exhibit focal neurological deficits and/or seizure disorders. The differential diagnosis with low-grade neuroglial tumors is usually made using MRI.[1]

Microsurgical cyst marsupialization is the treatment of choice. It is not necessary to remove the medial cystic wall, which is intimately connected with the underlying cerebral cortex. Shunt implantation is advised only in case of recurrences, although it has also been proposed as a primary procedure in infants with hemispheric cysts because of their immature absorptive ability and because of the related high risk of failure of open surgical procedures. In such cases, programmable valves are useful for better control of the intracystic pressure and for favoring the development of natural CSF pathways.[1,31]

29.7 Interhemispheric Fissure Cysts

Interhemispheric fissure cysts are rare, accounting for 5 to 8% of intracranial ACs in all age groups. According to the classification by Mori,[40] two main types of interhemispheric cysts are recognized:

- Intra-axial interhemispheric cysts.
- Extra-axial interhemispheric cysts.

Intra-axial cysts are associated with more complicated brain malformation, such as the dorsal cyst of holoprosencephaly, diencephalic cyst with upward extension of the third ventricle, and porencephalic cyst. In these cases, the cystic lesions are in communication with the ventricular system. Mori used the term *dorsal cyst malformations* to indicate these lesions. On the contrary, extra-axial cysts have no communication with the ventricles or with the subarachnoid space and may exert mass effect on the surrounding brain.[40] Distinction between communicating and noncommunicating cysts is usually easy on MRI. Noncommunicating cysts show a typical wedge-shaped appearance in coronal sections; differently from communicating cysts, the occipital horns of the lateral ventricles can be easily identified, even though they are displaced by the cystic lesion, and the basal ganglia are normally separated.

Mori distinguished two types of extra-axial cysts:

- Unilateral parasagittal cysts, with intact corpus callosum.
- Midline cysts, associated with (partial or total) agenesis of the corpus callosum and unilateral or bilateral extension (▶ Fig. 29.3).

Usually extra-axial midline interhemispheric cysts are associated with ventricular enlargement, often

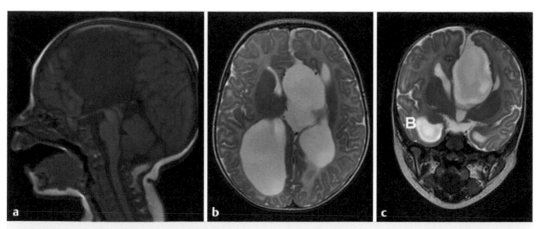

Fig. 29.3 (a) Extra-axial interhemispheric arachnoid cyst with agenesis of the corpus callosum and (b, c) prevalent left unilateral parafalcal extension.

asymmetrical: these cysts may distort the CSF pathways, displacing downward one or both the foramina of Monro, obstructing the aqueduct, or impairing the resorption mechanism over the convexity. Although interhemispheric cysts may be sporadically discovered in adulthood and in elderly patients, they are usually diagnosed in very young children. Macrocrania is the presenting sign in a large proportion of cases and symptoms of intracranial hypertension develop in about two-thirds of patients. Localized bulging of the skull is the second most common finding. Neuroendoscopic management of interhemispheric cysts has been proposed as first-line treatment in recent years. Preoperative planning is essential through careful evaluation of preoperative neuroradiological investigations (in particular MRI with 3D TSE techniques (DRIVE) sequences and CSF flow study) to detect the thinner point of the cyst walls where the stomy should be created with minimal brain damage. Neuronavigation is extremely helpful in placing a burr hole on the ideal trajectory and guiding the endoscope through the target. Neuroendoscopic management is able to obtain a reduction of the cyst volume and control of the hydrocephalus in up to 85% of the cases.[41,42]

Postoperative imaging is essential to assess the patency of the stomies and the patency of the subarachnoid spaces in which the CSF is diverted after the endoscopic procedure. They are also important to detect possible complications related to the rapid decrease of the cyst volume, such as subdural hygromas. Long-term radiological follow-up is mandatory to assess the decrease of the volume of the cyst, which in most of the cases is very slow.

Craniotomy with excision of the cystic linings is the treatment of choice. It allows the normalization of the ICP and brain expansion in the vast majority of affected patients. Because of the significantly high rate of related complications, shunting procedures should be considered only in cases refractory to endoscopic or craniotomic approach.[41]

29.8 Quadrigeminal Plate Region Cysts

Quadrigeminal plate cysts account for 5 to 10% of intracranial ACs. Most are diagnosed in children, with a slightly higher incidence in girls than in boys.

Like interhemispheric cysts, although less frequently, cysts originating in the quadrigeminal cistern may be associated with other central nervous system malformations such as holoprosencephaly, Chiari type II malformation, and encephaloceles, and tend to present in young children.[41] Clinical manifestations depend on the direction of expansion of the cyst growth. The largest proportion of these cysts develop upward into the posterior part of the interhemispheric fissure or downward into the cistern of the superior cerebellar vermis, with the possibility, in selected cases, of both a supratentorial and infratentorial extension. Because of their critical position along CSF pathways, these cases are usually diagnosed in infancy because of the secondary obstructive hydrocephalus (▶ Fig. 29.4).

Anomalies of pupillary reaction or eye movements owing to compression of the quadrigeminal

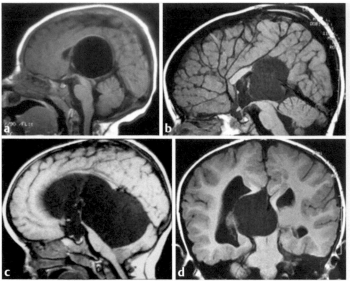

Fig. 29.4 Quadrigeminal cistern arachnoid cysts. **(a, b)** Interhemispheric fissure extension of the cyst and only partial obstruction of the sylvian aqueduct not associated with hydrocephalus. **(c, d)** Infratentorial extension of the cysts and complete obstruction of the aqueduct associated with secondary hydrocephalus.

plate or stretching of the trochlear nerve may be found; however, impairment of the upward conjugate gaze is relatively infrequent. When the direction of expansion is lateral in the cisterna ambiens, hydrocephalus is usually absent and focal signs can be found. Psychomotor retardation may be related to delay in the treatment of intracranial hypertension or to the rarely associated cerebral malformations. Quadrigeminal cysts are not homogeneous, but may have a different extension toward surrounding regions. Sagittal median and coronal MRI sequences clearly show the relationship of the cysts with supratentorial and infratentorial ventricular and neural structures[41,43] (▶ Fig. 29.4).

As for sellar region cysts, modern neuroendoscopy has significantly changed the management practice of this kind of lesion, once considered a technical challenge. In the case of small lesions (< 1 cm) causing secondary triventricular hydrocephalus, third ventriculostomy should be considered as the only surgical treatment needed. In larger lesions, ventriculocystostomy should be performed, possibly combined with third ventriculostomy in patients with associated hydrocephalus. The importance of third ventriculostomy associated with the simple opening of the cyst wall has been stressed by several authors.[41,43] In fact, extrinsic aqueductal stenosis arising from longstanding compression by the cyst may persist despite cyst opening. Approaching the ventricular system first and hence the cyst (transventricular ventriculocystostomy) appears to minimize the escape of CSF

into the subdural space, reducing the risk of postoperative subdural collections. Although limited series of patients appear in the literature, they univocally come to the conclusion that the endoscopic management of quadrigeminal plate cysts is safe and successful in almost all cases.[41,43]

29.9 Infratentorial Arachnoid Cysts

Posterior fossa ACs are rather uncommon, representing approximately 15% of all intracranial cysts. They should be distinguished from other cystic malformations of the posterior fossa, namely the Dandy–Walker malformation, the Dandy–Walker variant, and the cystic evaginations of the tela choroidea (i.e., the persistent Blake's pouch). The main differentiating features of these different pathological conditions are summarized in ▶ Table 29.2.

Three varieties of posterior fossa ACs are recognized:

- Midline cysts, which push the vermis anteriorly, while separating the two cerebellar hemispheres (▶ Fig. 29.5).
- Hemispheric cysts, overlying and compressing one cerebellar hemisphere.
- CPA cysts, displacing both the cerebellum and the brain stem contralaterally[44,45] (▶ Fig. 29.6).

Clinical manifestations depend on the cyst location and the age of the patient. In pediatric patients with midline or hemispheric cysts, macrocrania

Table 29.2 Main differentiating features of cystic malformations of the posterior cranial fossa and posterior fossa arachnoid cysts

	Dandy–Walker syndrome/variant (DWS/DWV)	Blake's pouch cyst	Posterior fossa arachnoid cysts
Relationship with the fourth ventricle	Cystic dilatation of the fourth ventricle: borders of the fourth ventricle not recognizable in DWS; roof and lateral borders present in DWV	Fourth ventricle separated in normal position or moderately dislocated	Fourth ventricle separated, compressed, and dislocated
Communication with the subarachnoid spaces	Absent in DWS, present in DWV	Present	Absent
Associated hydrocephalus	Present (distinguishing feature)	Absent	Common
Associated cerebellar anomalies	Partial or complete agenesis of the vermis	Absent	Absent
Associated cerebral anomalies	50–70% of the cases	Absent	Absent

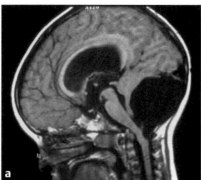
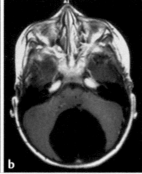

Fig. 29.5 (a) Midline retrocerebellar cyst, with anterior compression of the vermis and (b) separation of the two cerebellar hemispheres.

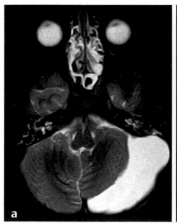
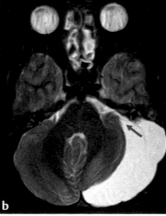

Fig. 29.6 (a) Left cerebellopontine angle arachnoid cyst, with clear compression of the left cerebellar hemisphere and (b) the presence of an evagination of the arachnoid wall (*arrow*) separating it from the cerebellopontine angle arachnoid cistern.

and symptoms of intracranial hypertension are the most frequent signs at presentation, in most instances because of the common association with hydrocephalus. Nystagmus and cerebellar signs may be associated in patients with hemispheric cysts. In adults, the clinical picture of a cerebellar cyst is that of a slowly developing posterior fossa mass, which usually has an intermittent course, suggesting periodic volume fluctuations of the lesion. The secondary development of a Chiari I malformation and syringomyelia has also been reported as a picture disclosing the presence of the AC.[44,45] Symptoms of CPA cysts include cochleovestibular dysfunction, cerebellar signs, and, less frequently, fifth and seventh cranial nerve deficits, as well as pyramidal signs. Papilledema is often observed.[45]

MRI is the diagnostic investigation of choice for posterior fossa cysts; flow-sensitive images have increased its sensitivity allowing a more complete preoperative diagnostic workup. CSF flow sequences are particularly important for patients who are occasionally discovered to harbor a posterior fossa AC or who present with aspecific clinical symptoms. Communicating ACs have in fact been demonstrated not to enlarge and hence to be considered for a conservative approach and a follow-up that might be limited in time.[27]

Direct microsurgical excision of the cyst walls is currently considered the most appropriate type of surgical management for patients with hemispheric and CPA cysts. In patients with midline cysts, relatively high rates of recurrence and persistent postoperative hydrocephalus have been reported, leading some authors to reconsider cyst and/or ventricular shunting to be the preferable surgical option/s. The main disadvantage of this approach is the high rate of shunt malfunctions that have been reported, with a frequency ranging from 10 to 26% in this specific subset of patients.[46] Neuroendoscopy has been recently introduced into the management of posterior fossa cysts. Successful endoscopic cyst marsupialization has been reported in limited series of patients.[46]

29.10 Common Clinical Questions

1. Does the risk of spontaneous/posttraumatic rupture of sylvian AC justify a preventive surgical treatment in asymptomatic children/children with aspecific clinical symptoms?
2. What is the actually considered optimal surgical management strategy for suprasellar ACs?

3. Is endoscopic cyst marsupialization of quadrigeminal plate ACs considered sufficient for the control of both the volume of the cyst and the associated hydrocephalus, when present?
4. Which are the radiological anatomical features which differentiate a Dandy–Walker syndrome from a posterior fossa retrocerebellar AC?

29.11 Answers to Common Clinical Questions

1. No, the risk of spontaneous/posttraumatic rupture of a sylvian AC is relatively low (3–5%); it is controversial if surgery can prevent following cyst rupture.
2. The optimal management strategy for suprasellar ACs is endoscopic marsupialization of the cyst to both the lateral ventricles and the interpeduncular arachnoid cisterns.
3. No, it cannot help in controlling the hydrocephalus in all cases; for this reason, endoscopic third ventriculostomy should be added to the endoscopic cyst marsupialization.
4. The main characteristic features of a retrocerebellar AC which are not present in Dandy–Walker syndrome are: (a) presence of the fastigium; (b) compression of the vermis, which is normally structured; (c) elevation of the tentorium; (d) scalloping of the occipital bone.

References

[1] Di Rocco C. Arachnoid cysts. In: Winn HR, Youmans JR, eds. Youmans Neurological Surgery. Philadelphia, PA: WB Saunders; 1996:967–994
[2] Mazurkiewicz-Bełdzińska M, Dilling-Ostrowska E. Presentation of intracranial arachnoid cysts in children: correlation between localization and clinical symptoms. Med Sci Monit. 2002; 8(6): CR462–CR465
[3] Tamburrini G, Dal Fabbro M, Di Rocco C. Sylvian fissure arachnoid cysts: a survey on their diagnostic workout and practical management. Childs Nerv Syst. 2008; 24(5):593–604
[4] Di Rocco F, R James S, Roujeau T, Puget S, Sainte-Rose C, Zerah M. Limits of endoscopic treatment of sylvian arachnoid cysts in children. Childs Nerv Syst. 2010; 26(2):155–162
[5] Ozek MM, Urgun K. Neuroendoscopic management of suprasellar arachnoid cysts. World Neurosurg. 2013; 79(2) Suppl:19.e13–19.e18
[6] Eskandary H, Sabba M, Khajehpour F, Eskandari M. Incidental findings in brain computed tomography scans of 3000 head trauma patients. Surg Neurol. 2005; 63(6):550–553, discussion 553
[7] Helland CA, Wester K. Intracystic pressure in patients with temporal arachnoid cysts: a prospective study of

preoperative complaints and postoperative outcome. J Neurol Neurosurg Psychiatry. 2007; 78(6):620–623

[8] Weber F, Knopf H. Incidental findings in magnetic resonance imaging of the brains of healthy young men. J Neurol Sci. 2006; 240(1–2):81–84

[9] Wester K. Peculiarities of intracranial arachnoid cysts: location, sidedness, and sex distribution in 126 consecutive patients. Neurosurgery. 1999; 45(4):775–779

[10] Galassi E, Tognetti F, Gaist G, Fagioli L, Frank F, Frank G. CT scan and metrizamide CT cisternography in arachnoid cysts of the middle cranial fossa: classification and pathophysiological aspects. Surg Neurol. 1982; 17(5):363–369

[11] Cress M, Kestle JR, Holubkov R, Riva-Cambrin J. Risk factors for pediatric arachnoid cyst rupture/hemorrhage: a case-control study. Neurosurgery. 2013; 72(5):716–722, discussion 722

[12] Krishnan P, Kartikueyan R. Arachnoid cyst with ipsilateral subdural hematoma in an adolescent—causative or coincidental: Case report and review of literature. J Pediatr Neurosci. 2013; 8(2):177–179

[13] Kertmen H, Gürer B, Yilmaz ER, Sekerci Z. Chronic subdural hematoma associated with an arachnoid cyst in a juvenile taekwondo athlete: a case report and review of the literature. Pediatr Neurosurg. 2012; 48(1):55–58

[14] Yamanouchi Y, Someda K, Oka N. Spontaneous disappearance of middle fossa arachnoid cyst after head injury. Childs Nerv Syst. 1986; 2(1):40–43

[15] McDonald PJ, Rutka JT. Middle cranial fossa arachnoid cysts that come and go. Report of two cases and review of the literature. Pediatr Neurosurg. 1997; 26(1):48–52

[16] Gelabert-González M, Castro-Bouzas D, Arcos-Algaba A, et al. Chronic subdural hematoma associated with arachnoid cyst. Report of 12 cases [in Spanish]. Neurocirugia (Astur). 2010; 21(3):222–227

[17] Seddighi A, Seddighi AS, Baqdashti HR. Asymptomatic presentation of huge extradural hematoma in a patient with arachnoid cyst. Br J Neurosurg. 2012; 26(6):917–918

[18] Tamburrini G, Caldarelli M, Massimi L, Santini P, Di Rocco C. Subdural hygroma: an unwanted result of Sylvian arachnoid cyst marsupialization. Childs Nerv Syst. 2003; 19(3):159–165

[19] Spacca B, Kandasamy J, Mallucci CL, Genitori L. Endoscopic treatment of middle fossa arachnoid cysts: a series of 40 patients treated endoscopically in two centres. Childs Nerv Syst. 2010; 26(2):163–172

[20] Fewel ME, Levy ML, McComb JG. Surgical treatment of 95 children with 102 intracranial arachnoid cysts. Pediatr Neurosurg. 1996; 25(4):165–173

[21] Gosalakkal JA. Intracranial arachnoid cysts in children: a review of pathogenesis, clinical features, and management. Pediatr Neurol. 2002; 26(2):93–98

[22] Raeder MB, Helland CA, Hugdahl K, Wester K. Arachnoid cysts cause cognitive deficits that improve after surgery. Neurology. 2005; 64(1):160–162

[23] Wester K, Hugdahl K. Arachnoid cysts of the left temporal fossa: impaired preoperative cognition and postoperative improvement. J Neurol Neurosurg Psychiatry. 1995; 59(3):293–298

[24] Zaatreh MM, Bates ER, Hooper SR, et al. Morphometric and neuropsychologic studies in children with arachnoid cysts. Pediatr Neurol. 2002; 26(2):134–138

[25] Hoffmann KT, Hosten N, Meyer BU, et al. CSF flow studies of intracranial cysts and cyst-like lesions achieved using reversed fast imaging with steady-state precession MR sequences. AJNR Am J Neuroradiol. 2000; 21(3):493–502

[26] Yildiz H, Erdogan C, Yalcin R, et al. Evaluation of communication between intracranial arachnoid cysts and cisterns with phase-contrast cine MR imaging. AJNR Am J Neuroradiol. 2005; 26(1):145–151

[27] Yildiz H, Yazici Z, Hakyemez B, Erdogan C, Parlak M. Evaluation of CSF flow patterns of posterior fossa cystic malformations using CSF flow MR imaging. Neuroradiology. 2006; 48(9):595–605

[28] Di Rocco C, Tamburrini G, Caldarelli M, Velardi F, Santini P. Prolonged ICP monitoring in Sylvian arachnoid cysts. Surg Neurol. 2003; 60(3):211–218

[29] Tamburrini G, Di Rocco C, Velardi F, Santini P. Prolonged intracranial pressure (ICP) monitoring in non-traumatic pediatric neurosurgical diseases. Med Sci Monit. 2004; 10(4):MT53–MT63

[30] Tamburrini G, Caldarelli M, Massimi L, et al. Prolonged ICP monitoring combined with SPECT studies in children with sylvian fissure arachnoid cysts. Childs Nerv Syst. 2005; 21:840

[31] Germanò A, Caruso G, Caffo M, et al. The treatment of large supratentorial arachnoid cysts in infants with cyst-peritoneal shunting and Hakim programmable valve. Childs Nerv Syst. 2003; 19(3):166–173

[32] Hund-Georgiadis M, Yves Von Cramon D, Kruggel F, Preul C. Do quiescent arachnoid cysts alter CNS functional organization?: A fMRI and morphometric study. Neurology. 2002; 59(12):1935–1939

[33] Kim DS, Choi JU, Huh R, Yun PH, Kim DI. Quantitative assessment of cerebrospinal fluid hydrodynamics using a phase-contrast cine MR image in hydrocephalus. Childs Nerv Syst. 1999; 15(9):461–467

[34] Martínez-Lage JF, Valentí JA, Piqueras C, Ruiz-Espejo AM, Román F, Nuño de la Rosa JA. Functional assessment of intracranial arachnoid cysts with TC99 m-HMPAO SPECT: a preliminary report. Childs Nerv Syst. 2006; 22(9):1091–1097

[35] Sgouros S, Chapman S. Congenital middle fossa arachnoid cysts may cause global brain ischaemia: a study with 99Tc-hexamethylpropyleneamineoxime single photon emission computerised tomography scans. Pediatr Neurosurg. 2001; 35(4):188–194

[36] Godano U, Mascari C, Consales A, Calbucci F. Endoscope-controlled microneurosurgery for the treatment of intracranial fluid cysts. Childs Nerv Syst. 2004; 20(11–12):839–841

[37] Invergo D, Tomita T. De novo suprasellar arachnoid cyst: case report and review of the literature. Pediatr Neurosurg. 2012; 48(3):199–203

[38] Mattox A, Choi JD, Leith-Gray L, Grant GA, Adamson DC. Guidelines for the management of obstructive hydrocephalus from suprasellar-prepontine arachnoid cysts using endoscopic third ventriculocystocisternostomy. Surg Innov. 2010; 17(3):206–216

[39] Ulmer S, Engellandt K, Stiller U, Nabavi A, Jansen O, Mehdorn MH. Chronic subdural hemorrhage into a giant arachnoidal cyst (Galassi classification type III). J Comput Assist Tomogr. 2002; 26(4):647–653

[40] Mori K. Giant interhemispheric cysts associated with agenesis of the corpus callosum. J Neurosurg. 1992; 76(2):224–230

[41] Spennato P, Ruggiero C, Aliberti F, Buonocore MC, Trischitta V, Cinalli G. Interhemispheric and quadrigeminal cysts. World Neurosurg. 2013; 79(2) Suppl:20.e1–20.e7

[42] Cinalli G, Peretta P, Spennato P, et al. Neuroendoscopic management of interhemispheric cysts in children. J Neurosurg. 2006; 105(3) Suppl:194–202

[43] Gangemi M, Maiuri F, Colella G, Magro F. Endoscopic treatment of quadrigeminal cistern arachnoid cysts. Minim Invasive Neurosurg. 2005; 48(5):289–292

[44] Arunkumar MJ, Korah I, Chandy MJ. Dynamic CSF flow study in the pathophysiology of syringomyelia associated with arachnoid cysts of the posterior fossa. Br J Neurosurg. 1998; 12(1):33–36

[45] Galarza M, López-Guerrero AL, Martínez-Lage JF. Posterior fossa arachnoid cysts and cerebellar tonsillar descent: short review. Neurosurg Rev. 2010; 33(3):305–314, discussion 314

[46] Cinalli G, Spennato P, Columbano L, et al. Neuroendoscopic treatment of arachnoid cysts of the quadrigeminal cistern: a series of 14 cases. J Neurosurg Pediatr. 2010; 6(5): 489–497

30 Neuroenteric Cysts

Peter A. Christiansen, John A. Jane, Jr

30.1 Introduction

Neurenteric cysts (NCs) are a rare spectrum of cystic lesions derived from embryologically displaced endodermal tissue that can present throughout the entire neuraxis in any age group.[1,2] With rare exceptions,[3,4] NCs are benign and slow-growing cysts suspected to arise from endodermal nests of the foregut that fail to separate from the notochord during excalation. NCs are most commonly found outside of the central nervous system (CNS) in the posterior mediastinum and abdominal viscera. Histologically, NCs resemble a simple cyst lined with gastrointestinal (50%) and/or respiratory (17%) type epithelium with ciliated and mucin-secreting components. Distinct from other neuraxis cysts, NCs contain a basement membrane and stain with carcinoembryonic antigen. Wilkins and Odom defined three groups of histological classification (▶ Table 30.1)[5]; however, there is no association with clinical outcomes or management. Extremely rare instances of adenocarcinoma have been reported in the setting of recurrence.[3]

Corresponding to their embryologic origin from primitive lung and foregut, NCs of the CNS usually develop ventrally near the cervicothoracic junction and become less frequent further along the neuraxis. Overall, spinal NCs are nearly 10 times more common than intracranial and represent 0.7 to 1.3% of spinal axis mass lesions and 0.01 to 0.35% of cranial mass lesions.[1,2,6,7]

Clinical presentation is primarily progressive local mass effect that is often fluctuant (e.g., myelopathy/radiculopathy, limb weakness, cranial nerve deficits, hydrocephalus) as well as focal pain.[6,8] Fluctuating symptoms are likely due to spontaneous leakage and reaccumulation of cyst contents. Accordingly, aseptic meningitis/meningmus and fevers are not unusual and spontaneous rupture can even lead to hydrocephalus.[8]

Since clinical presentation is usually secondary to mass effect, spinal NCs present earlier with a median age of diagnosis around 6 years, compared to the intracranial median age of diagnosis of 34 years.[2,6] Only around 20 intracranial NCs have been reported in patients younger than 14 years.[1] Gross total resection is recommended for symptomatic NCs.

30.1.1 Spinal

- Median age of diagnosis around 6 years.
- Ninety percent are intradural and extramedullary.
- Less than 5% have any intramedullary component.[9]
- Seventy percent found near the cervicothoracic junction with the majority ventral to the cord.[10]
- Mediastinal extension is possible.
- Bony vertebral anomalies characteristically occur in most cases including hemivertebrae, spina bifida, absence of vertebrae, kyphoscoliosis, Klippel–Feil syndrome, split cord malformation, and diastematomyelia.[2,10]

30.1.2 Cranial

- Median age of diagnosis in 30's.
- Seventy to ninety percent located in the posterior fossa in the prepontine, cerebellomedullary, or cerebellopontine angle cisterns.[1,11]
- Intraventricular, supratentorial, and intraparenchymal locations are possible.
- Often misdiagnosed as arachnoid or epidermoid cysts.

30.2 Radiographic Features

Due to variations in cyst contents, radiographic characteristics are unable to make a definitive

Table 30.1 Wilkins and Odom's histopathological classification of neurenteric cysts

Type A	Single-layer pseudostratified cuboidal or columnar epithelial cells mimicking the respiratory or gastrointestinal epithelium
Type B	Type A + glandular invaginations; mucinous or serous production; nerve ganglion, lymphoid, skeletal muscle, smooth muscle, fat, cartilage, bone elements
Type C	Type A + any associated glial elements or ependymal cells

Source: Information originally described in Wilkins and Odom.[5]

diagnosis of an NC. While there are exceptions to every characteristic, the classic depiction is a well-defined ovoid/lobulated homogenous nonenhancing cystic mass. A summary of the most frequent findings is listed in the following.[1,2,7,11,12,13]

30.2.1 Computed Tomography

- Hypodense.
- No contrast enhancement.
- Adjacent bony abnormality (spine).

30.2.2 Magnetic Resonance Imaging (MRI)

- T1: near-isointense to slightly hyperintense.
- T2: hyperintense.
- Fluid-attenuated inversion recovery (FLAIR): Hyperintense without surrounding edema.
- Diffusion-weighted imaging (DWI): Mild restriction.
- MR spectroscopy: A large peak at 2.02 ppm corresponding to *N-acetyl aspartate*-like compound not seen in other cystic lesions.[12,13]

The radiological differential includes arachnoid cysts, epidermoid or dermoid cysts, choroidal cysts, colloid cysts, Rathke's cleft cyst, ependymal cysts, cysts of parasitic or larval origin, and cystic tumors. Arachnoid, choroidal, and ependymal cysts suppress on FLAIR and have no DWI restriction. Rathke's and colloid cysts should be suspected based on location. Dermoid and epidermoid have more intense DWI restriction. Tumors and parasites tend to have contrast enhancement and surrounding edema.

30.3 Surgical Management and Outcome

Gross total resection is the treatment of choice for symptomatic NCs and can achieve a high frequency of neurological improvement with minimal morbidity. Neither radiation nor chemotherapy is recommended. Standard surgical approaches are used to adequately expose the cyst and its interface. Efforts to contain cyst contents will reduce postoperative chemical meningitis.[8] Some advocate aspiration of cyst contents prior to resection. Dissemination has been seen in a few instances.[14] Vertebral anomalies, extensive adhesions, and/or intramedullary components usually limit complete resection. Intramedullary cysts frequently lack a clear dissection plane; therefore,

cyst marsupialization should be attempted. Partial excision significantly increases the risk of recurrence and the need for further resection; however, it has not been associated with worse long-term outcomes.[10] The longest reported follow-up demonstrated a 37% recurrence rate,[15] all among those with partial resections. Recent studies have shown recurrences can occur even with gross total resection. Recurrences have appeared between 4 months and 14 years with a median of 36 months.[10] Long follow-up periods with repeat imaging are recommended.[6]

30.4 Common Clinical Questions

1. Why are cranial NCs seen more frequently in adults than pediatric patients?
2. What are the treatment options for NCs?
3. What radiographic characteristics would raise suspicion for an NC?

30.5 Answers to Common Clinical Questions

1. Presumably, NCs have been present since birth, growing slowly. They usually only become apparent when they begin to cause mass effect. Since most intracranial locations can accommodate mass more readily than the spinal canal, the presentation of intracranial NCs is typically delayed until the adult years.
2. Complete surgical resection is widely believed to be the ideal treatment as this relieves mass effect, minimizes the chance of recurrence, and reduces the chance of dissemination. Asymptomatic NCs have been followed with serial imaging to closely observe their growth. Not enough data are available to properly define their natural history. Chemotherapy is not a viable option since NCs are essentially hamartomas and slow growing. Radiation would have to target the thin cyst wall with high risk of damaging nearby normal tissue.
3. In pediatrics, NCs should always be in the differential with a cystic mass around the cervicothoracic junction, particularly if there are adjacent bony abnormalities. On MRI, a nonenhancing cystic mass that does not suppress on FLAIR and has slight DWI restriction should bring NCs to mind.

References

[1] Gauden AJ, Khurana VG, Tsui AE, Kaye AH. Intracranial neuroenteric cysts: a concise review including an illustrative patient. J Clin Neurosci. 2012; 19(3):352–359

[2] Savage JJ, Casey JN, McNeill IT, Sherman JH. Neurenteric cysts of the spine. J Craniovertebr Junction Spine. 2010; 1(1):58–63

[3] Dunham CP, Curry B, Hamilton M. Malignant transformation of an intraaxial-supratentorial neurenteric cyst–case report and review of the literature. Clin Neuropathol. 2009; 28(6):460–466

[4] Priamo FA, Jimenez ED, Benardete EA. Posterior fossa neurenteric cysts can expand rapidly: case report. Skull Base Rep. 2011; 1(2):115–124

[5] Wilkins RH, Odom GL. Tumors of the spine and spinal cord, part 2. In: Vinken PJ, Bruyn GW, eds. Handbook of Clinical Neurology. Amsterdam: North-Holland; 1976:55–102

[6] Al-Ahmed IH, Boughamoura M, Dirks P, Kulkarni AV, Rutka JT, Drake JM. Neurosurgical management of neurenteric cysts in children. J Neurosurg Pediatr. 2013; 11(5):511–517

[7] Preece MT, Osborn AG, Chin SS, Smirniotopoulos JG. Intracranial neurenteric cysts: imaging and pathology spectrum. AJNR Am J Neuroradiol. 2006; 27(6):1211–1216

[8] Choh NA, Wani M, Nazir P, et al. Intracranial neurenteric cyst: a rare cause of chemical meningitis. Ann Indian Acad Neurol. 2013; 16(2):286–288

[9] Lippman CR, Arginteanu M, Purohit D, Naidich TP, Camins MB. Intramedullary neurenteric cysts of the spine. Case report and review of the literature. J Neurosurg. 2001; 94(2) Suppl:305–309

[10] Garg N, Sampath S, Yasha TC, Chandramouli BA, Devi BI, Kovoor JM. Is total excision of spinal neurenteric cysts possible? Br J Neurosurg. 2008; 22(2):241–251

[11] Hingwala DR, Radhakrishnan N, Kesavadas C, Thomas B, Kapilamoorthy TR, Radhakrishnan VV. Neuroenteric cysts of the brain-comprehensive magnetic resonance imaging. Indian J Radiol Imaging. 2013; 23(2):155–163

[12] Candiota AP, Majós C, Bassols A, et al. Assignment of the 2.03 ppm resonance in in vivo 1 H MRS of human brain tumour cystic fluid: contribution of macromolecules. MAGMA. 2004; 17(1):36–46

[13] Periakaruppan A, Kesavadas C, Radhakrishnan VV, Thomas B, Rao RM. Unique MR spectroscopic finding in colloid-like cyst. Neuroradiology. 2008; 50(2):137–144

[14] Kimura H, Nagatomi A, Ochi M, Kurisu K. Intracranial neurenteric cyst with recurrence and extensive craniospinal dissemination. Acta Neurochir (Wien). 2006; 148(3):347–352, discussion 352

[15] Chavda SV, Davies AM, Cassar-Pullicino VN. Enterogenous cysts of the central nervous system: a report of eight cases. Clin Radiol. 1985; 36(3):245–251

31 Intracranial Lipomas

Tina Lovén, Mark A. Mittler

31.1 Introduction

Intracranial lipomas are rare benign lesions, considered to be congenital malformations rather than neoplasms or hamartomas. Lipomas make up less than 0.1% of all intracranial lesions.[1,2]

There are multiple theories about the etiology of intracranial lipomas. It is most commonly felt that a persistent focus of the meninx primitiva differentiates into adipose tissue and matures into lipoma. The meninx primitiva surrounds the developing brain. It represents the undifferentiated mesenchyme and typically differentiates to form the leptomeninges. This theory would explain the cisternal location lipomas, absence of other mesodermal derivatives, and intralesional location of blood vessels and nerves.[3] The majority of intracranial lipomas occur near the midline and at embryological sites of neural tube flexion.[4] More than half of identified intracranial lipomas are associated with brain malformations such as agenesis of the corpus callosum. This association may result from the persistence of the meninx primitiva at the location of lamina reuniens, blocking the formation of massa comissuralis. The effect on the development of the corpus callosum could depend on the timing of this process.[4]

Intracranial vessels and nerves were noted to course through the lipomas in 36% of the lesions.[4] The relative frequencies of the locations of the lipomas correspond to the temporal sequence of dissolution of the meninx primitiva—explaining the relatively high frequency of callosal lesions. Blood vessels and cranial nerves generally pass through, rather than be displaced by, the lipoma. Histology demonstrates mature adipose tissue with incorporated nerve fascicles, arteries, and veins.[5]

Intracranial lipomas can grow slowly as part of the general growth of the body.[3] While the natural history of these lesions is not fully known, the incidence of symptomatic compression from cerebellopontine angle (CPA) and dorsal brainstem lipomas suggests possibility of such growth.[3] These lipomas have generally not been shown to grow rapidly or undergo malignant change.[6,7]

31.2 Anatomy

Most intracranial lipomas are found in the midline or at embryologic sites of neural tube flexion.[4,5,8,9]

The anatomic distribution of intracranial lipomas was described by a retrospective review of 42 patients, identifying that 45% were interhemispheric, 25% were in the quadrigeminal cistern, 14% in the suprasellar/interpeduncular cistern, 9% laterally in the CPA, and only 5% more laterally in the sylvian fissure.[4] Other documented locations, although less common, include hypothalamus,[10] optic nerve,[11] interpeduncular fossa,[12] choroid plexus,[13] and cerebellar cortex.[14]

More than half of the patients with intracranial lipomas had other brain anomalies.[4] The most common associated anomalies included: agenesis or dysgenesis of the corpus callosum, cortical dysplasia, cerebral aneurysms, absence of septum pellucidum, spina bifida, subcutaneous lipoma, encephalocele, myelomeningocele, interhemispheric cyst, Dandy–Walker malformation, and craniovertebral anomalies.[8,13,15]

Certain congenital disorders are associated with intracranial lipomas. Pai's syndrome, for example, is a genetic disorder characterized by median cleft lip and palate, midline facial polyps, bifid nose, and midline lipoma particularly in the corpus callosum.[16] Other disorders include frontonasal dysplasia, epidermal nevus syndrome, congenital infiltration lipomatosis, and encephalocraniocutaneous lipomatosis.[17,18] Anatomically, lipomas tend to envelope adjacent nerves and vessels rather than displace them. For example, in CPA lipomas, the facial and vestibular nerves may course through the lipoma without any clear plane of dissection available to the neurosurgeon.[11,18] Histologically, a lipoma can contain elements of neuronal tissue, calcifications, bone, cartilage, vessels, or hematopoietic tissue but no ectodermal elements.[8]

Fat cells are mesenchymal type of mesoderm origin. They are widely distributed forming an intimate admixture with other mesenchymal cells in all body organs. Lipocytes are distinct from all epithelial cells of the ectoderm and endoderm, to which they become intimately related by apposition of growing epithelial cells with budding reticuloendothelial cells. Lipomas are trabeculated and fibrovascular, inseparable and indistinguishable from the arachnoid matter. When they extend into the underlying neural parenchyma, they do so along the Virchow–Robin spaces, outside the pia matter.[9] Lipomas are considered stable lesions; however, myelolipomatous change has been documented in

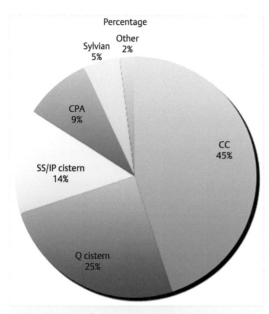

Percentage

Other 2%
Sylvian 5%
CPA 9%
CC 45%
SS/IP cistern 14%
Q cistern 25%

Fig. 31.1 Location of intracranial lipomas.

an interhemispheric lipoma associated with agenesis of corpus callosum (▶ Fig. 31.1).[19,20]

31.3 Presentation

Intracranial lipomas are generally incidental findings and asymptomatic. Symptomatic presentation is dependent on the location of the lesion. When symptomatic, lipomas may present with headache due to hydrocephalus, seizures, or vertigo.[21] Seizures are present in about half of the lipomas of the corpus callosum and are unlikely to be cured by surgical resection.[1]

CPA lipoma can present with hearing loss, vertiginous symptoms, trigeminal neuralgia, or hemifacial spasm.[22,23]

Seizures are common in lipomas located in the sylvian fissure.[13]

Lipomas of the quadrigeminal plate/ambient cistern may produce signs or symptoms in approximately 20% of the patients. These are most commonly seizures and hydrocephalus.[24]

There has been an association of severe obesity without hyperphagia in patients with hypothalamic lipoma. This highlights the importance of obtaining a magnetic resonance imaging (MRI) in children with otherwise unexplained morbid obesity.[25]

Few cases of lipomas affecting the optic nerve presenting with progressive visual loss have been described.[11]

31.4 Radiographic Imaging and Differential Diagnosis

MRI is often used to establish diagnosis of intracranial lipomas but a computed tomography (CT) scan can be helpful with achieving a diagnosis and differentiating from other similarly appearing lesions.[26,27]

Interhemispheric lipomas may be curvilinear or tubulonodular types. Curvilinear lipomas are thin and located along the longitudinal axis of corpus callosum. They are usually not symptomatic. Tubular lipomas are rounder, longer, and wider. They tend to be anterior near the genu or posterior near the splenium. Anterior subtype tends to be more problematic, with the associated structural abnormalities more likely to be responsible for the symptoms than the lipoma itself.[28]

Dermoids and teratomas prefer the third ventricle, invaded from the region of pineal body, and subfrontal and subtemporal area originating from the sphenoid bone.[1] CT appearance of a lipoma is homogenous low attenuation area.[27] Peripheral calcification can be seen and Hounsfield unit (HU) values range from −50 to −100 units. Lipomas do not enhance with intravenous contrast. MRI will often provide better anatomical information. Lipomas appear bright on T1-weighted imaging and dark on T2. They do not enhance with gadolinium, and occasionally vessels and nerves are seen traversing the lesion. Absence of peritumorous edema is also characteristic.[1]

Intracranial lipoma can be misinterpreted as dermoid based on MRI information or CT.[1] On CT, both can appear identical to the naked eye, but dermoid have Hounsfield values of −20 to −40 units.[1,2] From an MRI standpoint, fat-saturation or STIR (short tau inversion recovery) sequence demonstrates the suppression of signal within the lipoma, confirming fat within the lesions.[29]

Dermoids are less homogenous on both CT and MRI since they contain hair and other debris.

Epidermoids contain keratin and usually have HUs similar to CSF.[2,26]

Teratomas contain more than one tissue type and can vary in HUs and MRI relaxation parameters.[2,26]

Hamartomas have T1 similar to gray matter with slight increase in T2.[2]

Differential diagnosis also includes lipomatous transformation of neoplasm (primitive neuroectodermal tumor [PNET], ependymoma, glioma), myelolipoma, angiolipoma, choristoma,

Table 31.1 Differential diagnosis based on imaging findings

Imaging modality	Lipoma	Epidermoid	Dermoid	Hamartoma
MRI T1	Hyperintense	Slightly hyperintense (white epidermoid) to isointense	Hyperintense heterogenous	Isointense
MRI T2	Hypointense	Hypointense	Hypointense heterogenous	Iso- to slightly hyperintense
MRI FLAIR	Hyperintense	Hypointense	Hyperintense	Hyperintense
CT	Dark (low attenuation)	Dark	Dark	Dark or isointense
HU	−50 to −100	Similar to CSF	−25 to −30	
Contrast	Nonenhancing	Nonenhancing	Nonenhancing	Nonenhancing
Location	Midline, cisterns, CPA	Cisterns	Sellar or parasellar, frontonasal, posterior fossa, midline vermis, third or fourth ventricle	Hypothalamus Cortical in tuberous sclerosis
Shape	Tubulonodular or curvilinear	Well defined, lobulated	Round, lobulated, cystic	Variable
Calcifications	Yes, peripheral	Rarely	Yes	Yes

Abbreviations: CPA, cerebellopontine angle; CSF, cerebrospinal fluid; FLAIR, fluid-attenuated inversion recovery; HU, Hounsfield unit; MRI, magnetic resonance imaging.

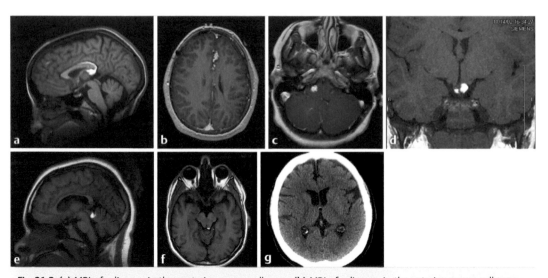

Fig. 31.2 **(a)** MRI of a lipoma in the posterior corpus callosum. **(b)** MRI of a lipoma in the anterior corpus callosum. **(c)** MRI of a suprasellar lipoma. **(d, e)** MRI of a cerebellopontine angle lipoma. **(f)** MRI of a lipoma in the quadrigeminal cistern. **(g)** CT image showing a typical sickle-shaped calcification.

and thrombosed berry aneurysm (▶ Table 31.1) (▶ Fig. 31.2).[1,2,11,26]

31.5 Surgical Considerations

Because surgical excision of intracranial lipomas carries a significant risk, medical management of potentially associated signs and symptoms should be maximized before consideration of operative intervention.[30] Seizures associated with intracranial lipomas typically respond to antiepileptic drugs.[15,24] Patients with hemifacial spasm with lipoma as the likely culprit should undergo medical treatment including Botox before surgical intervention is considered.[22,23] Lipomas associated with balance disorders (vertigo and dizziness) respond well to medical treatment.[24] Hearing loss or visual loss caused by compressive symptoms of lipoma is not likely to improve with medical or surgical treatment.[6,11,24] Treatment with steroids should be avoided as lipoma could potentially grow in response to steroids, inducing hypertrophy of the fat tissue.[31]

Limited surgery can be considered after conservative management has failed and patient continues to suffer from disabling neurological symptoms.

The management of asymptomatic incidentally found lipomas should include close follow-up of the patient and evaluation of a potential change in tumor size. The surgical management depends on the location of the lipoma. Total resection is usually quite difficult due to the deep location and adhesive nature of the lesion. They tend to envelop vessels and nerves and have attachments to the underlying parenchyma via Virchow–Robin spaces.[9,32] Lipomas in cisternal locations causing hydrocephalus are most often treated with shunts. Endoscopic third ventriculostomy (ETV) is an option in selected cases but to our knowledge in the literature there are no documented cases of treatment of hydrocephalus caused by intracranial lipoma with an ETV. Surgical management of CPA lipomas should be reserved for patients with intractable clinical symptoms due to tumor overgrowth.[24] Attempts at complete removal of CPA lipomas may result in severe neurological deficits; subtotal debulking of lipoma is often preferred.[6,22,23,32] Electrophysiologic intraoperative neuromonitoring can guide resection and help prevent injury to adjacent structures.[23]

Corpus callosum: Complete removal of lipoma from the corpus callosum should not be attempted as the fatty tissue is vascularized and interspaced with fibrous tissue that covers the pericallosal arteries and its branches.[1]

31.6 Surgical Pearls

- Caution against total resection as incorporation of neural and vascular structures makes risk of complications high and is not necessary for symptomatic relief.
- Use of intraoperative neuromonitoring may help prevent injury to adjacent structures and give information about when decompression in adequate.

- Management of hydrocephalus with shunts or for selected cases ETV.
- Seizures and vertiginous symptoms usually successfully controlled with medical management.
- Detection of intracranial lipomas is relevant because of their frequent association with other brain malformations.

31.7 Common Clinical Questions

1. What is the most common location of intracranial lipoma?
2. Do intracranial lipomas grow?
3. What are the operative indications for intracranial lipomas?

31.8 Answers to Common Clinical Questions

1. The most common location for intracranial lipoma is corpus callosum. The anatomic distribution of intracranial lipomas was described by a retrospective review of 42 patients, identifying that 45% were interhemispheric, 25% were in the quadrigeminal cistern, 14% in the suprasellar/interpeduncular cistern, 9% laterally in the CPA, and only 5% more laterally in the sylvian fissure.[4]
2. Intracranial lipomas are considered stable lesions. These tumors have generally not been shown to grow rapidly or undergo malignant change.[6,7]
3. Intracranial lipomas should be managed conservatively. Lipomas incorporate neural and vascular structures, making surgical excision risky. Limited surgery can be considered after conservative management has failed and patient continues to suffer from disabling neurological symptoms.

References

[1] Kazner E, Stochdorph O, Wende S, Grumme T. Intracranial lipoma. Diagnostic and therapeutic considerations. J Neurosurg. 1980; 52(2):234–245

[2] Friedman RB, Segal R, Latchaw RE. Computerized tomographic and magnetic resonance imaging of intracranial lipoma. Case report. J Neurosurg. 1986; 65(3):407–410

[3] Baeesa SS, Higgins MJ, Ventureyra EC. Dorsal brain stem lipomas: case report. Neurosurgery. 1996; 38(5):1031–1035

[4] Truwit CL, Barkovich AJ. Pathogenesis of intracranial lipoma: an MR study in 42 patients. AJNR Am J Neuroradiol. 1990; 11 (4):665–674

[5] Wolpert SM, Carter BL, Ferris EJ. Lipomas of the corpus callosum. An angiographic analysis. Am J Roentgenol Radium Ther Nucl Med. 1972; 115(1):92–99

[6] Jallo JI, Palumbo SJ, Buchheit WA. Cerebellopontine angle lipoma: case report. Neurosurgery. 1994; 34(5):912–914, discussion 914

[7] Pensak ML, Glasscock ME, III, Gulya AJ, Hays JW, Smith HP, Dickens JR. Cerebellopontine angle lipomas. Arch Otolaryngol Head Neck Surg. 1986; 112(1):99–101

[8] Kieslich M, Ehlers S, Bollinger M, Jacobi G. Midline developmental anomalies with lipomas in the corpus callosum region. J Child Neurol. 2000; 15(2):85–89

[9] Mattern WC, Blattner RE, Werth J, Shuman R, Bloch S, Leibrock LG. Eighth nerve lipoma. Case report. J Neurosurg. 1980; 53(3):397–400

[10] Kurt G, Dogulu F, Kaymaz M, Emmez H, Onk A, Baykaner MK. Hypothalamic lipoma adjacent to mamillary bodies. Childs Nerv Syst. 2002; 18(12):732–734

[11] Giannini C, Reynolds C, Leavitt JA, et al. Choristoma of the optic nerve: case report. Neurosurgery. 2002; 50(5):1125–1128

[12] Beşkonakli E, Cayli SR, Ergün R, Okten AI. Lipoma of the interpeduncular fossa: demonstration by CT and MRI. Neurosurg Rev. 1998; 21(2–3):210–212

[13] Yildiz H, Hakyemez B, Koroglu M, Yesildag A, Baykal B. Intracranial lipomas: importance of localization. Neuroradiology. 2006; 48(1):1–7

[14] Britt PM, Bindal AK, Balko MG, Yeh HS. Lipoma of the cerebral cortex: case report. Acta Neurochir (Wien). 1993; 121(1–2): 88–92

[15] Saatci I, Aslan C, Renda Y, Besim A. Parietal lipoma associated with cortical dysplasia and abnormal vasculature: case report and review of the literature. AJNR Am J Neuroradiol. 2000; 21(9):1718–1721

[16] Savasta S, Chiapedi S, Perrini S, Tognato E, Corsano L, Chiara A. Pai syndrome: a further report of a case with bifid nose, lipoma, and agenesis of the corpus callosum. Childs Nerv Syst. 2008; 24(6):773–776

[17] Karakas O, Karakas E, Boyacı FN, Celik B, Cullu N. Anterior interhemispheric calcified lipoma together with subcutaneous lipoma and agenesis of corpus callosum: a rare manifestation of midline craniofacial dysraphism. Jpn J Radiol. 2013; 31(7):496–499

[18] Fitoz S, Atasoy C, Erden I, Akyar S. Intracranial lipoma with extracranial extension through foramen ovale in a patient with encephalocraniocutaneous lipomatosis syndrome. Neuroradiology. 2002; 44(2):175–178

[19] Suri V, Sharma MC, Suri A, et al. Myelolipomatous change in an interhemispheric lipoma associated with corpus callosum agenesis: case report. Neurosurgery. 2008; 62(3):E745–, discussion E745

[20] Yalcin S, Fragoyannis S. Intracranial lipoma. Case report. J Neurosurg. 1966; 24(5):895–897

[21] Yilmaz N, Unal O, Kiymaz N, Yilmaz C, Etlik O. Intracranial lipomas–a clinical study. Clin Neurol Neurosurg. 2006; 108 (4):363–368

[22] Inoue T, Maeyama R, Ogawa H. Hemifacial spasm resulting from cerebellopontine angle lipoma: case report. Neurosurgery. 1995; 36(4):846–850

[23] Barajas RF, Jr, Chi J, Guo L, Barbaro N. Microvascular decompression in hemifacial spasm resulting from a cerebellopontine angle lipoma: case report. Neurosurgery. 2008; 63(4):E815–E816, discussion E816

[24] Ono J, Ikeda T, Imai K, et al. Intracranial lipoma of the quadrigeminal region associated with complex partial seizures. Pediatr Radiol. 1998; 28(9):729–731

[25] Puget S, Garnett MR, Leclercq D, et al. Hypothalamic lipoma associated with severe obesity. Report of 2 cases. J Neurosurg Pediatr. 2009; 4(2):147–150

[26] Feldman RP, Marcovici A, LaSala PA. Intracranial lipoma of the sylvian fissure. Case report and review of the literature. J Neurosurg. 2001; 94(3):515–519

[27] Ichikawa T, Kumazaki T, Mizumura S, Kijima T, Motohashi S, Gocho G. Intracranial lipomas: demonstration by computed tomography and magnetic resonance imaging. J Nippon Med Sch. 2000; 67(5):388–391

[28] Demaerel P, Van de Gaer P, Wilms G, Baert AL. Interhemispheric lipoma with variable callosal dysgenesis: relationship between embryology, morphology, and symptomatology. Eur Radiol. 1996; 6(6):904–909

[29] Given CA, Fields TM, Pittman T. Interhemispheric lipoma connected to subcutaneous lipoma via lipomatous stalk. Pediatr Radiol. 2005; 35(11):1110–1112

[30] Markou KD, Goudakos JK, Bellec O, et al. Lipochoristomas of the cerebellopontine angle and internal acoustic meatus: a seven-case review. Acta Neurochir (Wien). 2013; 155(3):449–454

[31] Haga HJ, Thomassen E, Johannesen A, Kråkenes J. Neural compressive symptoms appearing during steroid treatment in a patient with intracranial lipoma. Scand J Rheumatol. 1999; 28(3):184–186

[32] Zimmermann M, Kellermann S, Gerlach R, Seifert V. Cerebellopontine angle lipoma: case report and review of the literature. Acta Neurochir (Wien). 1999; 141(12):1347–1351

32 The Dandy–Walker Malformation: Disorders of Cerebellar Development and Their Management

Greg Olavarria

32.1 Introduction: Incidence, Genetics, and Evaluation

The Dandy–Walker malformation is an uncommon congenital syndrome associated with hydrocephalus and other cerebral and systemic anomalies. With a reported incidence of 1 in 25,000 to 35,000 live births, the malformation occurs early in intrauterine life (before the fourth week of gestation), often affecting multiple organ systems. Known etiologies include *in utero* exposure to toxins, drugs, or infectious agents, signaling pathway problems attributed to ciliary dysfunction, and abnormalities of chromosomes 3, 6, 9, 13, and 18.

The true Dandy-Walker malformation involves either agenesis of the fourth ventricle outlet foramina or lack of regression of fetal cystic structures, producing an enlarged fourth ventricle and posterior fossa displacing the tentorium and torcula superiorly. The majority of patients have hydrocephalus, vermian, and cerebellar hypoplasia, and the brainstem is often pushed anteriorly by the cyst (▶ Fig. 32.1 and ▶ Fig. 32.2). In most cases (60–70%), but not all, the fourth ventricle cyst communicates with the supratentorial ventricular compartment through a patent aqueduct and this has implications for management.[1,2]

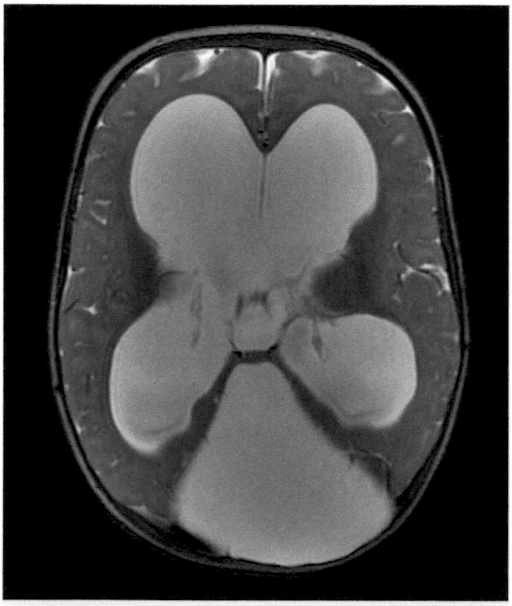

Children usually present early in life with an enlarging head circumference and signs of raised intracranial pressure (secondary to hydrocephalus). Hydrocephalus is present in the majority of patients (60–80% of cases), and other central nervous system (CNS) anomalies can be observed, such as callosal dysgenesis (in 32%), heterotopias, polymicrogyria (5–10%), and encephaloceles (16%).[3,4,5] A systemic workup should be initiated for associated cardiac and limb defects.

Magnetic resonance imaging (MRI) is the preferred imaging modality, and MR cine flow sequences can be used to determine flow across the aqueduct preoperatively. In the past, computed tomography (CT) contrast ventriculography has been used for this purpose.

32.2 Differential Diagnosis

The true Dandy–Walker malformation must be distinguished from other posterior fossa abnormalities such as varying degrees of vermian hypoplasia and less severe posterior fossa cystic collections (aka Dandy–Walker variant), persistent Blake's pouch, mega cisterna magna, and posterior

Fig. 32.1 True Dandy–Walker malformation with hydrocephalus.

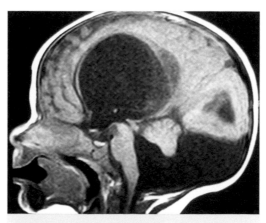

Fig. 32.2 The Dandy–Walker malformation with hydrocephalus, note brainstem displacement.

fossa arachnoid cysts. The variant, better considered the "Dandy–Walker spectrum" of disorders, may be seen with other CNS malformations (callosal dysgenesis) but without accompanying hydrocephalus (▶ Fig. 32.3). On the other hand, diffuse cerebellar hypoplasia is associated with metabolic disorders, trisomies, teratogens, and other *in utero* insults. A persistent Blake's pouch, an expansion of the embryonic posterior membranous area, leads to an enlarged fourth ventricle

and posterior fossa. It can be associated with vermian and cerebellar hypoplasia, and hydrocephalus can occur if there is no communication with the subarachnoid spaces.[5] This entity should also be included in the Dandy–Walker spectrum of abnormalities (▶ Fig. 32.4).

An enlarged cisterna magna does not compress cerebellar structures, and the vermis and fourth ventricle are normal. Hydrocephalus is absent, because the enlarged cistern communicates with the subarachnoid spaces.

Arachnoid cysts mimic the above entities, and can compress structures, but those structures themselves are not abnormal and the cyst itself does not communicate with the fourth ventricle. It is a separate entity from the subarachnoid space around it, and can be distinguished on imaging from the above cystic anomalies (▶ Fig. 32.5).

On imaging, the presence or absence of fourth ventricle choroid plexus can be useful. In the true Dandy–Walker malformation, it is absent, but in a Blake's pouch cyst, it is displaced superiorly in the cyst wall. Though the true malformation is usually evident (hydrocephalus is usually present), it is nearly impossible to distinguish the various Dandy–Walker spectrum disorders (the variant, Blake's pouch, and mega cisterna magna) from each other radiographically.[5,6]

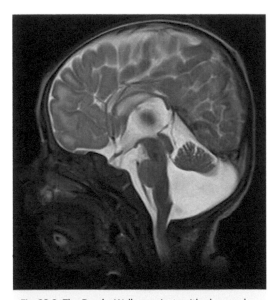

Fig. 32.3 The Dandy–Walker variant, with abnormal vermis, dysplastic corpus callosum without hydrocephalus.

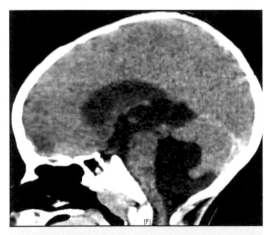

Fig. 32.4 A Blake's pouch cyst.

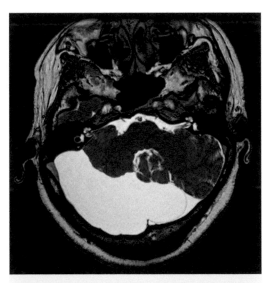

Fig. 32.5 Arachnoid cyst of the posterior fossa, note normal structures present but displaced by the cyst.

32.3 Management and Outcomes

Surgical treatment is indicated for large symptomatic cysts causing compression of the brainstem or hydrocephalus. Shunting the posterior fossa cyst, shunting the ventricles, shunting both, and/or endoscopic techniques are viable options tailored to each individual case. Controversy exists regarding best initial intervention, with the main goal of decompressing the cyst and reducing focal pressure. Management strategy depends on communication between the supratentorial ventricles and the posterior fossa cyst. Postshunting stenosis of the aqueduct and failure of the posterior fossa cyst to resolve has been described with lateral ventricular shunts, leading some authors to recommend cyst shunting primarily or connecting the two via a connector as the initial procedure.[1,3,7] Advocates of ventricular shunting as initial intervention cite numerous complications associated with posterior fossa shunts.[7] Endoscopy has been attempted, with third ventriculostomy procedures as sole treatment and/or combined with endoscopy-assisted stent placement. Third ventriculostomy can be tried if the aqueduct is open, although success rates in infants are less than with older patients.[8,9,10] Direct fenestration of the cyst, though mostly of historical interest, is still practiced by some, especially in patients presenting later in life.[7] A flexible approach should be taken, as the child's shunting needs may change over time.

The prognosis of children with Dandy–Walker malformation is largely dependent on other cerebral and systemic anomalies. At least half the children with the severe form of malformation have neurocognitive delays.[11] Complications associated with shunt surgery are also a factor, that is, infection, malfunction, and numerous surgical procedures, that can impact a child's intellectual functioning.

References

[1] Yüceer N, Mertol T, Arda N. Surgical treatment of 13 pediatric patients with Dandy–Walker syndrome. Pediatr Neurosurg. 2007; 43(5):358–363

[2] Detwiler PW, Porter RW, Rekate HL. Hydrocephalus clinical features and management: Dandy–Walker malformation and two compartment hydrocephalus. In: Choux M, ed. Pediatric Neurosurgery. Churchill Livingstone; 1999

[3] Hirsch JF, Pierre-Kahn A, Renier D, Sainte-Rose C, Hoppe-Hirsch E. The Dandy–Walker malformation. A review of 40 cases. J Neurosurg. 1984; 61(3):515–522

[4] Hart MN, Malamud N, Ellis WG. The Dandy–Walker syndrome. A clinicopathological study based on 28 cases. Neurology. 1972; 22(8):771–780

[5] Barkovich AJ. Congenital malformations of the brain and skull. In: Barkovich AJ, ed. Pediatric Neuroimaging. Philadelphia, PA: Lippincott, Williams and Wilkins; 2005: 291–439

[6] Wilkinson CC, Winston KR. Congenital arachnoid cysts and the Dandy–Walker complex. In: Albright, Pollack, Adelson, eds. Principles and Practice of Pediatric Neurosurgery. New York, NY: Thieme; 2008

[7] Kumar R, Jain MK, Chhabra DK. Dandy–Walker syndrome: different modalities of treatment and outcome in 42 cases. Childs Nerv Syst. 2001; 17(6):348–352

[8] Garg A, Suri A, Chandra PS, Kumar R, Sharma BS, Mahapatra AK. Endoscopic third ventriculostomy: 5 years' experience at the All India Institute of Medical Sciences. Pediatr Neurosurg. 2009; 45(1):1–5

[9] Faggin R, Bernardo A, Stieg P, Perilongo G, d'Avella D. Hydrocephalus in infants less than six months of age: effectiveness of endoscopic third ventriculostomy. Eur J Pediatr Surg. 2009; 19(4):216–219

[10] Mohanty A. Endoscopic third ventriculostomy with cystoventricular stent placement in the management of Dandy–Walker malformation: technical case report of three patients. Neurosurgery. 2003; 53(5):1223–1228, discussion 1228–1229

[11] Bindal AK, Storrs BB, McLone DG. Management of the Dandy–Walker syndrome. Pediatr Neurosurg. 1990–1991; 16 (3):163–169

33 Craniosynostosis

Christopher D. Kelly, Martin H. Sailer, Raphael Guzman

33.1 Introduction

Craniosynostosis is the premature ossification of the cranial sutures. Various nomenclatures are used, with craniostenosis and craniosynostosis often considered to be synonymous. Craniosynostosis can occur primarily as idiopathic craniosynostosis, may be syndromic or arise secondarily. By suture closure, a skull deformity arises. In addition to the deformity, the brain growth can be affected and intracranial pressure may increase, resulting in corresponding complications.[1] Even if there is no problem with intracranial pressure, the deformity may lead to psychosocial problems.[2] Surgery is therefore recommended, the optimum time of which is dependent on the affected suture and the surgical technique used. Surgical correction of craniosynostosis is not a new concept, but it was associated with a high morbidity and was very controversial in its early days. Almost simultaneously two surgeons reported their first experiences. In 1890, Odilon Lannelongue described the first incision of a suture, and in 1892 Lane described a technique for synostectomy.[3] The modern and successful treatment of cranial deformities and craniosynostosis was founded and decisively shaped by Tessier.[4]

In the following, we will discuss the various deformities, surgical techniques, and the expected results of treatment.

33.2 Classification

Craniosynostoses can be classified along several dimensions, which are now used in clinical assessment. Depending on the number of affected sutures, they may be described as "simple" or "isolated" if only one suture closes prematurely, or "complex" if more than one suture is affected.[5] Primary craniosynostosis describes the idiopathic premature closure of one or more cranial sutures without detectable genetic changes. Secondary craniosynostoses result from a number of pathologies and are often just an expression of the primary disease. Another possible classification is into syndromic or nonsyndromic types. The proportion of nonsyndromic is approximately 80 to 85%, with 15 to 20% correspondingly classified as syndromic.[6] In the latter, more than 100 known

syndromes are associated with craniosynostosis, the most important of which are listed in ▶ Table 33.1.

The phenotypic classification describes either the head shape or the underlying prematurely closed suture. The most frequently used terms are scaphocephaly in sagittal synostosis, brachycephaly with coronal synostosis, trigonocephaly in frontal (aka metopic) suture synostosis, and plagiocephaly in lambdoid synostosis (▶ Fig. 33.1).

33.3 Epidemiology

The incidence of craniosynostosis is estimated at 1 to 1.6 in 1,000 live births.[7] In England, it is estimated at 0.4:1,000, in Israel at 0.6:1,000,[8] and in France and in Holland at 0.47:1,000 and 0.64:1,000, respectively.[9] Similarly, the birth prevalence in a large U.S. cohort was estimated at 0.43:1,000.[10]

The frequency of each craniosynostosis is shown in ▶ Table 33.2. In most craniosynostoses, only one suture is affected, and in 5 to 15% of cases two or more sutures are closed prematurely.[11] Most craniosynostoses occur sporadically, with familial cases estimated to account for 7 to 14%,[7] which are mostly inherited in an autosomal dominant fashion. If one parent and one child are affected, the risk for craniosynostosis in the next child is

Table 33.1 Classification

Primary	Nonsyndromal (80–85%)	
	Syndromal (15–20%)	Apert's, Crouzon's, Pfeiffer's, Saethre–Chotzen
Secondary	Metabolic	Rickets, hyperthyroidism, hypophosphatemia
	Hematological	Polycythemia vera, sickle cell disease, thalassemia
	Pharmacological	Valproate, phenytoin, retinoids, methotrexate
	Structural	Microcephaly, shunt overdrainage

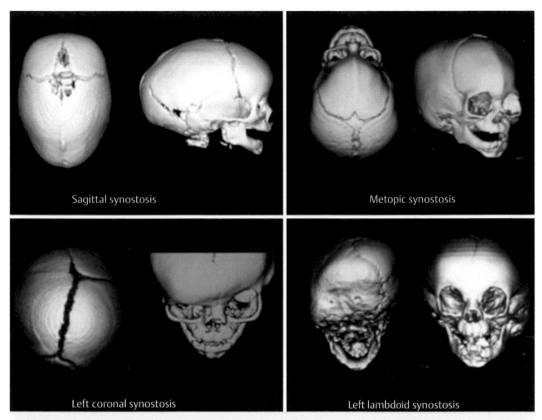

Fig. 33.1 3D computed tomography (CT) images of the typical bony changes in craniosynostosis.

Table 33.2 Epidemiology

Suture	Frequency	Male/female ratio	Familial
Sagittal	1/5,000	2–3:1 M:F	2–6%
Coronal	1/11,000	1:1–2 M:F	7–14%
Metopic	1/15,000	3:1 M:F	2–6%
Lambdoid	1/200,000	1:1–2 M:F	N/A

estimated to be 50%. If both parents are asymptomatic and two children are affected, the risk for the third child is estimated to be 25%.[12] Different family members may have involvement of different sutures.

33.4 Etiology and Genetic Factors

The etiology of craniosynostosis is unknown. However, some factors are known which may coincide with the occurrence of craniosynostosis. Multiple teratogens, hematological, and metabolic disorders have been associated with the early suture closure.

Also, maternal cigarette smoking during pregnancy leads to an increased risk of a single suture craniosynostosis.[13] Therefore, an accurate pregnancy and birth history is important. Specifically, intrauterine exposure to medicines, products of tobacco smoking, and drugs should be considered.[13,14,15,16] Further, intrauterine constriction in twin pregnancy,[7] abnormal position in the pelvis, amniotic bands, or oligohydramnios have been postulated as etiological factors[17] (▶ Table 33.1). Also, family history is important so that familial cases are not overlooked. Because of progress in molecular genetics, genetic mutations and interactions that are associated with premature suture closure have also been discovered. The physiology

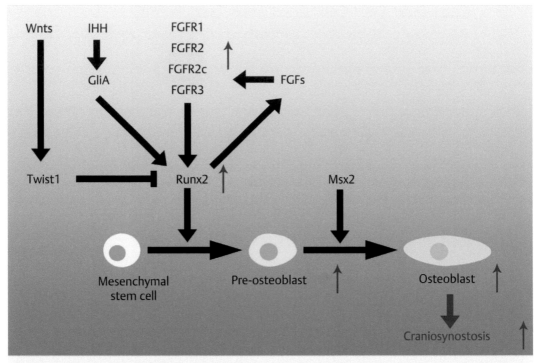

Fig. 33.2 Graphical illustration of the genes involved in craniosynostosis and their interactions. FGFR1, fibroblast growth factor receptor 1; FGFs, fibroblast growth factors.

of cranial suture growth and closure depends on a complex balance between the proliferation of mesenchymal stem cells within the cranial suture mesenchyme and their differentiation into osteoblasts at the osteogenic front[18] (▶ Fig. 33.2). Most syndromic craniosynostoses are caused by mutations in the genes that code for fibroblast growth factor receptors (FGFR1, FGFR2, and FGFR3) or the transcription factors Twist1, Runx2, and Msx2.[19,20,21] These mutations are the cause of approximately 20% of all craniosynostoses (▶ Table 33.3).

33.4.1 Clinical Disease and Radiological Investigation

The suspected diagnosis of craniosynostosis is primarily based on the presence of typical features on clinical examination, described in detail later. The deformity may be visible at birth, but often becomes apparent only within the first month of life. Persistent deformity 2 to 3 months after birth should be investigated. In children with syndromes, which can result in a secondary craniosynostosis, long-term follow-up should be performed.[22] The clinical examination must include a detailed neurological assessment to rule out associated pathologies. It is important to obtain a measurement of head circumference in order to exclude a microcephaly, which could indicate a secondary suture closure with underdevelopment of the cerebrum.

The diagnosis of craniosynostosis is primarily made clinically and confirmed by computed tomography (CT). If there is no clinical suspicion of a synostosis or the typical picture of positional plagiocephaly is observed, then CT is not indicated, in order to minimize radiation exposure. Therefore, medical assessment by a specialist with experience with this disease is important. In a clinically suspected craniosynostosis, further evaluation by cranial CT is indicated. This allows the determination of the prematurely closed suture and shows the characteristics of the deformity, including cranial contour and possible presence of thickening or ridging at the synostosis. Examples are shown in ▶ Fig. 33.1. The CT also serves to exclude other malformations[23] and may demonstrate hydrocephalus or indirect signs of increased intracranial pressure, the so-called thumb printing or beaten copper appearance of the tabula interna (▶ Fig. 33.3).

Table 33.3 Genetic factors

Gene	Mutation found in syndrome/symptom	Genetic alteration	Pathophysiological mechanism/gene function	Reference
FGFR1	Crouzon's, Pfeiffer's, Apert's, Beare–Stevenson, Jackson–Weiss	Gain-of-function	Activated FGF-signaling	5
FGFR2	Crouzon's, Pfeiffer's, Jackson–Weiss	Gain-of-function	Activated FGF-signaling	5
FGFR2c	Crouzon's, Apert's	Gain-of-function	Enhanced affinity for FGF7 and FGF10	5
FGFR3	Crouzon's, Muenke's	Gain-of-function	Activated FGF-signaling	5
Twist1	Saethre–Chotzen	Loss-of-function	Twist1 normal function: downregulation of Runx2	5,24
Msx2	Boston-type craniosynostosis	Gain-of-function	Promotes preosteoblast differentiation	25,26
Runx2/ Cbfa1	Pancraniosynostosis	Gain-of-function	Causes overossification. Runx2 deficient mice: complete bone loss	27
GliA	Greig's cephalopolysyndactyly with craniosynostosis	Unknown	Activated Gli3-signaling	28
NELL-1	Unilateral craniosynostosis	Gain-of-function	Unknown	29
FBN2, IGF2BP3, TINAGL1	Altered transcription in nonsyndromic craniosynostosis	FBN2, IGF2BP3: gain-of-function. TINAGL1: loss-of-function	In combination are associated with increased Runx2 expression	30

Abbreviation: FGFR, fibroblast growth factor receptor.

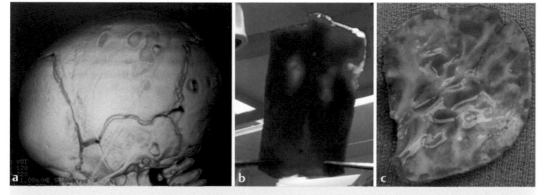

Fig. 33.3 Signs of a latent increased intracranial pressure. **(a)** 3D CT shows thinning of some sites of the inner surface of the skull ("thumb printing" or "beaten copper" appearance). Various pathologies with increased intracranial pressure can lead to this picture. **(b)** Example of a resected sagittal suture with some translucent patches. **(c)** Example of a resected coronal suture with "thumb printing" of the tabula interna.

33.5 Craniosynostoses and Their Treatment

33.5.1 Sagittal Craniosynostosis

The sagittal suture craniosynostosis, with an incidence of 1/5,000, is the most common craniosynostosis. The isolated premature ossification of the sagittal suture is found in 50 to 60% of craniosynostoses.[7] There are two to three times more boys than girls affected.[31] Because of the ossification of the sagittal suture, cranial growth is restricted in width, and there is a compensatory growth in length. This creates the head shape of scaphocephaly (boat-shaped skull), which is characterized by a narrow and elongated head with prominent occiput. The term *dolichocephaly* (elongated skull) describes the long head with a high forehead. In severe cases, there is a bifrontal prominent forehead (bifrontal bossing). In the clinical examination, suture ridging is apparent by palpation (▶ Fig. 33.4).

33.5.2 Coronal Craniosynostosis

With an incidence of 1/11,000, coronal craniosynostosis is the second most common craniosynostosis.[7] It accounts for approximately 20% of craniosynostoses. The ratio of girls to boys is 2:1.[32] The coronal synostosis may occur unilaterally or bilaterally. In the bilateral premature ossification of the coronal suture, the increased growth in cranial width and height is seen. This resulting brachycephaly (short skull) is characterized by a short head with a high forehead. Because of the bicoronal ossification, the anterior cranial fossa is shortened, resulting in shallow orbits with retracted orbital roof, which may be associated with hypertelorism, exophthalmos, and strabismus. Bicoronal synostoses are significantly more frequently familial than the unicoronal synostoses.[32] In the unilateral coronal synostosis (anterior plagiocephaly), an ipsilateral growth in width occurs, such that the ipsilateral forehead appears high and flat with a compensatory prominence of the contralateral forehead. Because of the restriction of the

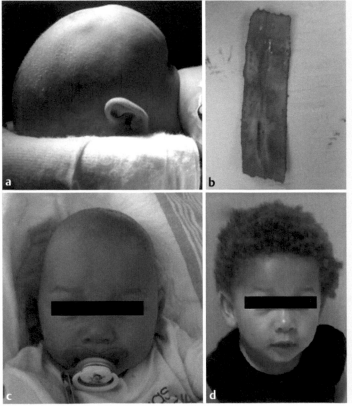

Fig. 33.4 Example of a child with sagittal craniosynostosis showing the typical head shape of scaphocephaly. **(a)** Characteristic long head shape with prominent occiput. **(b)** Example of an excised sagittal suture. **(c)** Preoperative image. **(d)** Two-year postoperative image.

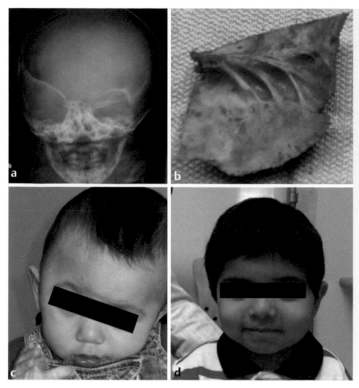

Fig. 33.5 Example of a child with unilateral coronal craniosynostosis on the right. **(a)** Characteristic harlequin eye on the ipsilateral right side with ipsilaterally strongly elevated lateral sphenoid wing. **(b)** Example of a fused coronal suture in the area of the lateral sphenoid wing. **(c)** Characteristic aspect of the anterior plagiocephaly with a right-sided coronal suture craniosynostosis with flattening of the ipsilateral forehead, lack of orbital roof protection on the right, and deviation of the nose to the opposite side. **(d)** Three-year postoperative control.

frontal growth on the side of the synostosis, there occurs an ipsilateral elongation of the sphenoid wing and the lower face, as well as elevation of the ipsilateral orbit, the classic image of the harlequin eye (▸ Fig. 33.5).

33.5.3 Metopic Craniosynostosis

The metopic craniosynostosis is the closure of the frontal suture (aka metopic suture). It occurs with an incidence of 1/15,000 live births, and is three times more common in boys than girls. The premature closure of the frontal suture results in a limitation of growth in width of the anterior cranial fossa and bilateral constriction of the frontal lobes. The phenotypic manifestation is a trigonocephaly, namely a triangular-shaped forehead (▸ Fig. 33.6). The reduction of growth in width often leads to hypotelorism and flattening of lateral orbital roofs. It is important to distinguish benign frontal suture prominence from a true metopic craniosynostosis. The frontal suture can ossify physiologically between 6 and 12 months, which may result in a so-called benign metopic ridge. Since in these cases the base of the skull develops normally, there is no hypotelorism and no limitation of the anterior cranial fossa. Benign

metopic ridging per se does not require treatment, but can be treated surgically for cosmetic reasons (▸ Fig. 33.6).

33.5.4 Lambdoid Craniosynostosis

The lambdoid suture is located between the occipital bone and the parietal bone. Lambdoid suture craniosynostosis is rare and manifests with an incidence of 1/200,000,[7] which is approximately 5% of all cases of craniosynostosis. When lambdoid craniosynostosis is unilateral, it results in ipsilateral posterior plagiocephaly. The one-sided flat back of the head ipsilateral to synostosis must be distinguished from postural plagiocephaly. In postural plagiocephaly, due to one-sided supine head posture preference, the ipsilateral ear shifts forward in relation to the contralateral ear and the ipsilateral forehead is prominent. In lambdoid craniosynostosis, there is a growth restriction of the lateral skull base so that the ipsilateral ear as well as the ipsilateral forehead is shifted to the rear in relation to the contralateral side (▸ Fig. 33.7 and ▸ Fig. 33.8). Thus, the head viewed from above resembles a parallelogram in postural plagiocephaly and a trapezoid in unilateral lambdoid craniosynostosis.

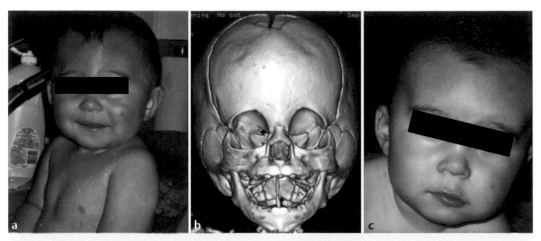

Fig. 33.6 Example of a child with metopic craniosynostosis. **(a)** Characteristic prominent frontal suture with triangular forehead shape and hypotelorism. **(b)** 3D CT of a metopic craniosynostosis. **(c)** Six-month postoperative control.

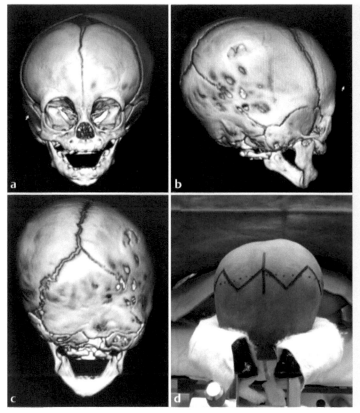

Fig. 33.7 Example of a child with lambdoid suture craniosynostosis. **(a–b)** 3D CT with characteristic posterior plagiocephaly due to early closure of the right lambdoid suture. **(c)** Noteworthy is the involvement of the entire skull base. **(d)** Patient positioning and skin incision for bilateral correction of posterior plagiocephaly.

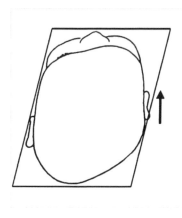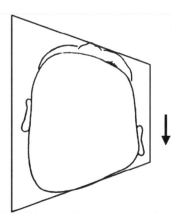

Fig. 33.8 Schematic illustration of head shape and ear positions in postural plagiocephaly (parallelogram, ipsilateral ear shifted forward) and unilateral posterior plagiocephaly in lambdoid suture craniosynostosis (trapezoid, ipsilateral ear shifted to the rear).

33.6 Surgical Treatment

33.6.1 Indication

Two main factors justify the indication to surgery. The first is correction of the skull deformity to prevent psychosocial disadvantages,[33] and the second is prevention of a potential increase in intracranial pressure.[34] Studies have demonstrated that up to 30% of children even with only single-suture craniosynostosis can present with an increased intracranial pressure.[35,36,37,38,39] Several studies were aimed to examine the neurocognitive development in children with single-suture craniosynostosis. Especially, reading and/or spelling learning disabilities were found in the long term in children with craniosynostosis compared to children without craniosynostosis.[40] It is debated whether an early operation can reduce the development of these deficits.[41]

33.6.2 Time of Treatment

The optimal time for surgical treatment of craniosynostosis is controversial. While older children better tolerate the surgery hemodynamically, the correction of the deformity and bone regeneration is better in younger children. Older children (> 6 months) tolerate the significant blood loss better than younger children. However, in children older than 12 months, the operation may take longer due to the more extensive bone reconstruction necessary to cover bone defects, which in turn is associated with increased blood loss.[42] Most surgeons prefer to operate on children with craniosynostosis between 3 and 12 months. We tend to perform surgery for sagittal suture synostosis between 4 and 6 months of age and all others (coronal, metopic, and

lambdoid) between 6 and 12 months.[42] It is also postulated that cognitive development is better if the child is operated before 12 months of age.[43] Timing is also dependent on the method of operation. The newer endoscopic procedures especially with sagittal craniosynostosis are performed between the ages of 1 and 4 months.[44,45]

33.6.3 Surgery

Numerous surgical techniques and nuances are described in the literature. The general principle is to allow free growth of the skull by opening or removing the closed suture. In the sagittal suture craniosynostosis, a so-called strip craniectomy is performed where the closed sagittal suture is removed (▶ Fig. 33.3b and ▶ Fig. 33.4b). Important for the preparation and planning of an operation is the presence of an open anterior or posterior fontanelle. These are exposed at the beginning of the operation and the sagittal synostectomy, extending from the anterior fontanelle (junction of the sagittal, coronal, and frontal suture) to the posterior fontanelle (interface of the lambdoid and sagittal suture), is performed. Subsequently, to correct the long and narrow head shape in scaphocephaly, lateral osteotomies are performed in the area of the parietal and frontal bone. This allows the biparietal diameter to increase and a wider head shape to develop. To reduce the elongated head shape, which is often associated with a pointed occipital bone, a remodeling of the occipital bone is carried out by multiple osteotomies. Usually, a fixation with resorbable plates or sutures is not necessary in the correction of sagittal synostosis. In older children (> 12 months), after the period of rapid head growth, fixation may be necessary to maintain the corrected head shape. In younger children, the modeling essentially takes places due to the physiological rapid head growth.

In metopic and coronal craniosynostosis, a fronto-orbital advancement is performed in most centers[42] (▶ Fig. 33.9). For that purpose, a bifrontal craniotomy is first performed with particular care to protect the superior sagittal sinus. Countless variations exist concerning the posterior and lateral extent of the craniotomy. This is then followed by the en bloc removal of the superior and lateral margins of the orbit. Osteotomies at the orbital roof, nasoethmoidal, and lateral in the area of sphenoid wing must be made to remove the so-called orbital bandeau (▶ Fig. 33.9b). Both bones, the frontal bone and the "orbital bandeau," are then reattached in an advanced position (▶ Fig. 33.9b) using resorbable plates and screws. This is done by placing the lateral orbital margins in a normal advanced position and thus correcting the entry angle of the orbit. The deformity of the forehead, which is either trigonocephalic or brachycephalic, is corrected by remodeling of the frontal bone.

In lambdoid suture synostosis, an occipital craniotomy is performed with correction of the posterior plagiocephaly (▶ Fig. 33.7). Again, there are countless variations with unilateral or bilateral correction, exchange of the affected occipital squama with the unaffected, and rotations of the bone plates.

In the endoscopic techniques, the correction is carried out primarily through small incisions in the region of the closed suture. Under endoscopic view, a subperiosteal preparation of the suture is performed followed by a synostectomy. The children then undergo helmet therapy for modeling of the head shape for 7 to 12 months, as is done for positional plagiocephaly. The average hospital stay is 3 to 5 days for the open technique and 1 to 2 days for the endoscopic method.

The most critical point and therefore also the most frequently cited complication is blood loss requiring transfusion. Meticulous hemostasis at each step of the operation is essential. Especially in the more complex fronto-orbital advancement surgery for coronal and metopic synostosis, the blood loss is significant. With a standard technique and an experienced team, the blood loss can be limited to a mean of 120 mL.[42] However, blood loss of about 250 mL, which corresponds to one-third to one-fourth of the total blood volume of the child, is often mentioned in the literature.[45] The amount of blood loss correlates with the operation time and the age of the patient.[42,45] Other surgical risks include intraoperative air embolism, which, however, can be well controlled with modern anesthesia, good patient positioning, and standard surgical techniques. Another avoidable complication with modern anesthesia is prevention of hypothermia. The risk of infection is reduced by prophylactic perioperative antibiotics.

33.6.4 Outcome

The mortality rate is now below 1% and the morbidity rate around 5%. Morbidity is especially due to infections, which are reported to be between 1 and 10%.[42,46] The risk is increased in reoperations or corrections of complex syndromes. The same applies to the risk of dural injury with cerebrospinal fluid fistula, also occurring especially in reoperations. Postoperative hyperthermia on day 2 to 3 is often observed but rarely associated with infection.[46,47]

A satisfactory correction in craniosynostosis surgery depends on multiple factors. An important factor is the age at correction. The head growth after correction of craniosynostosis is not different from the normal growth and a significant remodeling thereby takes place after the operation. Generally, a correction is recommended within the first year of life.[28] Corrections after the first year of life are more complex because the natural remodeling is limited and the capacity to grow bone is reduced. Especially in the correction of trigonocephaly and coronal craniosynostosis, the timing seems to be important. The highest relapse rates were shown for first operations before 6 months of age and after 12 months of age,[49] whereas the operations with the best outcomes were with patients aged between 6 and 12 months.[50] It is expected that after the first operation a satisfactory correction of the deformity can be reached in over 90% of patients.[42,47]

33.7 Conclusion

The treatment of craniosynostosis in the first year of life is essential to obtain good surgical results. Also, surgery is indicated to prevent a potential increase in intracranial pressure, which can occur in up to 30% of affected children. Craniosynostosis cannot be treated conservatively. The treatment should take place in a center with a specialized and experienced team of surgeons, anesthetists, and intensive care physicians.

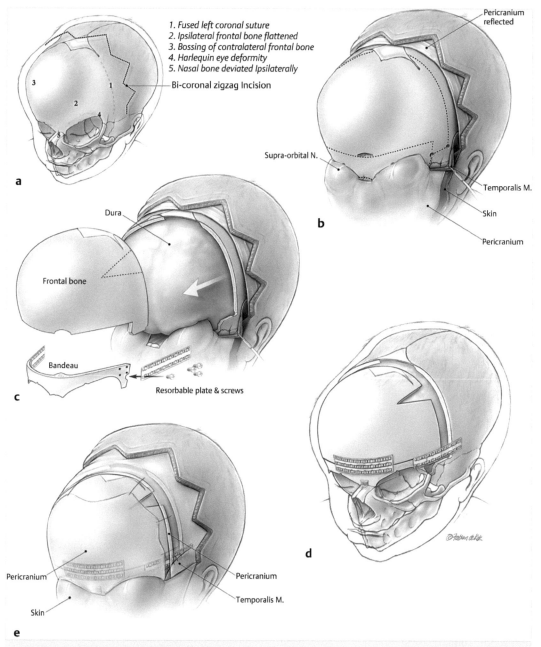

1. Fused left coronal suture
2. Ipsilateral frontal bone flattened
3. Bossing of contralateral frontal bone
4. Harlequin eye deformity
5. Nasal bone deviated Ipsilaterally

Bi-coronal zigzag Incision

Pericranium reflected

Supra-orbital N.

Temporalis M.

Skin

Pericranium

b

a

Dura

Frontal bone

Bandeau

Resorbable plate & screws

c

d

Pericranium

Pericranium

Temporalis M.

Skin

e

Fig. 33.9 **(a-e)** Illustration of the operating technique for **(a)** Fronto-orbital advancement with bifrontal craniotomy and removal of the orbital bandeau. **(b, c)** After the remodeling, the reconstruction with resorbable plates and screws is performed. (Reproduced with permission from Guzman et al.[42])

33.8 Common Clinical Questions

1. What is craniosynostosis and how are craniosynostoses classified?

2. What are the most common genetic causes of syndromic craniosynostoses?

3. How is craniosynostosis diagnosed, and what is "thumb printing" or "beaten copper" appearance?

4. What is the indication for surgery?

33.9 Answers to Common Clinical Questions

1. Craniosynostosis is the premature closure of one or more cranial sutures. Craniosynostoses can be classified as "simple" or "isolated" versus "complex," primary versus secondary, syndromic versus nonsyndromic (▶ Table 33.1), or by phenotypic classification (▶ Fig. 33.1) based on head shape or the underlying prematurely closed suture (since skull growth is restricted in the direction perpendicular to the prematurely closed suture).

2. See ▶ Table 33.3 and ▶ Fig. 33.2. Most syndromic craniosynostoses are caused by mutations in the genes that code for fibroblast growth factor receptors (FGFR1, FGFR2, and FGFR3 or the transcription factors Twist1, Runx2, and Msx2.

3. The suspicion of craniosynostosis is based on clinical evaluation. Typical sign is skull deformity persisting 2 to 3 months after birth and first occurring at birth or within the first month of life. Clinical evaluation includes a detailed neurological assessment to rule out associated pathologies, measurement of head circumference in order to exclude a microcephaly, and the exclusion of positional plagiocephaly by head shape and ear position (▶ Fig. 33.8). In a clinically suspected craniosynostosis, further evaluation by cranial CT is indicated. This will demonstrate the prematurely closed suture or sutures and the characteristics of the deformity with the cranial contour and/or ridging at the synostosis (▶ Fig. 33.1). "Thumb printing" and "beaten copper" describe the radiological evidence of increased intracranial pressure and are evident from the appearance of the tabula interna on skull CT or X-ray (▶ Fig. 33.3).

4. Two factors justify surgery: first, the correction of the skull deformity to prevent psychosocial disadvantages and, secondly, the prevention of a potential increase in intracranial pressure.

References

[1] Wiegand C, Richards P. Measurement of intracranial pressure in children: a critical review of current methods. Dev Med Child Neurol. 2007; 49(12):935–941

[2] Cloonan YK, Collett BR, Speltz ML, Anderka M, Werler MM. Psychosocial Outcomes in children with and without non-syndromic craniosynostosis: findings from two studies. Cleft Palate Craniofac J. 2013; 50(4):406–413

[3] Lane LC. Craniectomy for relief of mental imbecility due to premature sutural closure and microcephalus. JAMA. 1892; 18:49–50

[4] Tessier P. Treatment of facial dysmorphias in craniofacial dysostosis, Crouzon's and Apert's diseases. Total osteotomy and sagittal displacement of the facial massive. Faciostenosis, sequelae of Lefort 3 fracture [in French]. Dtsch Zahn Mund Kieferheilkd Zentralbl Gesamte. 1971; 57(9):302–320

[5] Kimonis V, Gold JA, Hoffman TL, Panchal J, Boyadjiev SA. Genetics of craniosynostosis. Semin Pediatr Neurol. 2007; 14 (3):150–161

[6] van Veelen ML, Mathijssen I, Arnaud E, Renier D. Craniosynostosis. Berlin: Springer; 2010

[7] Keating RF. Craniosynostosis: diagnosis and management in the new millennium. Pediatr Ann. 1997; 26 10:600–612

[8] Shuper A, Merlob P, Grunebaum M, Reisner SH. The incidence of isolated craniosynostosis in the newborn infant. Am J Dis Child. 1985; 139(1):85–86

[9] Kweldam CF, van der Vlugt JJ, van der Meulen JJ. The incidence of craniosynostosis in the Netherlands, 1997–2007. J Plast Reconstr Aesthet Surg. 2011; 64(5):583–588

[10] Boulet SL, Rasmussen SA, Honein MA. A population-based study of craniosynostosis in metropolitan Atlanta, 1989–2003. Am J Med Genet A. 2008; 146A(8):984–991

[11] Cohen MM Jr, MacLean RE.Craniosynostosis: Diagnosis, Evaluation, and Management. 2nd ed. New York, NY: Oxford University Press; 2000

[12] Cohen MM, Jr. Sutural biology and the correlates of craniosynostosis. Am J Med Genet. 1993; 47(5):581–616

[13] Alderman BW, Bradley CM, Greene C, Fernbach SK, Barón AE. Increased risk of craniosynostosis with maternal cigarette smoking during pregnancy. Teratology. 1994; 50(1):13–18

[14] Beeram MR, Abedin M, Shoroye A, Jayam-Trouth A, Young M, Reid Y. Occurrence of craniosynostosis in neonates exposed to cocaine and tobacco in utero. J Natl Med Assoc. 1993; 85 (11):865–868

[15] Gardner JS, Guyard-Boileau B, Alderman BW, Fernbach SK, Greene C, Mangione EJ. Maternal exposure to prescription and non-prescription pharmaceuticals or drugs of abuse and risk of craniosynostosis. Int J Epidemiol. 1998; 27(1): 64–67

[16] Lajeunie E, Barcik U, Thorne JA, El Ghouzzi V, Bourgeois M, Renier D. Craniosynostosis and fetal exposure to sodium valproate. J Neurosurg. 2001; 95(5):778–782

[17] Higginbottom MC, Jones KL, James HE. Intrauterine constraint and craniosynostosis. Neurosurgery. 1980; 6(1): 39–44

[18] Lenton KA, Nacamuli RP, Wan DC, Helms JA, Longaker MT. Cranial suture biology. Curr Top Dev Biol. 2005; 66:287–328

[19] Du X, Xie Y, Xian CJ, Chen L. Role of FGFs/FGFRs in skeletal development and bone regeneration. J Cell Physiol. 2012; 227(12):3731–3743

[20] Melville H, Wang Y, Taub PJ, Jabs EW. Genetic basis of potential therapeutic strategies for craniosynostosis. Am J Med Genet A. 2010; 152A(12):3007–3015

[21] Bellus GA, Gaudenz K, Zackai EH, et al. Identical mutations in three different fibroblast growth factor receptor genes in autosomal dominant craniosynostosis syndromes. Nat Genet. 1996; 14(2):174–176

[22] Currarino G. Sagittal synostosis in X-linked hypophosphatemic rickets and related diseases. Pediatr Radiol. 2007; 37(8):805–812

[23] Boop FA, Chadduck WM, Shewmake K, Teo C. Outcome analysis of 85 patients undergoing the pi procedure for

correction of sagittal synostosis. J Neurosurg. 1996; 85(1): 50–55

[24] Yousfi M, Lasmoles F, Lomri A, Delannoy P, Marie PJ. Increased bone formation and decreased osteocalcin expression induced by reduced Twist dosage in Saethre-Chotzen syndrome. J Clin Invest. 2001; 107(9):1153–1161

[25] Bernardini L, Castori M, Capalbo A, et al. Syndromic craniosynostosis due to complex chromosome 5 rearrangement and MSX2 gene triplication. Am J Med Genet A. 2007; 143A(24):2937–2943

[26] Ma L, Golden S, Wu L, Maxson R. The molecular basis of Boston-type craniosynostosis: the Pro148->His mutation in the N-terminal arm of the MSX2 homeodomain stabilizes DNA binding without altering nucleotide sequence preferences. Hum Mol Genet. 1996; 5(12):1915–1920

[27] Greives MR, Odessey EA, Waggoner DJ, et al. RUNX2 quadruplication: additional evidence toward a new form of syndromic craniosynostosis. J Craniofac Surg. 2013; 24(1): 126–129

[28] Tanimoto Y, Veistinen L, Alakurtti K, Takatalo M, Rice DP. Prevention of premature fusion of calvarial suture in GLI-Kruppel family member 3 (Gli3)-deficient mice by removing one allele of Runt-related transcription factor 2 (Runx2). J Biol Chem. 2012; 287(25):21429–21438

[29] Ting K, Vastardis H, Mulliken JB, et al. Human NELL-1 expressed in unilateral coronal synostosis. J Bone Miner Res. 1999; 14(1):80–89

[30] Stamper BD, Park SS, Beyer RP, Bammler TK, Cunningham ML. Unique sex-based approach identifies transcriptomic biomarkers associated with non-syndromic craniosynostosis. Gene Regul Syst Bio. 2012; 6:81–92

[31] Lajeunie E, Le Merrer M, Bonaïti-Pellie C, Marchac D, Renier D. Genetic study of scaphocephaly. Am J Med Genet. 1996; 62 (3):282–285

[32] Lajeunie E, Le Merrer M, Bonaïti-Pellie C, Marchac D, Renier D. Genetic study of nonsyndromic coronal craniosynostosis. Am J Med Genet. 1995; 55(4):500–504

[33] Pertschuk MJ, Whitaker LA. Psychosocial considerations in craniofacial deformity. Clin Plast Surg. 1987; 14(1):163–168

[34] Tamburrini G, Caldarelli M, Massimi L, Santini P, Di Rocco C. Intracranial pressure monitoring in children with single suture and complex craniosynostosis: a review. Childs Nerv Syst. 2005; 21(10):913–921

[35] Renier D, Sainte-Rose C, Marchac D, Hirsch JF. Intracranial pressure in craniostenosis. J Neurosurg. 1982; 57(3):370–377

[36] Whittle IR, Johnston IH, Besser M. Intracranial pressure changes in craniostenosis. Surg Neurol. 1984; 21(4):367–372

[37] Shipster C, Hearst D, Somerville A, Stackhouse J, Hayward R, Wade A. Speech, language, and cognitive development in children with isolated sagittal synostosis. Dev Med Child Neurol. 2003; 45(1):34–43

[38] Baird LC, Gonda D, Cohen SR, et al. Craniofacial reconstruction as a treatment for elevated intracranial pressure. Childs Nerv Syst. 2012; 28(3):411–418

[39] Bristol RE, Lekovic GP, Rekate HL. The effects of craniosynostosis on the brain with respect to intracranial pressure. Semin Pediatr Neurol. 2004; 11(4):262–267

[40] Magge SN, Westerveld M, Pruzinsky T, Persing JA. Long-term neuropsychological effects of sagittal craniosynostosis on child development. J Craniofac Surg. 2002; 13(1):99–104

[41] Lekovic GP, Bristol RE, Rekate HL. Cognitive impact of craniosynostosis. Semin Pediatr Neurol. 2004; 11(4):305–310

[42] Guzman R, Looby JF, Schendel SA, Edwards MS. Fronto-orbital advancement using an en bloc frontal bone craniectomy. Neurosurgery. 2011; 68(1) Suppl Operative: 68–74

[43] Arnaud E, Meneses P, Lajeunie E, Thorne JA, Marchac D, Renier D. Postoperative mental and morphological outcome for nonsyndromic brachycephaly. Plast Reconstr Surg. 2002; 110(1):6–12, discussion 13

[44] Jimenez DF, Barone CM. Early treatment of anterior calvarial craniosynostosis using endoscopic-assisted minimally invasive techniques. Childs Nerv Syst. 2007; 23(12):1411–1419

[45] Seruya M, Oh AK, Rogers GF, et al. Factors related to blood loss during fronto-orbital advancement. J Craniofac Surg. 2012; 23(2):358–362

[46] Esparza J, Hinojosa J. Complications in the surgical treatment of craniosynostosis and craniofacial syndromes: apropos of 306 transcranial procedures. Childs Nerv Syst. 2008; 24(12): 1421–1430

[47] Esparza J, Hinojosa J, García-Recuero I, Romance A, Pascual B, Martínez de Aragón A. Surgical treatment of isolated and syndromic craniosynostosis. Results and complications in 283 consecutive cases. Neurocirugia (Astur). 2008; 19(6): 509–529

[48] Marchac D, Renier D. Craniosynostosis. World J Surg. 1989; 13(4):358–365

[49] Selber JC, Brooks C, Kurichi JE, Temmen T, Sonnad SS, Whitaker LA. Long-term results following fronto-orbital reconstruction in nonsyndromic unicoronal synostosis. Plast Reconstr Surg. 2008; 121(5):251–260

[50] Foster KA, Frim DM, McKinnon M. Recurrence of synostosis following surgical repair of craniosynostosis. Plast Reconstr Surg. 2008; 121(3):70–76

34 Management of Craniofacial Syndromes

Miguel A. Medina III, Gerhard S. Mundinger, Amir H. Dorafshar

34.1 Introduction

Roughly 15% of patients with craniosynostosis present with an underlying syndromic condition. The presence of associated syndromic anomalies, coupled with the rarity of these disorders and the relatively increased severity of synostosis, makes surgical management of patients with most syndromic craniosynostosis, such as Apert's and Pfeiffer's syndrome, more challenging and nuanced when compared to patients with nonsyndromic synostosis. In contrast, many patients with unilateral coronal synostosis may have underlying identifiable mutations, as in Muenke's syndrome, that confer relatively mild phenotypes and offer targets for early pharmacological intervention. The craniofacial surgeon may be the first person to thoroughly examine a child with craniofacial anomalies and must endeavor to identify associated abnormalities and anomalies that may be present. By definition, syndromes are a pattern of anomalies that occur across noncontiguous embryological sites; however, they are pathogenically related.[1]

34.2 Embryology/Development

The developing skull and face is derived from three tissue lines: the membranous neurocranium, the cartilaginous neurocranium, and the visceral splanchnocranium. Facial development occurs between 3 and 8 weeks of gestation. Screening ultrasound can reliably identify craniofacial abnormalities between 14 and 28 weeks.[2]

34.2.1 Calvarial Skeletal Ossification

The fetal calvarium (membranous neurocranium) ossifies through intramembranous ossification (bone develops directly from mesenchymal precursor). The dura and the periosteum together provide osteogenic signals for the growing calvarium; however, unlike the periosteum, the dura loses its osteogenic potential in late infancy/early childhood.[3] The cranial base is composed of cartilaginous neurocranium and ossifies through endochondral ossification. These tissues are first cartilaginous structures before undergoing progressive replacement by bone. In the infant craniofacial skeleton, the margins of the cranial base form synchondroses allowing continued growth. Restriction of growth at these interfaces result in many types of midfacial chondrodysplasias. The cranial vault in particular grows in response to brain growth. These bones grow in a perpendicular fashion to their sutures. The cranial base responds with cartilaginous growth followed by ossification creating a malleable base that responds to calvarial growth.

Herniation of the cerebellar tonsils occurs in a significant percentage of children with syndromic craniosynostosis, and is thought to be an acquired anomaly resulting from downward pressure on the cerebellar tonsils due to relatively decreased intracranial volume. By increasing intracranial volume, anterior vault decompression has proven effective in correcting tonsilar herniation in asymptomatic patients, though herniation may recur over time.[4] Posterior vault remodeling with suboccipital decompression is recommended for symptomatic patients with cerebellar tonsillar herniation and for patients with syndromic Chiari malformations.[5] Additionally, in children with bicoronal craniosynostosis, turribrachycephaly, and evidence of elevated intracranial pressure (ICP), posterior expansion becomes the surgical priority. This may be achieved through a single operation or through distraction.

34.2.2 Facial Skeletal Ossification

The facial skeleton is derived from the visceral splanchnocranium. The midfacial skeleton and mandible both undergo intramembranous ossification. Final facial skeletal growth is not achieved until late adolescence/early adulthood.

34.2.3 Facial Clefting

Orofacial clefting may result in cranial base defects, encephaloceles, and hypertelorism. The most commonly accepted classification scheme for facial

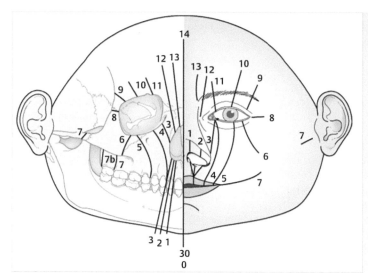

Fig. 34.1 Tessier classification. (Reproduced with permission from Anatomical classification of facial, cranio-facial and latero-facial clefts. J Maxillofac Surg. 1976.)

clefting was described by Tessier (▶ Fig. 34.1). Clefts 10 to 14 are most likely to require a combined neurosurgical and plastic surgical approach.

34.3 Genetics

34.3.1 Syndromic

- FGFR: Mutations of genes in the fibroblast growth factor receptor (FGFR) family account for the majority of known mutations in syndromic craniosynostosis. These mutations are generally activating, which accounts for observed autosomal dominant transmission patterns of all craniofacial syndromes caused by FGFR mutations.[6] FGFR1, FGFR2, and FGFR3 signaling modulates osteoblast activity in both endochondral and intramembranous bone ossification.[7] These receptors contain three major immunoglobulinlike regions with variable binding affinity for 22 known FGF ligands.[6] Activation and homodimerization of receptors facilitate downstream signaling via the MAP/ERK and PI3K/AKT signaling cascades.[8] Mutations in FGFR genes account for Apert's, Cruzon's, Pfeiffer's, and Muenke's syndromes, among others.[9]
- MSX: A gain-of-function mutation in the muscle segment homeobox 2 (MSX2) accounts for Boston-type craniosynostosis,[10] which has been identified in one cohort in the Boston, MA, area.[6] Expression and suture involvement is variable, accounting for variable phenotypes, from fronto-orbital recession to cloverleaf skull deformities.[9]
- TWIST1: Over 100 mutations of the helix-loop-helix transcription factor TWIST1, accounting for Saethre–Chotzen syndrome, have been identified.[7] Mutations include nucleotide substitutions (missense and nonsense), deletions, insertions, duplications, and complex rearrangements. These loss-of-function mutations result in haploinsufficiency, and cluster at the DNA binding and dimerization domains of the protein.

34.3.2 Associated Disorders/Anomalies

It would be beyond the scope of this chapter to provide an exhaustive list of associated anomalies in children with syndromic craniofacial disorders. However, it is important to note the other dysmorphisms are common in the extremities (syndactyly is especially common). Additionally, cardiac defects such as patent ductus arteriosus (PDA), conotruncal defects, and atrial septal defects (ASDs) are common with frontonasal dysplasias. Other overlooked affected areas in syndromic children are genitourinary dysmorphologies and vertebral anomalies.[1] It is also worth noting many children will fall into the unnamed syndrome category where syndromic pathology is present but has yet to fall into a well-described pathogenic/genetic mechanism.

34.3.3 Craniofacial Syndromes

As over 180 syndromes involve craniosynostosis[11] or craniofacial dysplasia, only the most common and well characterized will be discussed here. There is significant overlap between Apert's and Crouzon's syndrome (this at one time were thought to be the same entity), while Muenke's, Pfeiffer's, and Sathre–Chotzen syndromes are similar with distinctions in associated anomalies and facial dysmorphology patterns.

Apert's Syndrome

Apert's syndrome (1 in 60,000–90,000 births) is characterized by turribrachycephaly, forehead retrusion, midface retrusion, exorbitism, beaked nose, lateral canthal dystopia, downward slanting palpebral fissures, trapezoidal upper lip, eyebrows with a break in continuity,[12] and open mouth breathing.[7] Cleft palate and hearing loss due to fused ossicles may also be present. Central to the clinical diagnosis is complex symmetric acrocephalosyndactyly of the hands and feet. Radiohumeral fusion is variably present. Malformations of the central nervous system are numerous, and include hydrocephalus, ventriculomegaly, megalencephaly, gyral malformations, and defects in the corpus callosum, septum pellucidum, hippocampus, and cerebral cortex.[13] Skeletal pathology includes bilateral coronal synostosis. Initially, there may be a wide calvarial defect from the posterior fontanel to the glabella, but this typically closes over time. Patients have variable degrees of neurodevelopmental delay. Two mutations, FGFR2 S252 W and P253 R, account for 71 and 26% of cases, respectively.[11] Inheritance is autosomal dominant. Management of children with Apert's syndrome is complex, including surgical correction of craniosynostosis, cleft palate, and midface hypoplasia. Treatment typically includes a combination of calvarial vault remodeling, monobloc advancement with distraction,[14] Le Fort III[15] osteotomies, facial bipartition,[16] and/or midface distraction,[17] depending on the severity and location of vault and midface deformities.[18,19]

Crouzon's Syndrome

Crouzon's patients (1 in 65,000 births) typically demonstrate hypertelorism, divergent strabismus, midface hypoplasia, proptosis, relative mandibular prognathism, and a beaked nose.[7] Optic atrophy, found in approximately 20% of Crouzon's patients, and the lack of hand and foot syndactyly, distinguishes this syndrome from Apert's syndrome.[12] Craniosynostosis is typically bicoronal, with occasional early pansynostosis.[7] Crouzon's patients appear to have the highest incidence of cerebellar tonsilar (non-Chiari) herniation, with up to 71% of patients affected in some series.[4] There are no associated limb features, and intelligence is normal. Features of the disorder are frequently seen in relatives. Crouzon's is typically caused by FGFR2 mutations. Crouzon's syndrome with acanthosis nigricans of the axilla and groin (<5% of cases) is caused by the FGFR3 (A391E) mutation.[7] Goals of surgery are aimed at correction of turricephaly, and include bifrontal advancement with anterior vault remodeling between 6 months and 2 years of age.[9,19] In particular, most institutions now initially perform posterior vault expansion, followed by anterior vault remodeling, then in later childhood address facial deformity through monobloc advancement or Le Fort III advancement.

Pfeiffer's Syndrome

Phenotypic presentation of Pfeiffer's syndrome (1 in 100,000 births) is variable: patients typically have turribrachycephaly, hypertelorism, strabismus, choanal stenosis, midface hypoplasia, short, broad thumbs and toes, auditory canal atresia, airway obstruction, variable brachydactyly, and variable craniosynostoses.[7] Anomalies of the thumbs and toes can aid in clinically distinguishing Pfeiffer's syndrome from Crouzon's syndrome. The posterior skull may develop a "swiss cheese" appearance due to increased intracranial pressure in the setting of multisuture synostosis.[20] Central nervous system anomalies are common, and acquired Chiari malformations may be present in as many at 50% of cases.[21] Generally, bicoronal craniosynostosis is present, with multiple other sutures variably involved.[19,20] Pfeiffer's syndrome has been divided into three subtypes based on calvarial and midface severity as follows[7]: type 1: mildest and most common clinical presentation, and with least intellectual impairment; type 2: more severe, with cloverleaf skull, severe proptosis, medially deviated toes and thumbs, hydrocephalus, seizures, and intellectual disability; type 3: similar to type 2, but without cloverleaf skull, yet more severe mental disability and nonsynostotic anomalies. Greater than 95% of patients with this syndrome have FGFR2 mutations.[11] The remainder have FGFR1 mutations. Inheritance is autosomal dominant. Goals of craniofacial surgery include correction of proptosis, reduction of ICP, correction of airway obstruction, and anterior cranial vault remodeling.[19] Choice of surgical procedure is based on presenting symptoms and morphology, with probable benefits to earlier surgery in types 2 and 3 patients, and posterior decompression with symptomatic Chiari malformations in patients greater than 1 year of age.[20] As with Apert's patients, surgical management is complex and highly tailored to patient needs, with debate regarding timing and indications for specific procedures.[9,19,20]

Saethre–Chotzen Syndrome

Saethre–Chotzen syndrome (1 in 25,000–50,000 births) is characterized by a low-set hairline, deviated nose with beaked appearance, prominent chin, ptosis, and small ears with a prominent horizontal Cruz. Syndactyly of the index and long fingers is variably present. Less common features include cleft palate, maxillary hypoplasia, and hearing loss. Intelligence is typically normal, but may be abnormal with complete TWIST1 deletion. Phenotypic presentation may be mild and mimic nonsyndromic coronal synostosis. Patients typically have unicoronal or bicoronal synostosis, but may have metopic and sagittal synostosis as well. The majority of Saethre–Chotzen cases (40–80%) are caused by variable TWIST1 mutations, including substitutions, deletions, and rearrangements.[11] Inheritance is autosomal dominant. Goals of surgery include correction of facial asymmetry in unicoronal synostosis, reduction of ICP, and correction of midfacial hypoplasia.[22] Cleft palate repair typically follows cranial vault remodeling.

Muenke's Syndrome

Similar to Saethre–Chotzen, patients with Muenke's syndrome (1 in 30,000 births) display great clinical variability, and may have only mild unicoronal synostosis.[9] Phenotypes range from mild anterior plagiocephaly to brachycephaly, to cloverleaf skull deformity from multisuture synostosis.[7] Craniosynostosis is typically uni- or bicoronal. Patients may also have midface hypoplasia and ocular hypertelorism, though this is less common. Associated findings may include Klippel–Feil cervical anomaly, brachydactyly, and carpal bone fusion. Intelligence is usually normal. Muenke's syndrome is caused by a single FGFR3 mutation (P250R).[11] Inheritance is autosomal dominant. Variable expression accounts for the wide range of clinical findings, and this mutation may account for 20% of coronal synostosis cases. All patients with uni- or bicoronal synostosis should therefore be screened for this mutation,[9] and screening of patients with unclassified brachycephaly may result in increased diagnoses of this

syndrome.[23] Goals of surgery include correction of facial asymmetry, correction of turribrachycephaly in bicoronal synostosis, and reduction of ICP.[9,24]

Carpenter's Syndrome

Carpenter's syndrome (1 in 1,000,000 births) is characterized by any combination of multiple suture craniosynostosis in association with polydactyl, syndactyly, obesity, hypogenitalism, and congenital heart disease.[9] The degree of developmental delay is variable.[11] Loss-of-function RAB23 mutations disrupting vesicular transport protein cascades and sonic hedgehog signaling are thought to account for this syndrome.[11] Inheritance is autosomal recessive. Given the variable phenotypic presentation of this disorder, corrective surgery is dependent on suture involvement and deformation severity, and generally involves correction of anterior fossa underdevelopment.[25]

Craniofrontonasal Dysplasia

Patients with craniofrontonasal dysplasia (1 in 100,000–120,000 births) demonstrate brachycephaly or plagiocephaly due to coronal synostosis, hypertelorism (frequently asymmetric), cleft lip–cleft palate, limb abnormalities, frizzy curled hair, and longitudinal ridging and splitting of nails.[9,26] Mutations of the EFNB1 gene on Xq12, encoding a transmembrane protein, are responsible.[11] Transmission is X-linked, females are more severely affected than males, and severity increases with increased parental age.[9] Surgical correction typically includes staged four-wall orbital box osteotomies or facial bipartition (depending on degree of bimaxillary cant and occlusal plane deformities).[19,26]

Cranial Clefts

These are clefts of the superolateral orbit and extend through the frontal bone and/or the cranial base. They are usually associated with lower orofacial clefting as described by Tessier. Clefts 10 to 14 may result in hypertelorism and/or encephaloceles are repaired with respect to closure of the encephalocele and correction of the hypertelorism. These clefts tend to be rare and can in many cases be associated with severe central nervous system (CNS) anomalies and poor life expectancy.

34.4 Surgical Approaches

The standard craniofacial approaches are the fronto-orbital advancement (FOA), the monobloc/

Le Fort III advancement, facial bipartition, and orbital box osteotomies. These operations and variations of them form the basic foundation for correction of all craniofacial dysplasias.

- Indications: Elevated ICP, exorbitism/corneal exposure, normalization of craniofacial morphology, and airway obstruction.
- Typical timing and staging of procedures:
  - 6–8 months: Posterior vault remodeling if required (elevated ICP, severe turribrachycephaly).
  - 7–12 months: FOA, with calvarial remodeling for associated craniosynostosis deformities.
  - 7–10 years of age: Midfacial advancement and correction of orbital dystopias with treatment options including onobloc advancement, extracranial Le Fort III advancement, facial bipartition, or orbital box osteotomies, depending on type and degree of deformity. Midfacial correction is greatly individualized to each patient's particular dysmorphology.
  - 15–18 years of age: Orthognathic surgery for correction of final occlusion at skeletal maturity.

34.4.1 Fronto-Orbital Advancement

Indications/Procedure

The most common intracranial craniofacial procedure is the FOA. A common feature among many craniofacial dysmorphologies is a retrusive frontal bar. In addition, the osteotomies for the FOA form the foundation for all other craniofacial advancement procedures. In particular, it is critical to understand the cranio-orbital relationship in major craniofacial malformations; the majority of these disorders will exhibit some degree of hyper- or hypotelorbitism, vertical dystopia, or frank exorbitism.[27] The degree of frontal bar retrusion is measured from the anthropometric points orbitale superius (os) to apex corneae (ACOR). Os is the anterior most soft tissue projection of the superior orbital rim and ACOR is the anterior most corneal projection. Normal os to ACOR is 8 to 10 mm dependent on age.[27] Indications for FOA are dictated by degree of orbital retrusion, in severe craniofacial cases os-ACOR is often a negative value demonstrating exorbitism. FOA is also indicated as part of secondary correction of frontal craniosynostotic plagiocephaly resulting in distortion of the frontal bar and upper midfacial symmetry.[28] Patients with severe exorbitism, corneal exposure, elevated ICP, or changes in vision require earlier operations. Those patients requiring nonfunctional advancement can be delayed till the child is older. The approach to an FOA forms the basis for all other intracranial craniofacial operations (▶ Fig. 34.2▶ Fig. 34.3).

- A standard oral endotracheal intubation is performed. After induction of anesthesia, a Foley catheter is placed, in a central venous line, and in an arterial line. Additionally, it is standard at our institution to place a precordial Doppler probe to monitor for air embolus.
- The child is prepped and draped in the supine position, the head is placed in a padded horseshoe Mayfield; typically, the head is shaved or a coronal strip is shaved. The scalp is injected with a dilute epinephrine solution with or without dilute topical anesthetic (similar to tumescent solution). The eyes are protected with

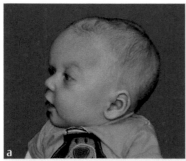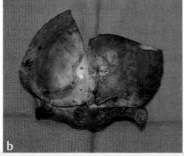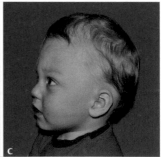

Fig. 34.2 Before and after fronto-orbital advancement in patient with multisuture synostosis. **(a)** Pre-operative lateral image demonstrating severe frontal bar retrusion secondary to coronal synostosis. **(b)** Intraoperative frontal bar and frontal bone unit after recontouring. **(c)** Postoperative result after advancement.

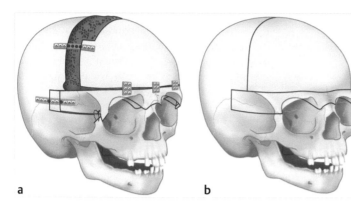

Fig. 34.3 (a,b) Fronto-orbital advancement.

a   b

tarsorrhaphy sutures. Either a straight line or a z-type incision is used for the frontal bone exposure. In males it is best to place the incision as far posterior as possible to avoid visibility with male pattern baldness.

- After the scalp incision, the exposure is carried down through the pericranium. The pericranium is carried attached to the scalp flap, thereby preserving pericranium for pericranial flaps if necessary. The temporalis muscle is raised in a subperiosteal plane attached to anterior skin flap.

- Throughout the exposure management of blood loss is essential, and every attempt made to control skin edge bleeding with bipolar cautery and the use of bone wax or other commercial hemostatic agents for control of bony blood loss. In addition, active communication between the operating surgeon and the anesthesia staff must be maintained with regard to resuscitation. The two points of maximum blood loss are the elevation of the scalp flaps and the elevation of the bony flaps. During this period, hemodynamic end points must be actively monitored and warm colloid resuscitation through a large-bore intravenous (IV) catheter is performed. At our institution, these children are resuscitated with packed red cells and fresh frozen plasma in either 1:1 or 2:1 ratios with minimal use of crystalloid. Once the craniotomies are complete, the blood tends to be minimal for the remainder of the case and blood products should be used judiciously from this point dictated by objective end points: urine output, central venous pressure, hemoglobin trend, base deficit, etc.

- The dissection must be carried in a subperiosteal plane to expose the nasal radix, the superior and lateral orbit and orbital rims. Often a 2-mm osteotome is often required to free the superior orbital neurovascular bundle from its ostia.

- This exposure forms the basis for all subsequent craniofacial procedures.

- After exposure for the upper midface and frontal bone, markings are made for the advancement and removal of the frontal bone and frontal bar. The burr hole sites are placed with care to avoid the sagittal sinus.

- Once the frontal bone has been removed, the osteotomies for the FOA may be performed. Typically, the frontal lobe is retracted and the temporal lobe is dissected free from the dural attachments to the middle cranial fossa in preparation for the osteotomies (inadvertent injury to the temporal lobe is possible during the lateral releasing osteotomies if attention is not paid to the middle cranial fossa). First a medial to lateral osteotomy is made in the anterior cranial fossa into the superior orbit. These osteotomies are made, using a reciprocating saw or a side cutting drill bit, across the superior orbit and laterally along the temporal bone. Once the lateral orbital wall is encountered, the osteotomy is deepened into the temporal fossa and carried out to the distal temporal bar (as marked). Care is taken to protect the temporal lobe with a retractor in the middle temporal fossa during the lateral most osteotomy, as the saw can inadvertently enter the middle cranial fossa with a long temporal bone extension. Next, attention is turned to completion of the lateral orbital rim osteotomy with connection to the superior orbital osteotomy completely the lateral dissociation of the frontal bar from the calvarium. Lastly, in order to release the frontal bar, a central osteotomy through the frontal bone above the cribiform plate is made, superior to the nasofrontal suture.

- After advancement and contouring of the frontal bone and frontal bar, they are rigidly fixated with absorbable plates and screws (▶ Fig. 34.3).

Common complications include frontal bar relapse, cerebrospinal fluid (CSF) leak secondary to dural tears, and residual cosmetic deformity.

34.4.2 Le Fort III/Monobloc Advancement

Indications/Procedure

Syndromic patients often suffer from midfacial dysplasia or hypoplasia. In particular, children with Apert's, Crouzon's, and Pfeiffer's[14,16,17,18,19] syndromes may present with severe exorbitism exacerbated by underdeveloped midfacial structures. Thus, advancement of the supraorbital bar alone would not correct the exorbitism because of concurrent maxillary hypoplasia that is best addressed in unison.[15] In these children, a monobloc advancement allows correction of the frontal bone and can help treat the bicoronal synostosis, frontal bar position, inferior orbit, and maxillary position. In patients that do not require early correction (i.e., they are able to protect their globes, and do not have evidence of optic nerve strain) of the superior orbit and inferior orbit, midfacial advancement may be delayed into mid childhood (7–10 years of age) (▶ Fig. 34.4). Additionally, a less well identified but emerging indication for midfacial advancement in these children is obstructive sleep apnea and tracheostomy dependence in severe cases.

- Initial preparation and exposure is performed as with FOA procedures. The endotracheal tube may be orally placed and is often secured to the mandible with a circumandibular wire or wired to the central mandibular incisors for older children (teeth should be wired in pairs to prevent accidental extraction via the wire).
- After exposure for FOA, the lateral extent is carried down to the zygomatic arches and complete exposure of the lateral orbital rim and inferior orbital rim is obtained. A second transconjuctival incision may be utilized to assist in the orbital floor exposure and inferior orbital rim exposure (this is surgeon and center specific). The orbit must be circumferentially freed in a subperiosteal plane.
- Additionally, the lower midface is also exposed using an upper gingivobuccal incision in order to free the lower midfacial periosteal attachments if necessary. This exposure in particular is used for an intraoral pterygomaxillary osteotomy. Or, if a gingivobuccal incision is not required, a posterior upper sulcal incision may be made for the intraoral pterygomaxillary disimpaction. This osteotomy may also be made through a superior temporal approach without intraoral incisions (these decisions are often case and surgeon specific).
- A frontal bone craniotomy is performed as with an FOA; however, in a monobloc advancement, the frontal bar is left attached to the midface. The same osteotomies are performed initially to free the superior orbital roof and lateral wall; however, the nasofrontal buttress is left intact preserving the frontal bar as an attached unit of the midface. The midline osteotomy is instead perpendicular to the FOA approach and placed in the anterior most cribriform plate through the

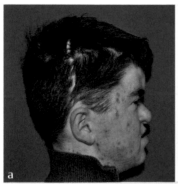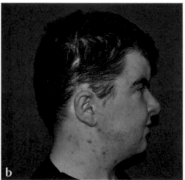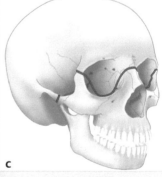

Fig. 34.4 Patient with Apert's syndrome with midfacial retrusion. **(a)** Preoperative appearance. **(b)** Postoperative results after extracranial Le Fort III midfacial advancement. **(c)** Illustration of Le Fort III advancement.

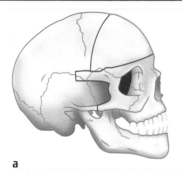
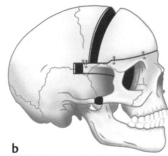

Fig. 34.5 (a, b) Monobloc advancement.

a

b

cranial base into the primitive nasoethmoid sinuses.

- Next, the orbital osteotomies are continued through the medial wall and orbital floor connecting to the lateral wall osteotomies performed earlier. Additionally, separate anterior zygomatic arch osteotomies are also performed. Once the orbits and the cranial base have been separated and the zygomatic arches have been cut, the face is only held to the calvarium via the pterygomaxillary buttress. This osteotomy is typically addressed intraorally with a curved osteotome but may also be approached through the temporal exposure. Care must be taken not to injury the internal maxillary artery. Injuries to this vessel may cause life-threatening hemorrhage and frequently require endovascular embolization for control.
- Monobloc advancements are typically used with distraction osteogenesis and placement of distractors. In cases where advancement of less than 10 to 15 mm may be performed a single stage with rigid fixation. In these cases, placement of pericranial flaps in the cranial base is critical to preventing CSF leaks and nasocranial communications with a risk of secondary meningitis (▶ Fig. 34.5).[15,29,30]

Complications include relapse, CSF leak, epidural abscess, meningitis, malocclusion, and endotracheal tube dislodgement/injury.

34.4.3 Facial Bipartition and Box Osteotomies

Indications/Procedure

Hypertelorism or orbital dystopia is common in patients with craniofacial anomalies. In these cases, the facial skeleton must be split either into halves or into separate orbital segments. Normal adult intercanthal distance is less than 35 mm, measured from medial canthus to medial canthus. For most cases this measurement provides the approximate degree of hypertelorism, but true measurement for repair can be derived from measurement of the bony dacryon–dacryon on imaging. The bony dacryon is a cephalometric point defined as the junction of the maxillary, lacrimal, and frontal bone. Normal distances are 25 to 30 mm. For symmetric hypertelorism with a narrow palate, the face may be addressed as a split monobloc advancement with removal of the portions of the central frontal bone, nasal skeleton, and maxilla.[29] This constitutes a facial bipartition (▶ Fig. 34.6). If the maxilla does not require widening and the child's occlusion is unaffected, box osteotomies are performed leaving the maxilla unchanged (▶ Fig. 34.6). These procedures are usually deferred until approximately 5 to 7 years of age because the tooth roots of the permanent dentition before this reside at or just below the inferior orbital rim.

- Surgical approach and preparation is the same as with monobloc advancement.
- Once dissection is complete, a portion of the central face is removed corresponding to the degree of hypertelorism and necessary palatal widening. The frontonasoethmoidal resection is planned by degree of widening (or degree of bimaxillary cant) seen clinically and on imaging.
  - Most significantly the decision whether to proceed with a facial bipartition versus a box osteotomy is decided by evaluation of the maxilla. If the maxilla is widened or canted, a facial bipartition is performed. If the maxilla is normal, then only box osteotomies are necessary. In facial bipartition, the maxilla is cut in the midline and realigned. For box osteotomies, a Le Fort I level cut is made to free the orbits from their attachment to the maxilla.
- This resection leaves the potential for a central facial dead space and oronasal communication with the meninges and thus

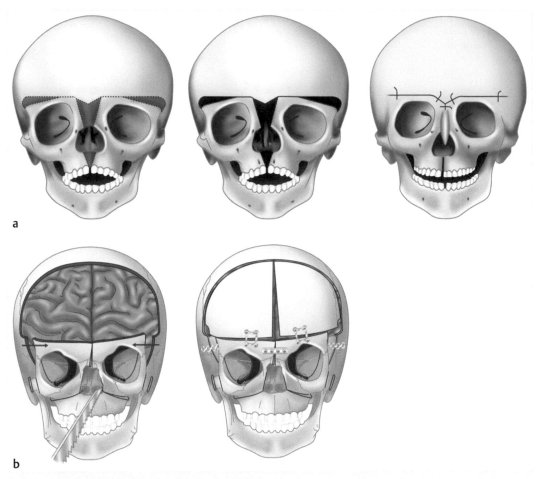

Fig. 34.6 (a, b) Facial bipartition and four-wall box osteotomies.

the anterior cranial base should be lined with a pericranial flap.[29,30]

- Preoperative imaging may play a critical role in these cases, as often encephaloceles and other sphenoethmoidal abnormalities are present. The location and types of abnormalities will affect placement of cranial base osteotomies and repair.

- Box osteotomies follow a similar approach but allow for preservation of the maxillary occlusion and can be used to address both vertical and horizontal asymmetries. Instead of a central maxillary osteotomy, the box osteotomies are carried out along the upper maxilla just inferior to the infraorbital nerve out laterally to the zygomas (in a Le Fort I fashion) and connected to the lateral orbital osteotomies allowing the anterior orbit to be positioned as a single unit (▶ Fig. 34.7).

Complications are typically the same as for monobloc advancement.

Postoperative Care

Every effort is made to extubate children at the conclusion of the procedure. In the pediatric intensive care unit (ICU), blood gases and chemistries are rechecked and the level of resuscitation evaluated. In addition, it is critical to limit excessive crystalloid resuscitation; if additional volume is necessary, an additional unit of blood is often given. The use of warm colloid resuscitation prevents postoperative third spacing, coagulopathies, and development of significant craniofacial edema. Typically, a drain is left under the scalp flaps and removed once it is draining less than 20 to 30 mL per day. The patient is observed overnight in the pediatric ICU and hourly neuro checks are

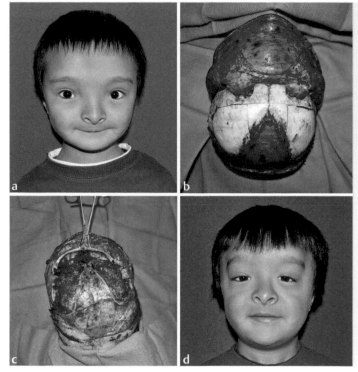

Fig. 34.7 Hypertelorism correction for severe orbital hypertelorism with frontal bone clefting. **(a)** Preoperative image demonstrating severe hypertelorism. **(b)** Intraoperative image of frontal bone and supraorbital bar markings prior to osteotomies of box orbital segments. **(c)** Intraoperative advancement and medialization of box orbital segments with central fixation. **(d)** Postoperative result demonstrating significant improvement in orbital hypertelorism and frontal bone contour.

performed during this period. For patients with an intraoral incision, a liquid diet is started, those without oral incisions are typically advanced as tolerated. On postoperative day 1, patients are usually transferred to the floor and are discharged on average on postoperative day 3 to 5 from the hospital. The dressings are removed on the first postoperative day and antibiotic ointment is then used once daily on the incision for approximately 1 week.

34.5 Summary

Craniofacial syndromes present complex anomalies of the craniofacial skeleton requiring a combined plastic and neurosurgical approach for repair. Many syndromes have readily identifiable clinical phenotypes that determine indications for surgery, and the genetic underpinnings of these syndromes are increasingly well characterized. The understanding of the timing of repair and the surgical indications are critical to successfully addressing craniofacial dysmorphologies. Typical first repair addresses the calvarium and supraorbital bar (after posterior distraction in cases with turribrachycephaly). The timing of repair is usually between 6 and 10 months of age but may

be sooner in cases of elevated ICPs or severe exorbitism with the threat of corneal exposure. Midfacial dysmorphologies and orbital dystopias are addressed in midchildhood because of the potential risk to facial growth. Thus, age of repair is typically reserved until 7 to 10 years of age. Final orthognathic procedures, which do not require a combined intracranial approach, are addressed when final facial skeletal maturity has been achieved (15–18 years old). Computer-aided design and preoperative modeling provide a window into the future of craniofacial surgery with preplanned operations based on objective cephalometric data and preoperative 3D CT imaging to guide in precise placement of osteotomies and degree of advancement. It is also crucial in the evaluation of syndromic children to assess for other anomalies and genetic counseling and analysis will be important factors in future understanding of the root causes of these syndromes.

34.6 Common Clinical Questions

1. When can significant craniofacial anomalies be diagnosed with prenatal ultrasound?

2. What are the major operative indications for craniofacial dysmorphologies?
3. When should craniofacial dysplasias be addressed, what are indications for urgent intervention?
4. How should craniofacial operations be staged for repair?

34.7 Answers to Common Clinical Questions

1. Typically, major craniofacial anomalies may be diagnosed by the 16- to 18-week ultrasound.
2. Major indications for operation are evidence of elevated ICP, corneal exposure for severe exorbitism, and significant facial deformity.
3. Urgent intervention is dictated by elevated ICP leading often to early (4–6 month posterior vault expansion), and FOA for severe exorbitism with threatened corneal exposure, temporizing tarsorrhaphy sutures may be placed for corneal protection. Additionally, tracheostomies may be necessary.
4. Syndromic craniofacial operations are staged by order of urgency and skeletal age of the child. They start with early posterior vault expansion. Next, the frontal bone and superior orbit are addressed, followed by midfacial procedures once the child is older, and orthognathic surgery and final rhinoplasty at completion of skeletal growth.
   - Typical timing and staging of procedures:
     - 6–8 months: Posterior vault remodeling if required (elevated ICP, severe turribrachycephaly).
     - 7–12 months: FOA with calvarial remodeling for associated craniosynostosis deformities.
     - 7–10 years of age: Midfacial advancement and correction of orbital dystopias with utilization of monobloc advancement, extracranial Le Fort III advancement, facial bipartition, or orbital box osteotomies, depending on type and degree of deformity. Midfacial correction is greatly individualized to each patient's particular dysmorphology.
     - 15–18 years of age: Orthognathic surgery for correction of final occlusion at skeletal maturity. Rhinoplasty can also be performed at this stage depending on surgical indication.

References

[1] Mulliken JB. The craniofacial surgeon as amateur geneticist. J Craniofac Surg. 2002; 13(1):3–17
[2] Hunt JA, Hobar PC. Common craniofacial anomalies: the facial dysostoses. Plast Reconstr Surg. 2002; 110(7):1714–1725, quiz 1726, discussion 1727–1728
[3] Maarse W, Bergé SJ, Pistorius L, et al. Diagnostic accuracy of transabdominal ultrasound in detecting prenatal cleft lip and palate: a systematic review. Ultrasound Obstet Gynecol. 2010; 35(4):495–502
[4] Fearon JA, Swift DM, Bruce DA. New methods for the evaluation and treatment of craniofacial dysostosis-associated cerebellar tonsillar herniation. Plast Reconstr Surg. 2001; 108(7):1855–1861
[5] Scott WW, Fearon JA, Swift DM, Sacco DJ. Suboccipital decompression during posterior cranial vault remodeling for selected cases of Chiari malformations associated with craniosynostosis. J Neurosurg Pediatr. 2013; 12(2):166–170
[6] Melville H, Wang Y, Taub PJ, Jabs EW. Genetic basis of potential therapeutic strategies for craniosynostosis. Am J Med Genet A. 2010; 152A(12):3007–3015
[7] Cunningham ML, Seto ML, Ratisoontorn C, Heike CL, Hing AV. Syndromic craniosynostosis: from history to hydrogen bonds. Orthod Craniofac Res. 2007; 10(2):67–81
[8] Turner N, Grose R. Fibroblast growth factor signalling: from development to cancer. Nat Rev Cancer. 2010; 10(2):116–129
[9] Forrest CR, Hopper RA. Craniofacial syndromes and surgery. Plast Reconstr Surg. 2013; 131(1):86e–109e
[10] Jabs EW, Müller U, Li X, et al. A mutation in the homeodomain of the human MSX2 gene in a family affected with autosomal dominant craniosynostosis. Cell. 1993; 75 (3):443–450
[11] Kimonis V, Gold JA, Hoffman TL, Panchal J, Boyadjiev SA. Genetics of craniosynostosis. Semin Pediatr Neurol. 2007; 14 (3):150–161
[12] Kreiborg S, Cohen MM, Jr. Ocular manifestations of Apert and Crouzon syndromes: qualitative and quantitative findings. J Craniofac Surg. 2010; 21(5):1354–1357
[13] Quintero-Rivera F, Robson CD, Reiss RE, et al. Intracranial anomalies detected by imaging studies in 30 patients with Apert syndrome. Am J Med Genet A. 2006; 140(12):1337–1338
[14] Allam KA, Wan DC, Khwanngern K, et al. Treatment of Apert syndrome: a long-term follow-up study. Plast Reconstr Surg. 2011; 127(4):1601–1611
[15] Wolfe SA, Morrison G, Page LK, Berkowitz S. The monobloc frontofacial advancement: do the pluses outweigh the minuses? Plast Reconstr Surg. 1993; 91(6):977–987, discussion 988–989
[16] Greig AV, Britto JA, Abela C, et al. Correcting the typical Apert face: combining bipartition with monobloc distraction. Plast Reconstr Surg. 2013; 131(2):219e–230e
[17] Hopper RA, Kapadia H, Morton T. Normalizing facial ratios in Apert syndrome patients with Le Fort II midface distraction and simultaneous zygomatic repositioning. Plast Reconstr Surg. 2013; 132(1):129–140
[18] Fearon JA, Podner C. Apert syndrome: evaluation of a treatment algorithm. Plast Reconstr Surg. 2013; 131(1):132–142
[19] McCarthy JG, Glasberg SB, Cutting CB, et al. Twenty-year experience with early surgery for craniosynostosis: II. The craniofacial synostosis syndromes and pansynostosis—results and unsolved problems. Plast Reconstr Surg 1995; 96:284–295; discussion 296–288
[20] Fearon JA, Rhodes J. Pfeiffer syndrome: a treatment evaluation. Plast Reconstr Surg. 2009; 123(5):1560–1569

[21] Cinalli G, Spennato P, Sainte-Rose C, et al. Chiari malformation in craniosynostosis. Childs Nerv Syst. 2005; 21(10):889–901

[22] Gallagher ER, Ratisoontorn C, Cunningham ML. Saethre-Chotzen Syndrome. 1993

[23] Mulliken JB, Steinberger D, Kunze S, Müller U. Molecular diagnosis of bilateral coronal synostosis. Plast Reconstr Surg. 1999; 104(6):1603–1615

[24] Agochukwu NB, Doherty ES, Muenke M. Muenke Syndrome. 1993

[25] Perlyn CA, Marsh JL. Craniofacial dysmorphology of Carpenter syndrome: lessons from three affected siblings. Plast Reconstr Surg. 2008; 121(3):971–981

[26] Kawamoto HK, Heller JB, Heller MM, et al. Craniofrontonasal dysplasia: a surgical treatment algorithm. Plast Reconstr Surg. 2007; 120(7):1943–1956

[27] Mulliken JB, Godwin SL, Pracharktam N, Altobelli DE. The concept of the sagittal orbital-globe relationship in craniofacial surgery. Plast Reconstr Surg. 1996; 97(4):700–706

[28] Greenwald JA, Mehrara BJ, Spector JA, et al. Immature versus mature dura mater: II. Differential expression of genes important to calvarial reossification. Plast Reconstr Surg. 2000; 106(3):630–638, discussion 639

[29] Fearon JA, Whitaker LA. Complications with facial advancement: a comparison between the Le Fort III and monobloc advancements. Plast Reconstr Surg. 1993; 91(6):990–995

[30] Marchac D, Sati S, Renier D, Deschamps-Braly J, Marchac A. Hypertelorism correction: what happens with growth? Evaluation of a series of 95 surgical cases. Plast Reconstr Surg. 2012; 129(3):713–727

35 Germinal Matrix Hemorrhage in Premature Infants

Moise Danielpour, Lindsey Ross

35.1 Introduction

Despite advances in prenatal care and sophisticated postnatal monitoring, the incidence of major neurodevelopmental deficits in very-low-birth-weight infants remains unacceptably high.[1] National outcomes data show that almost one-fourth of these children suffer major neurological deficits, with nearly one-fifth requiring some form of special education at school age.[2] Germinal matrix hemorrhage (GMH) is the most common diagnosed brain lesion in preterm infants and is often seen in the sickest and most premature. GMH with intraventricular extension and the resultant complication, of posthemorrhagic hydrocephalus of prematurity (PHH), is one of the most dreaded myriad of diseases that plague the premature infant. Despite numerous prevention and intervention trials, GMH occurs in up to 20% of preterm infants less than 1,500 g birth weight and is the predominant cause of neurodevelopmental disability in these infants.[3,4,5]

35.2 Pathophysiology of Germinal Matrix

The germinal matrix and the ventricular germinal zones are the sites of neuronal and glial proliferation from immature radial glia. The majority of the developing cortical neurons complete generation by 25 weeks' gestational age. During the late second and early third trimester, the germinal matrix gives rise to cortical neuronal and glial cell precursors, which involute and migrate toward the caudothalamic groove. By 32 weeks' gestation, the cellular component of cerebral cortex has nearly completely populated the appropriate layers. During this time there is an abundance of cortical axonal and dendritic activity with exponential increase in synaptic contacts. Thus, GMH, which most commonly occurs prior to 32 weeks of gestation, can have dramatic effects on cortical development and ultimately cognitive maturity.

More specifically, during the late second and early third trimesters, the microvasculature of the brain undergoes dramatic expansion to meet metabolic needs of the germinal matrix and cortex.[6] The capillary beds of the germinal matrix are composed of large and irregular vessels that are not yet identifiable as arterioles, venules, or capillaries. Additionally, there are luminal areas, which are significantly larger than the cortical vessels and these areas lack the traditional components of the blood–brain barrier, and may be more susceptible to disruption.[7]

Animal studies have demonstrated that autoregulation of cerebral blood flow matures with increasing gestation. During the late second and early third trimester, cerebral autoregulation is *inefficient*. This leaves the region susceptible to fluctuations of systemic blood pressure and cerebral blood flow. The germinal matrix and periventricular white matter are watershed zones at high risk for hypotensive injury. Because the germinal matrix is a metabolically active area, it tends to be exceptionally sensitive to hypoperfusion and hypotension. All these factors lead to extreme susceptibility to infarction and/or hemorrhage in the premature infant.

Pathogenesis of perinatal factors and comorbidities associated with an increased risk of hemorrhage.

35.2.1 Comorbidities

- *Postnatal hypoxia* because of any cause including respiratory distress syndrome, pneumothorax, anemia, or sepsis.
- *Hypercapnia* maximally dilates the thin-walled vasculature. If this is followed by increases in volume or perfusion of the tissue, this can result in hemorrhage.
- *Increased venous pressure* (i.e., positive pressure ventilation, stimulation, endotracheal suctioning) can result in hemorrhage.
- *Dehydration* followed by rapid resuscitation with hyperosmolar fluids encourages osmotic flow of fluids out of the tissue and into the vascular space resulting in rapid changes in transmural pressure and vascular rupture.

35.2.2 Risk Factors

- Weight less than or equal to 1,500 g.[5,8,9]
- Early gestational age (EGA) (< 28 weeks).
- Increased cerebral perfusion pressure (CPP), decreased tissue oxygenation or hypoxia, and increased cerebral blood flow.
  - Asphyxia or hypercapnia
  - Rapid volume expansion

- Seizures
- Pneumothorax
- Cyanotic heart disease
- Mechanical positive pressure ventilation anemia
- Decreased blood glucose on arterial catheterization
- Blood pressure fluctuations
- Acidosis
- Chorioamnionitis
- Coagulopathies, maternal aspirin use
- Extracorporeal membrane oxygenation (ECMO)
- Maternal cocaine abuse
- General anesthesia for cesarean section
• Failure to give antenatal steroids 48 hours prior to preterm delivery.
• Low Apgar's scores at 1 minute (< 4) or 5 minutes (< 8).

35.3 Epidemiology

35.3.1 Incidence

GMH is thought to affect 15 to 20% of infants with birth weights less than 1,500 g.[10] Nevertheless, many preterm patients are asymptomatic following GMH and may not be detected if routine surveillance is not instituted. In 1978, Papile utilized computed tomography (CT) to find that GMH occurred in 43% of extremely low-birth-weight infants with a mortality of 55% compared to mortality rate of 23% for premature infants without GMH.[11] Ultrasonography is the study of choice for detection of GMH in premature infants with a sensitivity of 90%.[12]

35.3.2 Timing

GMH has a bimodal distribution with 50% of hemorrhages occurring within 12 hours of birth and 45% of hemorrhages occurring by postnatal days 3 to 4. GMH may develop after day 4 in approximately 5% of these infants. Progression is documented in up to 20% of patients, which most frequently occurs within the first week of the initial hemorrhage.[13]

35.4 Etiology of Posthemorrhagic Ventricular Dilation

Following are the three main etiologies:
1. *Communicating* hydrocephalus from GMH with ventricular extension, which results in *scarring* of cerebrospinal fluid (CSF) flow pathways,

impeding CSF circulation, and decreasing CSF reabsorption by the arachnoid granulations. Transforming growth factor-β and other cytokines, which are released into the CSF following GMH, appear to stimulate extracellular matrix protein deposition, impeding the process of CSF absorption.
2. *ex vacuo* hydrocephalus from encephalomalacia and periventricular leukomalacia. GMH destroys repository stem cells in the germinal matrix, resulting in decreased number of neurons and myelinated oligodendrocytes.

Late-onset *obstructive* hydrocephalus may occur following CSF diversion procedure in a patient with communicating hydrocephalus, leading to an isolation of the fourth ventricle. This phenomenon has mostly been documented as a late finding in patients with intraventricular hemorrhage (IVH) of prematurity following a fluid diversion procedure such as placement of a ventriculoperitoneal shunt, where the infant appears to develop secondary aqueductal stenosis.

35.4.1 Etiology of Postperiventricular Hemorrhagic Infarction

• Ventricular hemorrhage evolves to compress and occlude the terminal veins, which serve to drain the internal cerebral veins into the vein of Galen. This leads to subsequent venous infarct and secondary hemorrhage.[4,14]

35.5 Clinical Presentation

It follows one of three following patterns[4]:
1. *Catastrophic*—Rapid neurological demise requiring aggressive neurosurgical intervention. Rare; carries a dismal prognosis.
2. *Salutatory*—Evolution over hours to days in stepwise fashion associated with decreased activity, abnormal eye movements, respiratory discordance, and hypotonia.
3. Clinically *silent*—Which may present as slight decrease in hematocrit and may be diagnosed via cranial ultrasound.

35.5.1 Grading System

The most commonly used grading system is based on CT or ultrasound. There is a direct correlation between the Papile grading system, gestational age, and neurological outcome (▶ Table 35.1).[11]

The incidence of grade IV germinal matrix hemorrhage is inversely proportional to gestational age, that is, 30% of GMH patients are grade IV at 22 weeks and only 3% are grade IV at 28 weeks.[15] Among the severely premature infants (24–26 weeks' gestational age), 32% will have a grade III (▶ Fig. 35.1) and 19% will have grade IV, as compared to the premature infants at 31 to 32 weeks'

gestational age, where 11% will have a grade II and 5% will suffer from a grade IV (▶ Fig. 35.2).[15]

35.6 Diagnosis

Routine head circumference measurements and examination of the anterior fontanel should be part of the daily examination performed on the premature infant. However, when there is a suspicion of possible germinal matrix injury, the diagnosis is best made via bedside cranial ultrasound.

35.6.1 Ultrasound

Cranial ultrasound is the standard diagnostic tool used for diagnosis and follow-up of premature infants with GMH. The accuracy is approximately 88% (91% sensitivity, 85% specificity).

The main advantages of using cranial ultrasonography (CUS) are as follows:

- CUS is performed at the bedside, obviating the need to transport a fragile infant.

Table 35.1 Papile grading system

Grade	Extent of hemorrhage
I	Restricted to germinal matrix
II	Intraventricular hemorrhage without ventricular dilation
III	Intraventricular with ventricular dilation
IV	IVH with parenchymal involvement

Abbreviation: IVH, intraventricular hemorrhage.

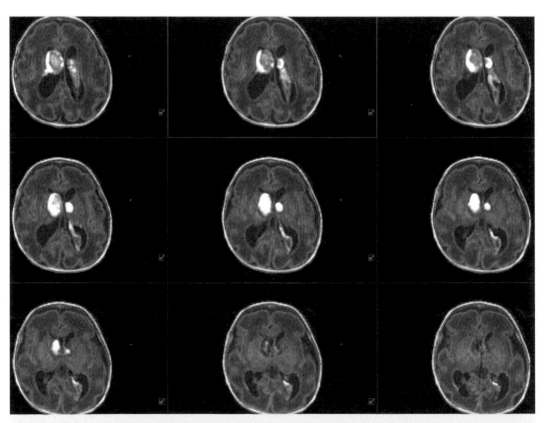

Fig. 35.1 Neonatal cranial ultrasound series exhibiting a left-sided grade III premature intraventricular hemorrhage.

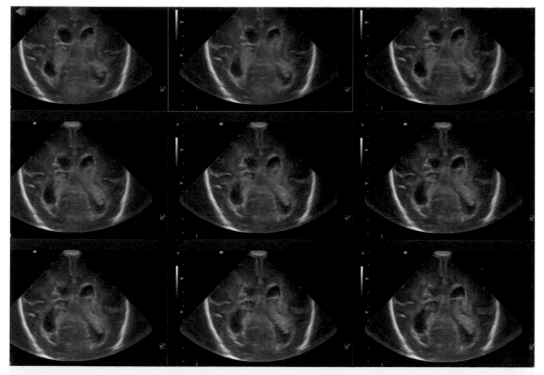

Fig. 35.2 CT scan serial images of the neonatal brain exhibiting a right-sided grade IV premature intraventricular hemorrhage.

- It is noninvasive test.
- Sedation is not required as occasional movements are well tolerated.
- There is no exposure to ionizing radiation.
- CUS demonstrates the size and location of hemorrhage, size of the ventricles, and thickness of the cortical mantle.
- CUS can be followed serially with relative ease.

The main disadvantage of using cranial ultrasound is poor visualization of the posterior fossa.

Determining severity of hydrocephalus in the preterm infant is objectified by calculation and knowledge of the following:

- *Levene's ventricular index*—Midline falx to lateral anterior horn in coronal view at foramen of Monro. Normal ventricular index + 4 mm is used as criteria for surgical intervention.[14,16]
  - Normal 27-week EGA ventricular index at 97th percentile = 14 mm + 4 mm = 18 mm would meet criteria for intervention.
- *Anterior horn width (AHW)* may be an even more effective way to measure early ventricular expansion. Normal AHW in a neonate is less

than 3 mm and a greater than 6 mm is grossly abnormal.[16]

35.6.2 Computed Tomography

It may be helpful in complex cases where anatomy is difficult to characterize, or there is need for better visualization of the contents of the posterior fossa. Use is limited given associated risks of radiation in the brain of a premature infant.

35.6.3 Magnetic Resonance Imaging

It is uncommonly used secondary to poor visualization of acute hemorrhage. This is reserved for cases where there is a need for detailed imaging of the brain such as in patients with aqueductal stenosis or isolated fourth ventricle. This modality often requires sedation and significant time away from the neonatal intensive care unit. Use of ultrafast imaging and MRI compatible incubators have increased the utility of MRI scans in these patients.

35.7 Pathology Associated with IVHp

Cystic periventricular leukomalacia with IVH grade III is often misdiagnosed as grade IV GMH. Although, they may share similar pathophysiological features, they are separate processes with likely different etiologies.[17] Often cerebellar hemorrhage can coexist with GMH as well. However, this is difficult to diagnose on magnetic resonance imaging (MRI) (10%) and even more difficult via ultrasound (~2%).[18] The presence of cerebellar hemorrhage also increases the risks of neurological complications by fivefold.[18]

35.8 Treatment

The goal of treatment is to optimize cerebral perfusion pressures without excessive elevation of cerebral blood flow, while carefully maintaining mean arterial pressures, normalizing Pco_2, and reducing ventriculomegaly. With recent evidence of the possible detrimental effects of blood breakdown products, as a consequence of methemoglobin-inducing expression of proinflammatory cytokines, there are ongoing discussions of the role of early ventricular drainage to reduce secondary injury.[19]

35.8.1 Ventriculomegaly

- *Transient* ventriculomegaly (may occur in the first few days of life, often not associated with raised intracranial pressure).
- *Progressive* ventriculomegaly occurs in 20 to 50% of cases as a result of decreased CSF reabsorption or obstruction of CSF flow versus hydrocephalus ex vacuo due to loss of brain tissue. If associated with increasing head circumference or physiological changes, it will require intervention.

35.8.2 Lumbar Puncture

Lumbar punctures can be effective at controlling the deleterious effects of posthemorrhagic hydrocephalus, but does not appear to reduce the frequency of long-term permanent shunting. Serial lumbar punctures in neonates can be cumbersome and difficult to perform, and have a variable success rate. As a result, they are usually used as a short-term temporizing or diagnostic measure. About 25% of patients with GMH with PHH will

have *progressive* ventriculomegaly. In 60% of these progressive patients, early temporization will lead to arrest of ventriculomegaly over several days to weeks.[20,21]

35.8.3 Ventricular Puncture

Multiple ventricular punctures can result in poor outcome and carry an increased risk of complications.[20] Ventricular punctures should be reserved for a neonate in extremis, as an initial temporizing event, or for diagnostic purposes.

35.8.4 External Ventricular Drain

Use of an external ventricular drain (EVD) is limited by technical difficulty secondary to small ventricular size, mobility of neonatal skin, and susceptibility to dislodging. Additionally, most neonates will require an extended period of drainage, which carry an unacceptably high risk for infection. Although theoretical advantages include decreased risk of overdrainage and subsequent formation of subdural hygromas, ability to monitor intracranial pressure, and continuous removal of CSF protein and blood products, evidence suggests that the increased risk of infection from CSF drainage catheters are an independent predictor of poor neurodevelopment and this risk far outweighs the benefits attained from use of external drains.[21]

35.8.5 Medical Therapy

Antenatal betamethasone (a corticosteroid) reduces the incidence of IVH in preterm infants.[22] Medical CSF diversion through acetazolamide and/or furosemide has not shown to decrease need for permanent shunting and has been shown to increase the incidence of neurological morbidity.[23] Intraventricular fibrinolytic therapy results in an increased risk of rehemorrhage and death.[24] Nevertheless, studies show that patients who survive the perinatal period have improved neurological function on long-term follow-up.[20] Fibrinolytic therapy is currently **not used as standard therapy** and in fact may be associated with mild motor delays at 1 year of age.[21,23]

35.8.6 Surgical Therapy

About 34% of IVHp infants less than 1,500 g require CSF drainage after failed medical management. In infants with grade III and IV IVH greater than 70% will develop progressive ventriculomegaly and **32** to 47% of these patients will ultimately require a shunt.[25]

Following are two surgical techniques for temporary CSF diversion/removal:
- Ventriculosubgaleal (VSG) shunt.
- Ventricular reservoir.

35.9 There is no Data to Prove Superiority of Either VSG Shunt or Reservoir Placement

Subcutaneous reservoir placement was first used for treatment of IVHp by McComb and colleagues in 1983 and originally had a 20% mortality rate, 10% infection rate, and was associated with an ultimate need for permanent CSF diversion of 75% of neonates with progressive ventriculomegaly.[26] The quantity of CSF that is removed is adjusted to opening pressure. In our practice, we limit number of CSF taps to three times per day to minimize the risk of secondary infections. Historically, infection has been the most common complication, although the infection rates have decreased dramatically. Other complications include skin necrosis, CSF fistula, or development of subdural hygromas.

VSG shunting involves placement of reservoir with a piece of shunt tubing attached to the reservoir outlet, which allows for redirection of CSF to subgaleal pocket where it collects and slowly reabsorbed. This allows for continuous CSF diversion, with a theoretically decreased risk of developing increased fluctuations in intracranial pressure and size of the cerebral ventricles. There does not appear to be any appreciable difference in the incidence of shunt placement or complications when compared to a CSF reservoir. Additionally, this technique allows for real-time observation in variance of CSF resorption overtime. One is able to easily ascertain if the patient is improving resorption capacity. Nevertheless, this also appears to be associated with a greater amount of parental anxiety as the pouch is a dysmorphic feature (▶ Table 35.2).

35.9.1 Neuroendoscopy

The use of endoscopy in GMH with PHH is limited but may allow for dilution of hemosiderin products and in special cases allows for single clot removal and relief of obstructive hydrocephalus. Gudegast et al published a series of seven patients with complex hydrocephalus defined by recurrent

Table 35.2 Benefits of VSG versus SQ reservoir placement

Benefits	VSG	SQ reservoir
Less CSF aspiration	+	–
Permanent decompression	+	–
Less electrolyte and fluid shifts	+	–
Conserves cerebral pressure	+	–
Dynamic observation	+	–

Abbreviations: CSF, cerebrospinal fluid; SQ, subcutaneous; VSG, ventriculosubgaleal.

infections and subsequent multiple shunt revisions that showed neuroendoscopy to be essential in clean up and communication of isolated compartments.[27]

35.9.2 Endoscopic Technique for Placement of a VSG Shunt, Ventricular Irrigation, and Aqueductoplasty

Technique for placement of CSF reservoirs and VSG shunts has been reported previously.[28] Since 2004, we have employed the endoscopic method for placement of the majority of our VSG shunts and ventricular reservoirs, and ventriculoperitoneal shunts (VPSs) in children with progressive ventriculomegaly following IVHp. This has allowed us both visualization of the cerebral aqueduct and decreased incidence of poorly placed ventricular catheters.

35.9.3 Postoperative

Patients are monitored daily by examining the anterior fontanel, vital signs, incidence of apnea and bradycardia, and accumulation of CSF in the subgaleal pocket when applicable. Weekly head ultrasounds can be used to monitor ventricular size.

35.9.4 Complications of VSG Shunt

- Readhesion of subgaleal pocket especially with lying on ipsilateral hemisphere. This can also be a sign of resolution of hydrocephalus.
- Increase in occipital frontal diameter of cranium. Risk decreases with immobilization and cranial padding.

- CSF leakage at attachment of reservoir to catheter; CSF leak from incision site occurred 4.7 to 32% of the time in the Koksal series and has a 0 to 10% risk of ventriculitis or meningiti.[28] We have not experienced any cases of CSF leaks in our patients, or an increased risk of infection.

35.9.5 Tapping for CSF Removal

Removal of CSF via a reservoir or by lumbar puncture plays an important role in not only relieving intracranial pressure, but also decreasing the proinflammatory byproducts of IVH. Nevertheless, there is little evidence showing that frequent tapping reduces the risk of shunt dependence, morbidity, or mortality. In fact, repeated taps are associated with an increased risk of central nervous system infection.[20,29] CSF tapping is performed on an as needed basis to prevent progressive ventriculomegaly. The frequency and quantity should vary based on evidence of intracranial pressure commonly measured through daily head circumference, fontanel characteristics and physiological changes, and direct measurements during the removal of spinal fluid. In patients where larger volumes of CSF have to be removed on a daily basis, there may be a need for replacement in the form of IV or PO isotonic fluids, especially in children who weigh less than 1 kg.

35.9.6 Permanent Shunting

Delayed insertion of permanent shunting in this population can result in decreased incidence of early VPS revisions. Permanent CSF diversion is required in 32 to 85% of patients following IVH of prematurity.[28,30] Most pediatric neurosurgeons also advocate waiting until an infant is greater than 2.5 kg and CSF protein is less than 1.5 g/L before placing a permanent shunt as this has also been shown to decrease surgical complications.[29] CSF removal through tapping is thought to remove hemosiderin blood products, thereby decreasing risk of obstructive hydrocephalus. Additionally, with delayed shunting, the infant is able to mature, gain weight, and improve immunity and skin integrity, which will improve overall ability to recover from surgical procedures.[29] Approximately, 45% of infants who receive VPS insertion before 1 year of age require revision within 9 months.[31]

Endoscopic third ventriculostomy (ETV) is used to treat patients with an obstructive component of hydrocephalus, which may be currently under-diagnosed in the GMH population. The role of ETV in GMH with PHH remains controversial. ETV provides high success rates (77%) for patient with pure aqueductal stenosis.[32] However, due to the complexity of IVHp and large component of communicating hydrocephalus multicenter trials have shown a poor success rate for IVHp patients undergoing ETV.[33] Theoretically, there is less risk of infection and a very low subsequent shunt placement rate.[32] ETV can be successful for a small and select group of patients following IVH of prematurity.[34]

35.10 Prognosis

Neurological complications of GMH include cerebral palsy, seizures, and cognitive delay. Multicenter studies have shown that premature neonates with IVH of prematurity have poorer neurofunctional outcomes at 5-year follow-up regardless of surgical management.[35] Often resolution of hydrocephalus is associated with normal cerebral cortex functioning and is often a good prognostic indicator.[30] Positive prognostic indicators of GMH include antenatal corticosteroid treatment, cesarean delivery, and prophylactic intravenous indomethacin treatment[36][37,38]. Several studies including a recent meta-analysis exhibited few very poor prognostic indicators including presence of chorioamnionitis, which increased the risk of cerebral palsy by 140%.[39]

Term-equivalent MRI scan of the brain appears to be the most effective imaging modality available at this time to provide a relative indication of long-term neurological prognosis.[14] This is primarily determined through measurement of summation of white matter thinning, delayed gyral maturation, and gray or white matter signal abnormalities.[14] However, MRI continues to be very poor predictor of cognitive outcomes.

35.11 Conclusions

Neurosurgeons have a unique perspective with respect to care of patients with IVH of prematurity; this is not simply a disease of the premature infant, but a lifelong disease with perpetual opportunities for complications including shunt dependency, repeat surgeries, and neurodevelopmental sequelae.

One of the most promising studies include the use of biologics to ameliorate the delayed effects of IVH on brain development. One recent study utilized intraventricular administration of a tumor necrosis factor-α (TNF-α inhibitor in a rabbit pup model. This was associated with decreased periventricular cell death, gliosis, and neuronal degeneration.[40] Additionally, promising research in the use of stem cells retrieved from umbilical cord blood at birth, which may differentiate to pluripotent neuronal stem cells in vitro, may have a role in the treatment of these infants. Studies thus far have shown that stem cells assist in anti-inflammation and restoring normal milieu, rather than replacement of injured cells.[41] Although such stem cell therapies may not ultimately replace the cells lost, but they may reduce the secondary injury to the remaining healthy neural tissue.[42]

Germinal matrix hemorrhage with subsequent posthemorrhagic hydrocephalus is the most common disease process the pediatric neurosurgeon will encounter among the preterm neonatal population. Although the incidence has continued to decline with technological advancements in perinatal care and improved understanding of molecular and cellular pathophysiology, there may be significant new therapies looming in the horizon for these infants.

References

[1] World Health Organization. Child Health Development: Health of the Newborn. Geneva: World Health Organization; 1991

[2] McCormick MC, Workman-Daniels K, Brooks-Gunn J. The behavioral and emotional well-being of school-age children with different birth weights. Pediatrics. 1996; 97(1):18–25

[3] Shankaran S, Bauer CR, Bain R, Wright LL, Zachary J, National Institute of Child Health and Human Development Neonatal Research Network. Prenatal and perinatal risk and protective factors for neonatal intracranial hemorrhage. Arch Pediatr Adolesc Med. 1996; 150(5):491–497

[4] Volpe JJ. Intraventricular hemorrhage in the premature infant—current concepts. Part I. Ann Neurol. 1989; 25(1):3–11

[5] Perlman JM, McMenamin JB, Volpe JJ. Fluctuating cerebral blood-flow velocity in respiratory-distress syndrome. Relation to the development of intraventricular hemorrhage. N Engl J Med. 1983; 309(4):204–209

[6] Breier G, Albrecht U, Sterrer S, Risau W. Expression of vascular endothelial growth factor during embryonic angiogenesis and endothelial cell differentiation. Development. 1992; 114(2):521–532

[7] Ment LR, Stewart WB, Ardito TA, Madri JA. Germinal matrix microvascular maturation correlates inversely with the risk period for neonatal intraventricular hemorrhage. Brain Res Dev Brain Res. 1995; 84(1):142–149

[8] Dykes FD, Lazzara A, Ahmann P, Blumenstein B, Schwartz J, Brann AW. Intraventricular hemorrhage: a prospective evaluation of etiopathogenesis. Pediatrics. 1980; 66(1):42–49

[9] Volpe JJ. Effect of cocaine use on the fetus. N Engl J Med. 1992; 327(6):399–407

[10] du Plessis AJ. Cerebrovascular injury in premature infants: current understanding and challenges for future prevention. Clin Perinatol. 2008; 35(4):609–641, v

[11] Papile LA, Burstein J, Burstein R, Koffler H. Incidence and evolution of subependymal and intraventricular hemorrhage: a study of infants with birth weights less than 1,500 gm. J Pediatr. 1978; 92(4):529–534

[12] Bejar R, Curbelo V, Coen RW, Leopold G, James H, Gluck L. Diagnosis and follow-up of intraventricular and intracerebral hemorrhages by ultrasound studies of infant's brain through the fontanelles and sutures. Pediatrics. 1980; 66(5):661–673

[13] Volpe JJ, Perlman JM, Hill A, McMenamin JB. Cerebral blood flow velocity in the human newborn: the value of its determination. Pediatrics. 1982; 70(1):147–152

[14] El-Dib M, Massaro AN, Bulas D, Aly H. Neuroimaging and neurodevelopmental outcome of premature infants. Am J Perinatol. 2010; 27(10):803–818

[15] Stoll BJ, Gordon T, Korones SB, et al. Late-onset sepsis in very low birth weight neonates: a report from the National Institute of Child Health and Human Development Neonatal Research Network. J Pediatr. 1996; 129(1):63–71

[16] Brouwer MJ, de Vries LS, Pistorius L, Rademaker KJ, Groenendaal F, Benders MJ. Ultrasound measurements of the lateral ventricles in neonates: why, how and when? A systematic review. Acta Paediatr. 2010; 99(9):1298–1306

[17] Kusters CD, Chen ML, Follett PL, Dammann O. "Intraventricular" hemorrhage and cystic periventricular leukomalacia: how are they related? J Child Neurol. 2009; 24(9):1158–1170

[18] Tam EW, Rosenbluth G, Rogers EE, et al. Cerebellar hemorrhage on magnetic resonance imaging in preterm newborns associated with abnormal neurologic outcome. J Pediatr. 2011; 158(2):245–250

[19] Gram M, Sveinsdottir S, Ruscher K, et al. Hemoglobin induces inflammation after preterm intraventricular hemorrhage by methemoglobin formation. J Neuroinflammation. 2013; 10:100

[20] Whitelaw A. Repeated lumbar or ventricular punctures in newborns with intraventricular hemorrhage. Cochrane Database Syst Rev. 2001; 1(1):CD000216

[21] Volpe JJ. Neurology of the Newborn. 5th ed. Philadelphia, PA: Saunders Elsevier; 2008

[22] Crowley PA. Prophylactic corticosteroids for preterm birth. Cochrane Database Syst Rev. 2000;(2):CD000065

[23] Kennedy CR, Ayers S, Campbell MJ, Elbourne D, Hope P, Johnson A. Randomized, controlled trial of acetazolamide and furosemide in posthemorrhagic ventricular dilation in infancy: follow-up at 1 year. Pediatrics. 2001; 108(3):597–607

[24] Whitelaw A, Evans D, Carter M, et al. Randomized clinical trial of prevention of hydrocephalus after intraventricular hemorrhage in preterm infants: brain-washing versus tapping fluid. Pediatrics. 2007; 119(5):e1071–e1078

[25] Robinson S. Neonatal posthemorrhagic hydrocephalus from prematurity: pathophysiology and current treatment concepts. J Neurosurg Pediatr. 2012; 9(3):242–258

[26] Brockmeyer DL, Wright LC, Walker ML, Ward RM. Management of posthemorrhagic hydrocephalus in the low-birth-weight preterm neonate. Pediatr Neurosci. 1989; 15(6):302–307, discussion 308

[27] Gudegast C, Niesytto C. Outcome of endoscopic therapy of complex hydrocephalus. Neuropediatrics. 2008:39–P080

[28] Köksal V, Öktem S. Ventriculosubgaleal shunt procedure and its long-term outcomes in premature infants with posthemorrhagic hydrocephalus. Childs Nerv Syst. 2010; 26(11):1505–1515

[29] Whitelaw A, Aquilina K. Management of posthaemorrhagic ventricular dilatation. Arch Dis Child Fetal Neonatal Ed. 2012; 97(3):F229–F3

[30] Kazan S, Güra A, Uçar T, Korkmaz E, Ongun H, Akyuz M. Hydrocephalus after intraventricular hemorrhage in preterm and low-birth weight infants: analysis of associated risk factors for ventriculoperitoneal shunting. Surg Neurol. 2005; 64 Suppl 2:S77–S81, discussion S81

[31] Sciubba DM, Noggle JC, Carson BS, Jallo GI. Antibiotic-impregnated shunt catheters for the treatment of infantile hydrocephalus. Pediatr Neurosurg. 2008; 44(2):91–96

[32] Oertel JM, Mondorf Y, Baldauf J, Schroeder HW, Gaab MR. Endoscopic third ventriculostomy for obstructive hydrocephalus due to intracranial hemorrhage with intraventricular extension. J Neurosurg. 2009; 111(6):1119–1126

[33] Siomin V, Cinalli G, Grotenhuis A, et al. Endoscopic third ventriculostomy in patients with cerebrospinal fluid infection and/or hemorrhage. J Neurosurg. 2002; 97(3):519–524

[34] Warf BC, Campbell JW, Riddle E. Initial experience with combined endoscopic third ventriculostomy and choroid plexus cauterization for post-hemorrhagic hydrocephalus of prematurity: the importance of prepontine cistern status and the predictive value of FIESTA MRI imaging. Childs Nerv Syst. 2011; 27(7):1063–1071

[35] Vassilyadi M, Tataryn Z, Shamji MF, Ventureyra EC. Functional outcomes among premature infants with intraventricular hemorrhage. Pediatr Neurosurg. 2009; 45 (4):247–255

[36] Shooman D, Portess H, Sparrow O. A review of the current treatment methods for posthaemorrhagic hydrocephalus of infants. Cerebrospinal Fluid Res. 2009; 6:1

[37] Linder N, Haskin O, Levit O, et al. Risk factors for intraventricular hemorrhage in very low birth weight premature infants: a retrospective case-control study. Pediatrics. 2003; 111(5 pt 1):e590–e595

[38] Been JV, Degraeuwe PL, Kramer BW, Zimmermann LJ. Antenatal steroids and neonatal outcome after chorioamnionitis: a meta-analysis. BJOG. 2011; 118(2):113–122

[39] Shatrov JG, Birch SC, Lam LT, Quinlivan JA, McIntyre S, Mendz GL. Chorioamnionitis and cerebral palsy: a meta-analysis. Obstet Gynecol. 2010; 116(2 pt 1):387–392

[40] Vinukonda G, Csiszar A, Hu F, et al. Neuroprotection in a rabbit model of intraventricular haemorrhage by cyclooxygenase-2, prostanoid receptor-1 or tumour necrosis factor-alpha inhibition. Brain. 2010; 133(pt 8):2264–2280

[41] Tanaka N, Kamei N, Nakamae T, et al. CD133 + cells from human umbilical cord blood reduce cortical damage and promote axonal growth in neonatal rat organ co-cultures exposed to hypoxia. Int J Dev Neurosci. 2010; 28(7):581–587

[42] Pimentel-Coelho PM, Mendez-Otero R. Cell therapy for neonatal hypoxic-ischemic encephalopathy. Stem Cells Dev. 2010; 19(3):299–310

36 Surgical Management of Hydrocephalus

Martina Messing-Jünger

36.1 Introduction

Hydrocephalus is a complex multifactorial disorder and can be congenital or acquired. The most important prognostic factors are age of onset and etiology.[1,2] The earlier a developing brain is confronted with problems leading to hydrocephalus, the greater will be the negative impact. Whenever a hydrocephalic disorder is associated with other brain malformations, there is an increased risk of neurodevelopmental problems. Besides these pre-existing facts, the treatment of a hydrocephalic child and potential complications are additional risk factors for the long-term course. Adequate treatment indication, thorough surgery, and follow-up concepts play an important role in order to provide the best neurological and developmental outcome.

36.2 Surgical Indications

According to the child's age and the given pathology, the treatment of choice can either be shunt implantation or endoscopic third ventriculostomy (ETV). In some cases, endoscopic-assisted shunt surgery might be appropriate as well. A posthemorrhagic hydrocephalus in a preterm infant most often requires a temporary reservoir or other drainage device before a definite shunt implantation is indicated. Not all cases of childhood hydrocephalus need to be treated surgically at the time of diagnosis. Besides meticulous clinical investigations, invasive intracranial pressure (ICP) measurements can be helpful. It is recommended, for example, in low-pressure entities, to record the pressure overnight. This can be realized by using a simple ventriculostomy, which is connected to a pressure monitoring system or by a telemetric probe.

36.2.1 Imaging

In order to precisely define a potential indication for endoscopic surgery, magnetic resonance imaging (MRI), preferably with high-resolution T2 sequences (CISS or TRUFI) in all three dimensions, is mandatory. For simple shunting, ultrasound or computed tomography (CT) scans are sufficient.

Because of the increased risk of acquired cancers after CT scans in childhood, this imaging method should only be reserved for emergency cases.[3,4]

36.2.2 ETV versus Shunting

Numerous publications exist regarding ETV indications,[5,6,7] probably the most practicable and evaluated one is the ETV success score (ETVSS). This score describes the patient's age, hydrocephalus etiology, and the fact whether a previous shunt surgery was performed or not.[8] Young age and a previous shunt are related to a low success rate. Postinfectious etiology also bears a high failure rate, whereas nontectal brain tumor, myelomeningocele, and history of intraventricular hemorrhage (IVH) have a medium risk. Aqueductal stenosis and tectal tumors as well as other typical occlusive three-ventricular entities are good risk indications for ETV.

There is still an ongoing discussion regarding long-term outcome of low-pressure ventriculomegaly in children, for example, after ETV, since normalization of the ventricular width is a rare exception in these cases.[7]

The immediate surgical risk for both methods—shunting and ETV—is considerably low in skilled hands. The mortality rate for the shunting procedure is less than 0.1%, for ETV up to 1%. During long-term follow-up, the shunt mortality rate raises substantially due to late fatal shunt failure. Also, the overall complication rate is higher in shunted patients and can be expected to be greater than 40%, although exact figures are missing. The most important failures are obstruction and infection. Children younger than 12 to 18 months of age have the highest complication rates, although in this age group also the highest failure rate of ETV is found and indications are less frequent. The overall complication rate of ETV is 6 to 20%. Infection rate after ETV is 1 to 5% and 1 to 20% after shunting. Infections after ETV are less severe. Generally, the major advantages of ETV are avoidance of foreign body implantation and a more physiological cerebrospinal fluid (CSF) circulation. But still, most of all hydrocephalus cases require shunting, either primarily or secondarily after ETV, due to the nature of the disease.[5,9,10,11,12,13,14,15]

Box 36.1 Shunting protocol with important rules

- Shunt surgery, if possible, no.1 on schedule
- Experienced surgeon at the table
- Doors of operating room closed
- As few staff as possible
- Thorough and repeated skin disinfection by surgeon
- Antiseptic hair washing (in theater)
- Keeping hardware in sterile inner packing as long as possible
- After unwrapping, hardware flushing and keeping in fluid
- Don't touch hardware with sharp instruments or fingers (if avoidable)
- Use of antimicrobial sutures

For both types of procedures, it could be proven that a specifically experienced surgeon and a standardized protocol are able to significantly reduce immediate and long-term complication rates.[16,17] Therefore, it is one of the most important surgical rules in pediatric neurosurgery that shunting and endoscopic procedures are no surgeries for beginners! (Box 36.1).

36.3 Shunt Implantation

36.3.1 Preparations

In elective shunt cases, preparations start already on admission. Systemic infection should be ruled out clinically and by assessing specific blood parameters (C-reactive protein [CRP], white blood cell [WBC]). Head and hair as well as the whole body are washed with an antiseptic solution prior to transportation to the operating room. Preoperative antibiotic prophylaxis and potentially necessary antiepileptic drugs are administered at least 30 minutes before starting surgery. The second-generation cephalosporin cefuroxime is recommended (30 mg/kg body weight), since it is passing the blood–brain barrier and has a wider gram-negative spectrum compared to first-generation cephalosporins.

Shunt operations should be on the first position of the operation list.[17]

Anesthesia introduction is conducted in a separate room and the intubated child will be transported into the operating room after preparation of all surgical tables and coverage of the instruments.

The child is positioned on a heating mattress. The final positioning using adequate positioning materials such as horseshoe headrest, silicone pads, and padding bandages is realized by the surgeon. Talking and air movements leading to particle turbulences should be avoided when silicone implants are used. Therefore, the number of individuals inside the operation room should be restricted.

It is necessary to stretch the patient's neck in order to avoid skin folds and to facilitate tunneling during the catheter implantation. The hairy head and the whole surgical field are prewashed with alcoholic disinfectant. Then the hair is combed and divided in the area of planned incisions. If necessary, a small hairy area is shaved as late as possible and adjacent hair clipped away. After surgical hand disinfection using an alcoholic solution, the surgeon performs the surgical skin disinfection, which covers usually the entire hairy head and the exposed half of the neck, anterior part of the chest, and the abdomen. If the child has bright skin and hair, the use of an undyed solution is recommended.

After a second surgical hand disinfection, the surgeon is dressed and places the surgical drapes, using impregnated incision drapes for the skin and hairy scalp as well as adhesive drapes to cover the body outside the surgical field.

36.3.2 Shunt Surgery

In virgin cases or new shunt insertions, the procedure starts with skin incisions for the burr hole and the peritoneal opening. Two standard burr hole sites do exist: a frontal precoronal one (Kocher's point) and a parieto-occipital one (Frazier's point). The choice depends on the ventricular shape and the surgeon's preference (▶ Fig. 36.1 and ▶ Fig. 36.2).

Positioning and draping must allow palpation of important landmarks (tip of the nose, ipsilateral eye, and ear) through the entire surgical procedure. The sagittal midline is preferably marked by a drape along its margin.

The abdominal incision can be made in one of the quadrants or directly at the umbilicus. The patient's conditions must be carefully considered before the incision is planned. If the umbilicus is deep and irregularly shaped, adequate disinfection may be a problem. Former abdominal interventions or diseases need to be explored in advance and abdominal ultrasound is recommended. The less affected quadrant is chosen. Some neurosurgeons prefer the left abdominal half in infants due

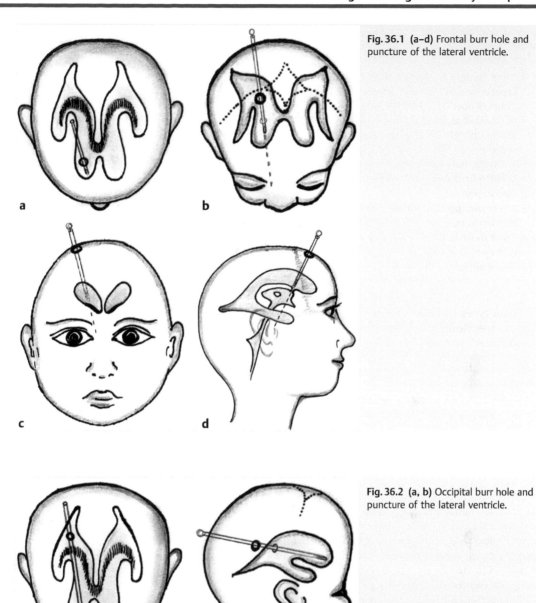

Fig. 36.1 (a–d) Frontal burr hole and puncture of the lateral ventricle.

a

b

c

d

Fig. 36.2 (a, b) Occipital burr hole and puncture of the lateral ventricle.

a

b

to a regular large liver in this age group. Does the child have a laparotomy history abdominal catheter insertion together with an experienced pediatric surgeon and with endoscopic assistance can be an option.

The first step is the opening of the peritoneal cavity, which is performed via an incision as small as possible depending on the thickness of the abdominal wall. The single layers will be opened according to their grain directions. The peritoneum itself can be punctured bluntly (trocar) or by a small incision just allowing to insert the catheter. If the catheter is not easily gliding into the cavity, or in cases of expected adhesions, a wider opening is mandatory in order to visualize or digitally explore the peritoneal cavity. In order to avoid early reoperation due to insufficient catheter length, as much catheter length as possible should be put into the cavity.

The next step is to perform a burr hole. In young infants, this is easily done by using a dissector or a knife as a drill. The periosteum is not detached from the skull in order to avoid ingrowth of the shunt components into the bone.

All shunt components have been kept in the sterile inner packaging on the instrumentation table. Now the catheters and the valve are unwrapped and put into Ringer's solution in order to avoid particle contamination from air. Flushing is recommended according to the manufacturer's prescription.

The next step is the tunneling of the peripheral catheter, which may already been connected to the valve and a possible pumping or flushing chamber. It is recommended to implant such a flushing reservoir, whenever possible. It helps to identify certain shunt malfunctions and allows aspiration of CSF.

If necessary, small skin incisions are made in the episternal, subclavian, or retroauricular region to allow staged tunneling. During the whole tunneling maneuver, the silicone components are not touched by the surgeon's gloves. Instead, blunt instruments or wet gauze pads are used. All open silicone parts are immediately covered with wet pads. It is also recommended to use iodine swabs, for example, when silicone tubes are in contact with skin edges.

At the end, the dura is opened using a knife or a small bipolar forceps, and the brain surface is coagulated. The central catheter with a guidewire and a rectangular deviation positioned at the planned intradural catheter length is inserted into the ventricle.

It is important that the central catheter is situated deeply enough inside the ventricle, and does not interfere with the choroid plexus in order to avoid plexus ingrowth and early obstruction. Ideally a parieto-occipital central catheter is placed with the tip in the frontal horn. In this case, the catheter is aimed toward the ipsilateral pupil and bluntly forwarded inside the ventricle until about 10 cm of length is inside the dura (▶ Fig. 36.2). In order to place a frontal catheter exactly, the dura is penetrated perpendicular aiming at the inner cantus of the ipsilateral eye (▶ Fig. 36.1). The median depth is 5 cm, depending on the size of the head. After 3 to 4 cm, a change in resistance indicates ependymal penetration, and in normal or increased intraventricular pressure, CSF flow is observed at the open catheter end. If no spontaneous CSF flow occurs, the catheter end is hold down in order to produce a negative pressure. If there is still no visible flow, aspiration or flushing is not recommended. Another trial or better, the use of a navigation tool should be considered.

It is recommended to use navigation, like ultrasound devices or standard neuro-navigation systems for adequate central catheter placement, for example, in narrow ventricles.

Now, all components will be connected and put in place. It is advisable to perform a pocket between the epicranium and the periosteum for valve body and flushing chamber. In infants, all components may easily pass through the soft tissue layers. All connector points will be secured with non-resorbable ligatures. The knots are placed towards the skull in order to avoid skin erosions. Generally, the shunt hardware should not be placed underneath a skin incision and no connectors or additional valves are allowed below the level of the skull. This prevents rupture or disconnection of the shunt catheter, reactive scar formation, and pain.

Finally, the skin is closed in a two-layer fashion. Intracutaneous stitches are allowed and in children with a thin skin layer, additional liquid bandage with or without steri-strip augmentation is recommended.

36.3.3 Postoperative Follow-up

Postoperative clinical monitoring includes electrocardiogram (ECG) and oxygen saturation during sleep, and when the child is without surveillance, regular neurological and abdominal checks and daily wound inspections. A final CRP is taken before discharge.

In young children, the wound healing process, for example, in silicone implantations, should be controlled 2 weeks before exposure to water and physical stress is allowed.

All children will be provided with a shunt pass and parents are informed regarding an appropriate follow-up program.

Postoperative imaging depends on the intraoperative course and the specific patient condition. In general, ultrasound of the brain in an infant is easy to obtain and is recommended as soon as possible. Abdominal ultrasound is able to detect the position of the peripheral catheter and free intraperitoneal fluid as sign of a functioning shunt. Early MRI or CT scans are indicated after complicated surgery or in older children when they are symptomatic for shunt malfunction. Otherwise, it is recommended to perform sectional imaging after 3 months, when the expected drainage effect is visible. These scans will serve as baseline pictures for future follow-up.

36.3.4 Variations of Shunt Surgery

Variations of this shunting procedure are frequent and depending on the patient's condition.

Whenever multiple compartments need to be drained, first a possible indication for endoscopic fenestration must be considered (▶ Fig. 36.3). It is essential to keep the number of hardware components as low as possible, since each of them may cause complications. If it is unavoidable to put more than one central catheter, it is generally recommended to connect those in front of the valve, otherwise differential ICP can cause problems. One exception from this rule is an intended differential pressure, for example, when a subdural hygroma is drained together with a ventricular hydrocephalus. In secondary shunt procedures, often only single components are revised. Because of the fact that in secondary shunt procedures not all steps

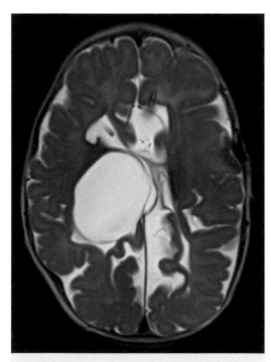

Fig. 36.3 Cystic posthemorrhagic hydrocephalus with two central catheters in place prior to endoscopic fenestration.

are clear in advance, a general informed consent for an entire shunt procedure should be obtained.

36.3.5 Ventriculoatrial Shunt

Ventriculoatrial shunting is becoming rare. A disadvantage of atrial shunting is the relatively high peripheral revision rate in young children in order to keep the catheter tip in the atrium.[13] However, some children with a complicated abdominal history may benefit from such a procedure. The peripheral catheter is placed into the right atrium. Venous access is performed on the ipsilateral side of the central catheter by open venisection of the facial vein or one of the jugular veins. A special atrial catheter with a tapered pliant tip facilitates the intravenous insertion and intra-atrial catheter movement. The tip position must be checked intraoperatively by fluoroscopy. In order to avoid thrombotic ingrowth of the catheter tip, the intra-atrial position is mandatory. There the catheter tip is in constant moving. ECG monitoring is important during surgery to indicate that there is no persistent arrhythmia. Like in central venous line insertion, it is important to ensure that no air is getting into the venous system. Increase of positive end-expiratory pressure (PEEP), flushing and aspiration of the catheter, and clamp occlusion are necessary steps.

In small infants and after a prolonged intensive medical treatment, access to peripheral or even central veins can be a major problem. In these cases, instead of open venesection regular central venous puncture and insertion of the peripheral catheter via Seldinger's technique is recommended. Postoperative imaging should include chest X-ray to verify atrial catheter position.

36.3.6 General Considerations

Further alternatives are peripheral catheter placement into the gallbladder, the ureter, and the pleural space. Disadvantages are the necessity of a special surgical expertise and a limited resorption capacity of the pleural space.

A broad variety of shunt devices and additional valve systems is on the market. So far, there is no proof that one of the devices is superior.[18] Overdrainage and slit-ventricle complications are well-known late sequelae mostly occurring years after primary shunting. It is assumed that standard differential pressure valves do not properly address the phenomenon of overdrainage in upright position. Therefore, special valve components like antisiphoning or antigravity devices are in use. In order to prevent shunt infections, the use of antibiotic-impregnated systems (AIS) is recommended. There is growing evidence that these materials are preventive against shunt infections. Whether this justifies a general usage is not yet proven statistically.[19,20,21,22] There is some evidence that antimicrobial sutures are also able to reduce wound and shunt infections.[16]

36.4 Endoscopic Third Ventriculostomy

ETV is an easy and elegant way to reestablish intracranial CSF circulation. It was originally invented to cure a typical occlusive three-ventricular hydrocephalus. However, more indications have been proven of being successfully addressed by this method.

It is essential to perform a brain MRI with T2-weighted images in all three dimensions, for example, a midsagittal slice, for evaluation of the inner CSF spaces and basal cisterns, and potential variations of brain structures and vessels. Normally, access is planned through the nondominant hemisphere. In cases with a small foramen of Monro, the contralateral side should be preferred.

Although the procedure itself is not difficult, potential damage can result to brain structures and adjacent vessels leading to devastating complications. Therefore, conduction of a highly standardized procedure with a four-handed well-trained surgical staff is mandatory.

Anesthesia introduction is realized in a separate room. Parallel to this, the instrumentation tables and necessary settings (positioning of endoscopy tower, endoscopy, and flushing system) are arranged and checked according to a strict protocol. Only when all components are checked of being fully functioning, the surgical procedure itself can start. The patient's head is positioned in a straight, slightly inclined fashion on a horseshoe headrest and securely fixed or in a Mayfield clamp. General hygienic and disinfection rules as well as draping are comparable to the shunt-implantation process. Again, landmarks like nose and ears as well as the sagittal midline must be identifiable after draping. A straight or curved skin incision just in front of the nondominant coronal suture in the middle of the median third of the suture is performed and the periosteum is cut and shove off. A burr hole wide enough to let the endoscope trocar easily pass through is placed just underneath. After

cutting the dura and coagulating the brain surface, the obturated trocar of the endoscope (or a peel-away sheath in case of using a small endoscope) is gently moved forward the same direction as puncturing the lateral ventricle in shunt surgery. After approximately 4 cm, the resistance changes and the ventricle is entered. After removal of all obturators, first the endoscope (0-degree optic) is inserted. Then the flushing line is attached. From now on, the whole team is watching the monitor pictures for intraventricular control. The endoscope/trocar can be steered freehand or using a supporting arm. Ideally, the tip of the endoscope directly points at the ipsilateral foramen of Monro. All landmarks will be identified. The choroid plexus is diving into the third ventricle, laterally the superior thalamostriate vein (terminal vein) is running over the thalamus and medially the septal vein points into the direction of the foramen (▶ Fig. 36.4). The endoscope is gently forwarded through the foramen. After this step, the fornix cannot be visualized any longer and must be kept in mind in order to avoid lesions. The floor of the third ventricle should be thinned out showing a grayish color and resembles a triangle. The tip of the basilar artery and the posterior cerebral arteries can be surmised just in front of the mammillary bodies at the base of the triangle. At the tip tiny vessels create a red dot and most often the infundibular recess can be identified. Ventrally the

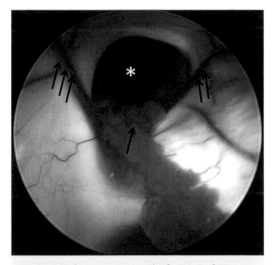

Fig. 36.4 Endoscopic view on the foramen of Monro (*), the choroid plexus (↑), on the lateral aspect the superior thalamostriate vein (↑ ↑), and medially the septal vein (↑ ↑ ↑).

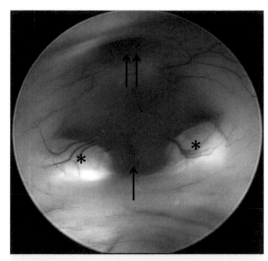

Fig. 36.5 Endoscopic view on the floor of the third ventricle: mammillary bodies (**), basilar tip (↑), infundibular recess (↑↑).

clivus becomes visible (▶ Fig. 36.5). In a markedly enlarged ventricle the third cranial nerves can be identified as well as white linear structures. Only in the middle of the membranous floor the opening is safe. It is important to use only blunt instruments without force and to avoid coagulation in order to create an opening of the sometimes resistant membrane. Otherwise, cisternal structures can be injured. Once the opening is performed, a 3-French Fogarty catheter, which is slowly inflated only at the level of the floor, is used as a bougie. An eventual bleeding is controlled best by flushing and compressing with the Fogarty catheter itself. During the whole procedure, gentle flushing is possible. It is important to keep the outflow (suction) channel open. This helps to keep an optimum pressure and filling inside the ventricles. Ringer's solution is less pyrogenic compared to physiological NaCl solution and should have body temperature.

For a few minutes, the intraventricular site is watched without flushing to detect minor bleedings. In case of no bleeding, the whole system will be removed under vision in order to detect hidden bleedings above the tip of the endoscope. The access is plugged with a piece of Gelfoam. The dura is closed and the periosteum can be sutured as well before the two-layer wound closure is performed. Some colleagues prefer to put a reservoir or a ventriculostomy inside the ventricle in order to control ICP during the first postoperative days.

We only consider these means in complicated cases due to the related risks, for example, infection and secondary wound healing disorders.

Postoperative monitoring is comparable to shunt surgery. Postoperative MRI should always include a midsagittal T2 sequence. A patent third ventriculostomy will be identified by a typical flow void through the floor into the prepontine cistern at the site of the fenestration.

36.4.1 Surgical Pearls

- Shunt surgery and ETV are supposed to be easy procedures. However, because of a significant intraoperative risk for ETV and high postoperative complication rates for shunting, only specifically skilled and experienced surgeons should perform this kind of surgeries.
- It is recommended to implement a standardized shunting protocol, since this has been proven to decrease shunt infection rates.
- In normal ventricular configurations, transfrontal puncture of the lateral ventricle is safe, when a precoronal, 2 to 2.5 cm parasagittal burr hole is performed and the direction of the puncture is perpendicular aiming at the inner cantus of the ipsilateral eye and the ipsilateral tragus.
- A long-persisting open exposure of the CSF system during surgery bears a high infection risk, therefore, placing the central catheter should be the last part of the surgery.
- Multiple punctures of the ventricle should be avoided.
- All kinds of connectors or inline components below the insertion of the nuchal muscles should be avoided in order to prevent rupture and scar formation.
- A flushing or pumping reservoir helps to identify potential complications during the further course.
- In order to prevent the child from early peripheral shunt revision, insertion of the entire catheter length is recommended.

36.5 Common Clinical Questions

1. Which patients will most likely benefit from ETV?
2. Which kind of diagnostic is mandatory to define ETV indication?

3. What are the most common complications after shunt surgery and which kind of patients are mostly affected?

4. What are the most important aspects regarding ventriculoatrial shunt placement?

36.6 Answers to Common Clinical Questions

1. The highest benefit from ETV will have hydrocephalus patients who are older than 1 year of age, suffering from a typical occlusive three-ventricular hydrocephalus, and never had a shunt before. The lowest success rate is to be expected in postinfectious hydrocephalus in very young infants, for example, when there was already a shunt in place.

2. Prior to any endoscopic procedure, MRI, for example, T2 with midsagittal projection and at least axial and/or coronal series are mandatory. Best demonstration of cystic components and membranes are provided by special T2 sequences like CISS or TRUFI.

3. The most common shunt complications do not occur intraoperatively but during follow-up. Obstruction and infection are by far the most common problems. Preterm infants with a history of posthemorrhagic hydrocephalus and myelomeningocele patients are mostly affected.

4. The most important points in ventriculoatrial shunting are the placement of the peripheral tip inside the right atrium in order to assure a constant movement and avoidance of air inside the venous system.

References

[1] Rashid QT, Salat MS, Enam K, et al. Time trends and age-related etiologies of pediatric hydrocephalus: results of a groupwise analysis in a clinical cohort. Childs Nerv Syst. 2012; 28(2):221–227

[2] Serlo W, Fernell E, Heikkinen E, Anderson H, von Wendt L. Functions and complications of shunts in different etiologies of childhood hydrocephalus. Childs Nerv Syst. 1990; 6(2):92–94

[3] Pearce MS, Salotti JA, Little MP, et al. Radiation exposure from CT scans in childhood and subsequent risk of leukaemia and brain tumours: a retrospective cohort study. Lancet. 2012; 380(9840):499–505

[4] Mathews JD, Forsythe AV, Brady Z, et al. Cancer risk in 680,000 people exposed to computed tomography scans in childhood or adolescence: data linkage study of 11 million Australians. BMJ. 2013; 346:f2360

[5] Di Rocco C, Massimi L, Tamburrini G. Shunts vs endoscopic third ventriculostomy in infants: are there different types and/or rates of complications? A review. Childs Nerv Syst. 2006; 22(12):1573–1589

[6] Kulkarni AV, Drake JM, Kestle JR, Mallucci CL, Sgouros S, Constantini S, Canadian Pediatric Neurosurgery Study Group. Predicting who will benefit from endoscopic third ventriculostomy compared with shunt insertion in childhood hydrocephalus using the ETV Success Score. J Neurosurg Pediatr. 2010; 6(4):310–315

[7] Kulkarni AV, Hui S, Shams I, Donnelly R. Quality of life in obstructive hydrocephalus: endoscopic third ventriculostomy compared to cerebrospinal fluid shunt. Childs Nerv Syst. 2010; 26(1):75–79

[8] Kulkarni AV, Riva-Cambrin J, Browd SR. Use of the ETV Success Score to explain the variation in reported endoscopic third ventriculostomy success rates among published case series of childhood hydrocephalus. J Neurosurg Pediatr. 2011; 7(2):143–146

[9] Durnford AJ, Kirkham FJ, Mathad N, Sparrow OC. Endoscopic third ventriculostomy in the treatment of childhood hydrocephalus: validation of a success score that predicts long-term outcome. J Neurosurg Pediatr. 2011; 8(5):489–493

[10] Lee JK, Seok JY, Lee JH, et al. Incidence and risk factors of ventriculoperitoneal shunt infections in children: a study of 333 consecutive shunts in 6 years. J Korean Med Sci. 2012; 27(12):1563–1568

[11] Paulsen AH, Lundar T, Lindegaard KF. Twenty-year outcome in young adults with childhood hydrocephalus: assessment of surgical outcome, work participation, and health-related quality of life. J Neurosurg Pediatr. 2010; 6(6):527–535

[12] Tuli S, Tuli J, Drake J, Spears J. Predictors of death in pediatric patients requiring cerebrospinal fluid shunts. J Neurosurg. 2004; 100(5) Suppl Pediatrics:442–446

[13] Vernet O, Campiche R, de Tribolet N. Long-term results after ventriculoatrial shunting in children. Childs Nerv Syst. 1993; 9(5):253–255

[14] Vinchon M, Baroncini M, Delestret I. Adult outcome of pediatric hydrocephalus. Childs Nerv Syst. 2012; 28(6):847–854

[15] Vinchon M, Rekate H, Kulkarni AV. Pediatric hydrocephalus outcomes: a review. Fluids Barriers CNS. 2012; 9(1):18

[16] Kestle JR, Riva-Cambrin J, Wellons JC, III, et al. Hydrocephalus Clinical Research Network. A standardized protocol to reduce cerebrospinal fluid shunt infection: the Hydrocephalus Clinical Research Network Quality Improvement Initiative. J Neurosurg Pediatr. 2011; 8(1):22–29

[17] Choux M, Genitori L, Lang D, Lena G. Shunt implantation: reducing the incidence of shunt infection. J Neurosurg. 1992; 77(6):875–880

[18] Kestle J, Drake J, Milner R, et al. Long-term follow-up data from the Shunt Design Trial. Pediatr Neurosurg. 2000; 33(5):230–236

[19] Kandasamy J, Dwan K, Hartley JC, et al. Antibiotic-impregnated ventriculoperitoneal shunts—a multi-centre British paediatric neurosurgery group (BPNG) study using historical controls. Childs Nerv Syst. 2011; 27(4):575–581

[20] Klimo P, Jr, Thompson CJ, Ragel BT, Boop FA. Antibiotic-impregnated shunt systems versus standard shunt systems: a meta- and cost-savings analysis. J Neurosurg Pediatr. 2011; 8(6):600–612

[21] Parker SL, Anderson WN, Lilienfeld S, Megerian JT, McGirt MJ. Cerebrospinal shunt infection in patients receiving antibiotic-impregnated versus standard shunts. J Neurosurg Pediatr. 2011; 8(3):259–265

[22] Steinbok P, Milner R, Agrawal D, et al. A multicenter multinational registry for assessing ventriculoperitoneal shunt infections for hydrocephalus. Neurosurgery. 2010; 67(5):1303–1310

37 Treatment of Hydrocephalus in the Developing World

Rodrigo Mercado, Jesus A. Villagómez, Luis A. Arredondo

37.1 Introduction

Hydrocephalus is a common clinical problem in pediatric neurosurgical practice in the developing countries. It is defined as a condition wherein the excess of cerebrospinal fluid (CSF) within the ventricular system and cisterns of the brain leads to increased intracranial pressure (ICP).[1] Hydrocephalus affects 1 to 2% of the general population.[2] It occurs due to subnormal reabsorption or overproduction of CSF. The etiologies can be described as either congenital or acquired.

37.1.1 Congenital

- Associated with myelomeningocele (MMC) with or without Chiari malformation. The hydrocephalus associated with MMC in developing countries represents the more common specific congenital etiology in children[3]; 11 to 16% of congenital hydrocephalus cases are associated with MMC. It is just second to infectious diseases in general infant populations and often associated with aqueductal stenosis.[4] Only one out six infants with MMC presents signs of ICP at birth and hydrocephalus is more commonly noticed at 2 to 3 weeks of age.[5]
- Perinatal germinal matrix hemorrhage. Intraventricular hemorrhages require definitive ventricular shunts in 15 to 35% of the cases.[6,7]
- Primary aqueductal stenosis.
- Chiari I. Chiari is associated with hydrocephalus in 14% of cases.[8] In patients with hydrocephalus, shunting is indicated prior to foramen magnum decompression.
- Dandy–Walker malformation.

37.2 Acquired

- Infectious: Infectious diseases are the most common specific etiology of hydrocephalus in infants.[4] It is not only observed as an acute complication of bacterial meningitis, but also associated with chronic granulomatous arachnoiditis observed in parasitic, mycobacterial, and fungal infections.
  - Postacute bacterial meningitis.
  - Tuberculosis. Signs of increased ICP are described in more than 70% of children with central nervous system (CNS) complications of tuberculosis. Hydrocephalus is a common radiological feature. Close to 17% of patients with tuberculosis (TB) and CNS involvement displayed this finding.[9]
  - Cysticercosis.
- Posthemorrhagic.
- Secondary to masses: Noncommunicating hydrocephalus secondary to obstruction of CSF flow inside or from outside the ventricle walls.
  - Neoplastic or no neoplastic
    - Posterior fossa lesions compressing or occupying the fourth ventricle.
    - Tumors occupying the third ventricle and obstructing the cerebral aqueduct arising either from the sellar or the pineal region.
    - Diencephalic lesions compressing or obstructing either the foramen of Monro or the third ventricle walls.
    - Overproducer CSF tumors such as the choroid plexus papilloma and choroid plexus carcinoma.
- Postoperative.
- Associated with spinal tumors.
- Constitutional ventriculomegaly.

37.3 Treatment

In spite of the growing experience with endoscopic procedures in many developing countries, ventricular shunts remain as the main treatment option in hydrocephalus, in particular, in pediatric populations.[10] Nulzen and Spitz introduced the use of internalized CSF derivative in the 50s. Most of the devices pose three components: ventricular catheter, valve, and peritoneal catheter. The components are made of Sylastic, impregnated with a radiopaque material for radiographic localization.

Either the location of the distal catheter or their hydrodynamic features can be used to classify shunts. Based on the location of the distal catheter, the *ventriculoperitoneal* (VP) shunt is the most widely used. It can be completed via two main approaches, the frontal precoronal and the posterior parietal. It uses the abdominal cavity as the recipient of the CSF, and it is contraindicated when there is an acute abdominal condition such as peritonitis, or the presence of adhesions or ineffective absorption secondary to prior abdominal surgeries. The *ventriculoatrial* (VA) shunt sends the CSF flow to the cardiac atrium through the internal jugular vein. It is indicated when the patient is not eligible for an abdominal derivative location. The rest of the probable locations are less common and are considered only when the VP and VA shunts are not defined as a therapeutic option: the distal catheter can be located at the subgaleal space, pleura, bladder, or biliary tract.[11]

Based on the mechanism of hydrodynamics, the valve can be described as:

Differential pressure valve (PS Medical Standard Valve, Medtronic). This is the most widely used valve. They work with a fixed opening pressure, which means that the valve will let the CSF flow out of the valve when the pressure difference drops below a predetermined pressure threshold.[11] They are available in three different opening pressures: low, medium, and high (▶ Table 37.1). The main disadvantage is the variation in CSF flow with position changes, and the probable need of repetitive revisions.

Flow-controlling shunts (Delta Valves, Medtronic; Orbits Sigma Valve). The progressive narrowing of the outflow orifice controls the flow of CSF, which increases in turn the pressure needed to increase the CSF flow.[12]

Adjustable valves. They permit the adjustment of valve opening pressures with an external controller.[13] There are four types of adjustable valves (▶ Table 37.2). They are considered the ideal shunting devices for their capacity to adjust to different CSF pressure requirements and control drainage-related complications. Their main disadvantages in developing countries are the elevated cost and the poor distribution of specialized centers for periodic revisions and pressure adjustments.

37.4 Surgical Indications and Contraindications

Ventricular shunts are indicated in cases of obstructive hydrocephalus such as in intraventricular or posterior fossa tumor cases, Chiari I malformation, and stenosis of the cerebral aqueduct, in particular, when an endoscopic third ventriculostomy (ETV) has failed, is contraindicated, or is not immediately available. It is also indicated in most cases of communicating hydrocephalus when the blood cell count and/or protein content of the CSF are not elevated. This concept is controversial in cases of chronic granulomatous meningitis due to neurocysticercosis or meningeal tuberculosis, conditions in which the elevations of both, white cells and protein content, are common CSF features.

An ongoing CNS infection is an absolute contraindication. Any infectious condition with no evidence of pharmacological control and persistent fever will increase the risk of a CNS infection facilitated by the opening of the blood–brain barrier or contamination of the components of the shunting device. The peritoneal approach is absolutely

Table 37.1 Main features of set pressure valves

	Low pressure	Medium pressure	High pressure
Dot code	□	□□	□□□
Closing pressure range	5–50 mm H_2O	51–110 mm H_2O	110–180 mm H_2O
Flow pressure	50–75 mm H_2O	50–140 mm H_2O	110–220 mm H_2O
Opening pressure	5	10	15 cm H_2O

Table 37.2 Features of programmable valves

	Codman–Hakim	Strata	Sophysa	Miethke ProGAV
Opening pressure (mm H_2O)	30–200	15–170	30–200	30–200
Antisiphon device	Yes	No	No	Gravitational unit
MRI compatibility	Yes	Yes	Yes	Yes

Abbreviation: MRI, magnetic resonance imaging.

contraindicated in the presence of severe abdominal acute conditions such as necrotizing enterocolitis and acute or chronic recurrent peritonitis. Repetitive abdominal surgeries should be considered as a relative contraindication due to the risk of a noneffective absorption of the peritoneal cavity. There is controversy about prematurity and body weight lower than 2,000 g.

37.5 Surgical Technique

37.5.1 Preparation

The most important preoperative issues we look at are directed toward the reduction of infection and contamination risks.
- When possible, schedule as the first case at the neurosurgery operating room.
- Limit the number of medical and paramedical personnel inside the operating room (OR) to the minimum required, and avoid in and out traffic from the OR.

Select the entry point and ventricular catheter location according to the anatomical features and etiology of the hydrocephalus described in the images, either computed tomography (CT) or magnetic resonance imaging (MRI).
- We prefer a right frontal horn location through an ipsilateral precoronal entry point.
- In the presence of significant ventricular asymmetry, it is important to identify the cause prior to the selection of the ventricular location. In the event of isolated segments of the lateral ventricles related to intraventricular or diencephalon tumors or ependymal scaring due to inflammatory or hemorrhagic conditions, a previous endoscopic septum fenestration or opening of the adherence walls might be suggested. When this is not possible, a complex trajectory directed toward the contralateral foramen of Monro through the septum will communicate both lateral ventricles. In isolated ventricles, direct the catheter to the isolated cavity, away from the scar or from the tumor wall.

37.5.2 Positioning

- Head over the horseshoe headrest or over a gel or cotton donut. We start with the head turned 45 degrees to the opposite side to facilitate the passer dissection, and then turn it back to neutral position for the catheter placement when a frontal approach is preferred. Take it

further lateral to 90 degrees when a posterior parietal approach is selected.
- Neck and ipsilateral shoulder elevated with a roll and pads in order to locate the clavicle and tip of the mastoid at the same level parallel to the floor. This will avoid the shunt passer stops and forceful manipulation of the skin.

37.5.3 Shaving and Skin Preparation

- Avoid the use of razor blades. Use a trimmer when necessary to shave the minimal required area. This is to avoid superficial cuts and abrasions that represent a risk for further skin opening and exposure of the shunt components.
- Perform a careful cleaning of the skin and place a drape over the surgical area before placing the operating cloths.

37.5.4 Ventricular Phase

We discourage the use of burr hole reservoir devices and prefer the flat base reservoir distal from the burr hole, therefore, the scalp incision can be drawn in a slightly curved or semilunar fashion with its base directed toward the distal catheter to avoid any suture line or incision scar over any of the components of the shunt. The size is related to the size of the cranial opening. We avoid the incisions over the burr hole and prefer to stay a few millimeters away from the border in order to reduce the risk of CSF fistula or the exposure of the catheter entry in the event of a defective scaring or incidental opening of the wound with scratching or mild trauma.

The burr hole is made with a hand perforator such as a Hudson tree, or a high-powered drill. In young children, it can be done with a surgical knife. Borders are regularized with curettes or roughers when necessary. The most common burr hole locations are:
- Frontal precoronal, also named the Kocher point.
  - It is 1 cm in front of the coronal suture in the mid-pupillary line, usually 3 cm lateral from midline in completely grown craniums (▶ Fig. 37.1).
- Posterior parietal, often misnamed as occipital, is also named the Frazier point.
  - It is 6 cm up from the inion and 3 cm from midline in older children, usually on the flat portion of the parietal boss in smaller children (▶ Fig. 37.2).

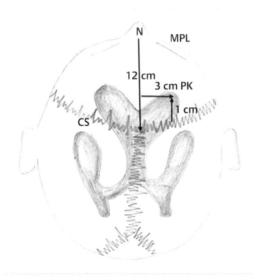

Fig. 37.1 Schematic drawing of the precoronal Kocher's point location. CS, coronal suture; MPL, mid-pupillary line; N, nasion; PK, point of Kocher. (Courtesy of Gutiérrez-Oliva K.)

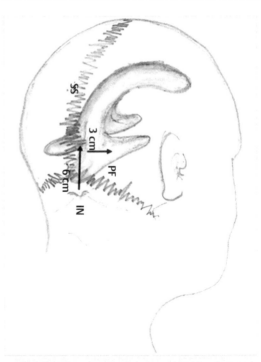

Fig. 37.2 Schematic drawing of the posterior parietal Frazier's point location. IN, inion; PF, point of Frazier; SS, sagittal suture. (Courtesy of Gutiérrez-Oliva K.)

The dura is not opened until the peritoneal phase is complete and the distal catheter has been passed completely. The dura is identified and cauterized with bipolar forceps before it is incised in a cruciate fashion. The pia is also cauterized and incised with the tip of the bipolar forceps.

37.5.5 Peritoneal Phase

A transverse 2- to 3-cm long linear incision, located on the ipsilateral abdominal quadrant, centered over the lateral border of the anterior rectus muscle, approximately 2 to 3 cm lateral and 1 to 2 cm above the umbilicus. Immediately after dissecting the subcutaneous fat, the anterior rectus sheath is identified and incised. The fibers of the rectus muscle are split following the direction of the fibers until the posterior rectus sheath is unveiled and incised. The peritoneum is identified and carefully grabbed with the tips of two mosquito forceps in a tent-like fashion, with great care to avoid any accidental lesion to the peritoneal cavity content. A purse-string suture is placed, either 3.0 Vicryl or 4.0 silk before the incision is done.

37.5.6 Shunt Tunneling Phase

A shunt passer is bent and advanced through the subcutaneous fat layer, from the abdominal incision all the way up to the scalp incision. Try to avoid a superficial tunnel trajectory. We usually do additional incisions where the passer stops, before traumatizing the skin when trying to force our dissector. A retroauricular incision over the tip of the mastoid is usually necessary. A subcutaneous pocket for the valve is dissected over the trajectory of the passer. The distal catheter is passed from the cephalic to the abdominal incision. We usually open the package containing the shunt components only after the incisions and dissection of the cephalic and distal wounds are complete. We manipulate the components with blunt or rubber-protected instruments.

37.5.7 Catheter Placement

Frontal Approach

- Relocate the head to neutral position.
- Use external cranial marks to define the trajectory of the ventricular catheter. This should end up being located at the ipsilateral foramen of Monro. On the coronal plane, the trajectory of the catheter is directed posteriorly towards the

outer ear, while the tip of the catheter, in the sagittal anteroposterior (AP) plane, is in line with the ipsilateral medial canthus.

- Should feel entering the frontal horn 3 to 5 cm deep. The catheter is advanced 1 cm further before the stylet is withdrawn. The rest of the catheter is advanced without the inner stylet at a depth of 5 to 6 cm from the cranial vault.

Posterior Parietal Approach

- Direct a parallel trajectory aiming for the ipsilateral medial canthus.
- Should feel entering the occipital horn by 3 to 4 cm from the cranial vault.
- The catheter is advanced 2 cm further before the stylet is withdrawn and the rest of the catheter is advanced to a depth of 6 cm, according to the preoperative measures.

The spontaneous flow of CSF is the commonest sign of a successful catheter location. The gentle aspiration of CSF without resistance trough a blunt needle connected to the catheter might be needed in cases when cerebral parenchyma or a blood clot blocks the catheter.

The most common devices come with a 90 degrees angle fixing attachment at the outer border of the burr hole, to stitch it to pericranium and to protect the catheter from the overbending. The proximal catheter is assembled with the reservoir shunt which has been previously attached the distal catheter. An arrow or arrowhead is usually drawn on the valve reservoir pointing at the direction of the flow, from cephalic to distal. The distal catheter is cut in a length that permits to locate the valve 2 to 3 cm distal from the burr hole, close to the incision and not far back in the neck. This will facilitate a revision procedure through only one incision when needed.

A final assessment of the catheter placement and of the correct assembly of the shunt, components should be done before placing the distal catheter inside the peritoneal cavity. CSF is aspirated from the distal catheter with a blunt needle through one of the distal catheter slits. There should be no resistance to gentle aspiration. Any difficulty suggests that the ventricular catheter has been retracted out of the ventricle, or cerebral parenchyma or a blood clot blocks the catheter, usually at the connections of the system, or that the assembly of the components have been erroneous.

The immediate postoperative care demands the continuous use of antibiotics for 24 hours, mobilization to be delayed for 6 to 12 hours, and discharge to home after 24 to 48 hours.

37.6 Complications

37.6.1 Transoperative

Cranial Complications

Erroneous Location of the Ventricular Catheter

- Too deep
- Misdirected trajectory

No spontaneous CSF flow through the catheter once inserted, or any resistance to gentle aspiration suggest blockade by a blood clot, brain parenchyma, or choroid plexus. Gently inject 2 cm of saline solution to unblock the flow. If there is no CSF flow and the resistance persists, parenchymal or cisternal location is suspected. The catheter has to be relocated.

Intracerebral or Intraventricular Hemorrhage

It is noticed when blood flows along with CSF through the catheter. It is especially common among patients with coagulopathies, which is a frequent complication of severe infectious disorders.

Usually, stops spontaneously or with saline solution instillation through the catheter. An immediate postoperative CT is mandatory to define the extent of the hemorrhage and decide whether to keep the shunt in place or change it for an external drainage. Rarely, an open craniotomy is required to explore and directly coagulate the injured vessel.

Abdominal Complications

Misplacement of the Distal Catheter

Preperitoneal location. Identified with resistance to pass the catheter into the abdominal cavity or the presence of CSF leaking through the abdominal wound.

Relocate the catheter.

Injury to Abdominal Viscera

Identified with the presence of intestinal fluid or hemorrhage from the injured wall.

Usually required assistance of a general pediatric surgeon. The peritoneal cavity might no longer be the option for CSF drainage. Select to either transform for an external drainage or modify the distal location of the catheter.

37.7 Postoperative

37.7.1 Shunt Malfunction

A mechanical obstruction is a common delayed complication. The overall failure rate during the first year of implantation is 35 to 40%.[14,15] Could be detected at the proximal catheter due to protrusion of the choroid plexus, infiltration from tumor, collapse of the ventricular walls, glial tissue from astrocyte proliferation, debris, or blood.[16] When the distal catheter is the site of the obstruction, consider preperitoneal migration or displacement and omentum obstruction.

37.7.2 Infections

Incidence of shunt infections ranges from 8 to 12%.[14,15,17,18,19] Shunt insertion at younger age, prematurity, and CSF leak are recognized risk factors.[20] Several bacterial pathogens have been described: *Staphylococcus epidermidis*, *Staphylococcus aureus*, *Klebsiella pneumoniae*, *Pseudomonas aeruginosa*, and *Candida albicans*.[19,20] The use of antibiotic-impregnated shunts lowers, but not abolishes, the infection rates. The infection rate in these shunts is 5%.[21] Great care should be taken during the preoperative phase to reduce the infection and contamination risks.

Shunt Erosion through Skin

To prevent this in malnourished and premature patients:
- Select the smallest shunt system available.
- Draw a larger scalp flap with extensive skin dissection.
- Avoid suture lines over any of the shunt components.

Catheter Migration

- Intestinal migration
- Rare migration sites

Identify the location and patency of the connections of the system by X-ray films.

Remove the system. Disarticulate the components and pull out the distal catheter from the exposed migration site. Never try to pull it out through the cephalic incision or along the subcutaneous trajectory.

Complication of Previous Abdominal Conditions Such as Hydrocele, Defects of the Abdominal Wall, or Ascites

Peritoneal Pseudocyst

Rare but recognized complication. Related to the presence of inflammatory cells and fibrous tissue lining on the surface of the distal catheter. Previous shunt infection or repetitive revisions are probable risk factors.[22] The removal of the whole system is advised, since it seems to be related to bacterial colonization of the distal catheter.

Seizures

The incidence of seizures in shunted children is reported to be quite high, ranging from 20% to approximately 50%.[23] Early shunting in patients younger than 2 years, history of shunt complications, shunt infection, and revisions are significant risk factors for developing post-shunt seizures.[24]

37.8 Common Clinical Questions

1. Which management strategy represents the optimal approach in Chiari I malformation with hydrocephalus?
2. Which is the best treatment for an infant with congenital hydrocephalus secondary to cerebral aqueduct stenosis?
3. Describe the management strategy that should be followed in order to reduce the risk of shunt infections.
4. Are the programmable valves more suitable than the set pressure valves in the developing world scenario?

37.9 Answers to Common Clinical Questions

1. In patients with Chiari I malformations and hydrocephalus, shunting or ETV is used to resolve hydrocephalus. It is recommended before trying foramen magnum decompression (FMD). Only if the symptoms and signs persist after the CSF shunt, a FMD should be considered.[8]

2. The overall success rates of ETV are 23 to 94%, with a mean of 68%. The success rate is homogeneous above 60% at any age in cases of obstructive hydrocephalus confined to the third and lateral ventricles. There is a trend in lower success rates in infants younger than 6 months of age.[25] In these patients, a low-pressure valve shunt is recommended. In a retrospective study, low-pressure shunts were effective in more than 80% of children under 2 years of age.[26]

3. Incidence of shunt infections ranges from 8 to 12%.[14,15,17,18,19] The use of antibiotic-impregnated shunts mildly lowers the infection rates. The infection rate in these shunts is 5%.[21] The most important preoperative issues are directed toward the reduction of infection and contamination risks especially in patients at higher risk such as young infants or premature newborns. We recommend to schedule as the first case at the neurosurgery operating room, limit the number of medical and paramedical personnel inside the OR, and avoid in and out traffic from the OR. Manipulate the components of the shunt as minimum required, with instruments rather than with your hands. We usually do additional incisions where the passer stops, before traumatizing the skin when trying to force our dissector. Since CSF leak is one of the recognized risk factors,[20] we avoid the incisions over the burr hole in order to reduce the risk of CSF fistula or the exposure of the catheter entry.

4. Several authors described safety and efficacy of programmable shunts as comparable with set pressure valves.[14,15] The main advantage of programmable shunts is reduced risk of overall shunt revision and proximal obstruction.[13] These arguments are in favor of programmable valves in developing countries, especially in areas with scarce distribution of neurosurgical services in large territories with poor means of transportation that demand long and complex journeys from their homes. The main obstacle is the cost-effectiveness relation when comparing to set pressure valves.

References

[1] Rekate HL. Hydrocephalus in children. In: Winn HR, ed. Youmans Neurological Surgery. 5th ed. New York, NY: Saunders Elsevier; 2004:3387–3404

[2] Bondurant CP, Jiménez DF. Epidemiology of cerebrospinal fluid shunting. Pediatr Neurosurg. 1995; 23(5):254–258, discussion 259

[3] Melo JRT, de Melo EN, de Vasconcellos AG, Pacheco P. Congenital hydrocephalus in the northeast of Brazil: epidemiological aspects, prenatal diagnosis, and treatment. Childs Nerv Syst. 2013; 29(10):1899–1903

[4] Warf BC. Hydrocephalus associated with neural tube defects: characteristics, management, and outcome in sub-Saharan Africa. Childs Nerv Syst. 2011; 27(10):1589–1594

[5] Tamburrini G, Frassanito P, Iakovaki K, et al. Myelomeningocele: the management of the associated hydrocephalus. Childs Nerv Syst. 2013; 29(9):1569–1579

[6] Robinson S. Neonatal posthemorrhagic hydrocephalus from prematurity: pathophysiology and current treatment concepts. J Neurosurg Pediatr. 2012; 9(3):242–258

[7] Behjati S, Emami-Naeini P, Nejat F, El Khashab M. Incidence of hydrocephalus and the need to ventriculoperitoneal shunting in premature infants with intraventricular hemorrhage: risk factors and outcome. Childs Nerv Syst. 2011; 27(6):985–989

[8] Lee S, Wang K-C, Cheon J-E, et al. Surgical outcome of Chiari I malformation in children: clinico-radiological factors and technical aspects. Childs Nerv Syst. 2014; 30(4):613–623

[9] Cho YH, Ho TS, Wang SM, Shen CF, Chuang PK, Liu CC. Childhood tuberculosis in southern Taiwan, with emphasis on central nervous system complications. J Microbiol Immunol Infect. 2014; 47(6):503–511

[10] Vinchon M, Rekate H, Kulkarni AV. Pediatric hydrocephalus outcomes: a review. Fluids Barriers CNS. 2012; 9(1):18

[11] Anderson RCE, Garton HJL, Kestle JRW. Treatment of hydrocephalus with shunts. In: Albright AL, Pollack IF, Adelson PD, eds. Operative Techniques in Pediatric Neurosurgery. New York, NY: Thieme; 2001

[12] Jain H, Sgouros S, Walsh AR, Hockley AD. The treatment of infantile hydrocephalus: "differential-pressure" or "flow-control" valves. A pilot study. Childs Nerv Syst. 2000; 16(4): 242–246

[13] McGirt MJ, Buck DW, II, Sciubba D, et al. Adjustable vs set-pressure valves decrease the risk of proximal shunt obstruction in the treatment of pediatric hydrocephalus. Childs Nerv Syst. 2007; 23(3):289–295

[14] Drake JM, Kestle JR, Milner R, et al. Randomized trial of cerebrospinal fluid shunt valve design in pediatric hydrocephalus. Neurosurgery. 1998; 43(2):294–303, discussion 303–305

[15] Pollack IF, Albright AL, Adelson PD, Hakim-Medos Investigator Group. A randomized, controlled study of a programmable shunt valve versus a conventional valve for patients with hydrocephalus. Neurosurgery. 1999; 45(6): 1399–1408, discussion 1408–1411

[16] Singh I, Rohilla S, Kumawat M, Goel M. Comparison of total versus partial revision of primary ventriculoperitoneal shunt failures. Surg Neurol Int. 2013; 4:100

[17] Eymann R, Steudel WI, Kiefer M. Pediatric gravitational shunts: initial results from a prospective study. J Neurosurg. 2007; 106 suppl 3:179–184

[18] Simon TD, Hall M, Riva-Cambrin J, et al. Hydrocephalus Clinical Research Network. Infection rates following initial cerebrospinal fluid shunt placement across pediatric hospitals in the United States. Clinical article. J Neurosurg Pediatr. 2009; 4(2):156–165

[19] Ahn ES, Bookland M, Carson BS, Weingart JD, Jallo GI. The strata programmable valve for shunt-dependent hydrocephalus: the pediatric experience at a single institution. Childs Nerv Syst. 2007; 23(3):297–303

[20] Lee JK, Seok JY, Lee JH, et al. Incidence and risk factors of ventriculoperitoneal shunt infections in children: a study of 333 consecutive shunts in 6 years. J Korean Med Sci. 2012; 27 (12):1563–1568

[21] Kan P, Kestle J. Lack of efficacy of antibiotic-impregnated shunt systems in preventing shunt infections in children. Childs Nerv Syst. 2007; 23(7):773–777

[22] Yuh SJ, Vassilyadi M. Management of abdominal pseudocyst in shunt-dependent hydrocephalus. Surg Neurol Int. 2012; 3:146

[23] Sato O, Yamguchi T, Kittaka M, Toyama H. Hydrocephalus and epilepsy. Childs Nerv Syst. 2001; 17(1–2):76–86

[24] Majed M, Andrabi Y, Nejat F, El Khashab M. Seizure risk factors in shunted hydrocephalic patients. Pediatr Neurosurg. 2012; 48(5):286–290

[25] Spennato P, Tazi S, Bekaert O, Cinalli G, Decq P. Endoscopic third ventriculostomy for idiopathic aqueductal stenosis. World Neurosurg. 2013; 79 suppl 2:21.e13–21.e20

[26] Breimer GE, Sival DA, Hoving EW. Low-pressure valves in hydrocephalic children: a retrospective analysis. Childs Nerv Syst. 2012; 28(3):469–473

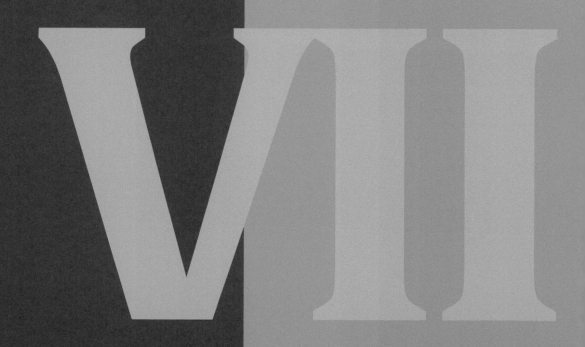

Section VII

Developmental and Congenital Spinal Disorders

38 Abnormalities of the Craniocervical Junction and Cervical Spine

Jared S. Fridley, Christina Sayama, Andrew Jea

38.1 Introduction

Abnormalities of the craniocervical junction (CCJ) and cervical spine (CS) can be seen in both adults and children. There is a wide spectrum of disorders that can affect the CCJ and CS. Their etiology may be developmental, congenital, or acquired. In the pediatric population, these abnormalities are often associated with a syndrome, such as Down's syndrome or Morquio's syndrome. Understanding the disease entities that underlie CCJ and CS abnormalities can help with identification of the underlying abnormal pathophysiology. Early identification and treatment of these patients may help prevent progression to more severe problems, such as basilar invagination or spinal cord injury/compression.

- Basilar invagination is a developmental anomaly of the CCJ in which the odontoid prolapses into the foramen magnum.[1]
- Atlantoaxial instability is present in 14 to 20% patients with Down's syndrome, due to ligamentous laxity.[2]
- Foramen magnum stenosis is seen in patients with achondroplasia, sometimes with cervicomedullary compression, which can lead to respiratory compromise.
- Odontoid anomalies include aplasia, hypoplasia, and os odontoideum, and are commonly seen in Morquio's syndrome (30–50% with combination of os odontoideum, atlantoaxial instability (AAI), and cervicothoracic abnormalities).[3]
- Klippel–Feil syndrome comprises a spectrum of CS osseous disorders often with congenital cervical fusion, limitation of cervical motion, and scoliosis in up to 50% of patients.[4]
- Majority of cervical spine injuries occur in children due to ongoing development of CS ossification centers, weak neck muscles with a relatively large head, ligamentous laxity, and angled facet joints.
- Patients with occipital–cervical synostosis have congenital fusion of the occiput to C1, which can lead to C1–C2 instability.
- Unilateral C1 absence can cause torticollis, and is associated with tracheoesophageal fistula.

38.2 Anatomy

- CCJ extends from the occipital bone to C2.
- Atlas develops from three ossification centers, the first of which (the body) appears at 1 year of age, completely fused and visible by 7 years of age.[5]
- Axis develops from five ossification centers; body fused to the dens by age 6.[5]
- Fifty percent of cervical spine rotation occurs at C1–C2.
- C2 is the first bifid process of the cervical spine.
- The superior and inferior obliques, levator scapulae, and rectus capitis muscles make up the musculature of the CCJ (▶ Fig. 38.1).
- Ligamentous structures of the CCJ include the anterior longitudinal ligament, the cruciate ligament (composed of the transverse and longitudinal ligaments), and the tectorial membrane (▶ Fig. 38.2).
- The hypoglossal nerve can be found exiting anterior and superior to the occipital condyle.
- The vertebral artery usually enters the transverse foramen of C6, ascends to the transverse foramen of C2, then travels through the C1 transverse foramen, and enters the sulcus arteriosus along the superior aspect of the C1 lamina, prior to piercing the dura.
- Borders of the suboccipital triangle include (1) obliquus capitis superior, (2) obliquus capitis inferior, and the (3) rectus capitis posterior major (▶ Fig. 38.3).
- The vertebral artery above C1 can be found within the suboccipital triangle.

38.3 Examination

Initial examination of the pediatric patient with a CCJ or CS abnormality must be comprehensive. This includes a thorough history of neurological and nonneurological systemic symptoms/signs. Physical examination should look for signs of an associated syndrome, looking for facial, neck, extremity, chest, back, and visceral abnormalities. Family history should be obtained in every patient.

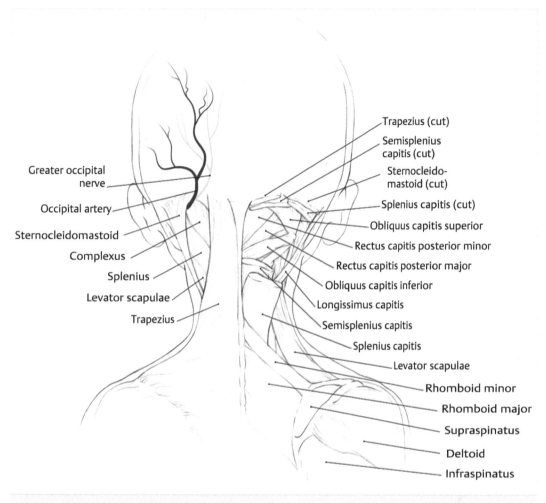

Greater occipital nerve

Occipital artery

Sternocleidomastoid

Complexus

Splenius

Levator scapulae

Trapezius

Trapezius (cut)

Semisplenius capitis (cut)

Sternocleido-mastoid (cut)

Splenius capitis (cut)

Obliquus capitis superior

Rectus capitis posterior minor

Rectus capitis posterior major

Obliquus capitis inferior

Longissimus capitis

Semisplenius capitis

Splenius capitis

Levator scapulae

Rhomboid minor

Rhomboid major

Supraspinatus

Deltoid

Infraspinatus

Fig. 38.1 The superior and inferior obliques, levator scapulae, and rectus capitis muscles make the musculature of the CCJ. (Courtesy of Katherine Relyea.)

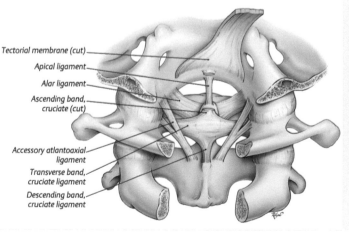

Tectorial membrane (cut)

Apical ligament

Alar ligament

Ascending band, cruciate (cut)

Accessory atlantoaxial ligament

Transverse band, cruciate ligament

Descending band, cruciate ligament

Fig. 38.2 Ligamentous structures of the CCJ include the anterior longitudinal ligament, the cruciate ligament (composed of the transverse and longitudinal ligaments), and the tectorial membrane. (Courtesy of Katherine Relyea.)

Boney landmarks

External occipital protuberence

Superior nuchal line

Inferior nuchal line

Posterior rim of foramen magnum

Suboccipital triangle

Obliquus capitis superior

Rectus capitis posterior major

Obliquus capitis inferior

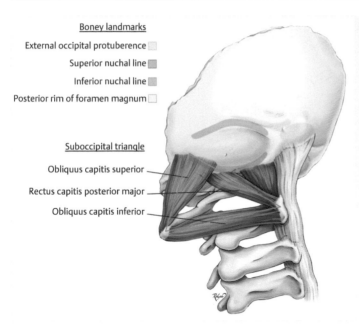

Fig. 38.3 Borders of the suboccipital triangle include obliquus capitis superior, obliquus capitis inferior, and the rectus capitis posterior major. (Courtesy of Katherine Relyea.)

Questions regarding developmental delay should be asked, especially with regard to motor function.

38.3.1 Physical Examination

- Up to 85% children with CCJ abnormality present with neck or occipital head pain.[3]
- Torticollis may be an important clinical sign of a CCJ abnormality in an infant or toddler.
- Cocking of the head to one side ("cock robin" deformity) in children can indicate atlantoaxial rotatory subluxation (AARS).
- Klippel–Feil syndrome classic clinical triad: (1) decreased neck range of motion, (2) short neck, (3) low posterior hairline.
- Myelopathy is the most common neurological deficit encountered in CCJ abnormalities.[3]
- In patient's suspected of Klippel–Feil syndrome, evaluate for associated renal abnormalities, congenital heart disease, and hearing impairment.
- "Basilar migraine" can be seen in 25% of patients with basilar invagination with compression of the vertebrobasilar arterial tree and/or medulla resulting in pain and neurological deficit.[6]

38.3.2 Radiographic Examination

- Flexion/extension lateral cervical X-rays can help screen for cervical instability.

- Computed tomography (CT) and magnetic resonance imaging (MRI) are useful to define bony anatomy/epiphyseal growth plates and ligamentous abnormalities prior to surgical intervention.
- The atlanto-dens interval (ADI) is normally less than or equal to 5 mm in children younger than 8 years; increased ADI can indicate atlantoaxial instability.
- Pseudosubluxation of the cervical spine at C2–C3 or C3–C4 occurs in 20 to 46% of children younger than 8 years.[7,8]
- Up to 6 mm of C1 lateral mass overhang on C2 can be seen in patients up to 8 years old, and is a normal variant.[9]
- If the tip of the dens is above a line (McRae's line) extending from the basion to opisthion, basilar invagination is present.
- Normal atlanto-occipital interval (AOI) is less than 2 mm in children and is strongly symmetric on the left and right sides[10]; an AOI greater than or equal to 4 mm has high sensitivity and specificity for atlanto-occipital dislocation.[11]
- Normal posterior interspinous distance should be less than or equal to 1.5 times the interspinous distance above or below the level being examined.[7]

38.4 Nonsurgical Management

- Mobile AARS man be treated conservatively with anti-inflammatory medications in patients where the cause is due to a post-inflammatory reaction, usually due to infection.[12]
- In AARS patients who undergo closed cervical reduction, collar immobilization may be considered.
- In neurologically intact patients with mild basilar invagination, clinical and radiographic follow-up may be tried.
- In children with Down's syndrome and radiographic concern for AAI, it is reasonable to manage them conservatively if there is no evidence of spinal cord injury.

38.5 Surgical Indications

A neurological deficit in a pediatric patient with either a CCJ or CS abnormality is an absolute indication for surgical intervention. Other indications for surgery include (1) AAI secondary to either acquired or congenital etiologies, (2) severe basilar invagination, (3) unilateral occipitocervical synostosis, (4) occipitocervical dislocation, (5) type II odontoid fractures, (6) occipitocervical instability secondary to acquired or congenital etiologies, and (7) iatrogenic kyphotic postoperative deformities.

Prior to surgical intervention, preoperative imaging must be obtained and reviewed. A thin-slice CT scan from occiput to lower cervical spine is useful to examine the bony anatomy of the pathology in general, but also for instrumentation planning.[13] The location of the vertebral artery must be identified as it courses from the cervical spine into the cranium. Patients with an abnormal course of the vertebral artery may preclude pedicle/pars or transarticular screws at C2. A CT sagittal view of the C2 pars is essential to identify the feasibility of a C2 pars screw. Screw lengths and widths should be discerned prior to entering the operating room. MRI examination is also useful to look for the extant of ligamentous instability and to identify any sites of neural compression.

38.6 Surgical Technique

The type of surgical approach chosen for patients with CS and CCJ pathologies is based on multiple factors including (1) level of the pathology, (2) whether neural compression is present and, if so, whether it is anterior or posterior, (3) site(s) of instability, (4) patient's age, weight, and comorbidities, and (5) bone quality. To access the anterior CCJ, a transnasal- or transoral–transpalatopharyngeal approach may be used. This allows access to the clivus, atlas, and axis. Posterior approaches will often involve posterior occipital and/or cervical decompression of neural elements followed by stabilization with instrumentation using various techniques.

- The anterior approach to the CCJ is useful for lesions causing cervicomedullary compression, especially nonreducible lesions, such as in cases of basilar invagination.
- The transoral–transpalatopharyngeal approach can be combined with palatal and/or mandibular splitting for further rostral or caudal exposure.
- The incision for the transoral approach is made in the midline posterior pharynx from the rostral clivus to the C2-C3 disc space to expose the prevertebral fascia and longus colli.
- Anatomical landmarks for the placement of occipital screws include (1) posterior rim of the foramen magnum, (2) superior nuchal line, (3) inferior nuchal line, and (4) external occipital protuberance (▸ Fig. 38.4).
- Drilling for occipital screws should be done in a stepwise fashion, in 2-mm increments, until the occipital bone inner cortex is penetrated to allow bicortical screw placement.
- When placing C1 lateral mass screws, the medial and lateral borders of the lateral masses should be palpated.
- Significant bleeding may be encountered due to the C1–C2 venous plexus, which can be avoided with careful subperiosteal dissection and bipolar cautery.
- The C2 nerve root can be transected if it is unable to be retracted for screw placement; this results in posterior scalp numbness.
- The entry point is in the center of the lateral mass, aiming toward the anterior arch of C1, 0 to 5 degrees medially.
- Placement of C1–C2 transarticular screws requires a steep insertion angle utilizing a posterior stab incision around T1, aiming for the medial border of the C2 pars.
- C2 pars screws are placed along a line running from the inferior articular process to the superior articular process, using a vertical trajectory.
- C2 pedicle screws utilize a more medial, horizontal trajectory, starting beneath the superior articular process, along the C2 superior laminar ridge.

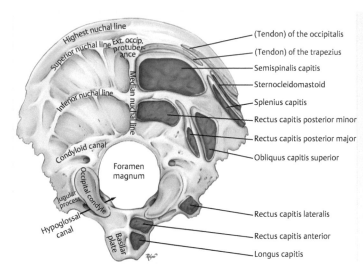

Fig. 38.4 Anatomical landmarks for the placement of occipital screws include (1) posterior rim of the foramen magnum, (2) superior nuchal line, (3) inferior nuchal line, and (4) external occipital protuberance. (Courtesy of Katherine Relyea.)

Labels in figure:
- Highest nuchal line
- Superior nuchal line
- Ext. occip. protuberance
- Inferior nuchal line
- Median nuchal line
- Condyloid canal
- Occipital condyle
- Jugular process
- Hypoglossal canal
- Basilar plate
- Foramen magnum
- (Tendon) of the occipitalis
- (Tendon) of the trapezius
- Semispinalis capitis
- Sternocleidomastoid
- Splenius capitis
- Rectus capitis posterior minor
- Rectus capitis posterior major
- Obliquus capitis superior
- Rectus capitis lateralis
- Rectus capitis anterior
- Longus capitis

- C2 translaminar screws have a high fusion rate, a low risk of vertebral artery injury, and are nearly always anatomically feasible.[14]
- The entry point for translaminar screw placement is made at the junction of the C2 spinous process and lamina.
- Subaxial cervical spine (C3–C7) lateral mass screw entry point is 1 mm medial and 1 mm inferior to the midpoint of the lateral mass, the trajectory is directed approximately 20 degrees cranial and 20 degrees lateral.
- Endoscopic endonasal approaches to the CCJ and upper cervical spine may offer improved visualization and decreased morbidity compared to the open transoral approach.[15]

38.7 Complications

- Complications associated with the transoral approach include posterior pharyngeal wound dehiscence, pharyngeal wound infection, velopharyngeal incompetence, dysphagia, odynophagia, and meningitis.[16,17]
- Anterior cervical approach dural tears should be primarily repaired or patched with a synthetic or fascial graft.
- There is an approximately 2.2% risk, per transarticular screw, of injuring the vertebral artery.[18]

38.8 Postoperative Care

All patients undergoing cervical spine surgery should be placed on analgesics and muscle relaxants postoperatively. Early mobilization and chemoprophylaxis to prevent deep venous thrombosis is instituted early after surgery. Posterior cervical patients have their diet advanced as tolerated, while special consideration is given to those patient's undergoing an anterior cervical approach, especially when significant laryngeal edema or dysphagia is present. Patients undergoing a transoral approach have a nasogastric tube and endotracheal tube left in place after surgery for one to several days to (1) protect airway and allow tracheal/airway edema to decrease, (2) provide nutrition, and (3) prevent gastric reflux into wound.[19]

38.9 Outcomes

- Pediatric patients undergoing a transoral approach usually experience neurological improvement and have an overall good neurological outcome despite a small but significant risk of morbidity/mortality.[17,20]
- Cervical spine instrumentation in the pediatric population has a high fusion rate (95–99%) with wiring constructs having higher morbidity than screw constructs.[13,21]
- Preoperative planning and review of patient's bony, neural, and vascular anatomy are critical to ensure the success of instrumentation constructs and avoidance of complications.[13]
- Bicortical occipital screw placement in children results in a higher fusion rate in occipitocervical constructs, but carries a small risk of dural venous sinus injury, and cerebrospinal fluid (CSF) leak.[22]

- Sectioning of the C2 nerve root for occipital mass screw placement in children enhances visibility of the C1 lateral mass, minimizes intraoperative complications, and does not lead to significant functional deficits.[23]

38.10 Surgical Pearls

- Always have a contingency plan determined preoperatively for placement of instrumentation if your first plan fails or is not feasible.
- Always look at the course of the vertebral artery, which may be anomalous in children with underlying disorders. Obtain preoperative vascular imaging if T2 flow void imaging is not sufficient.

38.11 Common Clinical Questions

1. What is the youngest age that a child has undergone craniocervical stabilization surgery?
2. How often should you image a child you are following conservatively for craniocervical instability?
3. Is there any utility in external cervical orthosis after fusion in the pediatric population?
4. What types of adjuvants are used to help aid in fusion?

38.12 Answers to Common Clinical Questions

1. 18 months. The surgeon must consider the individual child's anatomy, feasibility of hardware placement, bone maturity, and pathophysiology before committing the child to a fusion procedure.
2. Six- to twelve-month interval imaging with flexion and extension radiographs is sufficient unless the patient becomes symptomatic with neurological decline.
3. In special cases, there is a role for a rigid cervical collar after internal fixation, however, the senior author does not routinely use rigid cervical orthoses after cervical fusion.
4. Autograft when available, allograft based bone graft substitutes, rBMP-2, demineralized bone matrix, transforming growth factor-β (TGF-β), platelet-derived growth factor (PDGF), fibroblast growth factor (FGF). The senior author routinely uses the first three and has

had an excellent fusion rates with no untoward complications.

References

[1] Klimo P, Jr, Rao G, Brockmeyer D. Congenital anomalies of the cervical spine. Neurosurg Clin N Am. 2007; 18(3):463–478

[2] Menezes AH. Specific entities affecting the craniocervical region: Down's syndrome. Childs Nerv Syst. 2008; 24(10):1165–1168

[3] Menezes AH. Craniovertebral junction database analysis: incidence, classification, presentation, and treatment algorithms. Childs Nerv Syst. 2008; 24(10):1101–1108

[4] Herman MJ, Pizzutillo PD. Cervical spine disorders in children. Orthop Clin North Am. 1999; 30(3):457–466, ix

[5] O'Connor JF, Cranley WR, McCarten KM. Imaging of musculoskeletal disorders in children. Curr Opin Radiol. 1991; 3(5):727–736

[6] Menezes AH. Craniovertebral junction anomalies: diagnosis and management. Semin Pediatr Neurol. 1997; 4(3):209–223

[7] Lustrin ES, Karakas SP, Ortiz AO, et al. Pediatric cervical spine: normal anatomy, variants, and trauma. Radiographics. 2003; 23(3):539–560

[8] Cattell HS, Filtzer DL. Pseudosubluxation and other normal variations in the cervical spine in children. A study of one hundred and sixty children. J Bone Joint Surg Am. 1965; 47(7):1295–1309

[9] Suss RA, Zimmerman RD, Leeds NE. Pseudospread of the atlas: false sign of Jefferson fracture in young children. AJR Am J Roentgenol. 1983; 140(6):1079–1082

[10] Pang D, Nemzek WR, Zovickian J. Atlanto-occipital dislocation: part 1—normal occipital condyle-C1 interval in 89 children. Neurosurgery. 2007; 61(3):514–521, discussion 521

[11] Pang D, Nemzek WR, Zovickian J. Atlanto-occipital dislocation—part 2: the clinical use of (occipital) condyle-C1 interval, comparison with other diagnostic methods, and the manifestation, management, and outcome of atlanto-occipital dislocation in children. Neurosurgery. 2007; 61(5): 995–1015, discussion 1015

[12] Copley LA, Dormans JP. Cervical spine disorders in infants and children. J Am Acad Orthop Surg. 1998; 6(4):204–214

[13] Menezes AH. Craniocervical fusions in children. J Neurosurg Pediatr. 2012; 9(6):573–585

[14] Dorward IG, Wright NM. Seven years of experience with C2 translaminar screw fixation: clinical series and review of the literature. Neurosurgery. 2011; 68(6):1491–1499, discussion 1499

[15] Kassam AB, Snyderman C, Gardner P, Carrau R, Spiro R. The expanded endonasal approach: a fully endoscopic transnasal approach and resection of the odontoid process: technical case report. Neurosurgery. 2005; 57(1) Suppl: E213–, discussion E213

[16] Menezes AH. Surgical approaches: postoperative care and complications "transoral-transpalatopharyngeal approach to the craniocervical junction". Childs Nerv Syst. 2008; 24(10): 1187–1193

[17] Hadley MN, Spetzler RF, Sonntag VK. The transoral approach to the superior cervical spine. A review of 53 cases of extradural cervicomedullary compression. J Neurosurg. 1989; 71(1):16–23

[18] Wright NM, Lauryssen C, American Association of Neurological Surgeons/Congress of Neurological Surgeons. Vertebral artery injury in C1–2 transarticular screw fixation: results of a survey of the AANS/CNS section on disorders of the spine and peripheral nerves. J Neurosurg. 1998; 88(4):634–640

[19] Cheung KM, Mak KC, Luk KD. Anterior approach to cervical spine. Spine. 2012; 37(5):E297–E302

[20] Yang SY, Gao YZ. Clinical results of the transoral operation for lesions of the craniovertebral junction and its abnormalities. Surg Neurol. 1999; 51(1):16–20

[21] Hwang SW, Gressot LV, Rangel-Castilla L, et al. Outcomes of instrumented fusion in the pediatric cervical spine. J Neurosurg Spine. 2012; 17(5):397–409

[22] Hwang SW, Gressot LV, Chern JJ, Relyea K, Jea A. Complications of occipital screw placement for occipitocervical fusion in children. J Neurosurg Pediatr. 2012; 9(6):586–593

[23] Patel AJ, Gressot LV, Boatey J, Hwang SW, Brayton A, Jea A. Routine sectioning of the C2 nerve root and ganglion for C1 lateral mass screw placement in children: surgical and functional outcomes. Childs Nerv Syst. 2013; 29(1):93–97

39 Spina Bifida: Classification and Management

Lorelay Gutierrez, Luis A. Arredondo, Rodrigo Mercado

39.1 Introduction

Spinal dysraphism represents a constellation of clinical entities. The term covers a wide range of developmental conditions of the spinal cord and its surrounding structures. It is often referred as *spina bifida (SB) or neural tube defects.* Spinal dysraphism includes two conditions that may be present at birth or during linear growth:
- Spina bifida aperta (SBA), always evident at birth.
- Spina bifida occulta (SBO), or occult dysraphism. The congenital absence of the posterior vertebrae arches with no visible exposure of meninges or neural tissue.[1]

In recent years the prevalence of SB evident at birth appears to be reducing, due to better prenatal screening and nutrition programs. The causes of SB are multifactorial, with a significant genetic component. Familial tendency is probably due to a polygenic mechanism. Nutritional factors still play an important etiological role and is reflected in the higher incidence among the socioeconomical vulnerable segments of the population in developing countries. Low folate intake during preconception is the most common nutritional factor implicated in the etiology of SB. Several common medications such as anticonvulsants have also been implicated in animal models as teratogens.[2,3]

39.2 Spina Bifida Occulta

The prevalence in North America is 5 to 10%. In early ages, the most common finding is the presence of a cutaneous marker or *stigmata.* In older children, the symptomatology is often associated with tethered spinal cord syndrome (TSCS) and becomes more evident during linear growth.

Lesions associated with SBO:
- Lipomyelomeningocele.
- Conus medullaris lipoma.
- Dermal sinus.
- Split cord malformation.
- Filum terminale lipomas.
- Rare conditions include myelocystocele and neurenteric cyst, usually accompanied by genitourinary malformations.[4,5,6]

39.3 Spina Bifida Aperta

SBA encloses two main abnormalities (▶ Fig. 39.1):
- ***Meningocele.*** Congenital defect of vertebral arch with posterior distension of meninges with no

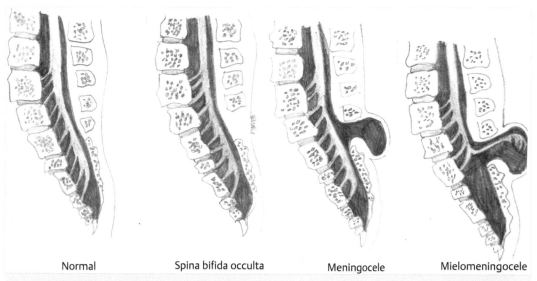

| Normal | Spina bifida occulta | Meningocele | Mielomeningocele |

Fig. 39.1 Schematic drawings of the anatomical features of common dysraphisms. (Courtesy of Gutiérrez-Oliva K.)

neural tissue included. About 30% could be associated to tethered spinal cord.

- *Myelomeningocele.* Congenital defect of vertebral arch with a cystic dilation of meninges including neural tissue and a placode.

39.4 Embryology

Three phases of the development of the embryonic spinal cord are described. This process begins around day 18 of gestation (▶ Table 39.1).

39.5 Clinical Presentation

The severity of the clinical presentation varies according to the type of dysraphism.

Myelomeningocele. The most severe defect is evident at birth. Characterized by:
- Presence of a midline cutaneous defect, more often lumbosacral.
- Protrusion of meninges and neural tissue enclosed in a cystic malformation.
- Neurological deficit is commonly associated with variable severity. Paraplegia with severe urinary dysfunction is the worst scenario.
- Associated nervous system developmental anomalies.
- *Hydrocephalus.*
- *Chiari II malformation.*
- Symptomatology related to SBO, such as urological, orthopedic, or neurological impairments, may be present at birth, but eventually will get worst or evident as the child grows.[4,6,7]

39.6 Prenatal Assessment

Prenatal assessment includes maternal ultrasonography, and biochemical markers such as high levels of alpha-feto protein in amniotic fluid at weeks 13 to 16, and amniotic acetycholinesterase levels greater than 500 ng/ml.

39.7 Postnatal Assessment
39.7.1 Imaging

- Magnetic resonance imaging (MRI) is the most reliable image study to determine the compromise of the neural structures. MRI is not mandatory in myelomeningocele cases, whereas it represents the gold standard when studying SBO cases.
- Plain X-ray and CT scan with 3D reconstruction are useful to evaluate the precise site of the dysraphism bone defect and to precise other orthopedic anomalies.

39.7.2 Electrophysiology

- Electromyography and motor- and sensory-evoked potentials are useful to evaluate the extent of neurological damage, especially in older children SBO cases.

39.7.3 Urodynamic Studies

- Serial urine test must be performed regularly in search of repetitive urinary tract infections. Retrograde cystourethrography to assess bladder function and to rule out the presence of cysto ureteral reflux. Urodynamic studies are of great value to select surgical candidates.[8]

39.7.4 Surgical Goals

Keep in mind that we are facing a malformation, so the primary goal is to achieve an anatomical environment as normal as possible.
- *Myelomeningocele.* Thoroughful reconstruction of the anatomical planes leads to a normal neural tube environment.
- *SBO.* Identify the anatomical features with attention to tethered cord.
- *Spinal lipomas* are complex lesions and its management remains controversial in the absence of symptoms.[9] Refer to Chapter 41

Table 39.1 Embryology of the spinal cord and closing failures

Spinal cord embryology	Main feature	Common failure
Primary neurulation	Closure of neural tube at day 21	Myelomeningocele
Secondary neurulation	Closure of the tail bud or posterior neuropore	Lipomas of the filum terminale
Regression of the caudal cell mass	Formation of sacral bone	Sacrum agenesis Myelocystocele

The dura is present in the majority of the malformations. Great care shall be observed when dissecting the dural layer. Watertight closure must be achieved in order to avoid cerebrospinal fluid (CSF) leaks.

39.7.5 Postoperative Care and Follow-up

Surgical repair does not represent the end of the treatment. A multidisciplinary team must be involved to evaluate and follow every case, optimizing functional recovery and looking for delayed complications and hidden associated anomalies.[10]

39.8 Common Clinical Questions

1. Which is the best timing for myelomeningocele repair?
2. Describe the best management strategy in patients with myelomeningocele and hydrocephalus.
3. Define the concept of occult tethered cord syndrome (OTCS).
4. Is surgery indicated for occult tethered cord?

39.9 Answers to Common Clinical Questions

1. Corrective surgery should be done as soon as possible. A retrospective study demonstrate that surgical intervention within the first 5 days was associated with a shorter duration of hospital stay, antibiotic therapy, and a lower complication rate.[11] Even more important are the results of a study on postoperative urological function, that showed an increased incidence of febrile urinary tract infections, vesicoureteral reflux, hydronephrosis, and secondary tethering of the spinal cord in children operated 72 hours after birth.[12]
2. Only one out six infants with myelomeningocele presents signs of intracranial pressure at birth. Hydrocephalus is commonly noticed at 2 to 3 weeks of age.[13] There is controversy over whether simultaneous CSF shunt insertion and repair of myelomeningocele increase shunt-related complications. One study concludes that there was no statistically

significant difference between complication rates in patients in whom the two procedures were performed concurrently and those who underwent separate operations.[14] A larger and more recent study described that patients shunted prior to, simultaneously, or within the first 4 days after SB closure had a fivefold higher shunt infection rate than those shunted 5 to 10 days following SB closure. Shunt malfunctions were also significantly higher in the group shunted prior to myelomeningocele closure.[15] We prefer to wait at least 5 days after the dysraphism is repaired, before placing a ventricular shunt.

3. In this condition, symptoms consistent with TCS are present and are thought to be related to tethering of the spinal cord by the filum, although the conus is in a normal position. Symptoms are classified into four main categories: neurological, motor or sensory dysfunction, urological, neurocutaneous, and neuro-orthopedic. The most common is urinary dysfunction, which is seen in 68 to 100% of the patients.[16]
4. The natural history of OTCS remains controversial. Some authors have suggested that neurological progression and deterioration occur in over 50% of patients with clinical tethered cord syndrome. A retrospective study compared OTCS patients undergoing surgery versus conservative treatment, found that 88% of patients improved with surgery and 29% of patients managed conservatively also had improvement in their symptoms.[17] The main surgical goal when operating OTCS is to disconnect the filum.

References

[1] Kumar R, Singhal N. Outcome of meningomyelocele/lipomeningomyelocele in children of northern India. Pediatr Neurosurg. 2007; 43(1):7–14
[2] MRC Vitamin Study Research Group. Prevention of neural tube defects: results of the Medical Research Council Vitamin Study. Lancet. 1991; 338(8760):131–137
[3] Laurence KM. A declining incidence of neural tube defects in the U.K. Z Kinderchir. 1989; 44 suppl 1:51
[4] Bui CJ, Tubbs RS, Oakes WJ. Tethered cord syndrome in children: a review. Neurosurg Focus. 2007; 23(2):E2
[5] McLone DG, La Marca F. The tethered cord: diagnosis, significance and management. Seminars in Pediatric Neurology. 1997; 4(3):192–208
[6] Huang SL, Shi W, Zhang LG. Surgical treatment for lipomyelomeningocele in children. World J Pediatr. 2010; 6 (4):361–365
[7] Blount JP, Elton S. Spinal lipomas. Neurosurg Focus. 2001; 10 (1):e3

[8] Nogueira M, Greenfield SP, Wan J, Santana A, Li V. Tethered cord in children: a clinical classification with urodynamic correlation. J Urol. 2004; 172(4 pt 2):1677–1680, discussion 1680

[9] Finn MA, Walker ML. Spinal lipomas: clinical spectrum, embryology, and treatment. Neurosurg Focus. 2007; 23(2):E10

[10] Wai EK, Owen J, Fehlings D, Wright JG. Assessing physical disability in children with spina bifida and scoliosis. J Pediatr Orthop. 2000; 20(6):765–770

[11] Oncel MY, Ozdemir R, Kahilogulları G, Yurttutan S, Erdeve O, Dilmen U. The effect of surgery time on prognosis in newborns with meningomyelocele. J Korean Neurosurg Soc. 2012; 51(6):359–362

[12] Tarcan T, Onol FF, Ilker Y, Alpay H, Simşek F, Ozek M. The timing of primary neurosurgical repair significantly affects neurogenic bladder prognosis in children with myelomeningocele. J Urol. 2006; 176(3):1161–1165

[13] Tamburrini G, Frassanito P, Iakovaki K, et al. Myelomeningocele: the management of the associated hydrocephalus. Childs Nerv Syst. 2013; 29(9):1569–1579

[14] Radmanesh F, Nejat F, El Khashab M, Ghodsi SM, Ardebili HE. Shunt complications in children with myelomeningocele: effect of timing of shunt placement. Clinical article. J Neurosurg Pediatr. 2009; 3(6):516–520

[15] Margaron FC, Poenaru D, Bransford R, Albright AL. Timing of ventriculoperitoneal shunt insertion following spina bifida closure in Kenya. Childs Nerv Syst. 2010; 26(11):1523–1528

[16] Tu A, Steinbok P. Occult tethered cord syndrome: a review. Childs Nerv Syst. 2013; 29(9):1635–1640

[17] Steinbok P, Kariyattil R, MacNeily AE. Comparison of section of filum terminale and non-neurosurgical management for urinary incontinence in patients with normal conus position and possible occult tethered cord syndrome. Neurosurgery. 2007; 61(3):550–555, discussion 555–556

40 Pathophysiology and Management of Tethered Cord (Including Myelomeningocele)

Eelco W. Hoving

40.1 Definitions

The word tether means to fasten, and it is used in the context of fastening an animal with a rope. The term tethered spinal cord was first used by Hoffman et al describing 31 patients with a thickened terminal filum.[1] The symptomatology of these patients resolved after sectioning the filum.

Tethered spinal cord is strongly associated with the morphology of spinal dysraphism. A distinction can be made between spina bifida aperta (SBA) and spina bifida occulta (SBO).

- In SBA, the cord is open (aperta) which means that the neural folds have not closed to a tube, and subsequently the lesion cannot be covered with skin. This is called a primary neurulation defect, and it results in a myelomeningocele (MMC).
- SBO refers to a variety of congenital anomalies that are all covered with skin (occult), but due to different pathophysiological disturbances during embryology. Premature disjunction between neuroectoderm (cord) and surface ectoderm (skin) may result in lipomyelomeningocele, while incomplete disjunction between these layers may lead to a dermal sinus fistula/cyst or limited dorsal myeloschisis (LDM) lesions.[2] SBOs of the most distal part of the cord, fatty terminal filum and terminal spinal lipomas, are associated with disturbances in secondary neurulation.[3]

The anatomy of spinal dysraphism will create a tethered cord (TC). As soon as clinical symptomatology arises, one speaks of tethered cord syndrome (TCS). These symptoms can be neurological, urological, orthopedic, and pain or a combination.

The pathophysiology of TCS is widely studied by Yamada et al, and it is considered to be a stretch-induced injury to the caudal end of the spinal cord up to the level of the dentate ligaments.[4] However, the symptomatology in TCS patients does not always resolve after surgical detethering and may even follow a progressive course. In this respect, myelodysplasia is considered to play an additional role in combination with TCS. In order to define clinical indications for surgical detethering in TCS patients, three different categories were proposed by Yamada and Won.[5]

- Category 1 represents TC patients with symptoms typically related to stretch-induced injury to the caudal spinal cord (inelastic terminal filum and caudal lipomyelomeningocele [LMMC]).
- Category 2 represents TC patients with similar symptoms, but due to additional local compression and subsequent ischemia to dorsal neural structures (MMC and dorsal or transitional LMMC).
- Category 3 represents patients with extensive and irreversible neurological and urological deficits due to myelodysplasia (large thoracolumbar MMC).

Based on these categories, a distinction can be made between true TCS (category 1) and relative TCS (category 2). Category 3 does not represent TCS patients. Only patients from categories 1 and 2 will benefit from surgical detethering.

40.2 Pathophysiology of TCS

TCS is a stretch-induced functional disorder of the spinal cord with its caudal portion anchored by an inelastic structure according to Yamada et al.[4] Extensive experimental work on TCS has been published by Yamada and his coworkers, and the following basic questions have been addressed on this topic:

- Experimental work in cats has shown that isotonic traction of the spinal cord results in different elongation of various cord segments. The viscoelasticity of the filum has the largest potential to elongate, and this protects the spinal cord from overstretching.
- The mechanism of TC dysfunction is related to electrical and metabolic changes in the interneurons of the cord that are located in gray matter. These changes could be recorded by measuring the redox shifts of cytochrome a,a3 as the final step of oxidative phosphorylation of adenosine diphosphate (ADP) to provide adenosine triphosphate (ATP) within the mitochondrion during traction of the distal cord.

Diminished spinal cord blood flow and altered glucose metabolism may play an additional role.

- These metabolic changes appeared to be reversible depending on the traction force and its duration. Excessive traction force of long duration will result in permanent neuronal damage within the caudal spinal cord.
- Permanent neuronal damage may also result from sudden stretching of the chronically tethered cord.
- Timing of detethering should preferably take place during the reversible phase of metabolic changes within the cord. Irreversible neuronal damage should be prevented.
- Early untethering, when only mild symptoms are present, warrants best results in TCS patients.

40.3 Pathophysiology of Recurrent Tethered Cord

Secondary deterioration of symptoms has been noticed in about one-third of MMC patients and about 10% of LMMC patients.[6]

In MMC patients, adhesions of the placode within a narrow spinal canal can hardly be prevented during primary surgical closure of the defect. Surgical aspects that may contribute to diminish the risk of secondary tethering are the remodeling of the neural placode into a neural tube and trying to create a dural sac as spacious as possible. The limited dimensions of the spinal canal at the site of the MMC cannot be changed, and most closed MMC will show the morphology of a TC.

The treatment of prophylactic LMMC patients has been controversial for many years because of the interpretation of secondary TCS. Some believed that the natural history would be responsible for secondary deterioration in 40% of patients during follow-up.[7,8] Others considered recurrent tethering to be the cause of progression of symptoms.[9] Pang et al have published extensively on these matters.[10,11] According to his data prophylactic detethering can be extremely effective in LMMC patients if one tries to resect the lipoma totally. The postoperative cord-sac ratio was found to be the most important prognostic factor in preventing secondary symptoms due to recurrent tethering. This finding was most apparent in the asymptomatic young LMMC patients.

The excellent lasting outcome after surgical detethering with complete resection of the lipoma corroborates the pathophysiological aspect of retethering in recurrent TCS.

40.4 Assessment of TCS

In MMC patients, any progression of neurological, urological, or orthopedic symptoms should be considered possibly due to TCS. The morphology of a surgically closed MMC is almost synonymous with a TC, and this may create additional damage to the cord. Most MMC patients will be followed in multidisciplinary spina bifida teams, and most changes of symptoms will be diagnosed. Since the majority of MMC patients belong to category 2 with relative TCS, the decision to propose surgical detethering should be judged per individual patient. A percentage between 10 and 30% of MMC patients is described to become symptomatic of a TCS.[6]

SBO patients are often diagnosed in a newborn when characteristic stigmata along the dorsal midline are present. These cutaneous manifestations are diagnosed in approximately 40% of patients, and they can be recognized as a tuft of hair, a lipomatous mass, a dimple or an abnormal coloring of the skin. The presence of musculoskeletal deformities such as a clubfoot may also indicate the presence of a TCS. Urological symptoms are prominent features of TCS, but they are not always recognized in young children. A history of a poor urinary stream or dribbling should be explored. Neurological symptoms may become apparent by an alteration of gait or motor strength in the legs. Sensory loss in the lower extremities is more seldom in a child.

The typical presentation of symptoms of TCS varies with age.[12]

- Children under 10 years often present with gait weakness, incontinence of reemergence of enuresis, or mild foot deformities.
- Teenagers tend to develop scoliosis or incontinence.
- In adults, pain is the most prominent symptom. The localization may be nonspecific but often within the perineal area.

Physical examination should include both a neurological and an orthopedic evaluation. Urological judgement often requires additional urodynamic tests by the urologist.

40.5 Imaging of TC

Magnetic resonance imaging (MRI) is essential in order to visualize TC. The morphology of TC can be clearly visualized on MRI in most cases of spinal dysraphism, but the degree of tension along the cord can only be postulated. In case of suspected tight filum terminale, sometimes only circumstantial evidence is present to support the diagnosis of TC. Therefore, the MRI should be examined systematically.[13]

- The position of the cord: A normal position of the conus is at the level of the L1–L2 disc. An abnormal caudal position of the conus may indicate a TC.
- The filum terminale may be thickened (wider than 2 mm) or fatty. The latter can be recognized by bright attenuation on T1-weighted MRI sequences.
- The position of the filum terminale may be posteriorly located within the dural sac because of covering the shortest distance between the dentate ligament and the tethering site.
- The presence of a syrinx within the distal cord.
- The presence of occult defects in the posterior elements of the spinal column (bifid lamina).
- The presence of additional congenital anomalies along the spine.
  Dysraphic anomalies with a classical appearance on MRI and that may cause a TC are as follows:
- Dermoid cyst/fistula that can often be visualized with a subcutaneous midline descending course and an intraspinal ascending course sometimes up to the level of the conus.
- Split cord malformations (SCMs) should be distinguished in type 1 (two hemicords within separate dural sheaths and a midline bony spur) and type 2 (two hemicords within one dural sac).[14] Type 1 is typically associated with TCS. SCM is often accompanied with vertebral anomalies (block or hemivertebrae).
- LMMCs can be subdivided in caudal, dorsal, or transitional lipomas.
- Limited dorsal myeloschisis may present with a subtle morphology of cord tethering along the dorsal midline in cervical, thoracic, or lumbar region.[2]

Ultrasonography can be used as a first evaluation of TC, but additional MRI will be indicated in case of its suspected presence.[15] The presence of pulsations of the cord may be useful in the evaluation of recurrent tethering in repaired MMC/LMMC patients.

40.6 Treatment of Tethered Cord

40.6.1 Myelomeningocele

Primary Closure

- Prenatal primary closure of the MMC has been developed in order to prevent secondary damage to the placode during gestation. The neural tube closes during the third and fourth gestational week. In MMC patients, the failure of closure creates a persistent neural placode with concomitant primary neurological damage. The exposure of the placode to the amniotic fluid during pregnancy has been found to lead to secondary neurological damage.[16,17]
- Intrauterine repair was also found to reduce the shunt insertion rate and to diminish hindbrain herniation.[18,19] These potential benefits must be considered in relation to the risk of surgery in a fetus and the maternal risks of hysterotomy. The Management of Myelomeningoceles Study (MOMS) has been designed to investigate in a randomized controlled fashion the benefit of reduction in shunt insertion and the neurological functional level after prenatal surgery.[20] The results showed a significant decrease in shunt-insertion rate in the prenatal group to 40% in relation to the postnatal group with 82% at 12 months. Improvements of mental developmental and motor function at 30 months were also significantly shown in the prenatal group. Hindbrain herniation and other secondary outcomes were also improved after prenatal repair. Only experienced surgical teams were involved in this trial, and the long-term risks for the development of a secondary TCS after prenatal repair have not been settled. Extensive prenatal counseling is required in order to discuss an individual benefit/risk profile.
- Postnatal primary closure of the MMC is meant to cover the unprotected neural placode and to prevent an infection of the central nervous system (CNS). The surgical aim is to create a watertight closure of dura, to provide a good skin cover, and to prevent secondary tethering.[21]
- Subsequent surgical steps can be distinguished: identification of the placode, resection of the surrounding thin epithelium; removal of cutaneous elements from the edges of the placode; transformation of the placode into a neural tube by approximation of the lateral

edges; mobilization of the underlying dura from the underlying fascial layer; creating a dural sac surrounding the neural cord as spacious as possible; an additional fascial layer to cover the dura is optional; closure of the skin (skin or musculocutaneous flap techniques may be used in case of large defects).

- Hydrocephalus is associated with most MMC patients (90%). Ventriculoperitoneal (VP) shunt insertion can be combined with closure of the MMC, if hydrocephalus is present at presentation. Most patients develop hydrocephalus after the defect has been closed, and a second surgery for shunt insertion will be needed.
- Chiari II is strongly associated with MMC, but only 10% of patients become symptomatic.
- Secondary TCS in MMC patients is present in 10 to 30% of patients.[6]

40.6.2 Spina Bifida Occulta

Tight Filum Terminale

- The viscoelasticity of the filum terminale is considered to protect the distal cord from stretch-induced injury. A loss of this viscoelasticity either due to a filum lipoma or to its shortness of length may result in a true TCS (category 1).[5] The tightness itself cannot be visualized. In case of a normal anatomy on MRI in conjunction with suspected symptoms, one may speak of an occult tethered cord syndrome.[22] Urological problems appear to be the most prominent initial symptoms in these patients.[23] The indication to treat these patients is questionable.[23,24] The surgical technique of cutting a tight filum is straightforward. After exposure of the caudal nerve roots intradurally at the level of the tight filum, one needs to identify the filum. The filum should be isolated from the caudal nerve roots, coagulated, and subsequently cut. Direct stimulation can be used to confirm the nonfunctional status of the filum.[25,26] The risks for surgical morbidity and for recurrent tethering are very low.

Limited Dorsal Myeloschisis

- LDM has been identified by Pang et al as a distinct form of spinal dysraphism with two distinct features: the presence of a fibroneural stalk connecting the skin and the cord

underneath an intact skin along the dorsal midline.[2] A wide variety of lesions have been described that can occur along dorsal spinal cord, and a classification is proposed in nonsaccular and saccular types. Surgical detethering is aimed at disconnection of the cord from the fibroneural stalk and reconstruction of the cord and/or dura in order to prevent recurrent tethering.

40.6.3 Lipomyelomeningocele

Split Cord Malformation

- SCM is strongly associated with concomitant congenital anomalies of the spine, and preoperative imaging of the complete spine with MRI is essential.[14] The presence of an additional filum terminale lipoma should be ruled out. The indication to treat is aimed at relieving symptoms of TCS and to prevent progression of symptoms. The exploration of the spinal canal may be complicated by the abnormal shape of the vertebrae and its posterior bony parts. In case of SCM type 1, the midline bony spur should be resected. After opening of the dural sacks, the cords can be detethered by dissecting the nonfunctional medial nerve roots that end blindly in the diastema. Subsequently, the medial parts of the dura at the site of the diastema can be resected, and one dural sac should be created containing both hemicords.[21] In SCM type 2, intradural detethering of both hemicords will suffice.

Spinal Inclusion Cysts

- Spinal inclusion cysts refer to dermoid fistulas/cysts, and should be treated to prevent accumulation of dermis within the spinal canal and secondary infection.[27] The close relationship of the dermis fistula/cyst with the cord may also result in a TCS. Radical excision is indicated, and a preoperative MRI is mandatory. The intradermal extension of the fistula is situated within the midline and may run in a rostrocaudal direction. The intradural extension is often present in a caudorostral direction up to the level of the conus. Total resection might require extensive multilevel intradural exposure of the fistula, and laminotomy with repositioning of the laminae is advised in children.

40.6.4 Miscellaneous

- Caudal spinal cord malformations may be associated with anorectal or urogenital anomalies like the caudal regression syndrome or the Currarino triad. These combinations of congenital disturbances might result in a TCS, but they always require an extensive diagnostic work-up and a multidisciplinary treatment strategy.[21]

40.7 Intraoperative Neuromonitoring in TCS

Intraoperative neuromonitoring (IONM) is meant to improve safety in TCS surgery by minimizing neurological morbidity.[25,26,28,29] The distinction between functional nerve roots and nonfunctional atretic nerve roots or fibrous bands may be difficult in various types of spina bifida. IONM has been used effectively in detethering of LMMC, LDM, tight filum terminale, and in recurrent TCS in MMC.

Three modalities of IONM are most widely used: direct nerve root stimulation (DNRS), transcranial electrical motor-evoked potentials (MEP) and bulbocavernosus reflex (BCR).[29]

- DNRS is used to discriminate between functional nerve roots and nonfunctional tethering structures. Multichannel electromyography (EMG) recording can be applied.
- MEP is utilized to identify the integrity of the motor pathways in the individual patient and to provide feedback on this during surgical detethering.
- BCR provides continuous feedback on the integrity of the sensory sacral nerve roots and the S2–S4 cord segments.
- IONM in small children is feasible, but preconditioning techniques might be required.[25,30]

40.8 Outcome in TCS

Considering the outcome in TCS surgery, one should realize that true TCS patients (category 1) represent the most reliable population concerning the evaluation of results of surgical detethering. Patients belonging to relative TCS (category 2) may also be symptomatic by other reasons than tethering like myelodysplasia or local compression.

Most TCS patient can be treated effectively and safely with the use of IONM.[2,10,25,29]

- True TCS in tight filum terminale is associated with excellent outcome and no surgical morbidity. The indication for treatment of occult TCS remains controversial, hence this affects evaluation of outcome.[23]
- LMMC can effectively be treated for TCS by radical excision of the lipoma creating an optimal cord-sack ratio with a low risk of recurrent TCS.[10,11,31]
- Prophylactic total resection appears to be the best option for the young child (< 2 years) with asymptomatic LMMC.[31]
- TCS surgery in adult patients can be quite effective, especially concerning improvement of pain.[32]
- Recurrent TCS in MMC patients can effectively be treated with improvement of symptoms in a majority of cases.[6]

40.9 Complications

- The use of IONM may contribute to minimize the chance of neurological morbidity especially in TCS patients with LMMC or in recurrent TCS patients with MMC.[21,26,28]
- Reversible surgical morbidity in TCS surgery is associated to disturbed wound healing, cerebrospinal fluid (CSF) leakage, pseudomeningocele, and infection.
- Recurrent TCS may occur after closure of MMC and after partial resection of LMMC.[6,7,10]

40.10 Surgical Pearls

- The primary goal of TCS surgery is to free the cord from its tethering structures and to create a spacious environment (dural sack) in order to prevent retethering.[10]
- IONM may contribute to the safety and efficacy of TCS surgery.[25,29]
- Timing of TCS surgery should take place before irreversible ischemic damage has occurred.[4]
- True TCS (category 1) includes tight filum terminale and caudal LMMC.[2]

40.11 Common Clinical Questions

1. Describe the pathophysiology in TCS.
2. Explain why the morphology of tight filum terminale and caudal LMMC are associated with true TCS.

3. What are the potential benefits of prenatal treatment of MMC?
4. Which surgical techniques can be used to potentially decrease the chance of recurrent TCS in MMC and LMMC treatment?

40.12 Answers to Common Clinical Questions

1. TCS is a stretch-induced functional disorder of the caudal portion of the cord due to anchoring by inelastic structures.[4] Repetitive strain to the cord will eventually lead to ischemic and metabolic injury to neurons located within the gray matter of the cord. The normal viscoelasticity of the terminal filum and the dentate ligaments protect the cord from repetitive strain injury.

2. A decreased viscoelasticity of the terminal filum or a caudal LMMC create repetitive stretch-induced injuries to the cord up to the level of the dentate ligaments.[4] The part of the cord distal to the dentate ligaments is most vulnerable to these forces. Since tight filum terminale and caudal LMMC are limited to the most caudal part of the cord as secondary neurulation disorders, additional aspects as an abnormal morphology of the cord due to primary neurulation or compression of the cord by the lipoma do not contribute to the symptomatology in these patients. In this respect, the symptomatology of these patients can be truly explained by tethering of the cord.

3. The MOMS trial has shown that a significant reduction in shunt insertion for hydrocephalus (40% instead of 80%), and a significant improvement of mental and motor score at 30 months had been achieved in the prenatally treated group of patients.[20] A reduction in hindbrain herniation as a result of prenatal treatment of MMC could also be confirmed.[19,20]

4. In order to prevent recurrent tethering, one should try to create a maximal cord-sack ratio. This means that in primary closure of MMC, it is advisable to reshape the placode into a cord and to make the dural sack as spacious as possible.[21] Because of the limited dimensions of the spinal canal at the site of the MMC, the morphology of a tethered cord can hardly be prevented in MMC patients. Only 10 to 30% of MMC patients become symptomatic and develop a TCS.[6] LMMC patients should be detethered by resecting the lipoma as radical as possible in order to create a maximal cord-sack ratio.[10,31] Reshaping the cord after resection of the lipoma (surgical neurulation) may also contribute to the prevention of recurrent tethering.[31]

References

[1] Hoffman HJ, Hendrick EB, Humphreys RP. The tethered spinal cord: its protean manifestations, diagnosis and surgical correction. Childs Brain. 1976; 2(3):145–155

[2] Pang D, Zovickian J, Wong ST, Hou YJ, Moes GS. Limited dorsal myeloschisis: a not-so-rare form of primary neurulation defect. Childs Nerv Syst. 2013; 29(9):1459–1484

[3] Dias MS, Rizk EB. Normal spinal cord development and the embryogenesis of spinal cord tethering malformations. In: Yamada S, ed. Tethered Cord Syndrome in Children and Adults. 2nd ed. New York, NY: Thieme; 2010:5–18

[4] Yamada S, Lonser RR, Won DJ, Yamada BS. Pathophysiology of tethered cord syndrome. In: Yamada S, ed. Tethered Cord Syndrome in Children and Adults. 2nd ed. New York, NY: Thieme; 2010:19–42

[5] Yamada S, Won DJ. What is the true tethered cord syndrome? Childs Nerv Syst. 2007; 23(4):371–375

[6] Caldarelli M, Boscarelli A, Massimi L. Recurrent tethered cord: radiological investigation and management. Childs Nerv Syst. 2013; 29(9):1601–1609

[7] Pierre-Kahn A, Zerah M, Renier D, et al. Congenital lumbosacral lipomas. Childs Nerv Syst. 1997; 13(6):298–334, discussion 335

[8] Kulkarni AV, Pierre-Kahn A, Zerah M. Conservative management of asymptomatic spinal lipomas of the conus. Neurosurgery. 2004; 54(4):868–873, discussion 873–875

[9] McLone DG, La Marca F. The tethered spinal cord: diagnosis, significance, and management. Semin Pediatr Neurol. 1997; 4(3):192–208

[10] Pang D, Zovickian J, Oviedo A. Long-term outcome of total and near-total resection of spinal cord lipomas and radical reconstruction of the neural placode, part II: outcome analysis and preoperative profiling. Neurosurgery. 2010; 66 (2):253–272, discussion 272–273

[11] Pang D, Zovickian J, Oviedo A. Long-term outcome of total and near-total resection of spinal cord lipomas and radical reconstruction of the neural placode: part I-surgical technique. Neurosurgery. 2009; 65(3):511–528, discussion 528–529

[12] Schneider S. Neurological assessment of tethered spinal cord. In: Yamada S, ed. Tethered Cord Syndrome in Children and Adults. 2nd ed. New York, NY: Thieme; 2010:43–50

[13] Hinshaw DB, Jacobson JP, Hwang J, Kido DK. Imaging of tethered spinal cord. In: Yamada S, ed. Tethered Cord Syndrome in Children and Adults. 2nd ed. New York, NY: Thieme; 2010:51–64

[14] Dias MS, Pang D. Split cord malformations. Neurosurg Clin N Am. 1995; 6(2):339–358

[15] Nelson MD. Ultrasonographic evaluation of tethered cord syndrome. In: Yamada S, ed. Tethered Cord Syndrome in Children and Adults. 2nd ed. New York, NY: Thieme; 2010:65–73

[16] Heffez DS, Aryanpur J, Hutchins GM, Freeman JM. The paralysis associated with myelomeningocele: clinical and experimental data implicating a preventable spinal cord injury. Neurosurgery. 1990; 26(6):987–992

[17] Meuli M, Meuli-Simmen C, Hutchins GM, et al. In utero surgery rescues neurological function at birth in sheep with spina bifida. Nat Med. 1995; 1(4):342–347

[18] Bruner JP, Tulipan N, Paschall RL, et al. Fetal surgery for myelomeningocele and the incidence of shunt-dependent hydrocephalus. JAMA. 1999; 282(19):1819–1825

[19] Tulipan N, Hernanz-Schulman M, Lowe LH, Bruner JP. Intrauterine myelomeningocele repair reverses preexisting hindbrain herniation. Pediatr Neurosurg. 1999; 31(3):137–142

[20] Adzick NS, Thom EA, Spong CY, et al. MOMS Investigators. A randomized trial of prenatal versus postnatal repair of myelomeningocele. N Engl J Med. 2011; 364(11):993–1004

[21] Hoving EW. Spinal anomalies. In: Lumenta CB, DiRocco C, Haase J, Mooij JJA, eds. Neurosurgery, European manual of Medicine. Heidelberg: Springer; 2010:493–499

[22] Drake JM. Occult tethered cord syndrome: not an indication for surgery. J Neurosurg. 2006; 104 suppl 5:305–308

[23] Tu A, Steinbok P. Occult tethered cord syndrome: a review. Childs Nerv Syst. 2013; 29(9):1635–1640

[24] Drake JM. Surgical management of the tethered spinal cord—walking the fine line. Neurosurg Focus. 2007; 23(2):E4

[25] Hoving EW, Haitsma E, Oude Ophuis CMC, Journée HL. The value of intraoperative neurophysiological monitoring in tethered cord surgery. Childs Nerv Syst. 2011; 27(9):1445–1452

[26] Kothbauer KF, Novak K. Intraoperative monitoring for tethered cord surgery: an update. Neurosurg Focus. 2004; 16 (2):E8

[27] Thompson DNP. Spinal inclusion cysts. Childs Nerv Syst. 2013; 29(9):1647–1655

[28] Dulfer SE, Drost G, Lange F, Journee HL, Wapstra FH, Hoving EW. Long-term evaluation of intraoperative neurophysiological monitoring-assisted tethered cord surgery. Childs Nerv Syst 2017;33(11):1985–1995

[29] Sala F, Squintani G, Tramontano V, Arcaro C, Faccioli F, Mazza C. Intraoperative neurophysiology in tethered cord surgery: techniques and results. Childs Nerv Syst. 2013; 29(9):1611–1624

[30] Journée HL, Polak HE, De Kleuver M. Conditioning stimulation techniques for enhancement of transcranially elicited evoked motor responses. Neurophysiol Clin. 2007; 37 (6):423–430

[31] Pang D, Zovickian J, Wong ST, Hou YJ, Moes GS. Surgical treatment of complex spinal cord lipomas. Childs Nerv Syst. 2013; 29(9):1485–1513

[32] Rajpal S, Lapsiwala SB, Iskander BJ. Tethered cord syndrome in adults with spina bifida occulta. In: Yamada S, ed. Tethered Cord Syndrome in Children and Adults. 2nd ed. New York, NY: Thieme; 2010:180–189

41 Intraspinal Lipomas

Rodrigo Mercado, Luis A. Arrendondo, Lorelay Gutierrez, Jesus A. Villagómez

41.1 Introduction

Spinal lipomas are the most common presentation of occult spinal dysraphism, term used to describe those malformations of the neural tube covered by skin. Represent a complex condition involving anatomical and clinical features and treatment decisions. The treatment options are controversial and the vast majority of neurosurgeons advocate for early treatment to avoid further complications during axial growth.

The neurosurgeon must keep in mind the fact that no lipoma is equal, and every case represents a new challenge. These lesions have similar embryology and can cause eventually, during aging, a wide spectrum of neurological, urological, or orthopedical deficits related to the tethered cord syndrome. Tethered cord syndrome develops during child growth, and the symptoms are mainly related to the effects of traction applied to the spinal cord from the anatomical location of the lipoma. Lipomas cause a fixed position of the spinal cord, and as the child grows, the spinal cord is stretched and suffers ischemic damage. This damage is more deleterious at the level of the conus medullaris.

41.2 Classification

The most accepted classification of the lesions divides the spinal lipomas into three major categories:
• Lipomas of the conus medullaris.
• Lipomas of the filum terminale.
• "Subpial" lipomas.

41.2.1 Lipomas of the Conus Medullaris

The most important group of malformations are the lipomas of the conus medullaris comprising more than 70% of cases among the lipomatous lumbosacral lesions. They are classified as dorsal, caudal, or transitional. This system is useful to define surgical extent and the main anatomical features. The variants are based on the situation of the lipoma related to the conus.
• *Dorsal conus medullaris* is attached to the dorsal aspect of the conus medullaris including the

cord, the dura, and the fat. It might include an associated thickened filum.
• *Caudal conus medullaris* describes a lipoma attached to the inferior aspect of the conus, extends to the central canal, and includes nerve roots within the lipoma.
• *Transitional conus medullaris lipomas* represent a combination of the two previous variants. The lipoma attaches to the dorsal aspect of the cord and extends into the central canal. It is commonly associated with a large placode–lipoma interface.

McLane and Naidich have proposed an interesting theory to explain the surgical anatomy of conus medullaris lipomas in which the anterior anatomy represents normal tissue and anatomical structures, whilst the posterior aspect represents the lipoma. They referred to a disjunction of the neural tube from the surrounding ectoderm leading to an opening of the neural plate posteriorly, while allowing mesenchymal cells to enter the cleft and being induced to form fatty tissue by the primitive ependymal. This is important to consider at the moment of the surgery because the dural border, the lipoma, and the nervous tissue coincide at the lateral edges of the placode.

Regarding the development of filum lipomas, most of the speculative theories center on the lack of retrogressive differentiation leading to a differentiation of pluripotent mass cells into adipocytes.

Lipomyelomeningocele is used often to describe all lumbosacral lipomas, however, it refers to a malformation including a neural placode lying outside the spinal canal attached to a fatty mass which extends to the subcutaneous tissue. This lesion should be considered as an open myelomeningocele due to the anatomical organization of the roots. The tethering site is often asymmetrical and leads to rotation of the cord. In a few cases, the sacral roots course inside the lipoma.

41.3 Clinical Presentation

There are two main findings:
1. Presence of *cutaneous marker*, which is evident early in life.
2. *Neurological deficits* that develop gradually related to the tethered cord.

Six different forms of cutaneous markers have been described:
1. Fatty lumbosacral mass in the midline or parasagittal plane
2. Hirsutism
3. Dermal sinus
4. Hemangiomas
5. Rudimentary tail
6. Atretic meningocele

Some patients present a coccygeal pit within the gluteal fold and the association with lipomas is considered to be rare. Patients having a cutaneous marker should be included in a tethered cord study protocol.

Neurological deficits are present in 70% of patients. Most of the lipomas are asymmetrical and the neurological deficit is related to the lipomatous attachment. Tethering of spinal cord leads to urological, orthopedical, and neurological dysfunctions. Infants at birth are often asymptomatic and the neurological sequelae may persist occult during infancy, whereas patient's symptomatology becomes evident throughout the years of growth. Urological manifestations affect 50% of patients including recurrent urinary tract infections, abnormal voiding, hyperactive bladder, and sphincter dysfunction. Urological signs can be reversible if detected early in infants, but prognosis in older children and adults is poor. Motor and orthopedic signs affect 33% of patients and may include progressive scoliosis, toes and lower limbs malformations, such as clubfoot and equinovarus. Sensitive symptoms may present as ulcerations and pain. Pain is a common symptom in older children and adults.

Patients with spinal lipomas will develop tethered cord syndrome eventually during aging. The most important factor to consider is the presence of tension and traction to the spinal cord. Mechanical stress represents the major risk during physical activity and leads to ischemic changes. Several studies have demonstrated an improvement in function after untethering, however, the results of the surgery are variable and the goal is to stabilize the symptoms.

41.4 Imaging

Magnetic resonance imaging (MRI) is mandatory in every patient with cutaneous markers or symptoms related to tethered cord syndrome is useful when planning the surgery to identify associated malformations and to evaluate the presence of syrinx. The position of the conus medullaris is often distal. An apparent "normal conus position" is not completely safe for patients who complaint of symptoms such as incontinence, gait disturbances, and scoliosis. Postoperative MR will always look tethered and must be interpreted with caution.

41.5 Surgical Treatment

The main goals are to preserve neurological function and to avoid delayed neurological decline. To achieve these goals, it is important to follow four important principles:
1. Untether the spinal cord
2. Preserve neurological tissue
3. Debulk the lipoma
4. Reconstruct neural tube and anatomical planes

The vast majority of studies advocate for surgical treatment in order to avoid potential deterioration during growth. The decision to operate in asymptomatic patients is still controversial.

41.5.1 Surgical Technique

- Patient in prone position.
- Intraoperative monitoring for continuous electromyography (EMG) and motor-evoked potentials. Avoid the use of muscular relaxants if possible during the procedure.
- A midline incision is centered from one or two normal spinous process rostral to the lipoma and extended caudal to the lesion.
- Debulking of the lipoma is done with monopolar electrocautery and the amount of lipoma excised must be planned to allow an adequate and cosmetic closure at the end of surgery.
- Dissection of the lipoma begins one level rostral and continues in a circumferential fashion until the pedicle of lipoma is apparent. The dissection must follow the bone plane to avoid dural damage.
- Dural opening starts after the removal of the lipoma. Rostral in the first upper normal level and continues caudally until the lipoma unites to the neural tissue.
- Disrupt any adhesion under continuous electrophysiological monitoring to preserve the normal neurological tissue.

- Remove the majority of fatty tissue attached to the neural tissue and reconstruct the placode when present with 5.0 nylon sutures to the pia.
- Finally, a thick filum terminal must be cut.

It is important to notice that the liberation of traction mechanisms interfere with the pathogenesis of tethering. Treatment of syringomyelia is controversial. Reoperation is considered when symptoms of tethered spinal cord reappear.

42 Scoliosis

Anthony J. Herzog, Paul D. Sponseller

42.1 Introduction

Scoliosis is defined as spinal curvature in the coronal plane greater than 10 degrees by Cobb's angle measurement. It can be caused by multiple etiologies, each with a different natural history of disease (▶ Table 42.1).

- Idiopathic scoliosis:
  - Infantile: Occurs in 0 to 3 years of age. Can rapidly progress and compromise cardiopulmonary function by adulthood. It is associated with a high risk of neural axis abnormalities. Left apex thoracic curves are more common in this form. There is a decreased risk of progression if the patient presents before the age of 1. Because of high risk of rapid progression and 20% risk of neural axis abnormality with curves greater than 20 degrees, obtain magnetic resonance imaging (MRI) during work-up.[1]
  - Juvenile: Occurs in 4 to 9 years of age. More commonly occurs in females. Right apex curves are more common, left apex curves warrant concern for neural axis abnormalities. There is a high rate of rapid curve progression and 21.7% risk of neural axis abnormality with curve greater than 20 degrees. Obtain MRI as part of work-up.[1]
  - Adolescent: Occurs in ages 10 and over. Larger curves over 40 degrees are nine times more frequent in girls. There is also an increased incidence with a positive family history, polygenic interaction is theorized. The risk of progression is based on size of curve and skeletal maturity (tanner stage, menarche, Risser's score, bone age).[2]
- Congenital: Scoliosis is caused by primary bony malformations of the vertebrae. There is no specific inheritance pattern but is associated with multiple syndromes. It occurs in 1% of the population. The greatest risk of progression is during rapid growth from 0 to 2 years of age or during the adolescent growth spurt.
  - Failure of segmentation: Bars present between vertebrae. Can be unilateral or bilateral bars (block vertebrae, best prognosis).
  - Failure of formation: May be in the form of hemivertebra or wedge-shaped vertebrae. These malformations can be segmented (open growth plates around malformed vertebrae), semisegmented, or unsegmented (nonprogressive with best prognosis).
  - Combinations: There may be different compositions of segmentation and formation defects. Hemivertebra with contralateral bar has worst prognosis and is rapidly progressive.
- Neuromuscular: Any disorder that disturbs balance of trunk can potentially cause scoliosis. Often presents as the rapid development of a large curve or with neurological symptoms.

Table 42.1 Etiological causes of scoliosis

Type	Etiology	Treatment
Congenital	Failure of segmentation (bars) Failure of formation (hemivertebra, wedges)	Bracing not effective. Can fuse in situ or excision with rod instrumentation over curve
Neuromuscular/syndromic	Syringomyelia, meningomyelocele, cord injury before puberty, Rett's, CP, CMTD, FA, MD, NF1, MS, LDS, EDS, OI	Bracing not effective. Curves often rapidly progressive. Likely need extended PSF
Idiopathic	Infantile Juvenile Adolescent	Can observe curves less than 20–25 degrees Curves 25–50 degrees, consider bracing Curves greater than 50 degrees, consider surgery Casting is an option in infantile for curves 30–50 degrees Infantile curves before 1 year or less than 30 degrees can be observed

Abbreviations: CMTD, Charcot–Marie–Tooth disease; CP, cerebral palsy; EDS, Ehlers–Danlos syndrome; FA, fractional anisotropy; LDS, Loeys–Dietz syndrome; MD, muscular dystrophy; MS, Marfan's syndrome; NF1, neurofibromatosis type 1; OI, osteogenesis imperfecta; PSF, posterior spinal fusion.

- Cerebral palsy (CP): Quadriplegic and totally involved CP have the highest incidence of scoliosis with over 50% of children developing it. Bracing is ineffective in preventing curve progression with CP, and often these curves will continue to progress even after skeletal maturity. Close follow-up is warranted.
- Rett's syndrome: Characterized by poor coordination and imbalance of muscles around spine. Scoliosis is more likely to develop in severe forms of the disease and less common in girls who continue to ambulate.
- Myelomeningocele: Often associated with multiple defects including scoliosis, tethered cord, and syringomyelia. Can be classified according to location, thoracic/high lumbar, low lumbar, or sacral involvement.
- Spinal cord injury before puberty: This often results in paralysis causing scoliosis of the growing spinal cord. Most of these children develop a progressive scoliosis that requires surgical correction.
- Friedreich's ataxia: Involves a genetic mutation resulting in progressive neurological damage, including poor muscle control often leading to scoliosis. Other findings include pes cavus, incoordination, speech problems, and diabetes.
- Charcot–Marie–Tooth disease: A progressive disease resulting from peripheral nervous system damage leading to loss of motor function. Cannot perform neuromonitoring during surgical repair of scoliosis in these patients due to damage to peripheral nervous system.
- Syringomyelia: Dilation of the canal of the spinal cord. The syrinx can disturb anterior horn cells affecting motor function and crossing fibers of the spinothalamic tract resulting in sensory deficits. Warning signs are rapidly progressive curve, asymmetrical abdominal reflexes, or left thoracic curve. It is detected with a MRI of the spinal cord.
- Syndromic: Disorders that disturb ligament integrity, growth, and balance are often associated with scoliosis.
  - Neurofibromatosis type 1: Mutation in neurofibromin 1 gene involved in the RAS cell signaling pathway. This mutation results in multiple benign tumors neural in origin. It is unknown how this disorder results in scoliosis. The curve seen can be a dystrophic type curve (sharply angulated) or nondystrophic curve.
  - Marfan's syndrome: Defect in connective tissue protein fibrillin resulting in ligamentous laxity and thin pedicles. Scoliosis occurs in 60% of these patients and if there is growth potential left there is a very high likelihood of curve progression even with bracing. Obtain MRI prior to surgery (dural ectasia may be seen which is important for surgical planning).
  - Loeys–Dietz syndrome: Transforming growth factor-β (TGF-β) mutation resulting in connective tissue disorder with many similar features to Marfan's syndrome, including progressive scoliosis.
  - Ehlers–Danlos syndrome: Multiple types of the syndrome classified according to collagen defect. Ehlers–Danlos type VI with a defect in lysyl hydroxylase commonly results in a progressive scoliosis. These patients often need longer fusions due to potential junctional complications.
  - Osteogenesis imperfecta: Defect in type 1 collagen resulting in weak bone with frequent breaks. Often have progressive scoliosis treated with extended posterior spinal fusion (PSF).
- Evaluation of scoliosis:
  - Family history: Positive in about 10% of scoliosis patients. Twin studies also suggest a polygenetic autosomal or sex-linked inheritance pattern. Scoliosis is three times more likely if a parent is affected and seven times more likely if sibling is affected.[2]
  - Growth history: Growth should be evaluated at every visit when following scoliosis. There is greatest risk for curve progression during growth spurts. The risk of progression decreases when growth slows to less than 1 cm in 6 months' time.
  - Motor evaluation: Evaluate for symmetric strength and reflexes. Asymmetry can indicate neural axis problem. Abdominal reflex asymmetry can indicate the level of a neural axis abnormality.
  - Balance/symmetry: Check for shoulder asymmetry which can indicate a rotational deformity of the spinal cord. If there is no shoulder asymmetry present but a thoracic curve is corrected, shoulder imbalance can result. Planning of more cephalad fusion levels is warranted in this case.[2,3] Plumb line can estimate head deviation from midline. Performed by drawing a vertical line from C7 to the gluteal cleft and visualizing distance from midline. Adams' forward bend test screens for thoracic and lumbar rotational deformity. Performed by evaluating the patient from behind with the patient bent at waist

attempting to touch toes. Can determine degree of rotation with scoliometer (5–7-degree scoliometer correlates roughly with 20–25 Cobb's measurement).
- Kyphosis: Often occurs with scoliosis. Can assess clinically by viewing the patient laterally with Adam's forward bend test or radiographically by measuring the curvature.
- Lower extremities/gait: Evaluate for symmetric gait, strength, coordination, and inspect feet for cavovarus deformity.

• Radiographs:
- Cobb's measurement: This is the angle between superior and inferior end plate vertebrae of the curve. To measure, draw lines parallel to the superior and inferior end plates. Can be measured directly with the difference between these lines, or geometrically by measuring the difference between lines perpendicular to the horizontal end plate lines.
- Risser's scale: Estimate of skeletal maturity that is measured radiographically on a scale of 0 to 5 based on the amount of calcification over the Ilium (▶ Table 42.2). Risser 0 indicates skeletal immaturity, 5 indicates skeletal maturity. Risser 0 has no ossification over the Ilium. Risser 1 is 25% ossification beginning with the lateral aspect of the Ilium, Risser 2 is 25%-50%, Risser 3 is 50%-75%, Risser 4 is 100%

and Risser 5 is 100% ossification with closure of the apophysis.
- Triradiate cartilage: Y-shaped ossification center on the floor of the acetabulum. Closes prior to calcification of ilium and just after period of peak growth velocity.
- MRI: Indicated for early-onset, congenital, significant pain, left main thoracic curves, or curves associated with neuromuscular conditions.

• Behavior and health effects of scoliosis:
- Progression rates: Idiopathic curve progression rate is related to the magnitude of the curve and skeletal maturity. Risser 0–1 with curve less than 20 degrees has less than a 25% risk of progression. Risser 0–1 with a curve greater than 20 degrees has a risk of progression of about 70%. Risser 2–4 with less than 20 degrees of curvature have less than 2% risk of progression. Patients who are Risser 2–4 with greater than 20 degrees of curvature have 23% risk of progression.[4] Congenital curve progression related to the type of malformation. Unsegmented bars with contralateral hemivertebra have the highest risk of being rapidly progressive. Unilateral unsegmented bar is rapidly progressive. Fully segmented hemivertebra is progressive at a constant rate. Partially segmented hemivertebra is less rapidly progressive. Incarcerated or unsegmented hemivertebra have little progression if any.
- Pulmonary function test (PFT): Thoracic curves approaching 90 degrees can compromise pulmonary function. Forced vital capacity and forced expiratory volume in one second decrease linearly when curves are greater than 100 degrees.
- Back pain: Increased incidence of back pain in scoliosis, but most of the back pain is rated as minimal and does not cause disability.[5]
- Appearance concerns: Cosmetic concerns regarding scoliosis are a legitimate reason to consider surgical options. Must balance appearance versus surgical risks and known consequences of surgery (decreased motion in fused segment of back).
- The majority of scoliosis cases are non–life threatening. In early-onset scoliosis, certain congenital scoliosis and scoliosis associated with neuromuscular conditions, the curve can be rapidly progressive with cardiopulmonary compromise when curve is greater than 100 degrees.

Table 42.2 Risser's scoring index

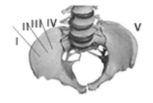

Risser 0	No calcification on iliac crest
Risser I	Lateral 25% of iliac crest ossified
Risser II	Lateral 25–50% of iliac crest ossified
Risser III	Lateral 50–75% of iliac crest ossified
Risser IV	Iliac crest 75–100% ossified
Risser V	Iliac crest 100% ossified with closure of the apophysis

42.2 Nonsurgical Treatment

There are multiple modes of treatment of scoliosis, ranging from observation to surgery. Different treatment options are considered in different curves. The best treatment is individualized to the patient and the curve.

- Physical therapy (PT): Very good for overall health and bone health. PT has not been shown to prevent curve progression.
- Observation: Initially indicated for most curves. It is important to determine rate of curve progression and overall growth rate. Curves less than 25 degrees should be monitored every 4 to 12 months with radiographic assessment. The curves should be monitored more frequently during periods of rapid growth rate. Curves greater than 30 degrees should continue to be monitored even after skeletal maturity.
- Mehta's casting: Indicated for infantile idiopathic scoliosis (IIS). The casting is not well tolerated in older children. If rib vertebra angle difference is greater than 20 degrees or curve is greater than 35 degrees in IIS, consider casting followed by bracing when the child becomes more mobile. If the curve is under 25 degrees or the child is under 1, there is a high probability that curve will spontaneously resolve. Follow-up in 4 months is acceptable.
- Brace treatment: Indicated for idiopathic scoliosis with 25 to 40 degrees of curvature. May also be used but with less success for nonidiopathic cases. Bracing does not correct the deformity; rather it slows the rate of curve progression. For adolescent idiopathic scoliosis (AIS), it has been shown that the more hours in the day you wear the brace, the better the results. For best results, the patient should wear the brace for 23 hours every day. The patient can stop wearing the brace at skeletal maturity, assessed by Risser's score and growth rate among other parameters. Bracing can be 65 to 75% effective with proper indications and compliance.[2,4]

42.3 Surgical Treatment

- Lenke's classification for AIS (▶ Table 42.3). Used for planning surgical treatment in AIS.[2,3,6,7]
  - Classifies curves into six major curve types with modifiers for the deviation of the apical vertebra and amount of kyphosis. The major curves are the largest curved vertebrae measured by the Cobb angle. They are classified as structural or nonstructural based on flexibility in lateral flexion. Structural curves do not bend out to less than 25 degrees in lateral flexion. The structural curves are classified according to location. Type 1 is main thoracic with a structural thoracic curve. Type 2 is double thoracic with two structural thoracic curves. Type 3 is double major with a structural thoracic and lumbar curve. Type 4 is a triple major with two structural thoracic curves and one structural lumbar curve. Type 5 is thoracolumbar/lumbar with a structural curve in the lumbar or thoracolumbar region. Type 6 is thoracolumbar/lumbar and thoracic with a structural thoracolumbar/lumbar and thoracic curves.
  - Lumbar modifiers are determined by the intersection of the stable vertebra with a line drawn vertically from the sacrum, the center sacral vertical line (CSVL). A modifier, the CSVL intersects between the pedicles of the stable vertebra. B modifier, the CSVL touches the pedicles of the stable vertebra. C modifier, the CSVL does not touch the pedicles of the stable vertebra.
  - Sagittal profile is modified according to the degree of kyphosis. Hypokyphotic is less than 10 degrees. Normal is between 10 and 40 degrees. Hyperkyphotic is greater than 40 degrees.
- PSF is the gold standard treatment. It is normally offered for curves greater than 50 degrees. The PSF varies according to the curve. Perform selective PSF of the structural curves in idiopathic scoliosis. Typically fuse from the neutral vertebra above to 1 to 2 levels below the stable vertebra.[2] Fuse selectively with congenital curves, modify according to the defect. Fuse more segments in neuromuscular and syndromic causes, often requiring pelvic fixation.
- Osteotomies: Ponte's osteotomy involves removal of facet joints which typically limit extension of the spine. This allows for correction of kyphosis. Indicated in rigid curves. Vertebral column resection (VCR) allows for the largest correction of kyphosis. Indicated for very large focal curves.
- Anterior spinal fusion (ASF): Indicated for skeletally immature patients and extreme lordosis. Skeletally immature patients, Risser 0 with triradiate cartilage open, are at greater risk for crankshaft phenomenon if PSF is performed. ASF can prevent this. ASF is also indicated for

Table 42.3 Lenke's classification of adolescent idiopathic scoliosis

Type	Lenke I	Lenke II	Lenke III	Lenke IV	Lenke V	Lenke VI
Curve type	Main thoracic curve	Double thoracic curve	Double Major curve	Triple major curve	Thoracolumbar/ lumbar curve	Thoracolumbar/ lumbar thoracic curve

Lumbar modifiers	A. CSVL intersects between pedicles of stable vertebra	B. CSVL touches stable vertebra	C. CSVL does not intersect stable vertebra

Sagittal modifiers	Hypokyphotic (−) < 10 degrees kyphosis	Normal kyphosis (N) 10–40 degrees kyphosis	Hyperkyphotic (+) > 40 degrees of kyphosis

lordosis as this approach allows direct access to the vertebra in the thoracolumbar and lumbar region. This approach can get similar correction with fusion of less vertebral levels. However, the surgery can increase thoracic kyphosis, and is a more difficult surgery that requires more time in the operating room.[7]

- Growing rod instrumentation: Indicated for young children with growth potential left with progressive curves that do not respond to bracing. Fuse proximally and distally to spinal curve with rods that distract across the curve. Perform growing rod distraction every 6 to 12 months until the patient is done growing. Eventually, the patient will need PSF. Another option is the vertical expandable prosthetic titanium rib (VEPTR). This device is attached to the ribs and distracted periodically in a spine-sparing approach. It is indicated in early-onset scoliosis and thoracic insufficiency.

- Innovative ideas: Anterior stapling/tethering involves attaching pedicle screws to the convexity of the curve connected by a cable that corrects the deformity. This method corrects deformity without fusion allowing the spine to grow and remain flexible. There is also no growing rod distraction periodically required with this technique. There is potential for overcorrection and no long-term follow-up with this technique.

- Neuromonitoring: Monitor both motor and sensory pathways during surgical correction of curves. Somatosensory-evoked potentials and motor-evoked potentials are generated by stimulating the torso and legs distally and measuring response in brainstem. Allows for rapid detection of any central nervous system (CNS) insult associated with correction of deformity. Many factors can interfere with neuromonitoring: inhalational anesthetics, hypothermia, hypotension, and technical malfunction. With a real deficit detected on neuromonitoring, a wake-up test should be performed. If a change in neuro status is real, steps to correct the deficit should be taken immediately including increase BP to a mean arterial pressure (MAP) greater than 90, decrease correction of spinal cord deformity, keep hematocrit above 30 (transfuse if necessary), administer high-dose intravenous (IV) steroids, and remove hardware if all else fails.

42.4 Complications

- Progression: Potential for failure of implants from fracture or dislodgement of implants leading to progression of the curve. Pseudoarthorosis formation can eventually lead to rod fracture. If spinal fusion is too short, it can lead to junctional problems at ends of the fused spinal segment, such as fracture or degenerative change, as these regions are subject to increased mechanical forces.
- Deep infection: Risk factors that are associated with increased rate of delayed infection include receiving blood transfusion, fusion into the lumbar region, significant medical history, and not using a drain postoperatively. Occurs roughly in 1 to 2% of patients. Requires instrument removal and antibiotic therapy. Early infection had the highest rate in neuromuscular curves at 9% and lowest in idiopathic scoliosis at 1.6%. Infection rate also varies according to the procedure performed being lowest for distraction procedures. Gram-negative bacteria are more commonly involved in infection in nonidiopathic curves, targeted antibiotics should be given in the perioperative period.[8,9]
- Neurological injury: Risk is less than 1% with typical AIS. The rate is higher with congenital or severe curves. Causes of neurological injury include correction of curvature leading to traction on the cord, offset at osteotomies,

hypotension, and direct contact with root or cord causing contusion (risk with hooks, screws).

42.5 Conclusion

Scoliosis may arise from any disturbance of the structure or regulation of spinal balance. It progresses most rapidly during growth but may slowly worsen at any time. It affects pulmonary function when the curve becomes substantial leading to cardiopulmonary compromise. There is an increased incidence of back pain associated with scoliosis. Bracing during growth, and surgery are the only methods proven to affect the natural history. Bracing prevents progression while surgery can correct the defect. The role of surgery depends on multiple factors. It must be performed with the utmost safety to maintain and improve quality of life.

42.6 Common Clinical Questions

1. When is it indicated to order an MRI in scoliosis?
2. Why is bracing the recommended treatment for scoliosis?
3. When is surgery the recommended treatment for scoliosis?
4. What are the steps to take if intraoperative neuromuscular monitoring changes during surgery?

42.7 Answers to Common Clinical Questions

1. MRI is indicated in congenital, infantile, and juvenile curves to rule out intraspinal pathology. These curves are at higher risk and warrant an MRI to rule out abnormalities such as tethered cord, syringomyelia, and spinal cord tumor. Specific curves that are alarming are left apex thoracic curve, short angular curves, patients less than 10 with a curve greater than 20 degrees, any neurological abnormality associated with a curve, excessive pain, or rapid progression of the curve.
2. Bracing is indicated in patients with idiopathic curves 25 to 40degrees. In IIS, bracing or casting is started when the curve is greater than 30 degrees. Many curves less than this in infantile

will spontaneously resolve. In juvenile and adolescent, bracing is considered when curves become greater than 20 to 25 degrees. The more the patient wears the brace, the more likely it is to be effective. Ideal treatment involves wearing the brace for 23 hours per day. Bracing should be continued until the patient is skeletally mature or until the curve progresses beyond 45 to 50 degrees.[4]

3. Surgery is indicated in idiopathic scoliosis when curve reaches 50 degrees. The curve is likely to continue progressing at this point and will not improve with bracing. It is indicated in congenital scoliosis when there is a curve known to be at high risk of progression (such as a unilateral bar with contralateral hemivertebra) or associated with severe pain, neurological defect, or pulmonary compromise.[2,7]

4. When intraoperative neurophysiological monitoring (IONM) changes first assess that it is a true neurological defect? Neuromonitoring changes can also be caused by hypotension, hypothermia, inhaled anesthetics, or technical errors such as monitor detachment. When a true neurological change is detected on IONM, perform a wake-up test, increase BP to a MAP greater than 90, keep hematocrit above 30 (transfuse if necessary), administer high-dose corticosteroids, reverse correction of spinal cord defect, and remove hardware as a last resort.

References

[1] Dobbs MB, Lenke LG, Szymanski DA, et al. Prevalence of neural axis abnormalities in patients with infantile idiopathic scoliosis. J Bone Joint Surg Am. 2002; 84-A(12): 2230–2234

[2] Rose PS, Lenke LG. Classification of operative adolescent idiopathic scoliosis: treatment guidelines. Orthop Clin North Am. 2007; 38(4):521–529, vi

[3] Lenke LG, Betz RR, Harms J, et al. Adolescent idiopathic scoliosis: a new classification to determine extent of spinal arthrodesis. J Bone Joint Surg Am. 2001; 83-A(8): 1169–1181

[4] Nachemson AL, Peterson LE. Effectiveness of treatment with a brace in girls who have adolescent idiopathic scoliosis. A prospective, controlled study based on data from the Brace Study of the Scoliosis Research Society. J Bone Joint Surg Am. 1995; 77(6):815–822

[5] Weinstein SL, Dolan LA, Spratt KF, Peterson KK, Spoonamore MJ, Ponseti IV. Health and function of patients with untreated idiopathic scoliosis: a 50-year natural history study. JAMA. 2003; 289(5):559–567

[6] Lenke LG. The Lenke classification system of operative adolescent idiopathic scoliosis. Neurosurg Clin N Am. 2007; 18(2):199–206

[7] Newton PO, Marks MC, Bastrom TP, et al. Harms Study Group. Surgical treatment of Lenke 1 main thoracic idiopathic scoliosis: results of a prospective, multicenter study. Spine. 2013; 38(4):328–338

[8] Ho C, Sucato DJ, Richards BS. Risk factors for the development of delayed infections following posterior spinal fusion and instrumentation in adolescent idiopathic scoliosis patients. Spine. 2007; 32(20):2272–2277

[9] Mackenzie WG, Matsumoto H, Williams BA, et al. Surgical site infection following spinal instrumentation for scoliosis: a multicenter analysis of rates, risk factors, and pathogens. J Bone Joint Surg Am. 2013; 95(9):800–806, S1–S2

43 Achondroplasia

Debraj Mukherjee, Moise Danielpur

43.1 Introduction

Achondroplasia is the most common of the skeletal dysplasia, occurring in approximately one of every 15,000 to 40,000 live births.[1] It is an autosomal dominant condition, with most cases due to new activating mutations in the *FGFR3* gene. The molecular defect in achondroplasia causes a quantitative decrease in the rate of endochondral bone formation, resulting in short and squat long bones, short stature, large calvarium, midface hypoplasia, short basicranium with narrowed foramen magnum and vascular channels, and small vertebral bodies with shortened pedicles and narrow spinal canals (▶ Fig. 43.1).[1,2,3] The most concerning neurological sequelae of achondroplasia that are important to the neurosurgeon include cervicomedullary compression, spinal stenosis, and hydrocephalus.

43.2 Cervicomedullary Compression

The most serious neurological complication in patients with achondroplasia is cervicomedullary junction (CMJ) compression caused by a tight deformed foramen magnum.[2] Compression at the foramen magnum can result in cervical myelopathy manifested as clonus and hyperreflexia, hypotonia, sleep apnea, and even sudden death.[2,3,4,5,6] Because of the potentially lethal complication associated with symptomatic disease, neurosurgical decompression has been used to widen the foramen magnum and relieve the pressure on the emerging cervical cord. Fortunately, most children with achondroplasia do not suffer neurological symptoms and achieve normal motor and intellectual development without surgical intervention.[6,7]

Criteria for decompression have been previously described in large surgical series, generally consisting of imaging and clinical findings consistent with symptomatic cervicomedullary stenosis.[3,8] Unfortunately, there has never been a study which provided a fail-safe method for prospectively identifying patients who are likely to die or experience severe neurological complications if decompression surgery was not performed. At our institution, we have used complete obliteration of cerebrospinal fluid (CSF) flow anterior to the spinal cord as an indication for decompression in symptomatic patients. Based on findings of our recent series, there may be a role for the use of dynamic cervical flexion/extension magnetic resonance imaging (MRI) and CSF flow studies in the evaluation of cervicomedullary compression among symptomatic patients with achondroplasia.

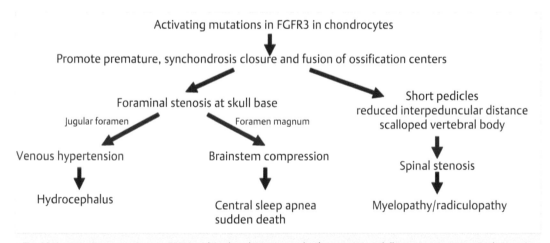

Fig. 43.1 Activating mutations in *FGFR3* within chondrocytes can lead to cervicomedullary compression, spinal stenosis, or hydrocephalus by decreasing the relative rate of endochondral bone formation.

43.3 Spinal Stenosis

Patients with achondroplasia are predisposed to spinal stenosis as a result of pedicles shortened in anteroposterior length and decreased interpedicular distance, leading to narrowed spinal canals.[9,10] The series of Jeong et al found that while the interpedicular distance widens from L1 to L5 in patients without achondroplasia, the interpedicular distance progressively decreases from L1 to L5 in patients with anchondroplasia.[11] Such patients often become symptomatic in young adulthood, when degenerative changes lead to thickening of the ligamentum flavum, limiting an already narrowed canal and causing symptomatic stenosis. It has been postulated that this stenosis is heightened by thoracolumbar kyphosis and compensatory lumbar hyperlordosis.[10,12] By the sixth decade of life, approximately 80% of patients will develop spinal stenosis, with approximately 10 to 20% requiring surgical intervention.[10,13]

Indications for surgery within their cohort remain broadly defined, but the largest series to date included the following operative criteria[14]:

- The presence of signs or symptoms of chronic spinal cord compression (weakness, bowel or bladder dysfunction, hyperreflexia or hypertonia, spastic gait, or clonus) or chronic nerve root compression (neurogenic claudication, weakness or sensory disturbance in a radicular pattern, or hyporeflexia).
- Neuroimaging evidence of spinal stenosis.

Once the decision has been made to pursue surgical intervention, the neurosurgeon must be aware of possible complications specific to this patient cohort.[15] Patients with achondroplasia are prone to have thinned dura, increasing the relative odds of an intraoperative durotomy. Additionally, the presence of scoliosis and thoracolumbar kyphosis is higher within this patient population and may require the use of either interspinolaminar decompression without laminectomy or use of concurrent or delayed instrumentation to prevent postoperative instability.

43.4 Hydrocephalus

Infants with achondroplasia commonly have an enlarged head; however, not all such patients require surgical intervention. All infants with achondroplasia should have head growth monitored at regular intervals using head circumference charts for achondroplasia, not charts for the general population.[16] The majority of patients with achondroplasia and macro-cephaly with mild to moderately enlarged ventricles have spontaneous stabilization of ventricular size. Patients with enlarging head circumference as well as signs or symptoms of increased intracranial pressure, such as a full fontanelle or dilated facial veins should be investigated with intracranial imaging, either ultrasonography or MR imaging. While cranial ultrasonography is thought to be an adequate screening test, MRI imaging allows for both assessment of ventricular size as well as evidence of transependymal flow. Ventriculoperitoneal shunting should be reserved for severely symptomatic patients with enlarging ventricles.[17] Although a specific mechanism has not been fully elucidated to explain the possible relationship between achondroplasia and hydrocephalus, previous authors have postulated that intracranial venous sinus hypertension secondary to jugular foramen stenosis, and in some cases jugular vein stenosis at the thoracic inlet within this patient population.[18,19]

References

[1] Rimoin DL. The chondrodystrophies. Adv Hum Genet. 1975; 5:1–118

[2] Hecht JT, Francomano CA, Horton WA, Annegers JF. Mortality in achondroplasia. Am J Hum Genet. 1987; 41(3):454–464

[3] Pauli RM, Horton VK, Glinski LP, Reiser CA. Prospective assessment of risks for cervicomedullary-junction compression in infants with achondroplasia. Am J Hum Genet. 1995; 56(3):732–744

[4] Bagley CA, Pindrik JA, Bookland MJ, Camara-Quintana JQ, Carson BS. Cervicomedullary decompression for foramen magnum stenosis in achondroplasia. J Neurosurg. 2006; 104 suppl 3:166–172

[5] Bland JD, Emery JL. Unexpected death of children with achondroplasia after the perinatal period. Dev Med Child Neurol. 1982; 24(4):489–492

[6] Francomano CA, Carson B, Seidler A, et al. Morbidity and mortality in achondroplasia: efficacy of prospective evaluation and surgical intervention. Am J Hum Genet. 1993; 53 3:112

[7] Reid CS, Pyeritz RE, Kopits SE, et al. Cervicomedullary compression in young patients with achondroplasia: value of comprehensive neurologic and respiratory evaluation. J Pediatr. 1987; 110(4):522–530

[8] Rimoin DL. Cervicomedullary junction compression in infants with achondroplasia: when to perform neurosurgical decompression. Am J Hum Genet. 1995; 56(4):824–827

[9] Dubosset J. Cervical abnormalities in osteochondroplasia. In: Nicoletti B, Kopits S, Ascani E, McKusick VA, eds. Human Achondroplasia: A Multidisciplinary Approach. New York, NY: Plenum Press; 1988:215–218

[10] Kopits SE. Orthopedic aspects of achondroplasia in children. Basic Life Sci. 1988; 48:189–197

[11] Jeong ST, Song HR, Keny SM, Telang SS, Suh SW, Hong SJ. MRI study of the lumbar spine in achondroplasia. A morphometric analysis for the evaluation of stenosis of the canal. J Bone Joint Surg Br. 2006; 88(9):1192–1196

[12] Lutter LD, Langer LO. Neurological symptoms in achondroplastic dwarfs—surgical treatment. J Bone Joint Surg Am. 1977; 59(1):87–92

[13] Hall JG. The natural history of achondroplasia. Basic Life Sci. 1988; 48:3–9

[14] Sciubba DM, Noggle JC, Marupudi NI, et al. Spinal stenosis surgery in pediatric patients with achondroplasia. J Neurosurg. 2007; 106 suppl 5:372–378

[15] King JA, Vachhrajani S, Drake JM, Rutka JT. Neurosurgical implications of achondroplasia. J Neurosurg Pediatr. 2009; 4 (4):297–306

[16] Horton WA, Rotter JI, Rimoin DL, Scott CI, Hall JG. Standard growth curves for achondroplasia. J Pediatr. 1978; 93(3): 435–438

[17] Pierre-Kahn A, Hirsch JF, Renier D, Metzger J, Maroteaux P. Hydrocephalus and achondroplasia. A study of 25 observations. Childs Brain. 1980; 7(4):205–219

[18] Yamada H, Nakamura S, Tajima M, Kageyama N. Neurological manifestations of pediatric achondroplasia. J Neurosurg. 1981; 54(1):49–57

[19] Mukherjee D, Pressman BD, Krakow D, Rimoin DL, Danielpour M. Dynamic cervicomedullary cord compression and alterations in cerebrospinal fluid dynamics in children with achondroplasia: review of an 11-year surgical case series. J Neurosurg Pediatr. 2014; 14(3):238–244

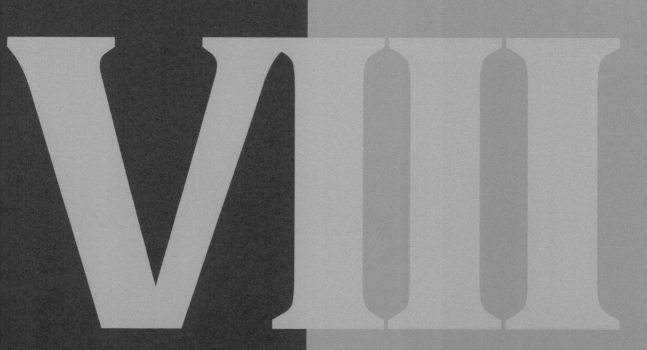

Section VIII

Functional Disorders

44 The Evaluation and Classification of Epilepsy

Sarah A. Kelley, Adam L. Hartman

44.1 Introduction

This chapter outlines epilepsy related definitions and classifications as put forth by the International League Against Epilepsy. Acquired forms of epilepsy and epileptic syndromes are then reviewed followed by a discussion of the evaluation of a patient with epilepsy.

44.2 Definitions

Recent updates to the International League Against Epilepsy classification scheme in 2017 are reflected here.[1]

A **seizure** is abnormal electrical activity in the brain that results in clinical signs and symptoms. These symptoms can range from motor or sensory symptoms to alternation in consciousness, and autonomic symptoms.

Epilepsy is two or more unprovoked (i.e., not provoked by fever, electrolyte abnormalities, drug withdrawal) seizures or one unprovoked seizure plus an electroencephalography (EEG) abnormality suggesting that the patient is at high risk for another seizure.

Incidence: About 10% of the population will have a single seizure at some point in life. The incidence of actively treated epilepsy is about 1% in the general population.[2]

Status epilepticus: Continuous seizure activity lasting 30 minutes or longer or more than one seizure without return to baseline cognition in between. Some have proposed using a shorter time frame because the vast majority of seizures last less than 5 to 10 minutes.

44.3 Classification of Epilepsy

44.3.1 Definitions

Generalized onset seizure: A seizure appearing to involve simultaneous abnormal firing of the whole brain and subsequent full body involvement and/or loss of awareness.

Focal Onset seizure: A seizure that involves abnormal neuronal firing of one part of the brain, which may or may not spread to involve the whole brain (focal to bilateral tonic-clonic—previously called secondary generalization) and subsequent localized symptoms as described below. If there is

loss of awareness with these seizures, they are described as focal with impaired awareness (previously complex partial seizure). If there is no loss of awareness, they are termed focal aware seizures (previously simple partial seizures).

Any patient with a focal seizure should get brain imaging (preferably magnetic resonance imaging [MRI]) unless the history and EEG are consistent with a benign epilepsy syndrome (see below).

44.3.2 Structural Abnormalities

Tumors: Common developmental tumors seen in pediatric patients include dysembryoplastic neuroepithelial tumors (DNET) and gangliogliomas. These may cause seizures while impinging on cortical tissue and are frequently associated with malformations of cortical development. MRI will identify these lesions as they may need to be resected if medication does not control seizures.

Cortical dysgenesis: Abnormalities in the formation of the cortex during development. In some cases, these may be easily demonstrated on MRI (lissencephaly, polymicrogyria) or less easily seen (such as in some syndromes where abnormal formation of the cell layers of the cortex may not be seen). These lesions may also be amenable to surgical resection.

- **Mesial temporal sclerosis** occurs when there is scarring of the temporal lobe for any number of reasons from infection to trauma. There is continuing debate as to whether it may be caused by febrile seizures. This, too, is often amenable to surgical resection with a temporal lobectomy and amygdalohippocampectomy.
- **Vascular malformations:** The most likely vascular malformations to lead to seizure are arteriovenous malformations and cavernous angiomas. They lead to epilepsy due to hemorrhage or surrounding brain tissue injury. Both are associated with focal epilepsy.

44.3.3 Posttraumatic Epilepsy

Posttraumatic epilepsy is a very common form of acquired epilepsy and is defined as recurrent seizures after a traumatic brain injury. These are divided into three main categories: immediate seizures, which occur within 24 hours of injury, early seizures, which occur within 1 week of injury and late seizures, which occur more than week after injury. An increased risk of developing epilepsy after head injury is noted if there is a depressed skull fracture, penetrating injury, intracranial hematoma, or early seizures.[3] Prophylaxis has been demonstrated to prevent early but not late posttraumatic seizures.[4] Posttraumatic seizures may be difficult to treat surgically due to coup–contrecoup injuries that may create multiple epileptogenic foci.

44.3.4 Epilepsy Syndromes

The diagnosis of epilepsy syndromes gives information as to how to best treat the patient as well as the likely prognosis.[5]

Neonatal

Neonatal seizures may be caused by all of the same etiologies as described above. In addition, there are a number of syndromes that are specific to the neonatal age group.

- Benign syndromes: Children most often grow out of these seizures. Benign idiopathic neonatal seizures and benign familial neonatal seizures both often occur within the first week of life.
- Other syndromes that occur early in the neonatal period including early infantile epileptic encephalopathy (Ohtahara's syndrome) and early myoclonic encephalopathy are refractory to treatment and the patients have poor outcomes. Both are characterized by a burst suppression pattern on the EEG.

Infant/Childhood

- **Febrile seizures** are the most common type of seizure in this age group, occurring in up to 5% of children between the ages of 6 months and 6 years in the US (this varies by country). These are typically developing children who have a fever over 38 °C without evidence of a central nervous system (CNS) infection. Febrile seizures are divided into two categories: simple and complex. Simple febrile seizures are relatively short (< 15 minutes), are generalized, and do not recur within a 24-hour period. Complex febrile seizures are longer (> 15 minutes), focal, or recur within 24 hours. Those with simple febrile seizures do not have an increased risk of later-developing epilepsy. The risk doubles for those who had complex febrile seizures. Those who

have simple febrile seizures do not require any additional work-up including EEG, brain imaging, or lumbar puncture. The source of the fever should be investigated and treated. Seizure prophylaxis is typically not recommended in these patients and studies have demonstrated that fever control does not reduce the risk of a subsequent febrile seizure.[6]

- **Infantile spasms** generally occur around 4 to 8 months of age. The triad of infantile spasms (flexor or extensor spasms often occurring in clusters often around sleep–wake transitions), a high voltage, chaotic, multifocal EEG (hypsarrhythmia), and developmental delay constitute West's syndrome. The vast majority of these patients (80–90%) have underlying brain pathology. Most have developmental delay and many go on to have other seizure types later in life.
- **Absence seizures** are divided into two types, childhood and juvenile, depending on the age of onset and associated seizure types. They develop between 4 and 14 years of age and are characterized by staring and behavior arrest lasting on average 10 to 12 seconds, sometimes associated with automatisms and often occurring very frequently throughout the day. These patients can also develop generalized tonic–clonic seizures and myoclonic jerks. Their seizures may be induced by hyperventilation and their EEG demonstrates generalized 3-Hz spike and slow-wave activity.
- **Benign epilepsy with centrotemporal spikes** (previously called benign rolandic epilepsy) is the most common focal epilepsy of childhood occurring between 3 and 13 years of age. These seizures often occur just after falling asleep and often involve one side of the face and tongue with inability to talk. They will often evolve into generalized tonic–clonic seizures. The EEG shows a classic centrotemporal spike distribution which may be unilateral. Children often grow out of these seizures around puberty.
- **Lennox–Gastaut syndrome** (LGS) is characterized by multiple seizure types including tonic, atonic, and absence seizures as well as focal and generalized tonic–clonic seizures. These children have very abnormal EEGs (slow spike wave and paroxysmal fast) and most have developmental delay. Children who have infantile spasms often go on to develop LGS.

Adolescent

- **Juvenile myoclonic epilepsy** is the most common generalized epilepsy in adolescents and often emerges in the teenage years. Usually, patients will experience early morning myoclonic jerks (although they can occur any time of day) prior to developing a generalized tonic–clonic seizure. Absence seizures may also be seen and the EEG typically shows a 4- to 5-Hz generalized spike and wave pattern. Most patients require lifelong treatment for this disorder.

44.4 Evaluation of Epilepsy

44.4.1 History

What happened to the patient during the seizure? This will vary depending on which part of the brain is involved. The initial clinical finding at the beginning of the seizure is often the most helpful in localizing the onset of the seizure within a specific anatomical location.

- **Generalized onset seizure:** Behavior arrest, staring, myoclonus, tonic posturing, tonic–clonic seizures
- **Focal onset seizure:** Localized motor, sensory or autonomic function, behavior arrest, or staring (the latter two can be seen with either generalized or focal seizures). Examples include left arm shaking, numbness on the side of the face, eye deviation, automatisms (chewing, lip smacking, picking behaviors). Auras also fall into this category. Auras consist of altered sensory function that start just before more obvious seizure activity. This can include an unusual feeling, sense of fear, unpleasant taste, or smell, among other symptoms.

After the Seizure (Postictal Signs and Symptoms)

- **Lethargy or confusion:** Unilateral weakness (Todd's paralysis) may indicate that a seizure was focal in nature.

Subtle Findings

Asking about more subtle clinical findings may help to determine how frequently the patient is having seizures. For example, asking about staring spells, myoclonic jerks, loss of time, unexplained nocturnal tongue biting, or enuresis.

Risk Factors

- Brain trauma, meningitis, encephalitis, febrile seizures as a child, or a complicated prenatal course are most likely to place a person at risk for future epilepsy.
- Other risk factors include a history of stroke, vascular malformations (if impinging on the cortex), cortical or developmental malformations, intracranial hemorrhage, and metabolic abnormalities.

44.4.2 Physical Examination

- Neurological deficits on physical examination may give clues as to an underlying lesion which could be the cause of the patient's seizures.
- A thorough skin examination may identify neurophokomatoses such as tuberous sclerosis, Sturge–Weber syndrome, or neurofibromatosis.

44.4.3 Diagnostic Studies

Characterization and Localization

1. **Electroencephalogram (EEG):** A routine (20–30 minutes) study will detect abnormalities even if no seizures are captured in about 90% of those with generalized epilepsy and half of those with focal epilepsy. Therefore, a normal routine EEG does not rule out the diagnosis of epilepsy. The interictal (between seizure) EEG may demonstrate a specific pattern which is diagnostic of a certain epilepsy syndrome (see below). Provocative tests such as hyperventilation and intermittent photic stimulation may bring out epileptiform discharges in certain types of epilepsy.
- When to get an EEG?
  - After a new onset, unprovoked seizure
  - If there is a change in seizure characteristics from the patient's baseline seizures
  - Concern for status epilepticus (clinical or subclinical)
2. **Epilepsy monitoring unit (EMU):** Extended monitoring of the EEG is often needed to further characterize seizure type to guide future treatment or localize a seizure focus for possible surgical resection. This also can be used to determine whether events are epileptic or nonepileptic in nature.
3. **Intracranial electrode monitoring:** Placing grids or strips of electrodes on the surface of the brain or depth wires with electrodes into the

brain parenchyma can better localize a seizure focus in preparation for surgical resection of this focus. These electrodes also allow functional mapping of potentially eloquent areas of cortex (via direct current stimulation during various motor, language, and sensory paradigms), which in turn allows for improved tailoring of resections.

4. **Magnetic resonance imaging:** MRI is helpful in identifying a lesion that may be the cause for focal epilepsy. This may be due to any number of lesions including tumors, strokes, cortical malformations, or vascular malformations. Obtaining a "seizure protocol" MRI that specifically acquires coronal slices along the long axis through the hippocampus is more sensitive in finding volumetric differences between mesial temporal structures than conventional MRI.

5. **Positron emission tomography (PET) scan:** This radioisotope study (typically using ^{18}F-deoxyglucose) evaluates metabolic activity within the brain. Regions with decreased metabolism may be abnormal and therefore have the potential to lead to seizures. Conversely, seizure activity may increase focal metabolism (an EEG should be recorded during PET studies to monitor for this potential confounder).

6. **Single-photon emission tomography (SPECT):** This radionuclide study may identify the region where seizures originate. It requires an injection of the isotope immediately after the onset of a seizure, followed by rapidly obtained nuclear medicine studies.

7. **Magnetoencephalography (MEG):** This type of study localizes magnetic dipoles, which, in combination with MRI (magnetic source imaging), can be useful in finding areas of cortical irritability. MEG is considered to be complementary to EEG.

Studies to Aid in the Determination of Risk of Surgical Resection

- **Neuropsychological testing:** Typically administered by a neuropsychologist, this testing may identify possible areas of dysfunction as well as the likelihood that the patient will have additional deficits if certain portions of the brain are resected.

- **Functional MRI (fMRI):** Performed using specific motor and language paradigms, fMRI may show specific regions of the brain that are activated during a task.
- **Wada test:** Using intracarotid amobarbital or methohexital, this study can lateralize language and memory function by anesthetizing half the brain and then testing with a neuropsychology battery of tests.
- **MEG:** This modality also can be used to localize neurological function.

Careful evaluation via history, physical examination, ancillary testing, and subsequent correct classification of seizure type and seizure syndrome is important to determine the correct treatment and likely outcome for a patient with epilepsy.

44.5 Common Clinical Questions

1. What criteria would you use to diagnose a patient with epilepsy?
2. What are the studies of choice for a patient who presents with right arm twitching that then spreads to entire body tonic–clonic activity with loss of consciousness?
3. Should a patient with a traumatic brain injury, who has not had a seizure, be treated prophylactically with anticonvulsant medications?
4. When would you refer a patient to the epilepsy monitoring unit for prolonged EEG monitoring?

44.6 Answers to Common Clinical Questions

1. Diagnose a patient with epilepsy if the patient has had two or more unprovoked seizures (i.e., not due to fever, metabolic abnormality, etc.) or has had one seizure and has epileptiform activity on the EEG that suggests they are likely to have another seizure.
2. This is a focal to bilateral tonic-clonic seizure (focal seizure with secondary generalization). An EEG and MRI of the brain would be appropriate studies to obtain at this time. Both of these studies will help to localize the epileptogenic zone and the MRI of the brain will help to determine if there is an underlying

structural pathology that is leading to the seizure.

3. Data demonstrate that prophylaxis does prevent early posttraumatic seizures (within the first 7 days of injury) but not late posttraumatic seizures (after 7 days). Therefore, the patient may be treated prophylactically for 7 days; however, treatment should be stopped if s/he has not developed seizures within the first week.

4. Refer to the epilepsy monitoring unit to further characterize seizure type, to guide future treatment, or localize a seizure focus for possible surgical resection. The monitoring may also be used to determine whether events are epileptic or nonepileptic in nature.

References

[1] Berg AT, Berkovic SF, Brodie MJ, et al. Revised terminology and concepts for organization of seizures and epilepsies: report of the ILAE Commission on Classification and Terminology, 2005–2009. Epilepsia. 2010; 51(4):676–685

[2] Hauser WA, Annegers JF, Kurland LT. Prevalence of epilepsy in Rochester, Minnesota: 1940–1980. Epilepsia. 1991; 32(4):429–445

[3] Lowenstein DH. Epilepsy after head injury: an overview. Epilepsia. 2009; 50 suppl 2:4–9

[4] Temkin NR, Dikmen SS, Wilensky AJ, Keihm J, Chabal S, Winn HR. A randomized, double-blind study of phenytoin for the prevention of post-traumatic seizures. N Engl J Med. 1990; 323(8):497–502

[5] Muthugovindan D, Hartman AL. Pediatric epilepsy syndromes. Neurologist. 2010; 16(4):223–237

[6] Rosenbloom E, Finkelstein Y, Adams-Webber T, Kozer E. Do antipyretics prevent the recurrence of febrile seizures in children? A systematic review of randomized controlled trials and meta-analysis. Eur J Paediatr Neurol. 2013; 17(6):585–588

45 Surgical Management of Childhood Epilepsy: Temporal and Extratemporal Pathologies

Aurelia Peraud

45.1 Introduction

In most patients, seizures can be well controlled with appropiate medication, but 20 to 30% of the patients are refractory to all forms of medical therapy. There has been increasing consensus on the efficacy of surgery to treat drug-resistant focal epilepsy in children. In addition to the control of disabling seizures, surgery may improve developmental, psychosocial, and behavioral impairment in children with early-onset epilepsy and those with long-standing antiepileptic medication. Brain maturation in infancy and early childhood leads to a complex evolution of seizure semiology, electroencephalography (EEG), and neuroimaging findings. Not surprisingly, developmental delay or progressive disturbances in cognition, behavior, and psychiatric state are common in pediatric epilepsy. Therefore, early surgical intervention is crucial in infants with catastrophic epilepsy to prevent such a developmental delay. Moreover, surgery in early childhood may take advantage of brain plasticity with chances for recovery from seizure-related damage and possible postsurgical neurological deficits. However, the clinical presentation and the etiology of medically refractory localized seizures can be rather heterogeneous.

45.2 Epilepsy Disorders in Childhood Epilepsy

45.2.1 Cortical Dysplasia

Cortical dysplasia is the most common neuropathological entity found in pediatric epilepsy and may be focal or multilobar. Neuroradiological alterations can be subtle or even absent, and if visible on MR images, the lesion may only be a small part of larger diffuse structural abnormality. Exact presurgical evaluation and surgical planning are of utmost importance to delineate the entire abnormal cortical area for complete resection yields the best seizure control.

45.2.2 Tuberous Sclerosis Complex

The evaluation of the epileptogenic focus in this patient groups can be challenging. These children may have a single epileptogenic region suitable for resection despite having multiple other tubers or a multifocal, rather diffuse, seizure onset.

45.2.3 Polymicrogyria

The clinical and eletrophysiological spectrum in this entity can be widespread and seizures may spontaneously remit. Polymicrogyria is commonly found in both hemispheres predominantely in the perirolandic or perisylvian region.

45.2.4 Hypothalamic Hamartoma

Seizures orginating from hypothalamic hamartomas are often pharmacoresistant and developmental and, behavioral problems as well as endocrinological disturbances are not uncommon. Several surgical approaches have been described including stereotactic, endoscopic, and radiosurgical procedures.

45.2.5 Hemispheric Syndroms

Congenital abnormalities affecting an entire hemisphere such as hemispheric dysplasia or hemimegalencephaly are summarized under this title. Surgical techniques include hemispherectomy or hemispherotomy procedures.

45.2.6 Sturge–Weber Syndrome

When seizures occur early in infancy or are associated with significant developmental delay or progressive focal deficits such as hemiparesis, urgent surgical intervention might be necessary. Depending on the seizure-onset zone, focal resection or hemispheric procedures are required. Operative risks are not only related to the size of resection but to the hemodynamic effects, which can compromise also the contralateral hemisphere.

45.2.7 Rasmussen's Syndrome

The etiology of Rasmussen's syndrome is still not understood (viral vs. autoimmune), but the severity of disabling seizures resistant to antiepileptic drugs makes surgical intervention necessary as early as possible to prevent other comorbidities. Hemispherotomies and other disconnection procedures are the treatment of choice. The risk–benefit assessment requires considerable clinical experience and these children should be evaluated in experienced pediatric epilepsy centers providing the whole armamentarium of medical and surgical management of this disease.

45.2.8 Tumors and Cerebrovascular Disorders

Seizures are a common initial presenting symptom of pediatric brain tumors especially of the cerebral hemispheres. However, brain tumors are a rare cause of childhood epilepsy and account for seizures in only 0.2 to 0.3% of the cases. However, in vascular problems, seizures can occur either as a presenting symptom or as a complication. Best examples are caveromas with sourrounding epileptogenic hemosiderin rims and large middle cerebral artery (MCA) aneurysms provoking temporal lobe epilepsy.[1,2]

45.3 Presurgical Evaluation

Surgical outcome in pediatric epilepsy is significantly correlated with correct patient selection (Is the patient truely refractory to medical treatment?) and presurgical assessment. This includes thorough neurological examination (clinical history and physical examination) by pediatric neurologists, electrophysiological assessment by pediatric epileptologists, cognitive evaluation by neuropsychiatrists, and finally the collaborative decision about the candidate and appropriate surgical procedure together with pediatric neurosurgeons. The presurgical evaluation should clarify whether the seizures are focal or generalized, and if focal, whether the origin is temporal or extratemporal. Is there a lesion visible on MR images that could be linked to the seizures? Are there functional important areas involved or close by the possible area of resection?

If the results of this noninvasive phase remain inconclusive, more invasive examinations are warranted.

45.4 Neuroimaging

In search for focal lesions, MR is the imaging modility of choice. Routine epilepsy protocols with additional special sequences (fluid-attenuated inversion recovery [FLAIR], magnetization-prepared rapid acquisition gradient echo [MP-RAGE], inversion recovery, diffusion tensor imaging [DTI]) in thin cuts and 3D reconstruction to existing MR protocols are capable to detect even small lesions such as focal cortical dysplasia (FCD), hamartomas, polymicrogyria, hippocampal sclerosis, and glial tumors.[3,4] Special MR sequences may be required in the first 2 years of life because of immature myelination, and serial scans may be necessary to identify abnormalities during early postnatal brain development.[5]

Other options are ictal and interictal single-photon emission computed tomography (SPECT) and positron emission tomography (PET) investigations and these analyses can be very helpful in nonlesional seizure foci especially in extratemporal epilepsy to identify the area of further invasive investigations.[6,7,8,9,10,11,12,13] Via substraction of ictal and interictal SPECT signal and by coregistration with MR images (SISCOM), the exact anatomical localization of the ictal seizure-onset zone can be highlighted. To determine hemispheric dominance for language, functional MR has been established in some centers to estimate the possible benefits of surgery against the risk of postoperative language deficits. Intracarotid amobarbital test (Wada's test) have been abandonned even in adult epilepsy surgical centers because of the risk of stroke and the more invasive nature of the procedure.[14,15]

45.5 EEG Investigations

The mainstay of presurgical evaluation is still the analysis of EEG activity between events (interictal) or of specific activity during events (ictal) which provides evidence of focal electrical dysfunction. Interictal EEG alterations such as spikes and slow-wave complexes can be of localizing value. Serial EEG studies may be necessary to document consistency or progression of epileptic area especially in infants and young children. Video EEG recordings are of utmost importance to simultaneously analyse seizure semiology during an epileptogenic event. Patients are hospitalized for video EEG monitoring and the antiepileptic medication is reduced or even withdrawn to provoke seizures. Patients' behavior during a seizure (semiology) allows an experienced epileptologist to gain an idea about the seizure origin in parallel to the EEG findings. Invasive electrode recordings are being performed more selectively and are indicated primarily to localize the epileptogenic region when alternative methods are nonconclusive.

45.6 Surgical Options

Surgical methods applied in epilepsy treatment can be roughly divided into diagnostic and therapeutic procedures.

45.6.1 Diagnostic Surgical Procedures

In case of nonconclusive results with regard to the seizure-onset zone obtained from noninvasive evaluations, further invasive EEG monitoring investigations have to be considered. Subdural strip electrodes are used to distinguish between cerebral lobes and can be very helpful in frontal interhemispheric ictal onset zones.[16] In recent years, stereotactically placed depth electrodes are more and more used because they can be precisely placed and allow recordings even from deep-seated locations such as the insula and the white matter.[17,18] When the area of seizure onset is known and the zone has to be further evaluated, subdural grid electrodes with EEG recordings directly from the cortex come into play.[16,19] In this way, the epileptogenic zone and the area of seizure propagation can be clearly discerned. The main goals of epilepsy surgery are to precisely localize the epileptogenic region and to resect the focus as completely as possible without causing further neurological or cognitive deficits. The proximity to functionally important, for example, eloquent areas may increase the risk of surgery and the resection has to be tailored accordingly. Although functionally important areas may be approximated with the help of anatomical landmarks, individual variations and distortion of these landmarks by the local pathology have to be taken into account. Therefore, mapping for functional important areas such as speech or motor function is crucial during invasive EEG monitoring prior to surgcial resection. During the resective procedure, these functional areas will be reidentified by direct cortical stimulation.[20,21,22]

45.6.2 Therapeutic Surgical Procedures

When the presurgical planning is finalized, the microsurgical resection can be accomplished in a subpial fashion. Cortical gray and white matter are carefully removed by suction and/or cavitron thereby leaving the adjacent gyri untouched. The vasculature and especially the large draining veins remain intact. The amount of scar tissue formation is minimal. Different types of surgical resections can be discerned such as lesionectomy, temporal lobe resection with selective amygdalohippocampectomy, extratemporal resections, and hemisperotomy or hemispherectomy. Other disconnective procedures include corpus callosotomy and multiple subpial transsections.

Lesionectomy

Lesions that are clearly identified as the cause of seizures can be of diverse histology. Cavernomas should be removed whenever safely possible including the hemosiderin-stained surrounding brain tissue.[23,24,25] Areas of focal atrophy or cortical dysplasia should be widely resected and the extent of cortical and subcortical resection is best determined by invasive monitoring for the epileptogenic area of these lesions tend to be larger than the morphological changes on preoperative MR images.[26,27,28,29] A recent retrospective study of Rowland and coworkers summarizing 37 studies with 2014 pediatric patients with FCD found that partial seizures, a temporal location, positive findings on MR images, complete margins of resection, and histological FCD type II were significantly associated with a seizure-free outcome, whereas age at surgery and the possibility to localize the epileptogenic region on EEG did not affect seizure freedom.[30] Brain tumors present in about 16% with seizures and as shown in a large series by the group of Constantini partial seizures were found in 85% of the cases. The tumors in this series of 48 children were all supratentorial mainly temporal in location and almost all gliomas frequently of low grade. A recent study suggests that glutamate secretion from gliomas may induce seizures.[31] Approximately, 92% of children in their study were seizure free for at least 2 years and significant pedictors were gross total tumor resection, seizure duration of less than 1 year, and temporal location. The same is true for dysembryoplastic neuroepithelial tumors with a predominant temporal location and good seizure control rates.[32] However, DNETs tend to be associated with focal cortical dysplasia with its own epileptogenic potential. Complete tumor resection along with the epileptogenic zone of cortical dysplasia is therefore important and intraoperative electrocorticography can be of immense value in this context.[33] Tuberous sclerosis is another well-known etiological entity leading to epilepsy in children. A recent paper from the Hospital of Sick Children in Toronto summarizes the results of 20 studies with 181 patients and determined that there was a nonsignificant trend on multivariate analysis for improved seizure outcomes over the last 15 years following resective surgery. The most likely reasons are advanced imaging and localization modalities introduced over the last years which help to discern between tubers responsible for epileptic discharges and those who are silent.[34,35] Most children do have multiple tubers and the challenge in epilepsy surgery is to identify those from which seizure originates. The resection of this lesion may have favourable outcome with regard to seizure control and only the concerted results from MR sequences, nuclear medicine studies, and electrocorticography are able to precisely define the epileptogenic tuber.

Temporal Resections

Hippocampal sclerosis is the most common pathology in adults undergoing surgery for temporal lobe epilepsy. In contrast, the majority of children receiving temporal lobe resection are found to have focal cortical dysplasia or low-grade gliomas as the primary underlying pathology. Hippocampal sclerosis prevails in 13 to 40% in children suffering from medically intractable epilepsy which is in contrast to 73% in adults. Seizure freedom after surgery is comparable and ranges between 66 and 80%.[4,36] While the sensitivity of MR images for the detection of hippocampal sclerosis in adults is high, this remains uncertain in children. Several studies agreed that the most reliable MR criteria for correct diagnosis are increased signal on T2-weighted MR images and reduced hippocampal volume. The presence of a dual pathology (hippocampal sclerosis and FCD) has been estimated to range between 12 and 79%.[37,38,39]

Selective Amygdalohippocampectomy/ Mesial Temporal Resection

Temporal lobectomies for mesial temporal sclerosis have been abandonned because of the inherent risk of injury to the optic radiation with quadrantanopsia. Several surgical approaches to the mesial temporal structures have been described via the temporal pole, transventricular subtemporal, or transylvian. Important in preoperative assessment is age-adapted neuropsychological testing because

of the risk of verbal memory deficits after resection in the dominant hemisphere. The younger the child's age, the less like is any neuropsychological deficit and it is speculated that these patients have poor verbal memory at baseline. Children appear to recover more quickly and completely than adults. Verbal memory deterioration in adults after left temporal resection prevails even 1 year after surgery, while the initial deterioration in children is recovered within 1 year.[40] Others even report on long-term follow-up (>5 years) a significant increase in intelligence quotient (IQ), psychosocial outcome, and quality of life in surgically treated children compared to those with only medical treatment for temporal lobe epilepsy.[39,41]

More extensive temporal resections may be useful in young children with epileptic encephalopathy and diffuse or multifocal epileptiform discharges on EEG but predominance for the temporal lobe. Recent date provide encouraging results in this catastrophic cases of epileptic encephalopathy. Seizures show an early onset during the first 3 months of life and are accompanied by an enormous developmental delay.[42]

Extratemporal Resection

More challenging than temporal epilepsy is the localization of a seizure focus in the frontal, frontoparietal of occipital lobe. Surgical outcome in general is by far better when a single seizure focus can be discerned than in cases with a more widespread epileptogenic zone requiring multilobar resections. A meta-analysis performed by Ansari and coworkers of 15 case series and two case reports confirmed that seizure type (complex partial seizures appear to have better outcomes) and pathological findings (patients with cortical dysplasia do better than those with other pathologies) are factors significantly associated with postoperative seizure outcome. Older children seem to benefit more most likely due to the greater difficulty in localizing the epiletogenic region in very young children.[43]

Hemispherectomy

Patients with Rasmussen's encephalitis or Sturge–Weber syndrome are the typical candidates for this type of procedure. The propagation of epileptogenic discharges from the pathological hemisphere to the opposite hemisphere should be impaired. The continuous seizure activity is provoking unilateral motor seizures and causing hemiparesis.

Also, patients with hemimegalencephaly and large areas of infarction or trauma or cerebral dysgenesis may benefit from this procedure. Functional hemispherectomy is very effective in seizure control with a success rate of more than 80% and in behavioral performance as well as cognitive function.[44,45,46,47]

Disconnective Surgical Procedures

Corpus Callosotomy

It is an option to alleviate seizure activity in children with different types of seizure, mainly in drop attacks or those in whom a single focus could not be identified or more than one focus seem to be present. Initially, the anterior two-thirds of the corpus callosum are sectioned and only when seizures persist, the remaining connective fibers are sacrificed in a second procedure. Apraxia and difficulties in bimanual tasks may be present following complete callosotomy but well compensated by improved seizure control.[48,49]

Multiple Subpial Transections

Rarely applied and thought to be effective in seizures originating from functional important areas. The vertical columnar arrangement of the cortex remains intact thereby preserving function.

Stereotactic Ablation

Stereotactic ablation has been described as an option for hypothalamic hamartomas. Stereotactic brachytherapy with radioactive seeds is a well estabilshed method in the treatment of low-grade gliomas even in children thereby possibly controlling seizures.

Neuroaugmentative Surgery

Vagus Nerve Stimulation

The vagus nerve stimulation (VNS) device consists of pliable, spiral-shaped electrodes that wrap around the vagal nerve and a generator implanted subcutaneously above the pectoral muscle. Typically, the left side is used to prevent disturbance of the cardiac electric current system. The efficiacy of this treatment modality has been tested in two trials and a reduction in seizure frequencey as well as intensity after an interval of 3 to 6 months. Seizure reduction has been described to be around 50%, complete seizure freedom is rare. Hoarseness

and dyspnea during stimulation and voice alterations can occur and are transient.[50,51] Fortunately, VNS has also a positive effect on depression and mood which might not be as important in infants but in older children.

Deep Brain Stimulation

More recently, deep brain stimulation (DBS) to the anterior thalamic nuclei has been attempted in order to ameliorate seizure activity in otherwise refractory patients. The success rate of 54% in seizure reduction is in the range of VNS.[51]

Radiosurgery

Gamma Knife radiosurgery is an effective tool in the treatment of refractory gelastic seizures due to hypothalamic hamartoma. A recent report with robotic-arm stereotactic radiosurgery in a teenager is very promising with complete absence of seizures after 12 months' posttreatment with a dose of 30 Gy in five fractions.[52]

45.7 Summary

In conclusion, the ultimate goal of epilepsy surgery would be a seizure-free state without significant neurological impairment. Once a child failed to respond to three antiepileptic drugs, surgical evaluation and intervention has to be considered. Proper selection and investigation of children is of utmost importance. With recent advances in neuroimaging, functional analysis, and video EEG monitoring in precisely localizing the seizure focus, the overall surgical results can be improved.

References

[1] Lad SP, Shannon L, Byrne RW. Incidental aneurysms in temporal lobe epilepsy surgery: report of three cases and a review of the literature. Br J Neurosurg. 2012; 26(1):69–74

[2] Wang X, Tao Z, You C, Li Q, Liu Y. Extended resection of hemosiderin fringe is better for seizure outcome: a study in patients with cavernous malformation associated with refractory epilepsy. Neurol India. 2013; 61(3):288–292

[3] Daghistani R, Widjaja E. Role of MRI in patient selection for surgical treatment of intractable epilepsy in infancy. Brain Dev. 2013; 35(8):697–705

[4] Kasasbeh A, Hwang EC, Steger-May K, et al. Association of magnetic resonance imaging identification of mesial temporal sclerosis with pathological diagnosis and surgical outcomes in children following epilepsy surgery. J Neurosurg Pediatr. 2012; 9(5):552–561

[5] Cross JH, Jayakar P, Nordli D, et al. International League against Epilepsy, Subcommission for Paediatric Epilepsy Surgery, Commissions of Neurosurgery and Paediatrics.

Proposed criteria for referral and evaluation of children for epilepsy surgery: recommendations of the Subcommission for Pediatric Epilepsy Surgery. Epilepsia. 2006; 47(6):952–959

[6] Bien CG, Raabe AL, Schramm J, Becker A, Urbach H, Elger CE. Trends in presurgical evaluation and surgical treatment of epilepsy at one centre from 1988–2009. J Neurol Neurosurg Psychiatry. 2013; 84(1):54–61

[7] Bilgin O, Vollmar C, Peraud A, la Fougere C, Beleza P, Noachtar S. Ictal SPECT in Sturge-Weber syndrome. Epilepsy Res. 2008; 78(2–3):240–243

[8] Desai A, Bekelis K, Thadani VM, et al. Interictal PET and ictal subtraction SPECT: sensitivity in the detection of seizure foci in patients with medically intractable epilepsy. Epilepsia. 2013; 54(2):341–350

[9] Fellah S, Callot V, Viout P, et al. Epileptogenic brain lesions in children: the added-value of combined diffusion imaging and proton MR spectroscopy to the presurgical differential diagnosis. Childs Nerv Syst. 2012; 28(2):273–282

[10] Fujiwara H, Greiner HM, Hemasilpin N, et al. Ictal MEG onset source localization compared to intracranial EEG and outcome: improved epilepsy presurgical evaluation in pediatrics. Epilepsy Res. 2012; 99(3):214–224

[11] Hur YJ, Lee JS, Lee JD, Yun MJ, Kim HD. Quantitative analysis of simultaneous EEG features during PET studies for childhood partial epilepsy. Yonsei Med J. 2013; 54(3):572–577

[12] Stanescu L, Ishak GE, Khanna PC, Biyyam DR, Shaw DW, Parisi MT. FDG PET of the brain in pediatric patients: imaging spectrum with MR imaging correlation. Radiographics. 2013; 33:1279–1303

[13] Widjaja E, Shammas A, Vali R, et al. FDG-PET and magnetoencephalography in presurgical workup of children with localization-related nonlesional epilepsy. Epilepsia. 2013; 54(4):691–699

[14] Norrelgen F, Lilja A, Ingvar M, Gisselgård J, Fransson P. Language lateralization in children aged 10 to 11 years: a combined fMRI and dichotic listening study. PLoS One. 2012; 7(12):e51872

[15] Wray CD, Blakely TM, Poliachik SL, et al. Multimodality localization of the sensorimotor cortex in pediatric patients undergoing epilepsy surgery. J Neurosurg Pediatr. 2012; 10 (1):1–6

[16] Wellmer J, von der Groeben F, Klarmann U, et al. Risks and benefits of invasive epilepsy surgery workup with implanted subdural and depth electrodes. Epilepsia. 2012; 53(8):1322–1332

[17] Kassiri J, Pugh J, Carline S. Depth electrodes in pediatric epilepsy surgery. Can J Neurol Sci. 2013; 40(1):48–55

[18] Taussig D, Dorfmüller G, Fohlen M, et al. Invasive explorations in children younger than 3 years. Seizure. 2012; 21(8):631–638

[19] Kalamangalam GP, Pestana Knight EM, Visweswaran S, Gupta A. Noninvasive predictors of subdural grid seizure localization in children with nonlesional focal epilepsy. J Clin Neurophysiol. 2013; 30(1):45–50

[20] Constant I, Sabourdin N. The EEG signal: a window on the cortical brain activity. Paediatr Anaesth. 2012; 22(6):539–552

[21] Elshoff L, Groening K, Grouiller F, et al. The value of EEG-fMRI and EEG source analysis in the presurgical setup of children with refractory focal epilepsy. Epilepsia. 2012; 53(9):1597–1606

[22] Fong JS, Alexopoulos AV, Bingaman WE, Gonzalez-Martinez J, Prayson RA. Pathologic findings associated with invasive EEG monitoring for medically intractable epilepsy. Am J Clin Pathol. 2012; 138(4):506–510

[23] Hugelshofer M, Acciarri N, Sure U, et al. Effective surgical treatment of cerebral cavernous malformations: a multicenter study of 79 pediatric patients. J Neurosurg Pediatr. 2011; 8(5):522–525

[24] Rydenhag B, Flink R, Malmgren K. Surgical outcomes in patients with epileptogenic tumours and cavernomas in Sweden: good seizure control but late referrals. J Neurol Neurosurg Psychiatry. 2013; 84(1):49–53

[25] Samii M, Gerganov VM, Freund HJ. Restorative neurosurgery of the cortex: resections of pathologies of the central area can improve preexisting motor deficits. Neurosurg Rev. 2012; 35(2):277–286, discussion 286

[26] Aubert S, Wendling F, Regis J, et al. Local and remote epileptogenicity in focal cortical dysplasias and neurodevelopmental tumours. Brain. 2009; 132(pt 11): 3072–3086

[27] Gaitanis JN, Donahue J. Focal cortical dysplasia. Pediatr Neurol. 2013; 49(2):79–87

[28] Hauptman JS, Mathern GW. Surgical treatment of epilepsy associated with cortical dysplasia: 2012 update. Epilepsia. 2012; 53 suppl 4:98–104

[29] Régis J, Tamura M, Park MC, et al. Subclinical abnormal gyration pattern, a potential anatomic marker of epileptogenic zone in patients with magnetic resonance imaging-negative frontal lobe epilepsy. Neurosurgery. 2011; 69(1):80–93, discussion 93–94

[30] Rowland NC, Englot DJ, Cage TA, Sughrue ME, Barbaro NM, Chang EF. A meta-analysis of predictors of seizure freedom in the surgical management of focal cortical dysplasia. J Neurosurg. 2012; 116(5):1035–1041

[31] Buckingham SC, Campbell SL, Haas BR, et al. Glutamate release by primary brain tumors induces epileptic activity. Nat Med. 2011; 17(10):1269–1274

[32] Zhang JG, Hu WZ, Zhao RJ, Kong LF. Dysembryoplastic neuroepithelial tumor: a clinical, neuroradiological, and pathological study of 15 cases. J Child Neurol. 2014(11): 1441–1447

[33] Wray CD, McDaniel SS, Saneto RP, Novotny EJ, Jr, Ojemann JG. Is postresective intraoperative electrocorticography predictive of seizure outcomes in children? J Neurosurg Pediatr. 2012; 9(5):546–551

[34] Ibrahim GM, Fallah A, Carter Snead O, Rutka JT. Changing global trends in seizure outcomes following resective surgery for tuberous sclerosis in children with medically intractable epilepsy. Epilepsy Res Treat. 2012; 2012:135364

[35] Koh S, Jayakar P, Dunoyer C, et al. Epilepsy surgery in children with tuberous sclerosis complex: presurgical evaluation and outcome. Epilepsia. 2000; 41(9):1206–1213

[36] Vadera S, Kshettry VR, Klaas P, Bingaman W. Seizure-free and neuropsychological outcomes after temporal lobectomy with amygdalohippocampectomy in pediatric patients with hippocampal sclerosis. J Neurosurg Pediatr. 2012; 10(2):103–107

[37] Mittal S, Montes JL, Farmer JP, et al. Long-term outcome after surgical treatment of temporal lobe epilepsy in children. J Neurosurg. 2005; 103 suppl 5:401–412

[38] Sinclair DB, Wheatley M, Aronyk K, et al. Pathology and neuroimaging in pediatric temporal lobectomy for intractable epilepsy. Pediatr Neurosurg. 2001; 35(5):239–246

[39] Terra-Bustamante VC, Inuzuca LM, Fernandes RM, et al. Temporal lobe epilepsy surgery in children and adolescents: clinical characteristics and post-surgical outcome. Seizure. 2005; 14(4):274–281

[40] Lee YJ, Lee JS. Temporal lobe epilepsy surgery in children versus adults: from etiologies to outcomes. Korean J Pediatr. 2013; 56(7):275–281

[41] Aaberg KM, Eriksson AS, Ramm-Pettersen J, Nakken KO. Long-term outcome of resective epilepsy surgery in Norwegian children. Acta Paediatr. 2012; 101(12):e557–e560

[42] Kayyali HR, Abdelmoity A, Baeesa S. The role of epilepsy surgery in the treatment of childhood epileptic encephalopathy. Epilepsy Res Treat. 2013; 2013:983049

[43] Ansari SF, Maher CO, Tubbs RS, Terry CL, Cohen-Gadol AA. Surgery for extratemporal nonlesional epilepsy in children: a meta-analysis. Childs Nerv Syst. 2010; 26(7):945–951

[44] Moosa AN, Gupta A, Jehi L, et al. Longitudinal seizure outcome and prognostic predictors after hemispherectomy in 170 children. Neurology. 2013; 80(3):253–260

[45] Moosa AN, Jehi L, Marashly A, et al. Long-term functional outcomes and their predictors after hemispherectomy in 115 children. Epilepsia. 2013; 54(10):1771–1779

[46] Schramm J, Kuczaty S, Sassen R, Elger CE, von Lehe M. Pediatric functional hemispherectomy: outcome in 92 patients. Acta Neurochir (Wien). 2012; 154(11):2017–2028

[47] Villarejo-Ortega F, García-Fernández M, Fournier-Del Castillo C, et al. Seizure and developmental outcomes after hemispherectomy in children and adolescents with intractable epilepsy. Childs Nerv Syst. 2013; 29(3):475–488

[48] Bower RS, Wirrell E, Nwojo M, Wetjen NM, Marsh WR, Meyer FB. Seizure outcomes after corpus callosotomy for drop attacks. Neurosurgery. 2013;73(6):993 – 1000

[49] Iwasaki M, Uematsu M, Sato Y, et al. Complete remission of seizures after corpus callosotomy. J Neurosurg Pediatr. 2012; 10(1):7–13

[50] Hauptman JS, Mathern GW. Vagal nerve stimulation for pharmacoresistant epilepsy in children. Surg Neurol Int. 2012; 3 suppl 4:S269–S274

[51] Rolston JD, Englot DJ, Wang DD, Shih T, Chang EF. Comparison of seizure control outcomes and the safety of vagus nerve, thalamic deep brain, and responsive neurostimulation: evidence from randomized controlled trials. Neurosurg Focus. 2012; 32(3):E14

[52] Susheela SP, Revannasiddaiah S, Mallarajapatna GJ, Basavalingaiah A. Robotic-arm stereotactic radiosurgery as a definitive treatment for gelastic epilepsy associated with hypothalamic hamartoma. BMJ Case Rep. 2013; 2013:2013

46 Surgical Management of Childhood Epilepsy: Corpus Callosotomy and Vagal Nerve Stimulation

Oguz Cataltepe

46.1 Introduction

Resective surgical procedures in epilepsy frequently provide seizure-free outcome and they are accepted as best surgical option for patients with epilepsy. However, resective surgery may not provide satisfactory seizure control in many patients. More significantly, resective surgery may not be feasible or preferable because of the location, extent, or multifocality of the epileptogenic focus. Resective surgical procedures are even not considered as an option in some cases such as atonic or multifocal, nonlocalizable seizures. Palliative epilepsy surgery techniques play significant role in the management of these patients. Although, palliative surgical interventions may not provide seizure-free outcome, they may still help the patient to have a better seizure control and improved quality of life. Corpus callosotomy (CC) and vagal nerve stimulation (VNS) are two most commonly used palliative epilepsy surgery interventions and we will review these techniques here.

46.2 Corpus Callosotomy

Corpus callosum is the largest and most critical commissure in propagation and generalization of the epileptogenic discharges to the contralateral hemisphere. Bilateral synchronization of epileptiform discharges, which is critical for generalization of seizures, also occurs primarily via corpus callosum. These anatomophysiological characteristics of corpus callosum makes it a very attractive surgical target to prevent atonic and secondarily generalized seizures and it is one of the oldest epilepsy surgery procedures.

46.2.1 History

Corpus callosotomy is used in treatment of intractable epilepsy first time by Van Wagenen and Herren in 1940.[1] Then Bogen et al published their corpus callosotomy series in 1960s, and Luessenhop et al and Wilson et al reported their experiences in several articles in 1970s.[2,3,4,5] Wilson et al have many contributions to this technique including introducing operating microscope to this procedure.[4,5] Surgical technique that was used initially included division of not only corpus callosum but also hippocampal and anterior commissures. Then, Wilson modified this technique in mid-70s and started not to divide anterior commissure and fornix and to leave the ependymal lining intact to avoid related complications. Then, he further modified his technique by applying two-stage sectioning of the corpus callosum with a few months interval.[4,5] Gradually, two-thirds anterior callosotomy became a standard CC technique and complete callosotomy was performed only if seizure control with two-thirds anterior callosotomy is not satisfactory. Although the early series had high morbidity and mortality rates, CC gradually became a safe, effective, and well-established procedure with the introduction and refinement of modern microsurgical techniques.[6,7,8,9,10] However, the number of CC surgeries dramatically decreased during the following decades in parallel to increasing popularity of vagal nerve stimulator placement procedures.

46.2.2 Anatomy and Physiology

Corpus callosum is the largest commissure and principal anatomical and neurophysiological connection pathway between the two hemispheres and consists of 180 to 200 million axons. Although it mostly links homotopic areas together, it also connects heterotopic areas.[7,11,12] Corpus callosum is frequently divided into four sections: rostrum, genu, body, and splenium. Anterior half of callosum (rostrum, genu, and anterior half of the body) includes decussation fibers from premotor, motor, anterior insular, and anterior cingulate cortical areas. Anterior half of corpus callosum is essential for the generalization of tonic, tonic-clonic seizures, and atonic drop attacks. The posterior half of the callosum includes posterior half of callosal body and splenium. Its fibers connect parietal, occipital, posterior insular, primary auditory area, and caudal portions of parahippocampus.

46.2.3 Surgical Indications

Corpus callosotomy is considered as a treatment option for patients with medically intractable generalized (primary or secondary) seizures that may frequently cause serious injuries secondary to drop attacks. Lennox–Gastaut is the most responsive epilepsy syndrome to callosotomy. The patients with atonic seizures, infantile spasms, unclear-onset epileptogenic abnormality with secondary widespread generalization, diffuse cortical malformations with generalized seizures might also be good candidates for CC.[9,13,14,15,16] CC may also have a diagnostic utility to define the seizure focus in patients with rapid generalization of epileptogenic activity.[17] In these patients, CC may be helpful to determine the focus of ictal onset by isolating the hemispheres and providing an opportunity for further diagnostic work-up to find a focus, which may be amenable for resective surgery.

46.2.4 Preoperative Assessment

Preoperative assessment of these patients is similar to other epilepsy surgery patients. First goal during the assessment of the patient is ruling out any lateralizable and localizable epileptogenic abnormality with a complete investigative work-up including brain magnetic resonance imaging (MRI), MR venography, video/electroencephalography (EEG) monitoring, and neuropsychological assessment. Video/EEG monitoring would provide a critical information regarding seizure semiology and electrophysiological characteristics of epileptogenic abnormalities. MRI is helpful to assess the structural abnormalities and MR venogram provides significant information for surgical planning of CC by showing location and distribution of parasagittal veins. Neuropsychological assessment is especially significant in these cases because presence of mixed cerebral dominance in complete CC cases may cause significant postoperative language deficits.

46.2.5 Surgical Technique

CC procedure has been generally performed as anterior two-thirds CC. Complete callosotomy is performed as a second step only if the patient does not benefit from the initial procedure.

The patient is placed in supine position and the head is secured with a pin head holder. Right-sided approach is used unless the patient has a pathology on the left hemisphere or has a right hemispheric dominance. The neck is flexed 20 degrees and is slightly tilted to right to use gravity for retraction during the procedure. A 6-cm length, lazy-S incision is marked 2 cm anterior and parallel to the coronal sutures. The incision crosses the midline to the left side about 2 cm. Two burr holes, 2 cm anterior and 3 cm posterior to coronal suture, are placed over the sagittal sinus and one burr hole is placed over the coronal suture about 4 cm lateral to midline. A triangular-shaped craniotomy flap is removed. Right-sided edge of the sagittal sinus is exposed and covered with Surgifoam and cottonoids. Dura is tented through the drill holes on surrounding bone edges. Intravenous mannitol can be administered at this point if needed. We do not use lumbar drain in these cases. Then the dura is opened U-shape and reflected over the sagittal sinus. MR venogram is reviewed carefully before surgery to determine the location of large bridging veins and/or dural venous lacuna. If there are large draining veins or venous lacuna, dural opening is made accordingly by leaving dural patches on them to work around these structures. Arachnoid granulations are gently dissected from the dura and sagittal sinus wall, then dural flap is further retracted, and interhemispheric fissure as well as falx are exposed. Cottonoid pledgets are placed over the exposed cortex. At this stage, surgical microscope is brought into the field and the remaining part of the surgery is continued under the microscope. If there are major bridging veins entering to the sagittal sinus, their arachnoid sleeves can be dissected as far lateral as possible to minimize their stretch during the retraction and surgical procedure can be carried out around these veins using separate surgical corridors anterior and posterior to them. However, if the bridging veins are well anterior to coronal suture and not draining from eloquent cortex, then they can be sacrificed if needed. Then the cortex is gently retracted away from the falx using a single retractor blade on the mesial frontal cortex. Arachnoid adhesions extending from cortex to sagittal sinus or falx can be easily dissected with bipolar and microscissors while sliding the retractor blade down. The inferior edge of the falx can also be seen at this stage. Then the retractor blade is gently slided further downward along a cottonoid until cingulate gyrus is seen. At this stage, arachnoid membrane over the mesial frontal cortex in interhemispheric fissure may be opened at a few separate points using a fine bipolar forceps and cerebrospinal fluid (CSF) is drained by suctioning it through the cotton balls. This maneuver provides a much relaxed exposure and the retractor can be removed at this stage and only used as needed to avoid unnecessary pressure over the cortex. Then dissection is further advanced downward to fully expose the cingulate gyri. Separation of cingulate gyri from each other can be difficult in some cases because of arachnoid adhesions and interdigitation of gyri. After finding a relatively free part, dissection of the cingulate gyri can be performed easily using bipolar forceps and Penfield #4 dissector. At this point, underlying glistening white corpus callosum is encountered with a very distinctive appearance and consistency. Next, the cortical ribbon is repositioned and further CSF drainage is obtained through supracallosal cistern. Then, fluffy small cotton balls are placed downward just over corpus callosum at both ends of the exposed area to keep cingulate gyri separated and to expose corpus callosum better. At this stage, pericallosal arteries are also seen. They frequently travel very close to each other with some tiny bridging vessels and sometimes they may even override. Then pericallosal arteries are mobilized and separated to have a wider exposure of the corpus callosum. This will provide a satisfactory exposure for performing planned CC. Corpus callosum division should be done between pericallosal arteries by staying strictly on the midline. Dividing corpus callosum lateral to pericallosal artery may cause injury to perforating vascular structures in the pericallosal sulcus and cause ischemic damage and edema. Corpus callosum is divided longitudinally using microdissectors and bipolar forceps. When the division of corpus callosum is deepened, a grayish color of the ependymal lining can be easily appreciated. Opening the ependyma and entering into ventricle should be avoided if possible to decrease the risk of chemical meningitis. CC is continued anteriorly around the genu until the visualization of anterior commissure between the fornices. Anterior commissure should be left intact. Then dissection continues posteriorly on the rostrum and anterior body of the corpus callosum. Posterior end of the callosotomy is determined based on surgical planning. If anterior two-thirds is aimed, then the length can be measured preoperatively using midsagittal MRI images. The measurement is translated onto the surgical field using a ruler or by using the thickness of the ribbon as measuring tool. Another practical and more reliable tool to use for this purpose is neuronavigator. After completing callosotomy as planned, meticulous hemostasis is obtained and the layers are closed appropriately.

If the goal is performing posterior callosotomy or completing the anterior two-thirds craniotomy to a complete callosotomy, a second incision, parallel to the first one, is placed at vertex level. The incision crosses the midline 2 cm to the left and the surgical field is exposed with self-retaining retractors. Targeted exposed area in midline extends from 4 cm anterior to lambda to just over or 1 cm behind the lambda posteriorly. The burr holes in midline are placed on sagittal sinus and the lateral burr hole is placed 4 cm lateral to midline on the right to remove a free bone flap. Using the same surgical technique described above, the dura is opened and the dissection is continued toward the posterior body of the callosum and splenium by following falx. It is very critical to stay on midline during this part of the procedure to avoid any injury to fornices. Neuronavigator would be very helpful in these cases. The division of the corpus callosum ends with the exposure of the arachnoid membranes covering the vein of Galen.

46.2.6 Surgical Complications and Side Effects

Complication rates for CC procedure have been reported 3 to 10% in different series. Most common complications are cerebral edema, infarction, meningitis (septic/aseptic), hydrocephalus, ischemia, and subdural/epidural hematoma originating from parasagittal veins.[8,9,18,19] Another well-know, although rare, issue is disconnection-related syndromes. This is closely related to the extent of callosotomy. Anterior two-thirds callosotomy may cause decreased spontaneity of speech that generally persists between a few days or weeks. In some cases, left-sided neglect, apraxia, various degrees of left leg paresis, hemiparesis, left-sided or bilateral forced grasp reflexes, bilateral extensor plantar responses, and urgency incontinence may be also seen.[8,9,18] Symptoms typically improve over days to weeks. Surgical retraction-related brain edema on nondominant parasagittal cortex, supplementary motor area, or premotor cortex might be responsible from these findings.

On the other hand, posterior callosotomy causes interhemispheric somatosensory, auditory, and visual disconnection syndromes, which are frequently temporary. However, permanent interhemispheric sensory disconnection can also develop and especially sectioning of splenium can result in visual and sensory disconnection syndromes with inability to describe the objects presented visually or tactilely on the nondominant side.[6,7,13,18]

Complete corpus callosotomy–related side effects include both anterior and posterior callosotomy–related findings which are described above. It may also infrequently cause interhemispheric antagonism. Split-brain syndrome can develop after complete callosotomy which involves language impairment, hemisphere competition, and disordered attention-memory sequencing. These findings generally improve with time.[7]

46.2.7 Outcome

One of the largest reviews on corpus callosotomy included 563 patients from multiple centers.[20] This study reported that 60.9% of the patients had worthwhile improvement with rare seizures, 7.6% of the patients had seizure-free outcome, and 31.4% had no improvement. Some other large series also provided similar results.[18,21]

The outcome of the corpus callosotomy has also been reviewed based on the extent of callosotomy.[8,10,17,22,23] Spencer et al reported better outcome with complete corpus callosotomy than partial callosotomy (80 vs. 50% satisfactory improvement).[21] Roberts and Siegel reported these rates as 81 and 38% in their series.[8] Some other authors also reported better outcome with complete corpus callosotomy in comparison to partial corpus callosotomy.[10,19,23,24,25,26,27,28] On the other hand, Jea et al reported that children in both anterior two-thirds and complete callosotomy groups achieved comparable improved seizure control, 80 and 87.5%, respectively.[16] Again, Fuiks et al did not find any significant difference between the two approaches.[22] Tanriverdi et al reported a large series that includes 95 patients and stated that complete callosotomy was not necessary at least initially and it should be reserved as a second stage in those cases in which anterior two-thirds resection fails.[29]

Outcome assessments based on seizure type were reported in several series. Roberts and Siegel published a detailed outcome analysis based on the seizure types.[8] They reported that atonic seizures responded best to corpus callosotomy with 72% significant improvement rate, 21% of them being seizure free. These authors observed 34% seizure freedom and 24% significant improvement (> 50% reduction in seizure frequency) in patients with generalized major motor seizures and 42% seizure freedom and 20% significant improvements in patients with complex partial seizures. The worst outcome was seen in the focal motor seizure group. According to Pinard et al, the best outcomes were associated with drop attacks with dramatical reduction in frequency in 90% of the children.[10] In another series, Kawai et al reported complete resolution of drop attacks in 80% of their patients.[14] In Tanriverdi et al series, the best response was achieved in generalized tonic–clonic seizures (77.3%), followed by drop attacks (77.2%), and generalized tonic seizures and simple partial seizures (71.4%).[29]

Overall, best response to corpus callosotomy is seen in patients with generalized tonic–clonic seizures with drop attacks, and patients with complex partial seizures with or without secondary generalization. Atypical absence seizures constitute the worst outcome group.[15,29]

46.3 Vagal Nerve Stimulation

VNS therapy has been used in the treatment of refractory epilepsy since 1988. Its effectivity and safety profile extensively tested since then and its efficiency is consistently demonstrated in many trials and series. Currently, VNS is one of the most commonly used adjunctive treatment modalities in epilepsy.

46.3.1 History

First study on the effect of VNS on cerebral activity was performed by Bailey and Bremer in 1938 in an animal model.[30] They demonstrated VNS-related changes in cortical EEG patterns using various animal models. Then in 1952, Zanchetti used a chemically induced seizure model in cats to demonstrate reduction in interictal epileptic activities by intermittent stimulation of vagal nerve.[31] Several decades later, Zabara conducted a series of animal studies to assess the effect of VNS on seizure control and published his findings in 1985.[32] Then, Zabara and Reese developed first vagal nerve stimulator model and then, first VNS implantation procedure in a patient was performed by Bell and Penry in 1988.[33,34] This was followed by a series of pilot studies with VNS Therapy System (Cyberonics Inc., Houston, Texas). VNS Study Group conducted five multicenter VNS clinical trials, the final one being in 1996, and published their results in a series of articles.[33,35,36,37] European community approved VNS therapy for epilepsy in 1994 and Food and Drug Administration (FDA) approved it in 1997.[33] Finally, American Academy of Neurology's Therapeutics and Technology Assessment Subcommittee reported that "sufficient evidence exists to rank VNS for epilepsy as effective and safe, based on a preponderance of Class I evidence."[38,39]

46.3.2 Vagus Nerve Anatomy

Vagus nerve is a mixed cranial nerve with both afferent and efferent fibers. Afferent fibers constitute approximately 80% of the vagus nerve which is composed of myelinated A, B, and nonmyelinated C fibers. Vagus nerve receives somatic sensory, visceral sensory, and special sensory afferent fibers and reaches to many parts of the brain with extensive projection fibers. Nucleus tractus solitarius (NTS) is the main recipient of the majority of afferent sensory fibers. Diffuse pathways originating from NTS are connected to dorsal raphe, locus coeruleus, the nucleus ambiguous, and reaches with extensive projection fibers to wide areas in the brain including cerebellum, hypothalamus, thalamus, and limbic structures. This anatomical and physiological characteristic of vagus nerve makes it a perfect pathway for neuromodulation.[40,41]

46.3.3 Mechanism of Action

Precise mechanism of seizure suppression of VNS therapy is still not completely understood. It was demonstrated that vagal nerve projections extend noradrenergic and serotonergic neuromodulatory systems of the brain via NTS through locus coeruleus and raphe nuclei. Some studies using animal models documented that activation of noradrenergic and serotonergic neurons has antiepileptic effects. It has also been demonstrated that VNS stimulation increases neuronal c-fos protein expression, increases regional blood flow in some areas such as thalamus, putamen, and cerebellum and again causes local or regional increase in GABA levels and decrease in glutamate aspartate levels.[40,41,42,43,44,45] Therefore, it is possible that action of VNS might be related to noradrenergic and serotonergic neuromodulatory systems, modulation of excitatory and inhibitory neurotransmitters, and also possibly by modified cerebral electrical activity through thalamocortical pathways.

46.3.4 Safety and Effectiveness

Series of large multicenter studies are conducted and many series are published to assess the safety and effectiveness of VNS since the first pilot study in 1998.[45,46,47,48,49,50,51,52,53] VNS Study Group conducted three open-label and two double-blind randomized controlled trials and results were published separately and also as a meta-analysis of five studies.[35,36,37,38,39] It was reported that although only 1 to 2% of patients became seizure free, many patients had significant long-term benefit from VNS with an average 50% seizure reduction in 43% of patients at 3 years after VNS placement. Although, there is no prospective, randomized controlled trial in pediatric age group, many pediatric series also consistently demonstrated sustained, long-term improvement in seizure control and quality of life after VNS placement.[46,50,51,52,53]

46.3.5 VNS Therapy System Components

The VNS Therapy System (Cyberonics Inc., Houston, Texas) composed of an implantable, programmable pulse generator and a bipolar lead. Nonimplantable components of the system are a programming wand and a handheld computer with software. The pulse generator delivers a biphasic current to the vagal nerve through the bipolar lead with cycles between on and off periods. Current generators are model 102/102 R 105 and 106 (25 g, 6.9-mm thickness) and smaller one, model 103 (16 g, 6.9-mm thickness) (▶ Fig. 46.1). There are two lead sizes (2- and 3-mm helix inner diameters). VNS lead has three helical (two electrodes and one anchor tether), which are wrapped around the vagal nerve and an extension cable ending with a connector pin for insertion into generator[47] (▶ Fig. 46.2 and ▶ Fig. 46.3).

46.3.6 Indications

VNS is used as an adjunctive therapy in patients with medically refractory epilepsy who are not candidates for resective epilepsy surgery or who

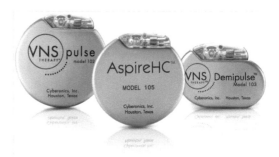

Fig. 46.1 Various VNS pulse generators: the models 102,103, and 105. (Reproduced with permission from Cyberonics.)

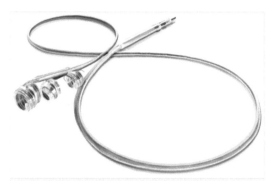

Fig. 46.2 VNS lead with helical electrodes. (Reproduced with permission from Cyberonics.)

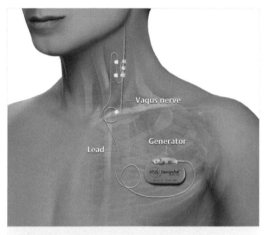

Fig. 46.3 Configuration of implanted VNS system. (Reproduced with permission from Cyberonics.)

have not responded to previous resective surgical interventions satisfactorily. Its effectiveness is demonstrated in generalized epilepsy, Lenox–Gastaut syndrome, and partial-onset seizures.[38,45, 46,47,48,49,50,53]

46.3.7 Preoperative Assessment

The patients have standard epilepsy surgery work-up. It needs to be demonstrated that patients' seizures are medically refractory and no resectable epileptogenic focus is present. History of cardiac dysfunction, apnea, and swallowing difficulties should also be questioned because of the possibility of worsening on these problems with VNS placement.

46.3.8 Surgery

VNS placement is typically performed under general anesthesia. Left vagal nerve is used for VNS placement because right vagal nerve innervates sinoatrial node and stimulation of left vagal nerve is less likely cause any cardiac problem.

The patient is placed in supine position with a shoulder role under the neck to give some extension. Head stays in neutral position or slightly turns to right. Left-sided neck and chest are prepped and draped as usual sterile manner. Intravenous antibiotic is given before skin incision. Surgery is performed under optic magnification. Two skin incisions on the left side are marked: one over the neck and the other is on chest. Neck incision is placed at midpoint of a line between mastoid tip and medial edge of the clavicula. A transverse, 2- to 3-cm length incision, preferably on a skin fold, is marked by centering the medial border of sternocleidomastoid muscle (SCM). Chest incision

is placed on anterior axillary line and the length is determined based on the generator size. While a small, 2 cm, incision might be sufficient for model 103 generators, a larger incision will be needed for models 101, 102/102 R. Neck incision is fashioned first. After skin incision on neck, platysma is sharply opened and undermined superiorly and inferiorly. Then cervical fascia is opened along the medial border of sternocleidomastoid muscle. Dissection continues along the medial border of SCM toward the neurovascular bundle. Carotid pulse is palpated to guide the dissection. After reaching the carotid sheath, it is opened sharply parallel to vascular structures. Internal jugular vein and carotid artery are easily exposed and gently separated by dissecting bluntly and holding separated with handheld retractors. Vagus nerve is generally located between these vessels posteriorly and frequently closer to jugular vein, although variations on the location of vagus nerve is not uncommon. Then about 3-cm length segment of vagus nerve is dissected proximally and distally and a vessel loop is passed underneath. Then chest incision is fashioned to create an appropriate size subcutaneous pocket for generator. This pocket is prepared in subclavicular area at left upper chest by exposing pectoralis fascia. Then a tunneler was inserted from chest incision and exited from neck incision. Lead cable is placed subcutaneously through the tunneler. Then helical electrodes and anchor tether are wrapped around vagal nerve one by one. First anchoring electrode, then positive electrode, and lastly negative electrode is placed. Anchor helix should be located farthest away from head and other two electrodes should be closer to head. All three helical electrodes should be coiled around vagal nerve segment below where the superior and inferior cardiac branches separate from the vagus nerve. All electrodes have attached sutures at the end and all manipulations during electrode placement should be done by holding these sutures, but not electrodes itself, with fine forceps. It is also very significant not to stretch or to devascularize vagus nerve or its branches during coiling the electrodes. Vagus nerve also should be kept moist throughout the procedure. After wrapping all three coils around the vagus nerve, it should be verified that lead cables exiting from coils are at the same direction and parallel to each other as well as to vagus nerve. After wrapping all three coils around the vagus nerve, coiled nerve is placed back to its original anatomical location without any stretch. Then a strain relief loop was created at the distal end by turning the cable upward. The lead is secured to deep fascia with a tie-down and nonabsorbable suture. Then another strain relief loop is created above the SCM and again it is secured to fascia with another tie-down. Then lead connector pin is inserted into pulse generator and connection is locked down by tightening the set screw with hex screwdriver. First intraoperative diagnostic testing of the system is performed at this stage to ensure the system integrity. Then pulse generator is inserted into subcutaneous pocket and extra lead is coiled and placed to the side of the generator. The generator is secured to pectoralis fascia with a silk suture. Surgical sites are irrigated with antibiotic-containing saline. Then all layers, platysma, subcutaneous tissue, and skin incision are closed with absorbable sutures. Second intraoperative diagnostic testing is again performed after skin closure using programming wand and handheld computer to confirm that the lead impedance is correct and the generator functions normally.

46.3.9 Surgical Complications and Side Effects

VNS procedure has relatively low rate of complications. Complications include infection, hoarseness of voice, temporary vocal cord paralysis, and, although much rare, nerve damage, vascular injury, bradycardia, asystole. Side effects typically occur during stimulation and improves over time. Most common side effects are voice alteration/hoarseness, throat paresthesia, cough, shortness of breath, and less frequently, drooling, and sleep apnea. Side effects can be frequently eliminated with some changes in stimulation parameters such as reducing the pulse width or signal frequency even without changes in output current.[36,37,38,45,46,50,51,52,53,54]

46.3.10 Postoperative Care

VNS system is generally activated 2 weeks after implantation to give some time to recover. Initial setting is typically 0.25-mA output current, 20- to 30-Hz frequency, 250 to 500 microseconds pulse width, on for 30 seconds, off for 5 minutes. The stimulation setting is readjusted by epileptologist over the weeks based on the patient's response and degree of side effects. The goal is obtaining maximum seizure control with minimal side effect.

Long-term follow-up is performed in epilepsy clinic with periodic diagnostic checks to determine the status of generator. Approximate battery life of the pulse generator is 5 to 6 years, depending on set stimulation parameters as well as extent of magnet use. It is always preferable to replace the generator before it is depleted.

46.3.11 Precautions

Patients with VNS should not receive shortwave diathermy or microwave diathermy. Again, therapeutic radiation therapy, external defibrillation, extracorporeal shockwave lithotripsy, or electrosurgery may damage the pulse generator. MRI can be performed with certain conditions. It should not be performed with MRI body coil in transmitter mode. 1.5 Tesla brain MRI with transmit-and-receive type head coils is considered as a safe procedure. The patient's VNS generator output current should be set to 0 mA before MRI and it should be tested and reprogrammed to original setting after MRI. Diagnostic ultrasound is a safe procedure for patients with VNS.[47]

46.3.12 Outcome

All published outcome studies regarding VNS in pediatric age group shows satisfactory benefit on seizure control.[36,37,38,45,46,50,51,52,53,55] Several large series reported about 50% responder rate with, again, about 50% decrease in overall seizure frequency. Elliott et al reported 56% seizure reduction and 64% responder rate in a series of 436 patients.[56] These rates were 51 and 59% (n:138

patients) in De Herdt, 51 and 59% (n: 269 patients) in Labar, 44% and 43% (n:440 patients) in Morris, 58% and 57% (n: 125 patients) in Helmers et al series.[37,57,58,59] It has been also consistently demonstrated in all these studies that response to VNS therapy improves with tolerance to side effects over time and is also sustains long term.

46.3.13 Failure and Removal

When necessary, both generator and lead can be removed. While generator removal is a simple procedure, removal of the lead is a challenging procedure with certain risks because of scarring of coil electrodes to vagus nerve and even to adjacent vascular structures. If removal of coil electrodes is not feasible, the lead might be removed by cutting the lead to leave only coils in place. In that case, no more than 4 cm of the lead wire should be left remaining.

46.4 Conclusions

Both corpus callosotomy and VNS therapy are effective palliative treatment options for patients with medically refractory epilepsy. Callosotomy is associated with greater efficacy in patients with drop attacks and Lennox–Gastaut syndrome, but it has higher risk for complications than VNS. Safety and effectiveness of VNS therapy have been confirmed with many studies including several randomized controlled trials and it has been used widely both in adult and pediatric patients. VNS became most commonly used palliative surgical procedure today. Although VNS has comparable results in most of the cases, corpus callosotomy is still a viable option in the patients with drop attacks and Lennox–Gastaut syndrome and also in patients who did not respond to vagal nerve stimulator. In general, VNS is considered as the initial approach in vast majority of cases because of better adverse event profile than corpus callosotomy which is still the more efficient treatment option for drop attacks and Lennox–Gastaut syndrome.[24,25,26,27]

46.5 Common Clinical Questions

1. What is the most common corpus callosotomy technique and which parts of the corpus callosum are divided?

2. Describe the most common complications of corpus callosotomy.
3. Which patient group responds better to corpus callosotomy?
4. What is the mechanism of action of VNS therapy?
5. Describe the most common complications and side effects of VNS therapy.

46.6 Answers to Common Clinical Questions

1. Partial or anterior two-thirds corpus callosotomy is the most common callosotomy technique today. Genu, rostrum, and anterior half of callosal body is divided and posterior end of the callosal body with splenium is spared in this technique.
2. Cerebral edema, meningitis (septic/aseptic), hydrocephalus, ischemia/infarction, subdural/epidural hematoma, and disconnection syndromes are most commonly seen complications of corpus callosotomy procedures.
3. Patients with generalized tonic–clonic seizures with drop attacks and Lennox–Gastaut syndrome respond better to corpus callosotomy.
4. We do not know the precise mechanism of action of VNS therapy. However, mechanism of action of VNS most likely related to noradrenergic and serotonergic neuromodulatory systems, modulation of excitatory and inhibitory neurotransmitters, and also possibly related to modification of cerebral electrical activity through thalamocortical pathways.
5. Voice alteration/hoarseness, throat paresthesia, cough, shortness of breath, and less frequently, drooling, and sleep apnea.

References

[1] Van Wagenen WP, Herren RY. Surgical division of the commissural pathways in the corpus callosum: relation to spread of an epileptic attack. Arch Neurol Psychiatry. 1940; 44:740–759

[2] Bogen JE, Sperry RW, Vogel PJ. Commissural section and propagation of seizures. In: Jasper HH, Ward AA, Pope A, eds. Basic Mechanism of the Epilepsies. Boston, MA: Little Brown and Company; 1969:439–440

[3] Luessenhop AJ, Dela Cruz TC, Fenichel GM. Surgical disconnection of the cerebral hemispheres for intractable seizures. Results in infancy and childhood. JAMA. 1970; 213 (10):1630–1636

[4] Wilson DH, Reeves A, Gazzaniga M. Division of the corpus callosum for uncontrollable epilepsy. Neurology. 1978; 28 (7):649–653

[5] Wilson DH, Reeves AG, Gazzaniga MS. "Central" commissurotomy for intractable generalized epilepsy: series two. Neurology. 1982; 32(7):687–697

[6] Spencer SS, Gates JR, Reeves AR, Spencer DD, Maxwell RE, Roberts D. Corpus callosum section. In: Engel J Jr, ed. Surgical Treatment of Epilepsies, New York, NY: Raven press; 1987:425–444

[7] Zentner J. Surgical aspects of corpus callosum section. In: Tuxhorn I, Holthausen H, Boenigk H, eds. Pediatric Epilepsy Syndromes and Their Surgical Treatment. London, UK: John Libbey; 1997;830–849

[8] Roberts D, Siegel A. Section of corpus callosum for epilepsy. In: Schmideck HH, Sweet WH, eds. Operative Neurosurgical Techniques. 4th ed. Philadelphia, PA: W. Saunders; 2000:1490–1498

[9] Menezes MS. Indications for corpus callosum section. In: Miller JW, Silbergerd DL, eds. Epilepsy Surgery: Principles and Controversies. London, UK: Taylor & Francis; 2006:556–562

[10] Pinard JM, Delalande O, Chiron C, et al. Callosotomy for epilepsy after West syndrome. Epilepsia. 1999; 40(12):1727–1734

[11] Tomasch J. Size, distribution, and number of fibres in the human corpus callosum. Anat Rec. 1954; 119(1):119–135

[12] Gazzaniga M, Ivry RB, Mangun GR. Cerebral lateralization and specialization. In: Cognitive Neuroscience: The Biology of the Mind. 2nd ed. New York, NY: WW Norton; 2002:405–410

[13] Sass KJ, Novelly RA, Spencer DD, Spencer SS. Postcallosotomy language impairments in patients with crossed cerebral dominance. J Neurosurg. 1990; 72(1):85–90

[14] Kawai K, Shimizu H, Yagishita A, Maehara T, Tamagawa K. Clinical outcomes after corpus callosotomy in patients with bihemispheric malformations of cortical development. J Neurosurg. 2004; 101(1) Suppl:7–15

[15] Bower RS, Wirrell E, Nwojo M, Wetjen NM, Marsh WR, Meyer FB. Seizure outcomes after corpus callosotomy for drop attacks. Neurosurgery. 2013; 73(6):993–1000

[16] Jea A, Vachhrajani S, Johnson KK, Rutka JT. Corpus callosotomy in children with intractable epilepsy using frameless stereotactic neuronavigation: 12-year experience at the Hospital for Sick Children in Toronto. Neurosurg Focus. 2008; 25(3):E7

[17] Clarke DF, Wheless JW, Chacon MM, et al. Corpus callosotomy: a palliative therapeutic technique may help identify resectable epileptogenic foci. Seizure. 2007; 16(6):545–553

[18] Wong TT, Kwan SY, Chang KP, et al. Corpus callosotomy in children. Childs Nerv Syst. 2006; 22(8):999–1011

[19] Maehara T, Shimizu H. Surgical outcome of corpus callosotomy in patients with drop attacks. Epilepsia. 2001; 42(1):67–71

[20] Engel J, Van Ness PJ, Rasmussen TB, Ojemann LM. Outcome with respect to epileptic seizures. In: Engel J, ed. Surgical treatment of the epilepsies. 2nd ed. New York, NY: Raven Press; 1993:609–621

[21] Spencer SS, Spencer DD, Sass K, Westerveld M, Katz A, Mattson R. Anterior, total, and two-stage corpus callosum section: differential and incremental seizure responses. Epilepsia. 1993; 34(3):561–567

[22] Fuiks KS, Wyler AR, Hermann BP, Somes G. Seizure outcome from anterior and complete corpus callosotomy. J Neurosurg. 1991; 74(4):573–578

[23] Rahimi SY, Park YD, Witcher MR, Lee KH, Marrufo M, Lee MR. Corpus callosotomy for treatment of pediatric epilepsy in the modern era. Pediatr Neurosurg. 2007; 43(3):202–208

[24] Nei M, O'Connor M, Liporace J, Sperling MR. Refractory generalized seizures: response to corpus callosotomy and vagal nerve stimulation. Epilepsia. 2006; 47(1):115–122

[25] You SJ, Kang HC, Ko TS, et al. Comparison of corpus callosotomy and vagus nerve stimulation in children with Lennox-Gastaut syndrome. Brain Dev. 2008; 30(3):195–199

[26] Lancman G, Virk M, Shao H, et al. Vagus nerve stimulation vs. corpus callosotomy in the treatment of Lennox-Gastaut syndrome: a meta-analysis. Seizure. 2013; 22(1):3–8

[27] Rosenfeld WE, Roberts DW. Tonic and atonic seizures: what's next–VNS or callosotomy? Epilepsia. 2009; 50 Suppl 8:25–30

[28] Jalilian L, Limbrick DD, Steger-May K, Johnston J, Powers AK, Smyth MD. Complete versus anterior two-thirds corpus callosotomy in children: analysis of outcome. J Neurosurg Pediatr. 2010; 6(3):257–266

[29] Tanriverdi T, Olivier A, Poulin N, Andermann F, Dubeau F. Long-term seizure outcome after corpus callosotomy: a retrospective analysis of 95 patients. J Neurosurg. 2009; 110 (2):332–342

[30] Bailey P, Bremmer FA. A sensory cortical representation of vagus nerve with a note on the low pressure in a surface electrogram. J Neurophysiol. 1938; 1:404–412

[31] Zanchetti A, Wang SC, Moruzzi G. The effect of vagal afferent stimulation on the EEG pattern of the cat. Electroencephalogr Clin Neurophysiol. 1952; 4(3):357–361

[32] Zabara J. Time course of seizure control to brief repetitive stimuli. Epilepsia. 1985; 26:518

[33] Lulic D, Ahmadian A, Baaj AA, Benbadis SR, Vale FL. Vagus nerve stimulation. Neurosurg Focus. 2009; 27(3):E5

[34] Penry JK, Dean JC. Prevention of intractable partial seizures by intermittent vagal stimulation in humans: preliminary results. Epilepsia. 1990; 31 Suppl 2:S40–S43

[35] Ben-Menachem E, Mann-Espaillat R, Ristanovic R, et al. VNS for treatment of partial seizures: 1. A controlled study of effect on seizures. First International Vagus Nerve Stimulation Study Group. Epilepsia. 1994; 35:616–626

[36] Handforth A, DeGiorgio CM, Schachter SC, et al. VNS therapy for partial-onset seizures: a randomized active control trial. Neurology. 1998; 51:48–55

[37] Morris GL, Mueller WM. Long-term treatment with VNS in patients with refractory epilepsy. VNS Study Group E01–E05. Neurology. 1999; 53:1731–1735

[38] Schachter SC. Vagus nerve stimulation therapy summary: five years after FDA approval. Neurology. 2002; 59(6) Suppl 4:S15–S20

[39] Fisher RS, Handforth A. Reassessment: VNS for epilepsy: a report of the Therapeutics and Technology Assessment Subcommittee of the American Academy of Neurology. Neurology. 1999; 53:666–669

[40] Fanselow EE. Central mechanisms of cranial nerve stimulation for epilepsy. Surg Neurol Int. 2012; 3 Suppl 4:S247–S254

[41] Krahl SE, Clark KB. Vagus nerve stimulation for epilepsy: A review of central mechanisms. Surg Neurol Int. 2012; 3 Suppl 4:S255–S259

[42] Henry TR. Therapeutic mechanisms of vagus nerve stimulation. Neurology. 2002; 59(6) Suppl 4:S3–S14

[43] Naritoku DK, Terry WJ, Helfert RH. Regional induction of fos immunoreactivity in the brain by anticonvulsant stimulation of the vagus nerve. Epilepsy Res. 1995; 22(1):53–62

[44] Vonck K, De Herdt V, Bosman T, Dedeurwaerdere S, Van Laere K, Boon P. Thalamic and limbic involvement in the

mechanism of action of vagus nerve stimulation, a SPECT study. Seizure. 2008; 17(8):699–706

[45] Amar AP, Heck CN, Levy ML, et al. An institutional experience with cervical vagus nerve trunk stimulation for medically refractory epilepsy: rationale, technique, and outcome. Neurosurgery. 1998; 43(6):1265–1276, discussion 1276–1280

[46] Healy S, Lang J, Te Water Naude J, Gibbon F, Leach P. Vagal nerve stimulation in children under 12 years old with medically intractable epilepsy. Childs Nerv Syst. 2013; 29 (11):2095–2099

[47] Cyberonics, Inc. VNS therapy product manuals and safety alerts. http://dynamic.cyberonics.com/manuals. 2013

[48] Labar D, Murphy J, Tecoma E. Vagus nerve stimulation for medication-resistant generalized epilepsy. E04 VNS Study Group. Neurology. 1999; 52(7):1510–1512

[49] Ben Menachem E, Hellstrom K, Runmarker B, Augustinsson LE. A prospective single-center open-label trial of VNS in 59 patients for the treatment of refractory epilepsy. Epilepsia. 1997; 38 suppl 8:208

[50] Alexopoulos AV, Kotagal P, Loddenkemper T, Hammel J, Bingaman WE. Long term results with VNS in children with pharmacoresistant epilepsy. Seizure. 2006; 15:491–503

[51] Benifla M, Rutka JK, Logan W, Donner EJ. VNS for refractory epilepsy in children: indications and experience in the Hospital for Sick Children. Childs Nerv Syst. 2006; 22:1018–1026

[52] Shermann EM, Connolly MB, Slick DJ, Eyrl KL, Steinbok P, Farrell K. Quality of life and seizure outcome after VNS in children with intractable epilepsy. J Child Neurol. 2008; 23: 991–998

[53] Elliott RE, Rodgers SD, Bassani EL, et al. VNS for children with treatment-resistant epilepsy: a consecutive series of 141 cases. J Neurosurg Pediatr. 2011; 7:491–500

[54] Ben-Menachem E. Vagus nerve stimulation, side effects, and long-term safety. J Clin Neurophysiol. 2001; 18(5):415–418

[55] Ben-Menachem E. Vagus-nerve stimulation for the treatment of epilepsy. Lancet Neurol. 2002; 1(8):477–482

[56] Elliott RE, Morsi A, Kalhorn SP, et al. VNS in 436 consecutive patients with treatment-resistent epilepsy: long-term outcome and predictors of response. Epilepsy Behav. 2011; 20:57–63

[57] De Herdt V, Boon P, Ceulemans B, et al. VNS for refractory epilepsy: a Belgian multicenter study. Eur J Paediatr Neurol. 2007; 11:261–269

[58] Labar D. VNS for 1 year in 269 patients on unchanged antiepileptic drugs. Seizure. 2004; 13:392–398

[59] Helmers SL, Wheless JW, Frost M, et al. VNS therapy in pediatric patients with refractory epilepsy: retrospective study. J Child Neurol. 2001; 16:843–848

47 Surgical Management of Pediatric Spasticity

Michael M. McDowell, Michelle Q. Phan, Richard C.E. Anderson

47.1 Introduction

Spasticity is a condition of hypertonia, causing hyperactive reflexes, poor coordination, and weakness that can greatly affect a child's comfort level and ability to perform daily activities. Spasticity is distinguished from other forms of childhood hypertonia, such as rigidity and dystonia, in that it is defined as hypertonia with velocity-dependent resistance to externally imposed movements.[1]

47.2 Epidemiology and Pathophysiology

In children, the most common cause of spasticity and motor disability is cerebral palsy. Cerebral palsy is not a discrete disorder, but a range of non-progressive syndromes of movement and posture due to static injuries to the developing fetal or infant central nervous system (CNS). Cerebral palsy is estimated to occur in 2 to 3 of every 1,000 live births, and in premature infants born before 28 weeks' gestational age, the incidence rises up to 100 per 1,000.[2] Advances in neonatal care have improved the survival in newborns of low birth weight and there has been a corresponding increase in the incidence of cerebral palsy.[3] Other factors that are linked to the development of cerebral palsy include multiple births, chorioamnionitis, antepartum vaginal bleeding, second stage of labor lasting longer than 4 hours, perinatal asphyxia, and perinatal infection.[2,4,5,6,7,8] Following cerebral palsy, common causes of childhood spasticity are traumatic brain injury, spinal cord injury, meningitis, encephalitis, stroke, and pediatric multiple sclerosis.

Spasticity can result from any disease process that impairs the upper motor neurons within the CNS, causing a decrease in descending inhibitory corticospinal and reticulospinal input to short-latency stretch reflexes and a loss of functionally important long-latency reflexes. Disinhibition of short-latency reflex arcs leads to the hyperexcitability of simple stretch reflexes. Combined with reduced facilitation of functional, polysynaptic, or long-latency reflexes, this results in a profound alteration of proprioception.[9] Initial maladaptive hypertonic movement patterns, with reduced proprioceptive feedback, lead to secondary viscoelastic changes in muscle fiber, collagen tissue, and tendon properties that propagate cycles of paresis, contracture, and spasticity (▶ Fig. 47.1).[10,11,12] Untreated, these changes can progress to joint and muscular contractures, bony deformations, joint subluxations and dislocations, and permanent loss of joint mobility, contributing to weight loss, skin breakdown, and chronic pain.[10,11,13,14,15,16]

47.3 Diagnosis and Examination

The clinical evaluation of spasticity requires a thorough accurate history with input from patient, caretakers, and therapists. The history should inquire about possible gestational and perinatal events, the patient's motor and cognitive milestones, potential triggers of spasticity, family history of motor disorders, patient's quality of life and functional limitations.[17,18] There are a variety of complementary global and specific functional measurement instruments; the gross motor performance measure and pediatric evaluation of disability index are generally considered the best standard measures of function.[19]

The physical examination should include assessments of motor power, muscle tone, active and passive range of motion (PROM) and joints, deep tendon reflexes, station, presence of limb deformities or contractures, and spinal alignment. Spasticity is differentiated from other causes of hypertonia by characteristic features including velocity dependence, the clasp-knife phenomenon, stroking affect, and differential distribution with antigravity muscles.[13,20] Spasticity can be quantified by rating systems such as the modified Ashworth scale, Tardieu scale, and pendulum test. The modified Ashworth scale is the most widely used in clinical practice and as an end point in clinical trials, it does not require additional instruments and is simple to administer (Box 47.1); however, it does not differentiate resistance due to spasticity and fibrotic changes in muscle.[21,22]

Supplementary testing may involve imaging studies such as cranial ultrasound, computed tomography (CT), or magnetic resonance imaging (MRI) in order to evaluate for hemorrhage, hydrocephalus, or other structural abnormalities of the CNS. A majority of cerebral palsy patients have MR

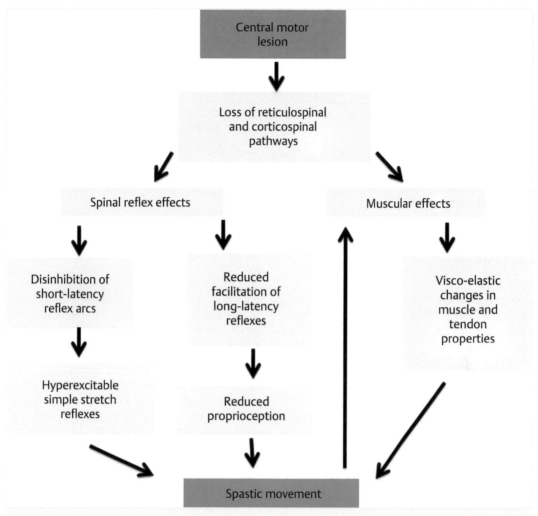

Fig. 47.1 Diagram depicting the cascade of mechanisms contributing to spastic movement disorders.

abnormalities, with general patterns of gyral anomalies, periventricular leukomalacia, and watershed cortical or deep gray nuclear damage.[23,24] Preoperative MR findings may help predict postoperative improvement, in particular, after selective dorsal rhizotomy.[25]

47.4 Nonsurgical Management

The goal of management is to reduce spasticity and halt the progression of contractures or deformities in order to improve the ease of caregiving, decrease pain, and increase quality of life.

47.4.1 Nonpharmacological Therapy

Nonpharmacological therapy is used to maximize range of motion, strengthen muscles, inhibit spastic agonist muscles, and encourage adaptive motor development. While controlled trials are limited, physical and occupational therapy are mainstays in the treatment of spasticity and are requisite for surgical and medical interventions to achieve their maximal benefit.[26,27,28] Specific exercises that have been shown to help reduce spasticity include cycling, strengthening exercises, and treadmill training.[29,30,31,32,33] Static weight-bearing exercises

Box 47.1 The modified Ashworth scale, measuring the relative spasticity in an individual muscle group

The individual muscle group scores and mean score for lower or upper extremities are frequently used both in clinical practice and research studies to approximate the objective outcome of spasticity-reducing operations.

0 = No increase in muscle tone.

1 = Slight increase in muscle tone.

1 + = Slight increase in muscle resistance throughout the range.

2 = Moderate increase in muscle tone throughout the range of motion; passive movement is easy.

3 = Marked increase in muscle tone throughout the range of motion; passive movement is difficult.

4 = Marked increase in muscle tone; affected part is rigid.

like standing with the assistance of tilt tables and standing frames can reduce spasticity, improve bone mineral density, prevent hip dislocation, and improve bowel and urinary functions. In contrast, passive stretching remains largely evidence-free despite its widespread popularity.[34,35,36] Constraint-induced therapy, in which temporary splinting or casting is used to encourage utilization and strengthening of less dominant muscle groups, has received renewed attention in the past decade due to positive results in adult stroke therapy; constraint in cerebral palsy patients showed better quality movements and structural neuro-

plastic changes.[37,38] While the evidence of upper extremity orthoses in children with cerebral palsy is inconclusive, ankle–foot orthoses are commonly used to treat dynamic equinus in cerebral palsy and can reduce ankle excursion and increase dorsiflexion in foot strike.[39,40] The use of orthotics for neurodevelopmental retraining are particularly important during the periods of weakness following botulinum toxin treatment.[41]

47.4.2 Oral Antispasticity Drugs

Oral antispasticity drugs can be used alongside an effective physical program or more invasive therapies. Use of these drugs is patient-centered as the drugs have different side effect profiles. Baclofen, diazepam, tizanidine, dantrolene, and gabapentin are the most prescribed oral antispastic drugs (▶ Table 47.1).

Baclofen is the most widely used antispastic drug in clinical practice, although most research involving oral use has been conducted in adults. Baclofen should be started at the lowest possible dose to minimize side effects such as sedation, somnolence, and vertigo. It must be carefully tapered when starting and discontinuing use in order to avoid central side effects of rebound spasticity, hallucinations, hyperthermia, and seizures.[42,43]

Diazepam is effective for short-term treatment of spasticity, but there are no studies formally addressing whether it improves motor function, and caution of physical dependence with prolonged use has limited its long-term use.[44] Clonazepam has been found to be particularly useful in treating nocturnal spasms.[13]

Sodium dantrolene is the only major antispastic drug that works at the muscle, rather than in the nervous system. Although it has been shown to

Table 47.1 Oral medications utilized in the treatment of spasticity

Drug	Mechanism of action	Adverse effects
Baclofen	GABA agonist	Drowsiness, respiratory depression, ataxia, confusion
Diazepam	Benzodiazepine receptor agonist	Lethargy, rapid tolerance and dependence
Dantrolene	Blocks calcium efflux from muscle sarcoplasmic reticulum	Weakness, hepatotoxicity, rash
Tizanidine	α_2 adrenergic agonist	Sedation, dizziness, hypotension
Gabapentin	Alters voltage-gated calcium channel traffic	Dizziness, somnolence, nystagmus
Cannabinoids	Cannabinoid receptor agonist	Palpitations, altered mentation, gastrointestinal distress

Abbreviation: GABA, γ-aminobutyric acid.

reduce spasticity in children with cerebral palsy, it is infrequently used chronically due to hepatotoxicity.[43,45]

Tizanidine has been found to be able to reduce spasticity in studies with adults with multiple sclerosis and spinal cord injury and in small studies with children with cerebral palsy. While muscle weakness may be seen less with tizanidine than baclofen, tizanidine may have cardiovascular, CNS, and hepatotoxic effects that must be taken into account.[46]

Gabapentin has been shown in small studies to have good tolerability and benefits for spasticity, but has mostly been investigated in the context of spinal cord injury or multiple sclerosis.[47] Cannabinoids have been of interest recently as a treatment for pain and spasticity in adults with multiple sclerosis, but have not been used in children.[47]

47.4.3 Intramuscular Injections

Intramuscular injections of alcohol, phenol, and botulinum toxin produce neuromuscular blockades that can help treat focal spasticity or manage problem muscle groups in more generalized spasticity.

Five to seven percent phenol or 45% alcohol injections perineurally or into the motor point of selected muscles induce necrosis of axons in hyperexcitable anterior horn cells. This produces a reduction in limb tone that can last up to 12 months when phenol is used and 2 to 5 months when alcohol is used. The sustained reduction in tone and relative low cost of phenol injections are balanced with side effects including pain and dysesthesia due to necrosis of secondary axons in the peripheral nerve, lethargy, and nausea due to systemic absorption, and potential necrosis at the injection site. Both treatments are rarely used today due to the advent of botulinum toxin therapy.[43]

Botulinum toxin acts to inhibit the release of acetylcholine at the neuromuscular junction, and today, it is the most commonly used pharmacological injection for the management of spasticity. The effects of botulinum toxin generally begin 1 to 3 days, peaking at 21 days, and dissipating by 3 to 4 months. It is licensed for the treatment of dynamic equinus foot in pediatric cerebral palsy, and there is good evidence for its use at calf, hip, adductor, hamstring, and upper limb levels.[48,49,50,51,52] Botulinum toxin is well tolerated, but has rare side effects that include respiratory infection, seizures, muscle atrophy, immunoresistance, and transient pain at injection site.[53,54,55] General dosing guidelines are 2 to 6 U/kg and should take into account the child's muscle bulk and degree of spasticity. The use of electromyography, muscle stimulators, or direct ultrasound guidance for the correct administration to targeted areas is increasingly common.[56] Postinjection care should include a comprehensive physiotherapy and follow-up for repeated or multilevel injections to accelerate functional outcomes and minimize the need for orthopedic intervention.[41,50,57]

47.4.4 Complementary Medicine

Complementary medicine, including hyperbaric oxygen, craniospinal osteopathy, and acupuncture has been used internationally for the management of spasticity in children; these treatments have been found to be useful in individual cases, but for most, there is little supportive evidence.[58,59]

47.5 Surgical Indications

A wide array of surgical options is available for the treatment of spasticity, allowing for various options based on the patient's clinical characteristics and the goals of treatment. Spasticity reducing operations will not resolve already established orthopedic issues such as contractures, joint subluxation, dislocation, or bony deformity. Early reduction in tone has been shown to reduce the development of orthopedic issues and, thus, operations to reduce tone should be considered prior to the onset of orthopedic problems when possible.[60,61]

Younger patients with the greatest amount of spasticity in the lower extremities are most likely to obtain the greatest functional benefit from selective dorsal rhizotomy (SDR), but functional benefit can be obtained at older ages as well.[61,62] Studies have also demonstrated that patients can have a reduction in spasticity and functional improvement in the upper extremities after SDR, but to a lesser extent than in the lower extremities.[63,64,65,66]

Intrathecal baclofen (ITB) pumps are most clearly indicated in patients with severe spastic quadriplegia that are dependent on caregivers. This therapy is also effective in older adolescents.[67] At some centers, patients being considered for baclofen therapy undergo a trial injection of 50 to 100 μg intrathecally. Antispastic effects are typically seen within 2 to 4 hours after lumbar puncture and wear off by 8 hours. A reduction in tone by one point or more on the Ashworth scale is considered a positive response, and is seen in the vast majority of patients undergoing trials.[17,68] Importantly, patients and caregivers can temporarily assess the realistic level of tone reduction and benefit from ITB on spasticity and joint mobility.

Patients in whom function-impairing spasticity is located to a single or a few muscle groups in an extremity may choose botulinum toxin injections as the best option.[52,69] There are few side effects due to its localized delivery, with the primary risk being an allergic reaction.[70,71] Botulinum toxin injections and baclofen pumps have largely supplanted the older technique of selective neurotomy. However, in contrast to botulinum toxin injections, selective neurotomy offers a longer-lasting reduction in tone and can also be performed to provide partial denervation of the muscle group based on intraoperative neurophysiologic monitoring and stimulation, allowing for a balance between spasticity and motor weakness.[72,73]

47.5.1 Surgical Technique

Selective Dorsal Rhizotomy

The patient is positioned prone and draped to allow adequate exposure of the lower back. Although this procedure is often performed with a five-level laminectomy or laminoplasty to expose the roots as they exit the spinal canal, we prefer the SDR through a single laminectomy as popularized by Park et al (▶ Fig. 47.2).[74] A single-level laminectomy at the L1 level is performed and access to the conus cauda

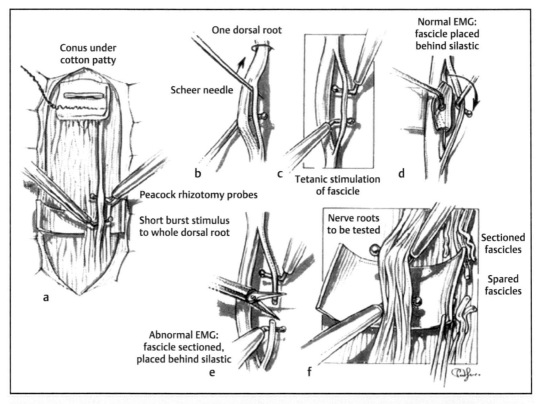

Fig. 47.2 Illustration of key steps during selective dorsal rhizotomy. **(a)** The innervation pattern of each dorsal root is examined using electrophysiogical stimulation using a threshold voltage. **(b)** The dorsal root is subdivided into three to seven smaller rootlets. **(c)** Each rootlet is tested to determine the relative level of spasticity generated with stimulation. **(d)** Rootlets to be preserved are placed behind the Silastic sheet. **(e)** Rootlets with the greatest spastic responses are sectioned. **(f)** The remaining dorsal roots to be examined are kept above the Silastic sheet. Section rootlets are displaced laterally. Spared rootlets are meticulously kept below the sheet. (Reproduced with permission from Oxford University Press.)

equina junction is confirmed via ultrasound prior to opening the dura.[74] Nerve roots are isolated and tested using electrical stimulation and neurophysiological monitoring. Ventral roots are separated from dorsal roots and each dorsal root is separated into four to eight rootlets. Individual dorsal rootlets are then stimulated to determine which should be transected based on the relative severity of the spasticity elicited. Stimulated sensory rootlets that demonstrate sphincter innervation or normal responses are preserved, while rootlets demonstrating spastic responses when stimulated are transected. Intraoperative palpation of muscle groups during rootlet stimulation by a physical and occupational therapy team or physiatrist is helpful in providing physiological feedback when determining which rootlets to transect based on the degree of spasticity elicited. With the single-level laminectomy surgical approach, ventral roots are easily identified via electrophysiological stimulation.[75] Many centers perform transection of 40% or less of rootlets due to concerns such as iatrogenic neurological deficits.[76, 77,78,79,80] However, other centers including ours support aggressively transecting up to 70% of rootlets based on data suggesting that relief of spasticity is proportional to the percent of dorsal nerve tissue transected.[63,78,81]

Intrathecal Baclofen Pump

The appropriate surgical techniques for ITB have been previously described.[82] Briefly, the patient is positioned in the lateral decubitus position to allow for both implantation of the pump in the anterior abdominal wall and insertion of the catheter tip into the subarachnoid space. The side of pump placement should be dictated by patient preference and existence of coexisting hardware such as a percutaneous gastrostomy tube. Both subcutaneous or subfascial placement are possible, with the latter favored in patients with low tissue volume that will be more prone to hardware erosion.[83] The abdominal incision is made and a subcutaneous plane is dissected and expanded for subcutaneous placement, if desired. For subfascial placement, the external oblique fascia and rectus abdominis fascia are identified and an incision is made followed by blunt dissection to develop a space between the fascial and muscle layers.

The location of catheter placement is dependent on the distribution of spasticity, with higher placement being indicated in the setting of increased upper extremity tone. For spastic diplegia, the catheter is threaded from insertion at L3–L4 or L4–

L5 to rest in the region of T10–T12. For spastic quadriparesis, the catheter can be threaded further upward to C5–T2.[82] Confirmation of placement is performed using fluoroscopic guidance. Flexible tubing is tunneled subcutaneously around the flank to the lumbar spine to connect the catheter and pump. Intermittent refilling is generally required every 2 to 6 months based on dosing parameters.

Selective Neurotomy

The patient is draped and positioned based on the muscle groups in question. Ideally, the limb being operated is sterilized and draped in such a way to allow intraoperative assessment of tone by the surgeon. Localization of the nerve is performed using anatomical landmarks and refined based on neurophysiological testing with a sharp probe (▶ Table 47.2). Temporary anesthetic blocks may be performed to determine the contribution of spasticity versus orthopedic complications for a given joint in order to determine the likely functional benefit of neurotomy.[84] Subsequent to incision and subcutaneous dissection, an operative microscope is used to identify individual motor nerve fibers. Nerve stimulation is then used to determine the most spastic fibers, which are then obliterated.

47.5.2 Complications
Selective Dorsal Rhizotomy

Selective dorsal rhizotomy is a well-tolerated procedure with a very low risk of permanent morbidity. Urinary retention from nerve root manipulation may be seen transiently, but permanent urinary dysfunction is rare.[85,86,87,88] Urinary catheterization from nerve room manipulation and anesthesia may be seen transiently. Transient dysesthesia and hypoesthesia are also frequently reported within the first few postoperative weeks, but permanent neurological complaints after SDR occur in less than 5% of patients. An even smaller percentage of patients have any type of functional decline after SDR.[88,89,90,91,92] Older studies have drawn attention to the possibility of an increased incidence of scoliosis after SDR.[93,94] As this is a common finding in children with spasticity without SDR, it is unclear what role SDR plays in the development of scoliosis and whether this relationship exists in the era of single-level laminectomy rather

Table 47.2 Indication, location of incision, and key anatomical landmarks for common nerves targeted with selective neurotomy

Nerve	Indication	Incision location	Nerve anatomical landmarks
Lateral pectoral nerve	Spasticity of shoulder with internal rotation and adduction	Curvilinear incision over infra-clavicular fossa in medial part of deltopectoral groove	Deep to partially reflected clavipectoral fascia and pec-toralis major
Teres major nerve	Spasticity of shoulder with internal rotation and adduction	Incision along inner border of teres major from lower border of posterior head of deltoid to lower extremity of scapula	In space separating teres ma-jor from teres minor and other infraspinatus muscles Midway between long portion of triceps brachii above and insertions of teres major on infraspinatus aponeurosis below
Musculocutaneous nerve	Spasticity of elbow with flexion	Longitudinal incision from in-ferior edge of pectoralis ma-jor, medial to biceps brachii muscle	Anterior and medial to bra-chialis muscle
Median nerve	Spasticity of forearm with pronation deformity, flexion deformity in wrist, swan-neck deformity of fingers	Curvilinear incision above flexion line of elbow, medial to biceps brachii tendon, through elbow and before junction of upper and middle third of anterior forearm	Medial to brachial artery, deep to lacertus fibrosus
Recurrent branch of median nerve	Thumb-in-palm deformity	Curvilinear carpal incision	Deep to transverse carpal ligament
Ulnar nerve	Spastic wrist flexion, adduc-tion/flexion deformity of thumb	Longitudinal or arched inci-sion between two heads of flexor carpi ulnaris	Medial to medial epicondyle between heads of flexor carpi ulnaris proximally
Obturator nerve	Spasticity of adductor muscles, diplegic children with scissoring, facilitation of perineal toileting and self-catheterization	Longitudinal incision ex-tended distally from point just below groin over belly of adductor longus Transverse incision in hip flexion fold centered on prominence of adductor lon-gus tendon (aesthetically preferred)	Anterior branch is lateral to adductor longus Posterior branch is deep and should be spared to preserve stabilizing muscles
Sciatic nerve	Spastic diplegia with flexion deformity of knees	Longitudinal straight incision on posterior thigh between ischial tuberosity and tip of femoral greater trochanter	Deep to gluteus maximus and biceps femoris
Femoral nerve	Spasticity of quadriceps, limited knee flexion during swing phase of gait	Horizontal incision in hip flex-ion fold, medial to sartorius muscle	Nerve to rectus femoris muscle is superficial to nerve to vastus intermedius
Tibial nerve	Spastic varus plantar flexion with or without claw toes	Z-shaped incision over popli-teal fossa	Deep to popliteal fascia, superficial to popliteal artery and vein Sensory medial cutaneous nerve is encountered first and should be spared Superior soleus nerve is mid-line and posterior to tibial nerve

than multilevel laminectomies. In addition, SDR does not eliminate the need for future orthopedic surgery. Approximately 34% of patients who are operated on between the ages of 2 and 5 years may ultimately still require surgery for orthopedic complications within 7.5 years after SDR.[95,96] However, this is in contrast to the approximately 60% of patients with spasticity at birth who without SDR will require an orthopedic procedure by the age of 8.[95,97]

Intrathecal Baclofen Pump

The body habitus and disability of patients undergoing pump placement contributes to a postoperative wound infection rate of 5 to 36%. More than half of these wound infections are severe enough to require removal of the pump hardware.[98,99,100] Cerebrospinal fluid (CSF) leakage occurs frequently, but can typically be resolved without operative repair or removal of the hardware.[98] Pump failure requiring replacement occurs in 5 to 10% of cases and failure of the catheter itself may occur as much as in 35% of early cases, though increased use and quality of the devices has lowered this to less than 10% in more recent studies.[98,99,101,102,103,104]

ITB infusions also harbor some risk. Most commonly, baclofen is often associated with mild sedation, which is easily resolved by lowering the does. More serious symptoms such dizziness, blurred vision, nausea, confusion, and slurred speech have also been reported on occasion.[102] Baclofen withdrawal is a serious condition resulting in rebound spasticity, tachycardia, hyperthermia, itching, paresthesias, and seizures. It is best managed through extensive education to the patient and family.[105,106] New-onset seizure or increased seizure frequency has been reported but typically resolve with repair of any device malfunction and short-term seizure prophylaxis.[101,107] Severe respiratory, neurological, or cardiovascular depression can occur during overdose scenarios and often are accompanied by weakness, flaccidity, and areflexia in all extremities. Reduction of the baclofen dose while supporting the patient's cardiovascular and respiratory status allows for continuation of the therapy after the crisis.[101]

Selective Neurotomy

Postoperative complications vary based on the specific location and nerve, but are typically transient in nature. Hematoma formation, infection, hypoesthesia, and weakness of the affected limb have been reported with rates ranging from 0 to 5%.[84,108,109]

47.5.3 Postoperative Care

Postsurgical pain from surgical exploration and pump implantation as well as laminectomy and nerve root manipulation is common. For postoperative pain following SDR, intravenous, epidural, and transthecal approaches to pain management have been reported, with morphine or fentanyl typically being the medication of choice in a survey of 59 centers worldwide. In more than half of cases, continuous infusion can be discontinued in 1 to 4 days, but may be required for up to 1 week followed by several additional days of oral opioids. The duration of pain management has not been found to be associated with drug of choice or mechanism of delivery.[110] In our center, we have had excellent results with the combination of intravenous toradol and diazepam, with additional morphine for breakthrough pain.[17,111]

As well as pain management, the primary goal of postoperative care is to maximize the long-term benefit from reduced spasticity and improved function.[26,76,112] Existing data suggest that patients may benefit from physiotherapy beyond the postoperative period.[26] Appropriate therapy is best obtained in conjunction with trained therapists who can accurately assess the physical presentation and key barriers to function, set appropriate goals, choose the appropriate intervention, and reassess following implementation.[113] These interventions typically focus on muscle lengthening, muscle strength, and motor memory, and planning. Temporary splinting and casting may assist patients in muscle lengthening between sessions when deemed necessary, as severely spastic children may require hours of stretching daily to prevent progression to contracture.[114] As well as traditional muscle strengthening exercises, high activity levels in daily life tapered to physical and mental disabilities should also be encouraged.[115]

47.5.4 Outcomes

Selective Dorsal Rhizotomy

There have been a number of excellent long-term outcome studies for selective dorsal rhizotomy. The outcome measures examined include muscle tone, flexibility, gait pattern, functional positioning, and the ability of the child to deal with his or her environment. Nearly all studies investigating SDR have demonstrated a significant and persistent decrease in spasticity without a return of hypertonicity over time. Improved function and ambulation are commonly seen regardless of the preoperative abilities.[116,117,118] After SDR, 50 to 78% of patients with impaired ambulation have been found to improve to a higher level of independence (e.g., walk with assistance to walk with walker alone).[119] More recently, long-term outcome data for children with spastic diplegia who underwent SDR in Capet own have been published.[117] In this prospective cohort study, the data demonstrated that significant improvements in both range of motion and quality of gait (cadence and step length) persisted over a 20-year period. Importantly, SDR did not abolish the need for subsequent orthopedic surgery, as approximately half of these children still required lengthening of the rectus femoris, hamstrings, and/or Achilles' tendon.

McLaughlin et al reported a comparative analysis and meta-analysis of three randomized clinical trials in 2002.[77,78] Eighty-two children with spastic diplegia received either SDR and physiotherapy or physiotherapy alone. Outcome measures were used for spasticity (Ashworth's scale) and function (gross motor function measure) and applied at a 12-month follow-up visit. Overall, selective dorsal rhizotomy with physical therapy was more effective than physical therapy alone in reducing spasticity and improving overall function in children with spastic diplegia.

Although many studies have documented the efficacy of SDR and ITB therapy on the treatment of spasticity, only recently has information comparing these treatments directly become available.[118] Kan and colleagues reported a consecutive series of 71 children who underwent SDR for spasticity and compared them with another group of 71 children who underwent ITB therapy matched by age and preoperative score on the gross motor function classification system (GMFCS).[118] At 1 year postoperatively, both SDR and ITB therapy decreased tone, increased PROM, and improved function. Compared with ITB therapy, however, SDR provided a significantly larger magnitude of improvement in tone, PROM, and gross motor function. In addition, fewer patients in the SDR group required subsequent orthopedic procedures (19.1 vs. 40.8%).

SDR has typically been only used for children with spastic diplegia due to the unpredictable effects of SDR on the upper extremities. However, numerous examples of suprasegmental improvements in the upper extremities have now been reported in patients with spastic quadriplegia undergoing SDR.[63,120] Most recently, Gigante et al demonstrated that over 90% of patients with upper extremity spasticity had a reduction in tone and over 70% had an increase in motor control or spontaneous movement of the upper extremities after SDR.[63]

Intrathecal Baclofen Pump

Multiple clinical trials have demonstrated that ITB therapy is effective at decreasing spasticity and improving functional outcome.[68,99,121,122] The degree of ambulation was found to be improved in 28 to 43% of patients.[123,124,125] In the original multicenter randomized controlled trial, 100% of patients randomized into the baclofen group were found to have at least a 1 point reduction on the mean Ashworth scale for their lower extremities.[122] This was subsequently supported in a predominantly pediatric trial of quadriplegic patients, all of which met the same criteria for reduced spasticity in upper and lower extremities on long-term follow-up. Further, it was found that, in all age groups, the required amount of baclofen needed to maintain this reduced spasticity tended to titrate upward toward twice the original dose during the initial 2 postoperative years, followed by a leveling off and stabilization of the dose.[121]

Perhaps the greatest benefit for ITB therapy is that it is a nondestructive procedure for which dosing can be adjusted to fit each patient's needs. However, vigilant maintenance is required with ITB therapy; as discussed above, patients may have a higher risk of complications and need for reoperations, particularly in patients under the age of 10 or with a mean Ashworth score of 3 or greater.[98]

Selective Neurotomy

Selective neurotomy is effective at increasing the postoperative passive and active range-of-motion of joints, and allows for a greater utilization of function of the limb, and reduces spasticity of the associated muscle groups.[72,84] However, most available data are in the form of small cohorts lacking in long-term follow-up. In contrast to SDR, there may be a higher rate of recurrence of spasticity following neurotomy. Approximately 15% of adult cases witness a partial or complete return of spasticity at 6 months and 37% at 17 months.[84,126]

Patients undergoing repeat neurotomy seem to benefit a similar degree as first time cases.[84] Data are lacking to support the widespread utility of this operation in children, in whom long-term reduction of spasticity is crucial given the number of years of expected life, and thus this technique is generally reserved for a highly select group of patients with focal spasticity.

References

[1] Sanger TD, Delgado MR, Gaebler-Spira D, Hallett M, Mink JW, Task Force on Childhood Motor Disorders. Classification and definition of disorders causing hypertonia in childhood. Pediatrics. 2003; 111(1):e89–e97

[2] O'Shea TM. Cerebral palsy in very preterm infants: new epidemiological insights. Ment Retard Dev Disabil Res Rev. 2002; 8(3):135–145

[3] Koman LA, Smith BP, Shilt JS. Cerebral palsy. Lancet. 2004; 363(9421):1619–1631

[4] Jarvis S, Glinianaia SV, Torrioli MG, et al. Surveillance of Cerebral Palsy in Europe (SCPE) Collaboration of European Cerebral Palsy Registers. Cerebral palsy and intrauterine growth in single births: European collaborative study. Lancet. 2003; 362(9390):1106–1111

[5] Nelson KB. The epidemiology of cerebral palsy in term infants. Ment Retard Dev Disabil Res Rev. 2002; 8(3): 146–150

[6] Yeargin-Allsopp M, Van Naarden Braun K, Doernberg NS, Benedict RE, Kirby RS, Durkin MS. Prevalence of cerebral palsy in 8-year-old children in three areas of the United States in 2002: a multisite collaboration. Pediatrics. 2008; 121(3):547–554

[7] O'Shea TM, Dammann O. Antecedents of cerebral palsy in very low-birth weight infants. Clin Perinatol. 2000; 27(2): 285–302

[8] O'Shea TM, Preisser JS, Klinepeter KL, Dillard RG. Trends in mortality and cerebral palsy in a geographically based cohort of very low birth weight neonates born between 1982 to 1994. Pediatrics. 1998; 101(4 pt 1):642–647

[9] Dietz V. Proprioception and locomotor disorders. Nat Rev Neurosci. 2002; 3(10):781–790

[10] Dietz V, Sinkjaer T. Spasticity. Handb Clin Neurol. 2012; 109:197–211

[11] Gracies JM. Pathophysiology of spastic paresis. II: Emergence of muscle overactivity. Muscle Nerve. 2005; 31 (5):552–571

[12] Gracies JM. Pathophysiology of spastic paresis. I: Paresis and soft tissue changes. Muscle Nerve. 2005; 31(5):535–551

[13] Kheder A, Nair KP. Spasticity: pathophysiology, evaluation and management. Pract Neurol. 2012; 12(5):289–298

[14] Burke D, Wissel J, Donnan GA. Pathophysiology of spasticity in stroke. Neurology. 2013; 80(3) suppl 2:S20–S26

[15] Ward T. Spasticity in children with non-progressive brain disorders. Nurs Times. 2012; 108(47):23

[16] Ward AB. A literature review of the pathophysiology and onset of post-stroke spasticity. Eur J Neurol. 2012; 19(1): 21–27

[17] Mandigo CE, Anderson RC. Management of childhood spasticity: a neurosurgical perspective. Pediatr Ann. 2006; 35(5):354–362

[18] Allen MC, Alexander GR. Using motor milestones as a multistep process to screen preterm infants for cerebral palsy. Dev Med Child Neurol. 1997; 39(1):12–16

[19] Ketelaar M, Vermeer A, Helders PJ. Functional motor abilities of children with cerebral palsy: a systematic literature review of assessment measures. Clin Rehabil. 1998; 12(5):369–380

[20] Capute AJ. Identifying cerebral palsy in infancy through study of primitive-reflex profiles. Pediatr Ann. 1979; 8(10): 589–595

[21] Bohannon RW, Smith MB. Interrater reliability of a modified Ashworth scale of muscle spasticity. Phys Ther. 1987; 67(2): 206–207

[22] Mutlu A, Livanelioglu A, Gunel MK. Reliability of Ashworth and modified Ashworth scales in children with spastic cerebral palsy. BMC Musculoskelet Disord. 2008; 9:44

[23] Truwit CL, Barkovich AJ, Koch TK, Ferriero DM. Cerebral palsy: MR findings in 40 patients. AJNR Am J Neuroradiol. 1992; 13(1):67–78

[24] Ashwal S, Russman BS, Blasco PA, et al. Quality Standards Subcommittee of the American Academy of Neurology, Practice Committee of the Child Neurology Society. Practice parameter: diagnostic assessment of the child with cerebral palsy: report of the Quality Standards Subcommittee of the American Academy of Neurology and the Practice Committee of the Child Neurology Society. Neurology. 2004; 62(6):851–863

[25] Grunt S, Becher JG, van Schie P, van Ouwerkerk WJ, Ahmadi M, Vermeulen RJ. Preoperative MRI findings and functional outcome after selective dorsal rhizotomy in children with bilateral spasticity. Childs Nerv Syst. 2010; 26(2):191–198

[26] Palmer FB, Shapiro BK, Wachtel RC, et al. The effects of physical therapy on cerebral palsy. A controlled trial in infants with spastic diplegia. N Engl J Med. 1988; 318(13): 803–808

[27] Cada EA, O'Shea RK. Identifying barriers to occupational and physical therapy services for children with cerebral palsy. J Pediatr Rehabil Med. 2008; 1(2):127–135

[28] Watanabe T. The role of therapy in spasticity management. Am J Phys Med Rehabil. 2004; 83 suppl 10:S45–S49

[29] Verschuren O, Ketelaar M, Gorter JW, Helders PJ, Uiterwaal CS, Takken T. Exercise training program in children and adolescents with cerebral palsy: a randomized controlled trial. Arch Pediatr Adolesc Med. 2007; 161(11):1075–1081

[30] Ada L, Dorsch S, Canning CG. Strengthening interventions increase strength and improve activity after stroke: a systematic review. Aust J Physiother. 2006; 52(4):241–248

[31] McBurney H, Taylor NF, Dodd KJ, Graham HK. A qualitative analysis of the benefits of strength training for young people with cerebral palsy. Dev Med Child Neurol. 2003; 45 (10):658–663

[32] Damiano DL, Arnold AS, Steele KM, Delp SL. Can strength training predictably improve gait kinematics? A pilot study on the effects of hip and knee extensor strengthening on lower-extremity alignment in cerebral palsy. Phys Ther. 2010; 90(2):269–279

[33] Dodd KJ, Taylor NF, Damiano DL. A systematic review of the effectiveness of strength-training programs for people with cerebral palsy. Arch Phys Med Rehabil. 2002; 83(8):1157–1164

[34] Ketelaar M, Vermeer A, Hart H, van Petegem-van Beek E, Helders PJ. Effects of a functional therapy program on motor abilities of children with cerebral palsy. Phys Ther. 2001; 81 (9):1534–1545

[35] Pin T, Dyke P, Chan M. The effectiveness of passive stretching in children with cerebral palsy. Dev Med Child Neurol. 2006; 48(10):855–862

[36] Pin TW. Effectiveness of static weight-bearing exercises in children with cerebral palsy. Pediatr Phys Ther. 2007; 19(1): 62–73

[37] Sterling C, Taub E, Davis D, et al. Structural neuroplastic change after constraint-induced movement therapy in children with cerebral palsy. Pediatrics. 2013; 131(5): e1664–e1669

[38] Taub E, Ramey SL, DeLuca S, Echols K. Efficacy of constraint-induced movement therapy for children with cerebral palsy with asymmetric motor impairment. Pediatrics. 2004; 113 (2):305–312

[39] Carlson WE, Vaughan CL, Damiano DL, Abel MF. Orthotic management of gait in spastic diplegia. Am J Phys Med Rehabil. 1997; 76(3):219–225

[40] Autti-Rämö I, Suoranta J, Anttila H, Malmivaara A, Mäkelä M. Effectiveness of upper and lower limb casting and orthoses in children with cerebral palsy: an overview of review articles. Am J Phys Med Rehabil. 2006; 85(1):89–103

[41] Leach J. Children undergoing treatment with botulinum toxin: the role of the physical therapist. Muscle Nerve Suppl. 1997; 6:S194–S207

[42] Delgado MR, Hirtz D, Aisen M, et al. Quality Standards Subcommittee of the American Academy of Neurology and the Practice Committee of the Child Neurology Society. Practice parameter: pharmacologic treatment of spasticity in children and adolescents with cerebral palsy (an evidence-based review): report of the Quality Standards Subcommittee of the American Academy of Neurology and the Practice Committee of the Child Neurology Society. Neurology. 2010; 74(4):336–343

[43] Papavasiliou AS. Management of motor problems in cerebral palsy: a critical update for the clinician. Eur J Paediatr Neurol. 2009; 13(5):387–396

[44] Verrotti A, Greco R, Spalice A, Chiarelli F, Iannetti P. Pharmacotherapy of spasticity in children with cerebral palsy. Pediatr Neurol. 2006; 34(1):1–6

[45] Krause T, Gerbershagen MU, Fiege M, Weisshorn R, Wappler F. Dantrolene—a review of its pharmacology, therapeutic use and new developments. Anaesthesia. 2004; 59(4): 364–373

[46] Wagstaff AJ, Bryson HM. Tizanidine. A review of its pharmacology, clinical efficacy and tolerability in the management of spasticity associated with cerebral and spinal disorders. Drugs. 1997; 53(3):435–452

[47] Stevenson VL. Rehabilitation in practice: spasticity management. Clin Rehabil. 2010; 24(4):293–304

[48] Russman BS, Tilton A, Gormley ME, Jr. Cerebral palsy: a rational approach to a treatment protocol, and the role of botulinum toxin in treatment. Muscle Nerve Suppl. 1997; 6: S181–S193

[49] Steenbeek D, Meester-Delver A, Becher JG, Lankhorst GJ. The effect of botulinum toxin type A treatment of the lower extremity on the level of functional abilities in children with cerebral palsy: evaluation with goal attainment scaling. Clin Rehabil. 2005; 19(3):274–282

[50] Ward AB. Spasticity treatment with botulinum toxins. J Neural Transm (Vienna). 2008; 115(4):607–616

[51] Sutherland DH, Kaufman KR, Wyatt MP, Chambers HG, Mubarak SJ. Double-blind study of botulinum A toxin injections into the gastrocnemius muscle in patients with cerebral palsy. Gait Posture. 1999; 10(1):1–9

[52] Koman LA, Mooney JF, III, Smith BP, Walker F, Leon JM, BOTOX Study Group. Botulinum toxin type A

neuromuscular blockade in the treatment of lower extremity spasticity in cerebral palsy: a randomized, double-blind, placebo-controlled trial. J Pediatr Orthop. 2000; 20(1):108–115

[53] Turkel CC, Bowen B, Liu J, Brin MF. Pooled analysis of the safety of botulinum toxin type A in the treatment of poststroke spasticity. Arch Phys Med Rehabil. 2006; 87(6): 786–792

[54] Hastings-Ison T, Graham HK. Atrophy and hypertrophy following injections of botulinum toxin in children with cerebral palsy. Dev Med Child Neurol. 2013; 55(9):778–779

[55] Goldstein EM. Safety of high-dose botulinum toxin type A therapy for the treatment of pediatric spasticity. J Child Neurol. 2006; 21(3):189–192

[56] Schroeder AS, Berweck S, Lee SH, Heinen F. Botulinum toxin treatment of children with cerebral palsy—a short review of different injection techniques. Neurotox Res. 2006; 9(2–3): 189–196

[57] Wallen M, O'Flaherty SJ, Waugh MC. Functional outcomes of intramuscular botulinum toxin type a and occupational therapy in the upper limbs of children with cerebral palsy: a randomized controlled trial. Arch Phys Med Rehabil. 2007; 88(1):1–10

[58] Hurvitz EA, Leonard C, Ayyangar R, Nelson VS. Complementary and alternative medicine use in families of children with cerebral palsy. Dev Med Child Neurol. 2003; 45(6):364–370

[59] Glew GM, Fan MY, Hagland S, Bjornson K, Beider S, McLaughlin JF. Survey of the use of massage for children with cerebral palsy. Int J Ther Massage Bodywork. 2010; 3 (4):10–15

[60] Tilton AH. Therapeutic interventions for tone abnormalities in cerebral palsy. NeuroRx. 2006; 3(2):217–224

[61] Tilton A. Management of spasticity in children with cerebral palsy. Semin Pediatr Neurol. 2009; 16(2):82–89

[62] Steinbok P. Selection of treatment modalities in children with spastic cerebral palsy. Neurosurg Focus. 2006; 21(2):e4

[63] Gigante P, McDowell MM, Bruce SS, et al. Reduction in upper-extremity tone after lumbar selective dorsal rhizotomy in children with spastic cerebral palsy. J Neurosurg Pediatr. 2013; 12(6):588–594

[64] Ghotbi N, Ansari NN, Naghdi S, Hasson S, Jamshidpour B, Amiri S. Inter-rater reliability of the modified Ashworth Scale in assessing lower limb muscle spasticity. Brain Inj. 2009; 23(10):815–819

[65] Loewen P, Steinbok P, Holsti L, MacKay M. Upper extremity performance and self-care skill changes in children with spastic cerebral palsy following selective posterior rhizotomy. Pediatr Neurosurg. 1998; 29(4):191–198

[66] Ojemann JG, McKinstry RC, Mukherjee P, Park TS, Burton H. Hand somatosensory cortex activity following selective dorsal rhizotomy: report of three cases with fMRI. Childs Nerv Syst. 2005; 21(2):115–121

[67] Armstrong RW, Steinbok P, Cochrane DD, Kube SD, Fife SE, Farrell K. Intrathecally administered baclofen for treatment of children with spasticity of cerebral origin. J Neurosurg. 1997; 87(3):409–414

[68] Awaad Y, Tayem H, Munoz S, Ham S, Michon AM, Awaad R. Functional assessment following intrathecal baclofen therapy in children with spastic cerebral palsy. J Child Neurol. 2003; 18(1):26–34

[69] Corry IS, Cosgrove AP, Walsh EG, McClean D, Graham HK. Botulinum toxin A in the hemiplegic upper limb: a double-blind trial. Dev Med Child Neurol. 1997; 39(3):185–193

[70] Baker R, Jasinski M, Maciag-Tymecka I, et al. Botulinum toxin treatment of spasticity in diplegic cerebral palsy: a

randomized, double-blind, placebo-controlled, dose-ranging study. Dev Med Child Neurol. 2002; 44(10):666–675

[71] Francisco GE. Botulinum toxin: dosing and dilution. Am J Phys Med Rehabil. 2004; 83 suppl 10:S30–S37

[72] Fitoussi F, Ilharreborde B, Presedo A, Souchet P, Penneçot GF, Mazda K. Shoulder external rotator selective neurotomy in cerebral palsy: anatomical study and preliminary clinical results. J Pediatr Orthop B. 2010; 19(1):71–76

[73] Sitthinamsuwan B, Chanvanitkulchai K, Nunta-Aree S, Kumthornthip W, Pisarnpong A, Ploypetch T. Combined ablative neurosurgical procedures in a patient with mixed spastic and dystonic cerebral palsy. Stereotact Funct Neurosurg. 2010; 88(3):187–192

[74] Park TS, Gaffney PE, Kaufman BA, Molleston MC. Selective lumbosacral dorsal rhizotomy immediately caudal to the conus medullaris for cerebral palsy spasticity. Neurosurgery. 1993; 33(5):929–933, discussion 933–934

[75] Steinbok P, Tidemann AJ, Miller S, Mortenson P, Bowen-Roberts T. Electrophysiologically guided versus non-electrophysiologically guided selective dorsal rhizotomy for spastic cerebral palsy: a comparison of outcomes. Childs Nerv Syst. 2009; 25(9):1091–1096

[76] Steinbok P, Reiner AM, Beauchamp R, Armstrong RW, Cochrane DD, Kestle J. A randomized clinical trial to compare selective posterior rhizotomy plus physiotherapy with physiotherapy alone in children with spastic diplegic cerebral palsy. Dev Med Child Neurol. 1997; 39(3):178–184

[77] McLaughlin JF, Bjornson KF, Astley SJ, et al. Selective dorsal rhizotomy: efficacy and safety in an investigator-masked randomized clinical trial. Dev Med Child Neurol. 1998; 40(4):220–232

[78] McLaughlin J, Bjornson K, Temkin N, et al. Selective dorsal rhizotomy: meta-analysis of three randomized controlled trials. Dev Med Child Neurol. 2002; 44(1):17–25

[79] Wright FV, Sheil EM, Drake JM, Wedge JH, Naumann S. Evaluation of selective dorsal rhizotomy for the reduction of spasticity in cerebral palsy: a randomized controlled tria. Dev Med Child Neurol. 1998; 40(4):239–247

[80] Nordmark E, Josenby AL, Lagergren J, Andersson G, Strömblad LG, Westbom L. Long-term outcomes five years after selective dorsal rhizotomy. BMC Pediatr. 2008; 8:54

[81] Newberg NL, Gooch JL, Walker ML. Intraoperative monitoring in selective dorsal rhizotomy. Pediatr Neurosurg. 1991–1992; 17(3):124–127

[82] Albright AL, Turner M, Pattisapu JV. Best-practice surgical techniques for intrathecal baclofen therapy. J Neurosurg. 2006; 104 suppl 4:233–239

[83] Kopell BH, Sala D, Doyle WK, Feldman DS, Wisoff JH, Weiner HL. Subfascial implantation of intrathecal baclofen pumps in children: technical note. Neurosurgery. 2001; 49(3):753–756, discussion 756–757

[84] Maarrawi J, Mertens P, Luaute J, et al. Long-term functional results of selective peripheral neurotomy for the treatment of spastic upper limb: prospective study in 31 patients. J Neurosurg. 2006; 104(2):215–225

[85] Deletis V, Vodusek DB, Abbott R, Epstein FJ, Turndorf H. Intraoperative monitoring of the dorsal sacral roots: minimizing the risk of iatrogenic micturition disorders. Neurosurgery. 1992; 30(1):72–75

[86] Fasano VA, Broggi G, Barolat-Romana G, Sguazzi A. Surgical treatment of spasticity in cerebral palsy. Childs Brain. 1978; 4(5):289–305

[87] Peacock WJ, Arens LJ. Selective posterior rhizotomy for the relief of spasticity in cerebral palsy. S Afr Med J. 1982; 62(4):119–124

[88] Steinbok P, Schrag C. Complications after selective posterior rhizotomy for spasticity in children with cerebral palsy. Pediatr Neurosurg. 1998; 28(6):300–313

[89] Abbott R, Forem SL, Johann M. Selective posterior rhizotomy for the treatment of spasticity: a review. Childs Nerv Syst. 1989; 5(6):337–346

[90] Abbott R, Johann-Murphy M, Shiminski-Maher T, et al. Selective dorsal rhizotomy: outcome and complications in treating spastic cerebral palsy. Neurosurgery. 1993; 33(5):851–857, discussion 857

[91] Arens LJ, Peacock WJ, Peter J. Selective posterior rhizotomy: a long-term follow-up study. Childs Nerv Syst. 1989; 5(3):148–152

[92] Fasano VA, Broggi G, Zeme S, Lo Russo G, Sguazzi A. Long-term results of posterior functional rhizotomy. Acta Neurochir Suppl (Wien). 1980; 30:435–439

[93] Mooney JF, III, Millis MB. Spinal deformity after selective dorsal rhizotomy in patients with cerebral palsy. Clin Orthop Relat Res. 1999(364):48–52

[94] Turi M, Kalen V. The risk of spinal deformity after selective dorsal rhizotomy. J Pediatr Orthop. 2000; 20(1):104–107

[95] Dudley RW, Parolin M, Gagnon B, et al. Long-term functional benefits of selective dorsal rhizotomy for spastic cerebral palsy. J Neurosurg Pediatr. 2013; 12(2):142–150

[96] O'Brien DF, Park TS, Puglisi JA, Collins DR, Leuthardt EC. Effect of selective dorsal rhizotomy on need for orthopedic surgery for spastic quadriplegic cerebral palsy: long-term outcome analysis in relation to age. J Neurosurg. 2004; 101 suppl 1:59–63

[97] Watt JM, Robertson CM, Grace MG. Early prognosis for ambulation of neonatal intensive care survivors with cerebral palsy. Dev Med Child Neurol. 1989; 31(6):766–773

[98] Motta F, Buonaguro V, Stignani C. The use of intrathecal baclofen pump implants in children and adolescents: safety and complications in 200 consecutive cases. J Neurosurg. 2007; 107 suppl 1:32–35

[99] Murphy NA, Irwin MC, Hoff C. Intrathecal baclofen therapy in children with cerebral palsy: efficacy and complications. Arch Phys Med Rehabil. 2002; 83(12):1721–1725

[100] Dickey MP, Rice M, Kinnett DG, et al. Infectious complications of intrathecal baclofen pump devices in a pediatric population. Pediatr Infect Dis J. 2013; 32(7):715–722

[101] Coffey JR, Cahill D, Steers W, et al. Intrathecal baclofen for intractable spasticity of spinal origin: results of a long-term multicenter study. J Neurosurg. 1993; 78(2):226–232

[102] Penn RD. Intrathecal baclofen for spasticity of spinal origin: seven years of experience. J Neurosurg. 1992; 77(2):236–240

[103] Gardner B, Jamous A, Teddy P, et al. Intrathecal baclofen—a multicentre clinical comparison of the Medtronics Programmable, Cordis Secor and Constant Infusion Infusaid drug delivery systems. Paraplegia. 1995; 33(10):551–554

[104] Taira T, Ueta T, Katayama Y, et al. Rate of complications among the recipients of intrathecal baclofen pump in Japan: a multicenter study. Neuromodulation. 2013; 16(3):266–272, discussion 272

[105] Watve SV, Sivan M, Raza WA, Jamil FF. Management of acute overdose or withdrawal state in intrathecal baclofen therapy. Spinal Cord. 2012; 50(2):107–111

[106] Gooch JL, Oberg WA, Grams B, Ward LA, Walker ML. Complications of intrathecal baclofen pumps in children. Pediatr Neurosurg. 2003; 39(1):1–6

[107] Kofler M, Kronenberg MF, Rifici C, Saltuari L, Bauer G. Epileptic seizures associated with intrathecal baclofen application. Neurology. 1994; 44(1):25–27

[108] Deltombe T, Gustin T. Selective tibial neurotomy in the treatment of spastic equinovarus foot in hemiplegic patients: a 2-year longitudinal follow-up of 30 cases. Arch Phys Med Rehabil. 2010; 91(7):1025–1030

[109] Kim JH, Lee JI, Kim MS, Kim SH. Long-term results of microsurgical selective tibial neurotomy for spastic foot: comparison of adult and child. J Korean Neurosurg Soc. 2010; 47(4):247–251

[110] Hesselgard K, Reinstrup P, Stromblad LG, Undén J, Romner B. Selective dorsal rhizotomy and postoperative pain management. A worldwide survey. Pediatr Neurosurg. 2007; 43(2):107–112

[111] Anderson RCMC, Pinkus DW. Spastizcity—selective dorsal rhizotomy. In: Jallo GI, ed. Controversies in Pediatric Neurosurgery. 1st ed. New York, NY: Thieme; 2012

[112] Engsberg JR, Ross SA, Wagner JM, Park TS. Changes in hip spasticity and strength following selective dorsal rhizotomy and physical therapy for spastic cerebral palsy. Dev Med Child Neurol. 2002; 44(4):220–226

[113] Richardson D. Physical therapy in spasticity. Eur J Neurol. 2002; 9 suppl 1:17–22, 53–61

[114] Tardieu C, Lespargot A, Tabary C, Bret MD. For how long must the soleus muscle be stretched each day to prevent contracture? Dev Med Child Neurol. 1988; 30 (1):3–10

[115] Damiano DL. Activity, activity, activity: rethinking our physical therapy approach to cerebral palsy. Phys Ther. 2006; 86(11):1534–1540

[116] Engsberg JR, Ross SA, Park TS. Changes in ankle spasticity and strength following selective dorsal rhizotomy and physical therapy for spastic cerebral palsy. J Neurosurg. 1999; 91(5):727–732

[117] Langerak NG, Lamberts RP, Fieggen AG, et al. A prospective gait analysis study in patients with diplegic cerebral palsy 20 years after selective dorsal rhizotomy. J Neurosurg Pediatr. 2008; 1(3):180–186

[118] Kan P, Gooch J, Amini A, et al. Surgical treatment of spasticity in children: comparison of selective dorsal rhizotomy and intrathecal baclofen pump implantation. Childs Nerv Syst. 2008; 24(2):239–243

[119] Steinbok P. Outcomes after selective dorsal rhizotomy for spastic cerebral palsy. Childs Nerv Syst. 2001; 17(1–2):1–18

[120] Mittal S, Farmer JP, Al-Atassi B, et al. Impact of selective posterior rhizotomy on fine motor skills. Long-term results using a validated evaluative measure. Pediatr Neurosurg. 2002; 36(3):133–141

[121] Albright AL, Gilmartin R, Swift D, Krach LE, Ivanhoe CB, McLaughlin JF. Long-term intrathecal baclofen therapy for severe spasticity of cerebral origin. J Neurosurg. 2003; 98 (2):291–295

[122] Gilmartin R, Bruce D, Storrs BB, et al. Intrathecal baclofen for management of spastic cerebral palsy: multicenter trial. J Child Neurol. 2000; 15(2):71–77

[123] Gerszten PC, Albright AL, Barry MJ. Effect on ambulation of continuous intrathecal baclofen infusion. Pediatr Neurosurg. 1997; 27(1):40–44

[124] Francisco GE, Boake C. Improvement in walking speed in poststroke spastic hemiplegia after intrathecal baclofen therapy: a preliminary study. Arch Phys Med Rehabil. 2003; 84(8):1194–1199

[125] Bleyenheuft C, Filipetti P, Caldas C, Lejeune T. Experience with external pump trial prior to implantation for intrathecal baclofen in ambulatory patients with spastic cerebral palsy. Neurophysiol Clin. 2007; 37(1):23–28

[126] Garland DE, Thompson R, Waters RL. Musculocutaneous neurectomy for spastic elbow flexion in non-functional upper extremities in adults. J Bone Joint Surg Am. 1980; 62 (1):108–112

Section IX

Trauma

IX

48 Neonatal Brachial Plexus Injury

Jonathan Pindrik

48.1 Introduction

Neonatal brachial plexus injury (nBPI) occurs within 0.4 to 4 newborns per 1,000 live births annually.[1,2,3] Shoulder dystocia indicates trapping of the anterior shoulder below the pelvic rim during delivery. While several obstetric maneuvers ameliorate passage of the neonate through the birth canal, mechanical or stretching forces jeopardize the structural and functional integrity of the brachial plexus. Temporary deficits that resolve completely represent a *neurapraxia*. Other injuries result in prolonged deficits that may improve with surgical intervention and/or spontaneous neural regeneration. The severity of nBPI typically relates to the number of nerves involved, degree of structural damage and functional impairment, and duration of neurological deficits.[3]

- Perinatal risk factors for nBPI: Fetal macrosomia, prior delivery history of nBPI, multiparity, and breech or complex deliveries (including those requiring vacuum or forceps assistance).[1,2]
- Nearly one-third of infants with mild nBPI exhibit incomplete recovery by 6 months of age.[1,2,3]
- Over 80% of infants with severe nBPI exhibit residual deficits by 6 months of age.[3]
- Neuropathological grading of nBPI severity is based on the Sunderland classification: I—neurapraxia; II—axonotmesis with myelin damage; III—axonotmesis with endoneurial damage; IV—axonotmesis with perineurial disruption; V—neurotmesis with nerve discontinuity.[1,4]

- Clinical grading system for nBPI severity: Narakas' classification[3] (▶ Table 48.1).
- Less severe nBPIs show a greater propensity for spontaneous neural regeneration and functional recovery.[3] More severe nBPIs typically result in permanent deficits and require surgical intervention.[2]

48.2 Anatomy

Originating from roots C5–T1, the brachial plexus represents an organized network of peripheral nerves ultimately innervating sensory dermatomes and muscle groups associated with the upper extremity. Most nBPIs occur proximally at the level of roots or trunks and affect the upper trunk (C5–C6) as in Erb–Duchenne palsy. The middle trunk (C7) also may sustain damage. Lower trunk (C8–T1) injuries, consistent with Klumpke's palsy, rarely occur in isolation but may appear in severe nBPI extending to the lower plexus.[2] Mild nBPIs involve stretch or traction injury with transient conduction impairment, while more severe nBPIs may result in neuroma formation or nerve root avulsion. A *neuroma* represents a focal collection of fibrosis and misdirected sprouting axons along the course of an injured peripheral nerve.[4]

- The proximal portion of the brachial plexus traverses the posterior cervical triangle, bordered by the sternocleidomastoid, trapezius, and clavicle.
- The hierarchical structure of the brachial plexus from proximal to distal: Roots → trunks → divisions → cords → branches (▶ Fig. 48.1).

Table 48.1 Narakas' classification for neonatal brachial plexus injury (nBPI) severity

Narakas' grade	Description of injury	Comment
I	Involves upper trunk (C5, C6)	- Classic Erb–Duchenne palsy[1,2] - Most common and least severe type[1] - Most favorable prognosis[1]
II	Involves upper and middle trunks (C5, C6, C7)	- Less severe than type III or IV lesions - Second most common type of nBPI[1]
III	Involves full plexus (C5–T1) with global impairment	- Type III and IV lesions account for nearly 25% of nBPIs
IV	Involves full plexus (C5–T1) with arm flaccidity and possible Horner's syndrome	- Most severe type of nBPI - Suggests presence of preganglionic nerve root avulsions[1]

Source: Data from Foad SL, Mehlman CT, Foad MB, Lippert WC. Prognosis following neonatal brachial plexus palsy: an evidence-based review. J Child Orthop 2009;3(6):459–463.

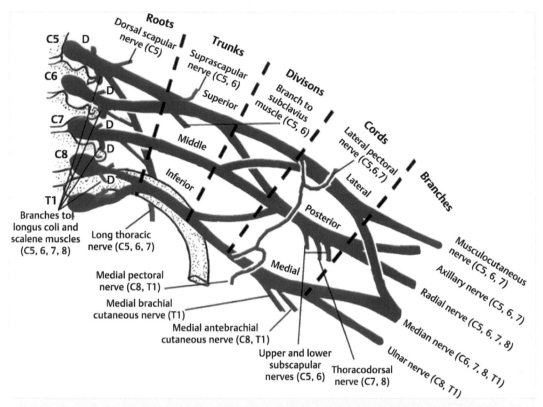

Fig. 48.1 Anatomical diagram of the brachial plexus. (Reproduced with permission from Figure 1–44. Brachial Plexus. Page 80. Comprehensive Neurosurgery Board Review by Citow, Macdonald, Kraig, Wollmann. Thieme 2000.)

- The nerve roots of the brachial plexus travel between the anterior and middle scalene muscles to form the upper, middle, and lower trunks.
- From their respective trunks, divisions and cords run inferolaterally between the clavicle and first thoracic rib into the axilla.
- The lateral, medial, and posterior cords are named anatomically with respect to the axillary artery.
- Inferior to the clavicle, the cords pass deep to the pectoralis major and minor muscles.

48.3 Examination

Physical examination of infants with nBPI evaluates passive and active movement and any asymmetries or deformities associated with the upper extremity. Examination involves observation of spontaneous activity and intentional reaching or grasping of presented objects.[1] Most nBPIs involve deficits of shoulder external rotation or abduction and elbow flexion. Middle trunk injury addition-

ally impairs extension about the elbow, wrist, and/or fingers. Lower trunk involvement causes deficits in hand or finger movement.

- Assessing the passive range of motion about the shoulder and elbow may reveal contractures.
- Palpation of the pectoralis major, latissimus dorsi, and teres major muscles may reveal tightness.[1]
- Glenohumeral subluxation or instability should be assessed visually and tactilely during rest and passive range of motion exercises.[1]
- Active movement about the shoulder, elbow, wrist, forearm, and fingers should be thoroughly assessed without and with gravity. Findings can be graded and recorded using the Toronto Obstetric Brachial Plexus Active Movement Scale (AMS).
- Examination of other systems may reveal neurological deficits. For instance, approximation of the diaphragmatic height or chest radiography may reveal hemidiaphragm elevation due to phrenic nerve dysfunction.

- Lesions extending inferiorly to the lower trunk may cause an incomplete Horner's syndrome with ptosis and myosis. This often suggests preganglionic nerve root avulsion of C8 and/or T1.[1]

48.4 Nonsurgical Management

Initial patient evaluation within 2 weeks of delivery helps establish a neurological baseline for later comparison in nBPI. The next follow-up appointment should occur at 3 months of age. Depending on the severity of nBPI and management strategy, reevaluation may occur at age 6 to 9 months or sooner. These serial examinations help track the progression of neurological deficits and functional impairment. Patients that exhibit adequate functional recovery (at least partial antigravity strength) in motion about the shoulder, elbow, and/or hand may be managed nonoperatively.[1]

Clinic visits provide the opportunity to link the patient and family with specialists trained in physiotherapy or physical medicine and rehabilitation. Physiotherapy exercises focus on passive range of motion and stimulation to encourage activity of the affected extremity. Furthermore, parents or caretakers may be coached regarding appropriate positioning strategies and activities to mobilize the affected extremity. Supervised home therapy may help reduce contracture formation about the shoulder or elbow, promote shoulder stability, and help prevent neglect of the paretic limb.[1,2] Physiotherapy and rehabilitative care also represent important adjuncts to operative management.

48.5 Surgical Indications

Serial evaluations and monitoring of nBPI allow sufficient time to observe spontaneous neural regeneration.[1] Inadequate functional recovery in shoulder external rotation or abduction, elbow flexion, and/or hand movement by age 3 months prompts surgical consideration during the 3- to 6-month age range.[1,2,5] Some peripheral nerve surgeons prefer surgical intervention at 9 months of age to allow longer observation periods for spontaneous recovery.[1] When nerve root avulsions are present, surgical intervention should occur at the earliest time point.

- Inadequate performance on objective measures such as the Toronto Obstetric Brachial Plexus Active Movement Scale (AMS) and the Cookie test may corroborate surgical decision making.

- The presence of Horner's syndrome on follow-up examination at age 3 months indicates severe nBPI likely spanning the full plexus. Extensive nBPIs usually require early surgical intervention.
- Additional diagnostic studies help investigate the severity of injury and corroborate surgical decision making. Cervical spine magnetic resonance imaging (MRI) may reveal pseudomeningoceles suggesting nerve root avulsion.
- Other ancillary studies include electromyography and nerve conduction studies, performed at or beyond 3 months of age.[2,4] These studies help identify the presence of regenerating motor units and conducting action potentials.

48.6 Surgical Technique

Most operative explorations and repairs of nBPI require a supraclavicular approach. Extension of the traumatic injury or neuroma along the divisions and cords may require the addition of an infraclavicular approach. Following exposure of normal anatomy, the injured elements of the brachial plexus can be identified through direct visualization and nerve stimulation. Depending on the extent of injury and function of donor nerves, various methods of repair may be employed. Different types of peripheral nerve repair include neurolysis, neuroma resection and grafting, and nerve transfers (with or without bridging grafts). The goals of surgery revolve around promoting neural regeneration and muscular reinnervation to improve elbow flexion and shoulder stability, abduction, and external rotation. Additional approaches target hand and finger functional recovery. For all nBPI explorations and repairs, anesthetic paralytic agents should be avoided.

- Patient position: Supine, head rotated contralaterally, with a rolled sheet or bump under the upper torso to elevate the supraclavicular region.
- Special lucent drapes or sterile preparation of the affected extremity within the surgical field allow intraoperative nerve stimulation and observation of muscular contractions.
- One or both lower extremities should be sterilely prepared from the popliteal fossa to lateral malleolus if surgical planning involves sural nerve harvesting.
- Skin incision for supraclavicular approach: Parallel to and one to two finger-breadths above

the clavicle, extending laterally toward the anterior border of the trapezius and medially along the posterior border of the sternocleidomastoid (as needed).[6]

- Skin incision for infraclavicular approach: Vertically oblique line along the deltopectoral groove, curving medially toward the clavicle.
- Relevant anatomical landmarks: See ▶ Table 48.2.
- Brachial plexus exposure requires careful division of the anterior scalene while protecting the phrenic nerve.
- Division of the anterior scalene first exposes the upper trunk and C5–C6 nerve roots. Gentle retraction of the upper trunk exposes the underlying middle and lower trunks.

- Fibrotic scarring and neuroma formation in nBPI may complicate plexus exploration. Neuroma formation typically occurs along the upper or middle trunks.
- Nerve stimulation and observation of muscle contraction aid identification of plexus elements and help investigate the presence of conduction across a neuroma or region of trauma.
- After identification of a neuroma or nonfunctioning plexus elements, several different methods of repair may be employed (▶ Table 48.3).
- Common examples of nerve grafting include cables between the C5 or C6 nerve roots and anterior or posterior divisions of the upper trunk or lateral cord, following neuroma resection.

Table 48.2 Anatomical landmarks in neonatal brachial plexus injury (nBPI) surgery

Anatomical structure	Location	Relevance/comments
Platysma mm.	First layer of mm. deep to skin during supraclavicular approach	Separated during exposure and reapproximated during closure
Sternocleidomastoid mm. (SCM)	Deep to platysma, along medial aspect of exposure	Dividing the lateral one-third of this mm. enhances exposure of the plexus
Supraclavicular fat pad	Deep to platysma, along inferior aspect of exposure	Careful dissection or retraction of the fat pad allows better visualization of deep structures
Omohyoid mm.	Inferior belly lies within lower region of neck, deep to the SCM	Division or retraction of this mm. helps expose deeper structures
Anterior scalene mm.	Deep to SCM and omohyoid, along medial aspect of exposure	• Brachial plexus travels between anterior and middle scalene mm. • Division of anterior scalene mm. exposes the proximal plexus
Phrenic n.	Ventral surface of the anterior scalene mm., running from lateral to medial as it descends	• Stimulation with low amplitude produces diaphragmatic contractions • Requires careful protection while dividing the anterior scalene mm.
Subclavian a. and v.	• Subclavian a. lies between anterior and middle scalene mm. • Subclavian v. lies ventral to anterior scalene mm. • Both lie near lower trunk and C7 transverse process	• Damage to either structure may require assistance from vascular surgery team
Clavicle	• Located between manubrium of the sternum and acromion of the scapula	• Typically hinders visualization and manipulation of underlying divisions or proximal cords of the plexus
Pectoralis major mm.	• Origin: medial clavicle, sternum, costal cartilage, aponeurosis of external oblique mm. • Insertion: proximal humerus	• Separation of fibers during an infra-clavicular approach allows exposure of underlying pectoralis minor mm. and distal brachial plexus
Pectoralis minor mm.	• Deep to pectoralis major mm. • Origin: ribs 3–5 (anterior surface) • Insertion: scapula (coracoid process)	• Division of this mm. exposes distal brachial plexus (cords, proximal branches)

Abbreviations: a., artery; mm., muscle(s); n., nerve; v., vein.

Table 48.3 Methods of repair neonatal brachial plexus injury (nBPI)

Method of repair	Description	Applicability/comments
Neurolysis	Dissection along the longitudinal axis of a nerve to expose fascicles	• Applicable to neuroma or fibrotic scarring along the course of a nerve • Release of scar tissue may enhance peripheral nerve regeneration
Neuroma resection	Division of a nerve segment proximal and distal to a region of obvious scarring and dysfunction	• Applicable to any neuroma, especially with poor conduction along the nerve • Requires grafting across the resultant defect
Nerve grafting	• Bridging the gap between proximal and distal portions of damaged nerve • Autologous grafts include MABCN and sural nerves • Artificial grafts include synthetic nerve guides typically approved for defects up to 30 mm in length[7,8]	• Applicable to gap between proximal and distal nerve stumps created by neuroma resection or nerve root avulsion • May also parallel a nonresected neuroma when affixed to nerve segments proximal and distal to the site of injury
Nerve transfer or neurotization	• Promotes neural regeneration by adjoining proximal end of functioning nerve to distal end of nonfunctioning nerve • Decrements the function of donor nerve, while favoring regeneration of damaged target motor nerves	• Applicable to nonfunctioning nerves distal to the level of injury (beyond a nerve root avulsion or neuroma) • Useful in preganglionic nerve root avulsions when proximal nerve ends are not available for grafting[5]

Abbreviation: MABCN, medial antebrachial cutaneous nerve.

Table 48.4 Different examples of nerve transfer for neonatal brachial plexus injury (nBPI)

Common nerve transfers	Ultimate goal	Comments
Spinal accessory n. → suprascapular n.	Shoulder stability, arm abduction	Spinal accessory n. is dissected along anterior border of trapezius mm.
Radial n. (triceps branch) → axillary n.	Shoulder stability, arm abduction	Usually requires dorsal approach to shoulder within quadrilateral space[5]
Ulnar n. → musculocutaneous n. (biceps branch)	Elbow flexion	Classic Oberlin technique[1,2,5]
Median n. → musculocutaneous n. (brachialis branch)	Elbow flexion	Modified Oberlin technique[1,2,5]
Intercostal n. → musculocutaneous n. (biceps branch)	Elbow flexion	Typically requires at least 3 intercostal nerve donors[5]
Medial pectoral n. → musculocutaneous n. or axillary n.	Elbow flexion or shoulder stability	

Abbreviations: mm., muscle; n., nerve(s).

• Synthetic nerve guides help reduce operative times and eliminate donor-site morbidity, but have shown encouraging results only for short gaps up to 30 mm in length.[7,8]
• Several options for nerve transfers (neurotization) exist depending on the function of plexus elements (▶ Table 48.4).
• Common targets of neurotization include the suprascapular, musculocutaneous, and axillary nerves. Ulnar nerve targeting helps recover hand function in nBPI involving the lower trunk.

• Complete nBPI with preganglionic avulsions may benefit from contralateral C7 nerve root transfer targeting elbow flexion or hand movement. This may additionally require a vascularized ulnar nerve graft due to large gap distances.[1,3,5]
• Grafting and neurotization require neurolysis to expose healthy-appearing fascicles in preparation for coaptation. Coaptation can be performed in end-to-end, end-to-side, or side-to-side fashion.

- Nerve grafts or transfers are secured with adhesive glue at the site of nerve coaptation. The junction can be reinforced with one to two low-caliber epineurial sutures prior to gluing.
- Free gracilis muscle transfers are employed in delayed fashion during secondary surgery to recapitulate elbow flexion. This technique requires neurotization from intercostal, spinal accessory, or ulnar nerves to the preserved recipient obturator nerve.[3,5]
- Other examples of secondary surgery for nBPI include attempts to improve shoulder stability with trapezius or latissimus dorsi tendon transfers or osteotomies.

48.7 Complications

Complications of nBPI exploration and repair may occur intraoperatively or postoperatively. Surgical risks include damage to nearby vasculature or nerves. Injury to the subclavian vessels may require assistance from a vascular surgeon, while trauma to the phrenic nerve may result in respiratory compromise or hemidiaphragm elevation. In more complicated repairs, harvesting intercostal nerves may cause violation of the pleura and pneumothorax. Occurrence of these latter events can be evaluated with plain chest radiography. Postoperative complications include delayed surgical site hematoma, wound infection or dehiscence, lack of functional recovery in targeted muscle groups, or decrement of function in a donor nerve used for neurotization.

48.8 Postoperative Care

Postoperative care for nBPI repair involves a combination of early immobilization to protect nerve grafts or transfers, wound monitoring, and eventual rehabilitative therapy. For the first 2 to 3 weeks following surgery, upper extremity immobilization and sling support ensure the continuity of nerve coaptations. Postoperative follow-up within 10 to 14 days allows adequate wound inspection and investigation of muscle groups potentially affected by nerve donor usage in neurotization. After immobilization, physiotherapy and rehabilitation represent important adjuncts in the management of nBPI. Patients and caretakers should be seen regularly for physiotherapy and guidance with passive and active motion exercises or rehabilitative devices.

48.9 Outcomes

The length of peripheral nerve regeneration required to reinnervate target muscles determines the anticipated duration of recovery.[2] Since peripheral nerve growth and regeneration occur at a rate of 1 mm/day, observing functional recovery requires prolonged follow-up.[4] Full realization of functional improvement may require up to 2 years following surgery due to the necessity of physiotherapy and adaptation following neurotization. Surgical success rates of functional recovery depend on the type of repair and vary between 67 and above 90%, with lower rates (< 50%) for contralateral C7 transfers.[2,5] Long-term morbidity most commonly relates to shoulder weakness or instability, affecting over one-third of nBPI patients.[1] Complications associated with the glenohumeral joint include contracture, subluxation, and deformity requiring surgical correction.

Surgical outcomes are influenced by location of the injury and timing of surgical intervention. While upper trunk injuries carry the best prognosis for functional recovery, lesions involving the lower trunk exhibit worse outcomes.[1] Additional poor prognostic factors include pan plexopathy and preganglionic avulsions.[1] Regarding timing, early surgical intervention maximizes recovery time. Surgical intervention for nBPI at 3 to 6 months of age typically offers better chances of functional recovery.[1] Primary exploration or repair in nBPI beyond 9 to 12 months of age may portend worse outcome due to target muscle fibrosis and scarring. Ideally, reinnervation of target muscle groups should occur by 18 months to provide the best chance for functional recovery.[4,7] Patients with unimproved deficits following primary surgery, failed conservative management, or delayed presentation may benefit from secondary surgery involving free muscle (e.g., gracilis) transfers.

48.10 Surgical Pearls

- Identification of a dorsal root ganglion (DRG) distal to its normal location within the neural foramen implies nerve root avulsion.
- The suprascapular nerve represents an important early branch of the plexus whose origin helps confirm the identity of the upper trunk.
- Vascular loops placed without tension around identified nerves help organize the surgical field.

- Nerve conduction across a neuroma with muscular contraction distally suggests some degree of spontaneous reinnervation. In this setting, less aggressive surgical techniques include neurolysis, side-to-side cable grafting along the neuroma, and/or distal nerve transfers. However, many peripheral nerve surgeons routinely advocate neuroma resection and grafting.[1]
- Nerve coaptation in grafting and neurotization should be accomplished without tension on the nerve segments.
- Testing for excursion involves observing nerve donor and recipient relative motion during upper extremity movement to estimate the length of nerve dissection required to prevent tension or separation following coaptation.
- Intraoperative nerve stimulation, harvesting nerve grafts, and division of nerves require careful attention. Respect the common adage: Measure/check twice, cut once.
- Specialized centers facilitating a multidisciplinary approach with peripheral nerve surgeons, pediatric neurologists, physiotherapists, and specialists in physical medicine and rehabilitation offer the best management strategy for patients with nBPI.

48.11 Common Clinical Questions

1. Describe the appearance of an upper extremity in nBPI involving the upper trunk (classic Erb–Duchenne palsy).
2. Which management strategy represents the optimal approach in nBPI with evidence of partial but incomplete biceps functional recovery at 3 months of age?
3. In the context of preganglionic nerve root avulsion, will the affected peripheral nerve conduct sensory nerve action potentials?
4. Can nerve grafting and transfers be combined within the same procedure?

48.12 Answers to Common Clinical Questions

1. Injuries confined to the upper trunk (C5–C6) cause weakness in the supraspinatus, infraspinatus, deltoid, biceps, and brachial muscles.[2] In this context, the upper extremity appears adducted, internally rotated, extended at the elbow, and pronated along the forearm.[2] Additional middle trunk (C7) involvement causes unopposed flexion of the wrist and fingers.[2]

2. The optimal treatment strategy in this situation has not been determined. No randomized, controlled clinical trial has compared nonoperative and operative management for incomplete functional recovery at 3 to 6 months following nBPI. Many authors advocate surgical intervention; however, case series have reported spontaneous recovery without operative intervention despite lack of elbow flexion at 3 months age.[2] Furthermore, controversy exists between different surgical approaches. Many peripheral nerve surgeons advocate neuroma resection and grafting, while newer approaches involve neurolysis or distal nerve transfers.

3. Yes. In the context of nerve root avulsion, sensory nerve action potentials may still conduct along the involved peripheral nerve due to continuity between axons and the neuronal cell body within the DRG. The differentiation between preganglionic and post-postganglionic injury represents an important distinction in nBPI. The presence of preganglionic nerve root avulsion carries significant implications for anticipated recovery and surgical planning. Without surgical intervention, spontaneous reinnervation will not occur in the distribution of avulsed nerves. To promote functional recovery, brachial plexus exploration and repair should be planned early (after 3 months of age). Without the presence of proximal nerve stumps for grafting, several types of nerve transfer can be employed.

4. Nerve grafting and transfers are commonly employed in the same surgical approach to the brachial plexus. These techniques can be combined on the same nerve construct, as with an ulnar or median nerve to musculocutaneous nerve transfer with an interpositional bridging nerve graft. The graft may be harvested from the medial antebrachial cutaneous nerve or sural nerve. Interpositional nerve grafts from a proximal intercostal nerve stump have proven less effective; therefore, direct intercostal nerve transfers to the musculocutaneous nerve are favored currently.[3,5] Alternatively, neurotization may reinforce nBPI repair separate from the site of grafting. For instance, nerve grafting from the C5 nerve root to the suprascapular nerve following neuroma resection can be supplemented by distal Oberlin's or modified

Oberlin's transfers. While the former approach promotes shoulder abduction and stability, the latter techniques provide for elbow flexion.

References

[1] Hale HB, Bae DS, Waters PM. Current concepts in the management of brachial plexus birth palsy. J Hand Surg Am. 2010; 35(2):322–331

[2] Malessy MJA, Pondaag W. Obstetric brachial plexus injuries. Neurosurg Clin N Am. 2009; 20(1):1–14, v

[3] Foad SL, Mehlman CT, Foad MB, Lippert WC. Prognosis following neonatal brachial plexus palsy: an evidence-based review. J Child Orthop. 2009; 3(6):459–463

[4] Belzberg AJ. Acute nerve injuries. Rengachary SS, Ellenbogen RG, eds. Principles of Neurosurgery. 2nd ed. Philadelphia, PA: Elsevier Mosby; 2005:387–395

[5] Shin AY, Spinner RJ, Bishop AT. Nerve transfers for brachial plexus injuries. Oper Tech Orthop. 2004; 14:199–212

[6] Laurent JP. Supraclavicular approach to birth-related brachial plexus injury. Albright AL, Pollack IF, Adelson PD, eds. Operative Techniques in Pediatric Neurosurgery. New York, NY: Thieme; 2001:219–225

[7] Siemionow M, Brzezicki G. Chapter 8: Current techniques and concepts in peripheral nerve repair. Int Rev Neurobiol. 2009; 87:141–172

[8] Dornseifer U, Matiasek K, Fichter MA, et al. Surgical therapy of peripheral nerve lesions: current status and new perspectives. Zentralbl Neurochir. 2007; 68(3): 101–110

49 Pediatric Spine Trauma

Douglas Brockmeyer

49.1 Introduction

Spine trauma is a common occurrence in the pediatric age group. This chapter will outline common spinal injuries in children, as well as their evaluation and management. Surgical approaches to the treatment of unstable pediatric cervical spine injuries are highlighted.

49.2 Epidemiology

Although less common than spinal trauma in other age groups, pediatric spinal injuries are not rare. The incidence of pediatric spine trauma within the overall population of spinal injuries ranges from 1 to 11%.[1,2,3] A reasonable estimate at most major pediatric trauma centers is that 5% of spinal column and spinal cord injuries will occur in the age group between 0 and 16 years of age. Males more frequently sustained spinal column and spinal cord injuries than females.[1] This statistic is influenced by an increased likelihood of vertebral column injury in adolescent males in the 10- to 16-year-old age group. The pediatric spine can be subjected to every pattern of force that its adult counterpart may see. The actual type of injury responsible for the mechanism varies according to the age of the patient.

- Differences in referral patterns, injury grading, and treatment and outcome measures between physicians all mask the true incidence and severity of pediatric spinal cord and spinal column injury.
- The lack of a standardized nationwide database for these injuries has hampered our understanding of this disease process. Until strict guidelines and a national database are established, our understanding of injury patterns and injury types will be incomplete.

49.3 Pathophysiology

- Pure forces of flexion, extension, rotation, axial loading, and distraction have all been documented and described, also combination forces, such as flexion/distraction injuries.
- Spinal cord ischemia either by compression or disruption has also been documented. Compression of the spinal cord from blood clots, fractured bones, bending or buckling of

ligaments, and angulation of the spinal column also occurs.

- Underlying congenital or developmental conditions of the patient, including os odontoideum, Down syndrome, Chiari malformations, congenital bone abnormalities, rheumatoid arthritis, ankylosing spondylitis, and other infections or tumors may contribute to the risk of spinal injury.
- The youngest patients (0–10 years) have a high incidence of falls and pedestrian/automobile accidents, while older children have a higher incidence of motor vehicle accidents, motorcycle accidents, and sports-related injuries.

49.4 Anatomy

The pediatric spine demonstrates significant anatomical and biomechanical differences from the adult spine. Many of the anatomical differences explain the different injury patterns seen in various age groups. The infant spine is very flexible and elastic because of its incomplete development. Between the ages of 2 and 10 years, tremendous changes occur in the supportive elements of the spinal column. Gradually, the spinal anatomy develops an adult configuration. Muscles and ligaments strengthen, bones grow and reach a mature shape and size, and areas of cartilage and soft bone are replaced with normal calcified bone. In addition, the body habitus changes so that the head is smaller in proportion to the torso. These changes shift the focus of injury from the upper cervical spine (skull-C1–C2) to the lower cervical spine (C5–C6).

- The spine of infants between 0 and 2 years of age has tremendous mobility and elasticity because of underdevelopment of the neck muscles; incompletely calcified, wedge-shaped vertebrae; and shallow, horizontally oriented facet joints. The relatively large head size in young patients with respect to the torso increases the likelihood of cervical spine injuries, especially between the skull and first two cervical vertebrae.
- Age-related maturation in the upper pediatric cervical spine is usually completed by approximately age 10, and the maturation of the lower cervical spine occurs by approximately age 14.

- The elasticity of the young spinal column probably allows some protection against spinal cord trauma that might cause fracture in older patients. This mobility and elasticity in the infant spine explains the relatively low incidence of spinal column injuries and the proportionately high incidence of spinal cord injuries without radiographic abnormalities (SCIWORA). In essence, the young spine will stretch, but not break, but this places the spinal cord at increased risk for stretching and disruptive injuries.

49.5 Specific Injuries

As described above, different patterns of spinal cord and spinal column injuries are seen in adult and pediatric patients. This section will expand on these differences in light of specific injury types.

49.5.1 Fractures and Dislocations

Fractures encompass all types of disruption of the bony vertebral column. Fracture types vary widely from simple linear fractures affecting the vertebral bodies or posterior portion of the spine to complex fractures involving several elements of the spine or possibly several vertebral levels. Specific fracture types, listed from least to most unstable, include compression fractures, burst fractures, and fracture/dislocations.

- A fracture may or may not make the spinal column unstable, depending on its type and severity. The AO/Orthopedic Trauma Association classification of spine fractures[4] developed for adults is a good general starting point in determining spinal stability, although it may not be completely applicable in children. Fractures may or may not compress the spinal cord and cause spinal cord injury.
- Dislocation refers to abnormal position and motion between vertebral levels in the spine. Typically, dislocations are caused by injuries of the bony–ligamentous complex that stabilizes each vertebral level. In addition to ligamentous injuries, intervertebral disk disruption may also contribute to spinal dislocation. Obviously, fractures and dislocations may exist either independently or in combination with each other.
- Complex fracture/dislocations are typically the worst type of vertebral column injury and imply both bony and ligamentous disruption. These

patients usually have the most severe neurological injuries as well.

49.5.2 Injuries Seen in Young Children

Young children (< 4 years of age) tend to sustain soft tissue injuries without incurring "true fractures," a finding that reflects hypermobility and skeletal immaturity. Most of the spinal injuries in the first decade of life affect the upper segments of the cervical spinal column. Young children are also prone to ligamentous injury without fracture. In these instances, a higher rate of persistent instability can occur than with fracture dislocation injuries.

Young children sometimes have traumatic growth plate fractures and separations, also known as "synchondrosis fractures." These fractures are highly likely to heal with immobilization; however, the chronic nonunion of an odontoid synchondrosis fracture is thought to be a possible etiological factor behind many cases of os odontoideum. Os odontoideum may lead to chronic instability and confer an increased risk of spinal cord injury.[5] In young patients, a C2 synchondrosis fracture is almost always treated with an external halo orthosis, although surgical stabilization might be needed in rare cases.[6]

49.5.3 Strains and Sprains

Muscular cervical sprains and strains are perhaps the most common type of spinal injury in young children but have been poorly documented because of their "trivial" status. More serious ligamentous injuries also probably have a much higher incidence than we realize, but are most often self-limited.

Cervical strains and sprains may sometimes be diagnosed using a combination of dynamic X-ray imaging and magnetic resonance imaging (MRI), although the diagnostic utility of these modalities is suspect because of the high rate of false-positive results, especially with MRI.[7]

49.5.4 Atlanto-Occipital Dislocation

Atlanto-occipital dislocation (AOD) is an injury of the supporting ligaments of the occipitocervical joint. Flexion, distraction, and rotational mechanisms are commonly involved. Unfortunately, a large proportion of AOD injuries are fatal; their overall incidence is probably underreported.

- Although injuries in this area can result in extreme instability at the craniocervical junction, many are less severe and patients may have little to no neurological deficit.
- Recently, the "condyle–C1 interval" (CCI) has been recognized as a useful measurement for diagnosing AOD.[8] A CCI of greater than 4.0 mm is generally accepted as diagnostic of AOD.

49.5.5 C1–C2 Injuries

Dislocations between C1 and C2 may occur alone or in combination with an O–C1 injury. They may sometimes be misdiagnosed as solely an AOD injury. They are usually due to flexion–distraction mechanisms and commonly occur when a young child restrained in child safety seat is involved in a motor vehicle accident.

49.5.6 Atlantoaxial Rotatory Subluxation

Because of its unique anatomy, the C1–C2 joint is prone to rotational injuries. Most atlantoaxial rotatory subluxation (AARS) injuries are mild and self-limited, but severe AARS injuries can occur, causing significant signs and symptoms, including neck pain and torticollis.

- A general rule of thumb is that if C1–C2 rotational angulation is greater than 30 degrees on axial computed tomography (CT) scan, then the C1–C2 joint capsule is likely incompetent and surgical fixation may be required.

49.5.7 Lower Cervical and Thoracolumbar Injuries

Fractures and dislocations of the lower cervical spine are relatively rare in young patients because of factors involving the maturing spine. Fractures involving the thoracolumbar spine in young children tend to involve the junction between the thoracic and lumbar spine where the relatively rigid thoracic segments join the more mobile lumbar segments. Again, the injuries of younger children tend to involve the soft tissues and ligaments resulting in cartilage or growth plate injuries. The AO classification is generally used to describe fracture types and determine stability.[9]

- In automobile accidents with frontal impact, children restrained by standard rear seat lap

belts can sustain mid lumbar spine fractures. Clues to an injury include lap belt abrasions across the abdomen or lower thorax.

49.5.8 Adolescent Injuries

Adolescents and young adults in the 16- to 24-year-old age group have the highest incidence of spinal injury in many studies. Once the patient's age reaches 15 to 16 years, injury mechanisms and patterns closely resemble those of adults. Typically, fractures are seen more often than soft tissue injuries. Combination fracture and dislocation injuries are seen more often as well. In this age group, the level of injury in the cervical spine is more evenly distributed throughout the entire neck, with the most common level of injury at the C5–C6 level. Spinal column injuries to the thoracic and lumbar levels assume greater importance in the adolescent age group.

- Changes in lifestyle patterns among adolescents account for a large part of the injury pattern differences. Drugs, alcohol, and motor vehicles are all important causative factors in this age group.
- Sports-related accidents also assume a higher prominence in the adolescent age group. In the United States, organized tackle football has the highest incidence of spinal column and spinal cord injury of any sport. In other countries, hockey and rugby account for a significant fraction of sports-related spinal column and spinal cord injuries. Other "at-risk" sports include wrestling and boxing. A more detailed discussion of sports-related spinal column injuries in adolescents is beyond the scope of this discussion.

49.5.9 Spinal Cord Injury without Radiographic Abnormality

SCIWORA is defined as a spinal cord injury that cannot be observed on normal plain radiographic studies and CT.[10,11] There are wide differences in the reporting of SCIWORA and its incidence ranges from 5 to 70% of all pediatric spinal cord injuries, depending on the study examined. A true incidence is probably close to 20% of all pediatric spinal cord injuries. Cervical and thoracic spinal levels are injured with almost equal frequency and lumbar levels are rarely involved. In all cases of suspected SCIWORA injury, an MRI should be performed. It is possible that compressive, treatable lesions may be identified that are not seen on X-ray or CT. Examples of such lesions include hematomas or ligamentous injury not shown on other studies.

SCIWORA is ultimately due to the ligamentous flexibility and elasticity of the immature spine. A young child's vertebral column can withstand elongation without evidence of deformity while the spinal cord is injured. The infant spine and cadaver specimens can withstand up to 2 in of stretch without disruption. In contrast, the spinal cord ruptures after only 1/4 in of stretching. This mismatch of elasticity response between the spinal column and spinal cord is the major factor contributing to the high incidence of SCIWORA injuries in young children.

- SCIWORA occurs almost exclusively among younger children. SCIWORA is very uncommon in adolescents and rare among adults. There are important differences in SCIWORA injury patterns between younger age groups (0–8 years) and older children (9–16 years). Younger patients account for two-thirds of all SCIWORA injuries and have a higher proportion of complete neurological injuries.
- Strict guidelines regarding treatment of this injury are lacking, and there is significant variability between physicians regarding the type of treatment necessary. In general, once a diagnosis of SCIWORA is made, most practitioners are very conservative in their approach, and some type of external immobilization is usually necessary for at least 1 to 2 months.

49.5.10 Birth Injuries

Spinal cord injury due to birth-related trauma is probably underdiagnosed and underreported because of the lack of radiographic findings in most instances. Typically, the upper cervical spine or cervicothoracic junction is affected; however, any level of the spinal cord can be involved and involvement in multiple levels is not uncommon. Two-thirds of all birth injuries accompany breech presentation and one-third occur with cephalic presentation or transverse lie. A wide variety of factors have been implicated in birth-related spinal cord trauma, including mechanical repositioning, breech presentation, and forceps extraction.

- The mortality for birth-related spinal cord injury is high, and survivors may have a poor prognosis. Improved prenatal monitoring and

obstetrical techniques have helped reduce these injuries over time.

49.6 Examination

The principles involved in treatment of pediatric spinal cord injury are similar to those established in adults. Spinal cord injury in the pediatric age group is usually caused by a traumatic insult, and the resulting neurological deficit ranges from an incomplete spinal cord injury with partial loss of function to complete spinal cord injuries where all function below the level of injury is lost.

- Injuries in the high cervical spinal cord affect muscles required for respiration as well as nerves responsible for motor strength and sensation in the arms or legs. In addition, bowel and bladder function is lost if the lesion is complete.
- Injuries to the lower cervical cord have varying degrees of sparing of arm strength depending on the level of the lesion. In these instances, lower extremity and bowel and bladder function are also lost. Injuries in the thoracic spine or in the upper lumbar areas have sparing of the upper extremities, but loss of function in the lower extremities and bowel and bladder.
- Injuries in the lower lumbar spine can show incomplete and patchy loss of function in the lower extremities as well as incomplete loss of function in the bowel and bladder, consistent with a cauda equina syndrome.
- Identifying the proper level and injury affecting the spinal column is important to determine the appropriate treatment protocol. This includes identification of the fracture type (if any), recognition of dislocation and instability, identification of any mass lesions that may be compressing the spinal cord (such as hematomas or ruptured disks), and identification of spinal cord injury.
- This evaluation is firmly based on adequate history and clinical examination as well as the acquisition of proper radiographic studies. Radiographic studies include plain films with or without dynamic (flexion/extension) views and CT and MRI scans.

49.7 Prehospital Management

The treatment of traumatic spinal cord injury should begin in the field shortly after the accident. Modern techniques of resuscitation and transport include complete spine immobilization, application of a rigid cervical collar, and prevention of hypotension. The high-dose methylprednisolone protocol has shown little or no benefit to patients with spinal cord injury,[12] and most major Level 1 trauma centers no longer use it routinely. In the intensive care unit, treatment should be directed at maintaining adequate blood flow and oxygenation to the spinal cord.

49.8 Nonsurgical Management

- There are certain instances in which spinal column injuries may be managed conservatively, often with a hard cervical orthosis. These situations generally include stable fractures and/or ligamentous injuries. Chip fracture, unilateral facet fractures, linear vertebral body fractures, and mild compression fractures are all examples of injuries that might be managed in a hard collar. The time required for hard collar immobilization varies between fractures, but typically is in the range of 1 to 2 months.
- The injury that most commonly requires an external halo orthosis in the pediatric population is a C2 synchondrosis fracture across the base of the odontoid. These fractures most often occur in young children, a population in which direct surgical repair is challenging, and the odds of successful healing across the fracture are high with a halo orthosis.
- The final step in nonsurgical management is close follow-up of the patient after treatment. For example, a patient who has not been operated on and is placed in an external cervical collar may develop progressive kyphotic instability over time. Serial follow-up X-rays are important to make sure that proper treatment is given. In the case of progressive cervical kyphosis, most patients go on to require operative fusion.

49.9 Surgical Indications

The surgical indications for a spinal column injury with or without spinal cord injury include spinal instability (i.e., radiographic demonstration of two-column injury of the cervical spine), the presence of a mass lesion such an epidural hematoma, and/or a traumatic disc rupture with neurological deficit. There are various published adult criteria[13] for predicting instability of the cervical spine, but these criteria have not been validated in children (▶ Table 49.1).

Table 49.1 Checklist for the diagnosis of clinical instability in the middle and lower cervical spine

Element	Point value
Anterior elements destroyed or unable to function	2
Posterior elements destroyed or unable to function	2
Positive stretch test	2
Radiographic criteria • Flexion/extension X-rays - Sagittal plane translation > 3.5 mm or 20% (2 points) - Sagittal plane rotation > 20 degrees (2 points) OR • Resting X-rays - Sagittal plane displacement > 3.5 mm or 20% (2 points) - Relative sagittal plane angulation > 11 degrees (2 points)	4
Abnormal disc narrowing	1
Developmentally narrow spinal canal • Sagittal diameter < 13 mm • 2. Pavlov's ratio < 0.8	1
Spinal cord damage	2
Nerve root damage	1
Dangerous loading anticipated	1
Total of 5 or more = unstable	

Source: Reproduced with permission from White and Panjabi.[14]

49.10 Surgical Technique

- Once the level and injury affecting the spinal column have been identified, the next step is correction of any spinal column deformity that is present. This may require the use of preoperative traction in either Gardner–Wells tongs or a halo ring. A general rule of thumb in children is to use 5 lb of traction per vertebral level.
- An anterior approach is commonly used for treating unstable pediatric cervical spine fractures. The approach is similar to those performed in adults, with minor variations. In children, with their long, slender necks, it is typically very easy to get from C2 all the way down to C7 with an anterior approach.
- The disc material in children is typically very hydrated and fibrous, making for a tedious resection. When preparing the vertebral bodies for fusion, it is very important to remove all of the cartilaginous end plate at each level to ensure bone-to-bone contact for the graft.

- An interbody allograft is commonly used both for discectomies and corpectomies in children.
- One of the most important surgical issues is finding an anterior cervical plating system that fits the patient. In young patients, an adult-sized implant may not fit and another solution must be found. Some device manufacturers make anterior cervical plates with only one fixation screw per level, which is a possible alternative in selected cases.
- Posterior cervical approaches are preferred for occipitocervical instability and atlantoaxial instability, both out of the scope of this chapter. Posterior approaches to subaxial instability in children are commonly performed and are similar to their adult counterparts. The biggest caveat for most posterior lateral mass fixation in children is the size of the lateral mass complex in a given patient. In our experience, after the age of 8 to 10 years, the lateral mass complex is of sufficient size to accept full adult-sized instrumentation.
- For cases involving extreme instability, such as traumatic spondyloptosis, a combined anterior and posterior approach is necessary. The general principles outlined above apply in these situations as well.

49.11 Complications

- Fortunately, complications after cervical spine surgery in children are rare. In general, the risk of surgical site infection is low, but it may be possibly higher for posterior approaches.
- Vascular injury, tracheoesophageal injury, spinal cord injury, and postoperative hematoma are the main complications of anterior cervical surgery.
- Posterior cervical surgery has a similar set of complications as anterior approaches.

49.12 Outcomes

- The rate of successful arthrodesis in the stabilization of traumatic cervical spine injuries is quite high, probably approaching 100%.
- The outcomes for pediatric spinal cord injuries depend primarily on the severity of the initial insult to the spinal cord, followed by the timing and quality of early management. In general, however, children tend to recover better and more quickly than their adult counterparts.

49.13 Postoperative Care and Rehabilitation of Spinal Cord Injury

Once a spinal cord and spinal column injury has been diagnosed and treated, rehabilitation begins. Some patients are lucky enough to have no neurological deficit and will just require close follow-up by their physicians. Other patients have significant neurological deficits and require intensive rehabilitation programs to maximize their potential for recovery of function or learn to function with their new neurological status. Many pediatric hospitals have in-house rehabilitation units where this may be done. Rehabilitation includes physical therapy, occupational therapy, speech therapy, as well as close follow-up by physiatrists and rehabilitation medicine specialists. Rehabilitation doctors typically work closely with the treating surgeons. Some rehabilitation centers are freestanding, offering many, if not all, of the same features of in-hospital rehabilitation centers.

49.14 Surgical Pearls

- Most unstable pediatric spinal column injuries can be managed with surgical instrumentation and fusion. The choice of approach (anterior vs. posterior) varies with surgeon training, preference, and experience.
- Removal of all the cartilaginous end plate and proper preparation of the vertebral body are critical for the success of an anterior interbody fusion.
- Preoperative traction should be used judiciously. The pediatric spine is in general very flexible, and even major deformities may be corrected with intraoperative reduction.

49.15 Common Clinical Questions

1. Is high-dose methylprednisolone indicated for spinal cord injury in children?
2. Why does SCIWORA happen so frequently in young children?
3. What age group has the highest incidence of upper cervical spinal injury?
4. What is the CCI for measuring AOD?

49.16 Answers to Common Clinical Questions

1. No, it is not.
2. The soft tissues and ligaments of the neck are more distensible than the spinal cord at that level.
3. 0 to 4 years old.
4. The CCI measures the distance between the occipital condyle and superior articular capsule of C1.

References

[1] Brown RL, Brunn MA, Garcia VF. Cervical spine injuries in children: a review of 103 patients treated consecutively at a level 1 pediatric trauma center. J Pediatr Surg. 2001; 36(8): 1107–1114

[2] Polk-Williams A, Carr BG, Blinman TA, Masiakos PT, Wiebe DJ, Nance ML. Cervical spine injury in young children: a National Trauma Data Bank review. J Pediatr Surg. 2008; 43 (9):1718–1721

[3] Eleraky MA, Theodore N, Adams M, Rekate HL, Sonntag VK. Pediatric cervical spine injuries: report of 102 cases and review of the literature. J Neurosurg. 2000; 92 suppl 1:12–17

[4] Cervical spine injuries—Orthopaedic Trauma Association (OTA) classification. OrthopaedicsOne Articles. OrthopaedicsOne—The Orthopaedic Knowledge Network. http://www.orthopaedicsone.com/x/TYEXBQ. Accessed April 1, 2014

[5] Klimo P, Jr, Kan P, Rao G, Apfelbaum R, Brockmeyer D. Os odontoideum: presentation, diagnosis, and treatment in a series of 78 patients. J Neurosurg Spine. 2008; 9(4):332–342

[6] Fassett DR, McCall T, Brockmeyer DL. Odontoid synchondrosis fractures in children. Neurosurg Focus. 2006; 20(2):E7

[7] Brockmeyer DL, Ragel BT, Kestle JR. The pediatric cervical spine instability study. A pilot study assessing the prognostic value of four imaging modalities in clearing the cervical spine for children with severe traumatic injuries. Childs Nerv Syst. 2012; 28(5):699–705

[8] Pang D, Nemzek WR, Zovickian J. Atlanto-occipital dislocation—part 2: the clinical use of (occipital) condyle-C1 interval, comparison with other diagnostic methods, and the manifestation, management, and outcome of atlanto-occipital dislocation in children. Neurosurgery. 2007; 61(5): 995–1015, discussion 1015

[9] Reinhold M, Audigé L, Schnake KJ, Bellabarba C, Dai LY, Oner FC. AO spine injury classification system: a revision proposal for the thoracic and lumbar spine. Eur Spine J. 2013; 22(10): 2184–2201

[10] Pang D. Spinal cord injury without radiographic abnormality in children, 2 decades later. Neurosurgery. 2004; 55(6): 1325–1342, discussion 1342–1343

[11] Pang D, Pollack IF. Spinal cord injury without radiographic abnormality in children—the SCIWORA syndrome. J Trauma. 1989; 29(5):654–664

[12] Walters BC, Hadley MN, Hurlbert RJ, et al. American Association of Neurological Surgeons, Congress of Neurological Surgeons. Guidelines for the management of acute cervical spine and spinal cord injuries: 2013 update. Neurosurgery. 2013; 60 suppl 1:82–91

[13] White AA, III, Johnson RM, Panjabi MM, Southwick WO. Biomechanical analysis of clinical stability in the cervical spine. Clin Orthop Relat Res. 1975(109):85–96

[14] White AA III, Panjabi MM. The problem of clinical instability in the human spine: a systematic approach. In: White AA 3rd, Panjabi MM, eds. Clinical Biomechanics of the Spine. 2nd ed. Philadelphia, PA: J.B. Lippincott; 1990:277–378

50 Pediatric Peripheral Nervous System Trauma

Kambiz Kamian, Andrew T. Healy

50.1 Introduction

The peripheral nervous system (PNS) has the capability to regenerate itself at a rate of 1 mm/day, afforded by the unique differences in contrast to the central nervous system (CNS), including a basal lamina provided by Schwann's cells and central inhibitory signals not present in the periphery.[1] Despite a rich blood supply and regenerative capacity, severe injury often yields poor recovery without intervention. In children, speed and extent of functional recovery is felt to exceed that of adults[2] given the lower likelihood of negative systemic factors, neuroplasticity, higher metabolic rates, and shorter distances to target organs.[3] Schwann's cells provide a scaffolding and a hospitable milieu to guide and support daughter axons emerging from endbulbs of the proximal stump of injured nerves, powered by a new regenerative neuronal phenotype, which become "regeneration units."[4]

Proceeding with operative intervention, interrupting this slow regenerative process is often the crucial decision point in treating PNS injury. Proximal injuries that are required to regrow long distances (hand intrinsic muscles) have poorer functional outcomes and target muscles will atrophy up to 80 to 90% in 3 months, undergoing fatty replacement[5,6] that is likely permanent beyond 1 year[7] and completely replaced by fibrosis in 2 years.[1] Proximal sciatic or brachial plexus lesions rarely restore distal limb function.[4] When operative intervention is decided upon, the most important factor is a tension-free approximation. Surgical strategies range from neurolysis in the setting of a spontaneously regenerating nerve, resection and reapproximation in a short segment of dysfunction, resection with donor grafting for long-segment dysfunction, and neurotization (sacrificing less important donor nerve function to transplant to more desired targets) in the setting of nerve root avulsion.

50.2 Peripheral Nerve Anatomy

The functional unit of the nerve, the neuron, is ensheathed by Schwann's cells (+/- myelin). Each axon with its Schwann's cells is enveloped by the endoneurium, which provides the loose connective tissue scaffolding and itself provides an endoneurial tube. Altogether the axon, Schwann's cells, and endoneurium are considered a single "nerve."[8] The perineurium is a thicker collagenous connective tissue sheath around a group of axons creating the fascicle, which includes tight junctions—forming the blood–nerve barrier.[1] Multiple fascicles travel within the epineurium, along with arteries and veins. The epineurium is dense and more fibrous connective tissue with both collagen and elastin and is contiguous with the dura matter proximally. Epineurial vessels provide collateral flow, which most often can be safely sacrificed without disrupting perineural/endoneurial blood supply.[1]

50.3 Mechanism of Neuronal Injury

Peripheral nerve injury occurs in 5% of multitrauma patients.[9] This underestimates the peripheral nerve injuries in patients who are not multiple trauma patients or who have other neural injuries that preclude the diagnosis of distal nerve injury.[4] After peripheral nerve axotomy, there is a period of anterograde and retrograde change.

- Anterograde: "Wallerian" degeneration detectable beyond 48 hours from injury:
  - Target organ denervation.
  - Schwann's cell scaffold remains.
- Retrograde:
  - Cell body change[10] or "chromatolysis".
    - Cell body swelling.
    - Upregulation of genes involved with regeneration.
    - Dissolution of the Nissl bodies.
    - Prominent migration of the nucleus toward the periphery.
    - Increase in the size of nucleolus and nucleus.
  - Proximal stump sprouts endbulbs (distal swellings of axoplasmic material), which yield daughter axons.[4]

Directed regrowth is guided by distal stump Schwann' cells, whereas misdirected regrowth can result in neuroma formation, or neuroma in continuity in partial injury.[4] Regrowth is limited by the rate of anterograde slow axonal transport (1–2 mm/day).[1] Mechanism of injury is one major determinant of recovery and also surgical management.

- **Sharp laceration:** Clean, sharp laceration (with predictable degree of neural damage) should be reapproximated within 72 hours.[11]
- **Blunt division:** Proximal and distal stumps appearing contused (with unpredictable length of neural injury) should be tagged and reapproximation planned in 3 to 4 weeks.[11]
- **Blunt injury/contusion/stretch:** Common, with a greater tendency to be nonfocal with multilevel plexal involvement,[11] more commonly, supraclavicular (72 vs. 28%)[12] with injury expected over longer segments. About 85% of gunshot wounds (GSWs) do not directly transect the nerve and result in this injury.[1] Managed expectantly for 3 to 4 months, if surgical repair is indicated, outcome is less favorable.[11,12]
- **Avulsion:** Often seen in perinatal and traction brachial plexus injuries. Recovery is not expected, however, with other functional plexal elements in children, some advocate longer expectant management[11] prior to neurotization procedures.

50.4 Sunderland's Classification

- **First degree (aka neurapraxia[13]):** Disturbance of axonal conduction (+/– demyelination) without significant damage to or degeneration of the nerve. Transient alteration of function usually lasts seconds to minutes, but more severe cases can last up to a few weeks. Electrophysiological evidence of denervation is absent when tested 18 to 21 days after the injury. Prognosis for full recovery is excellent.
- **Second degree (aka axonotmesis[13]):** Axonal injury (with wallerian degeneration) within an intact endoneurial tube. Electromyography (EMG) will show denervation and it may remain abnormal up to 1 year. Full recovery is expected.[7]
- **Third degree (aka axonotmesis[13] with endoneurial damage):** More severe axonal injury, which includes disruption of the endoneurium, conveying variability in the expected spontaneous regeneration.[8] EMG after 2 weeks will show fibrillation potentials reflecting wallerian degeneration. This injury is often managed expectantly but degree of recovery is unpredictable.[8]

- **Fourth degree (neurotmesis[13]):** Complete disruption of the nerve with degeneration. Clinical picture is consistent with "complete interruption of the nerve." Scarring is more severe with epineurial damage, some motor units may attempt to regenerate, but rarely of good quality.[8] EMG will be similar to axonotmesis; however, spontaneous recovery is unexpected.[1]
- **Fifth degree (avulsion):** Involves discontinuity of the nerve trunk yielding complete loss of its motor, sensory, and *autonomic function*. Dorsal horn injury predisposes to pain.

50.5 Examination

Physical examination of children is difficult to assess isolated motor function. In the older child, the preferred method is the British Council system used in adults (Medical Research Council) or the Louisiana State University (LSU) medical center system.[1] Gilbert described a more global system M0–M3 describing limb position to determine flexor, extensor, or total plexus involvement in perinatal neuronal injury.[14] Other important examination findings include phrenic nerve involvement (diaphragm paralysis), long thoracic nerve (serratus paralysis), or sympathetic involvement (Horner's syndrome), which likely indicate root avulsion.[7] Sensory preservation in motor-affected distribution is a good prognostic sign indicating neurapraxia.[15] See **Appendix A.1** and **Appendix A.2** for motor and sensory examination scales and peripheral nerve examination pearls.

Examining children is difficult. Other signs of neuronal injury other than volitional movement must be utilized: (1) skin changes: smooth, dry skin in the denervated digit; (2) fingerprints made on ninhydrin paper revealing anhydrosis; and (3) muscular atrophy. Anhydrosis may be the only indication of denervation in a child.[5] Under magnification, perspiration on the palmar surface can be detected by visual inspection alone. Another crude test is the O'Riain's wrinkle test, where digits are submerged in tepid water for 5 minutes and parasympathetic-injured digits will not wrinkle.[1] On sensory examination, 2-point discrimination should be 2 to 5 mm at fingertips and 7 to 12 mm at palmar base.[1] This can be tested with paper clips if calipers are not available. During the regeneration phase, a progressive Tinnel's sign can be seen with grade 2 or above as axon regenerates.[7]

Note: Rapidly advancing Tinnel's sign may be a positive prognostic factor for recovery, but is felt to have a less valuable positive predictive value. On the other hand, the lack of a Tinnel sign at 4 to 6 weeks is much more specific for poor regenerative potential.[1]

50.6 Neurophysiology

Neurophysiological tests are useful in determining whether the lesion is pre- or postganglionic, although not to replace computed tomography (CT) myelography (gold standard) for this purpose. EMG can be utilized in children with 80% sensitivity for root avulsion and can document subclinical recovery.

50.6.1 Electromyography

A normal muscle will generate the following:
- Insertional activity.
- Followed by absence of signal during rest.
- Electrical activity with voluntary/proximal neuronal activation.

A denervated muscle with axonal loss will generate the following:
- Spontaneous electrical activity at rest after 2 weeks from the injury that include the following:
  - Fibrillation potentials.
  - Positive sharp waves.

EMG is most useful 2 to 3 weeks after injury to permit denervation changes to occur in target muscles. Note: EMG will falsely show distal activation over the first 1 to 2 days prior to the onset of wallerian degeneration. Therefore, in the acute

setting, an absent response to proximal stimulus and *an intact response to distal stimulus cannot differentiate conduction block from axonal disruption.* An important sign of recovery at 6 weeks is denervation potential or nerve action potential (NAP) from neural stimulation.[1]

50.6.2 Nerve Action Potentials

Denote direct stimulation of the nerve proximal to a lesion and recording distal to that lesion. This test is more sensitive and will reveal neuronal regeneration prior to actual muscular activation, or EMG detection. NAPs may be conducted across lesions that do not permit voluntary signaling of muscle contraction. Intraoperative NAPs can determent if axonal regeneration has occurred across the site of injury. If not, grafting has been shown to improve outcomes (▶ Table 50.1).[1]

50.6.3 Somatosensory-evoked Potentials and Muscular-evoked Potentials (SSEPs/MEPs)

Useful to determine complete avulsions (absent motor but intact sensory nerve action potentials), however, clinically complete avulsions may have sparse sensory fiber connections resulting in false-negative results of SSEP. MEPs are useful in testing the ventral fibers. Electrodiagnostic is an important tool especially with function loss.[5] It is recommended that a baseline study be taken 1 week to 10 days and repeating at 3 to 4 weeks and 10 to 12 weeks.[5] A common protocol is as follows:
- Baseline (0–7 days).
- Initial Follow-up (10–21 days): Distinguish demyelination (preserved distal responses) from axonal loss.

Table 50.1 Brachial plexus outcomes (in-continuity lesions)

Injury type	Plexus elements with (+) NAP, neurolysis alone		Plexus elements with (−) NAP, nerve repair	
	Complete LOF preoperatively	Incomplete LOF preoperatively	Complete LOF preoperatively	Incomplete LOF preoperatively
Stretch/contusion	90.3	94.1	44.6	62.2
GSW	97.6	93.6	55.2	87.5
Iatrogenic	94.4	100	71.9	66.7
Laceration I/C	90.0	94.4	66.7	75.0
Totals	92.6	94.6	49.5	66.7

Abbreviations: GSW, gunshot wound; I/C, in-continuity, LOF, loss of function; NAP, nerve action potential.
Source: Adapted from Kline and Hudson.[1]
Note: Values represent percent of plexal elements gaining grade 3 function or better.

- Follow-up (3–6 months): Determine the extent of reinnervation +/– operative intervention.
- Follow-up (6–12 months): Documents extent of distal muscle reinnervation. Note: EMG recovery may take more than 12 months, however, waiting beyond this time frame may result in poorer outcomes due to target muscle loss and fibrosis.[6]

50.7 Imaging

50.7.1 X-Ray

In brachial plexus injury may be suggested by fracture. Transverse apophysis clavicular fracture or fracture of the first rib may suggest proximal lesions. Chest X-ray (CXR) may also reveal an elevated hemidiaphragm indicating phrenic nerve injury. Extremity fractures are also associated with peripheral nerve injury.

50.7.2 MRI

Noninvasive and more sensitive for BP injury, therefore examination of choice for children ahead of CT myelography.[16] T1 provides useful anatomical information outlining the neuronal adiposity with hyperintensity. Note: Coronal views for contralateral plexus comparison are important.[16] Short T1-inversion recovery (STIR) sequences to see pathological neuropraxic/inflammatory plexopathy and T2 is most useful for pseudomeningoceles with axial gradient recalled echo (GRE) for nerve root avulsions. In traumatic injury, imaging may reveal associated fractures.

50.7.3 CT Myelography

It may be more sensitive than MRI for detecting avulsions and is considered gold standard in this regard.[17,18] Sensitivity in perinatal Behavioral Problems Index (BPI) is 63%, whereas the specificity is about 85%. Nerve root integrity may be present in up to 18% of pseudomeningoceles and therefore CT is most sensitive when pseudomeningocele is combined with the absence of the respective nerve root.[16,18]

50.8 Nonsurgical Management

- **Bracing:** Prevents contracture, however, stresses the importance of range-of-motion (ROM)

exercises multiple times/day. Immobilized joints stiffen rapidly.
- **Physical therapy**: Full ROM exercises, prevents joint contracture.
- **Painkillers:** For the acute stage, avoid long-term use.
- **Neuropathic pain:** Neurontin, Lyrica, tricyclic antidepressants (TCAs), transcutaneous electrical nerve stimulation (TENS).
- **Frequent follow-up**.

50.9 Surgical Repair

50.9.1 Repair Types

- **Exploration:** If operation is required for another pathology (i.e., pseudoaneurysm, open fracture reduction, hematoma) or ongoing neuronal compression, the peripheral nerve surgeon may be needed for exploration alone.
- **Neurolysis:** Consists of decompressing neural elements. It is best served for injuries in continuity which reveal preexisting neuronal regeneration (intraoperative NAPs present).[1] Note: Neurolysis includes epineurial scar resection (external neurolysis) and even splitting fascicles to determine the need for a split repair (internal neurolysis).
- **Direct repair**.

Epineurial: Epineurial repair using neural vessels to help alignment[19] after injured nerve is sectioned back to healthy functioning nerve.

   Grouped fascicular or fascicular: Group fascicular repair or fascicular repair should be carried out when these groupings can be clearly identified.[20] Note that fascicular orientation can change along the length of a nerve every few centimeters.[1]
- Grafting:
  - Minimize number of sutures (4–10) with 8 to 11.0 monofilament nylon to limit scar formation.[21]
  - Harvested nerve should be 25% longer than what is needed due to nerve shortening and end preparation.[21]
  - Alternatives for repair (defects < 3 cm): Autologous vein grafts, perineurial tubes, silicone alloplastic tubes, and resorbable conduits (polyglycolic acid, collagen).
  - Graft should be as close to proximal nerve diameter as possible.
  - Graft should match the size and number of injured nerve fascicles as closely as possible.[21]

- Note: With distinct fascicles, cable grafting is an option to either match up clearly differentiated polyfascicular nerves or to better match the cross-sectional area of the injured nerve with a small nerve graft.[21]
- **Neurontization:** See brachial plexus section.

50.9.2 Repair Timing

- "Rule of 3s":
  - Sharp laceration: 3 days (72 hours, immediate repair)[22]—Rule out associated vascular injury (computed tomography angiography [CTA], angiogram); pseudoaneurysm, hematoma, or fistula, rule out and other organ damage (esophagus, trachea). Ask for help from other specialties, need immediate repair.[23]
  - Blunt laceration: 3 to 4 weeks (delayed)[22]: If during the primary repair for sharp laceration, any contusion or long-segment damage was noticed, tag the nerve with silk and wait 3 to 4 weeks.
  - Blunt injury/stretch/avulsion: 3 to 6 months with electrodiagnostic studies to distinguish neuropraxia from axonal loss +/– spontaneous recovery.[22]

50.10 Pearls

- Proximal injuries convey poorer prognosis.[24,25]
- Upper extremity injury recovers better than lower.[24,25]
- About 10% of an injured nerve's axons after simple transaction will reach a target after surgical approximation.[26]
- Tension-free approximation is best, avoid interposed graft as much as possible with long dissection and neurolysis especially when damage is proximal, but if not possible, interposed graft is acceptable.
- Primary approximation if the ends are within 2 cm.[5]
- Intraoperative NAPs: If present, leave them as is, if absent then reapproximation is best, nerve graft is second best and neural tubes are third.[1,27]
- Nerve growth occurs at 1 mm/day or 1 in/month, two more delays; (a) 3 to 4 weeks crossing any suture line, (b) 3 to 4 weeks for reaching the end plate and end plate maturation.[1,28]
- Proximal function has better chance of restoration of function, in follow-up, test the muscles proximal to distal.

- EMG recovery can be detected 3 to 4 weeks prior to clinical recovery.
- Grouped fascicular repair is favorable if components can be distinguished, if not, epineural repair with alignment based on epineural vessels and gross fascicular approximation.
- Sural nerve: 2.1 mm in diameter mark the direction of axoplasmic flow when harvesting (mark or tag it) and use it along the flow. Locate it lateral to gastrocnemius tendon.[1,21]
- Other grafts available: Lateral cutaneous nerve of the forearm.
- Open injury—explore. If the nerve cut is blunt, then tag it for delayed exploration.
- No long-acting paralytics from anesthesia!
- Use motor nerve graft for critical motor restoration.[29]
- Protecting the nerve from surrounding tissues during peripheral nerve surgery can improve outcomes by providing a protective barrier, reducing fibrosis, decreasing adhesions to surrounding tissues, and providing a vascularized wound bed.[30]

50.11 Postoperative Care/Follow-up

- Ensure dressings are not too tight, check distal vascular examination.
- CXR postoperative for brachial plexus.
- Immobilization temporarily after surgery for short period of time, 1 to 2 weeks.
- Start physical therapy 3 to 4 weeks after the surgery; full ROM exercises, prevent contracture and development of capsular contractures and muscular contraction.
- Painkillers; short period.
- Neuropathic pain; Neurontin, TCA, Lyrica, TENS
- Electrotherapy.
- Bracing; splints to encourage finger flexion.
- Treating contractures: Botox.
- As the patient ages, add physical activity such as swimming.
- Ancillary surgeries
  - Tendon transfer.
  - Free muscle transfer.
  - Joint fusion, open joint (glenohumeral) reduction.
  - Subscapular muscle release for fixed shoulder adduction.
  - Biceps tendon transfer brachioradialis tendon transfer for wrist extension.

- Biceps tendon transfer to remove it as a supinator, need to restore wrist extension.
- Osteotomies.
- Pain from sclerotic DREZ may be treated with ablation.[15]

50.12 Brachial Plexus

50.12.1 Epidemiology

Brachial plexus injuries are commonly associated with head trauma causing loss of consciousness (LOC) (72%) and coma (19%), upper extremity fracture dislocation (20%), and rib fracture in 41% of adult trauma populations. Subclavian artery (15–30%) and spinal cord injury (5%) are also associated with these high-velocity accidents.[15] Brachial plexus injuries in the pediatric population, compared to adults, are more often associated with skeletal injuries[31] and nerve root avulsion (63–80%),[32] as compared to the adult population (40 and 20%, respectively).[33] Children less frequently report denervation pain (0–5%).[32] Isolated infraclavicular injury (Klumpke's) is uncommon.[12,17]

Traumatic peripheral nerve injury in pediatrics is predominantly as follows:

1. **Perinatal** (obstetric brachial plexus palsy) with 0.8 to 2.5 in 1,000 live births[15,17] (covered separately).
2. **Trauma.** Pediatric brachial plexus injury outside of obstetrics is most often related to the following:
   - **Motor vehicle collisions** for only 1% of all brachial plexus injury.[33]
   - **Pedestrian accidents** predominate (67%).
   - **Road traffic injury**.
   - **Falls** from height, shoulder dislocation (4.5%).[17]
   - **Gunshot wounds/stabbing injuries**.[15]

Note: Contact sports. Less severe injuries to the plexus occur frequently, given the term "Burner," transient dysesthesias and even motor weakness can be the result of stretch injury or direct blunt trauma to Erb's point, a neuropraxia, which often resolves within minutes but rarely can persist.

50.12.2 Anatomy

Covered separately (see perinatal brachial plexus injury).

50.12.3 Distribution of Injury

- **Upper (Erb's): C5–C6 +/– C7:** Often exceeds lower BP injury 3:1 and is more often severe in trauma populations,[12,33] C5–7 results in the classic "waiters tip" position.
- **Intermediate: C7 +/– C8, T1:** Often the lower roots are more mildly affected in perinatal injury and may result in distal improvement greater than shoulder, however, recovery is variable.
- **Lower (Klumpke's): C8, T1:** Most commonly caused by stretch, GSW, and laceration. Exceedingly rare in neonatal Traumatic Brain Injury (nTBI) and less common than its supraclavicular counterpart in adult trauma populations and more often transient neuropraxia (50%).[33] Cord injuries at this level are associated with other injuries to greater extent than supraclavicular.[12] IE: shoulder dislocation, fracture, axillary artery injury. They are surgically more demanding given vasculature around the neural elements.
- **Total plexus palsy: (C5–C8 +/– T1):** Often associated with multiple avulsions to variable degree, often lower plexus avulsions. Poor recovery expected for distal extremity function, goal of surgery is proximal functional restoration.

50.12.4 Examination

There are reliable methods of quantifying upper extremity function in patients with brachial plexus palsy and may be used clinically and to assess functional outcomes. (Perinatal examination is covered separately.)
- The Modified Mallet Classification.[17]
- The Toronto Test Score.[34]
- The Active Movement Scale.[35]

The physical examination for brachial plexus injury must include the following:
- **Musculoskeletal palpation:** Trapezius, scapula, clavicle, shoulder, etc. may elicit tenderness or evidence of fracture/muscle spasm.
- **Cervical spine palpation** and neck clearance must be done to rule out cervical fracture.
- **Passive and active range of motion** testing.
- **Detailed dermatome and myotome-specific neurological examination**.
- **Imaging:** Evaluate for fracture.

See "examination" above for imaging and neurophysiological testing. See **Appendix A.1** and **Appendix A.2** for examination scoring and pearls.

50.12.5 Surgical Indications

Common indications include the following:
- **Clear-cut upper trunk lesions** (biceps function) with no recovery at 2 to 3 months.
- **Complete plexus injury** should be operated sooner.
- No functional recovery in the first 3 weeks should be further investigated with electrodiagnostic studies for consideration of exploration.[15]

In the presence of partial or minimal functional recovery, reexploration may mean an initial loss of function. This is especially challenging since most commonly the surgeon will find neuroma in continuity and must decide to leave it or perform resection.
- **Repair after 9 months** has success,[15] however, in perinatal injury some feel longer observation is warranted given dramatically improved rates of spontaneous recovery.[22]

50.12.6 Surgical Technique

- **Supraclavicular incision** It is most often used given the preponderance of upper injury.
- **Infraclavicular injury** will often need clavicle osteotomy and inferior clavicular incision (try to avoid cutting the clavicle because of the high risk of nonunion extending beyond deltopectoral triangle toward axilla. Division of pectoralis near the deltoid, often pectoralis minor will need division as well. Musculocutaneous and median nerve dissection are required, which lead to the deeper axillary artery, which may be gently retracted for exposure of the posterior cord. Sural nerve grafting is needed almost invariably with neuroma resection. Grafting procedure is often sutured but some authors utilize solely fibrin glue in neonatal injury.[17]
- If one functional root is found, goal is renervation of the lateral cord or anterior upper trunk for proximal restoration. A second target is the posterior cord for axillary/radial function.[15]
- In the setting of root avulsion, neurontization is necessary.[36]

Common Donor Nerves

- Intraplexal:
  - Medial pectoral nerve to axillary for upper trunk lesion C5 to musculocutaneous.[32]
  - Suprascapular nerve.[37]
  - Partial ulnar.[38]
- Extraplexal:
  - Accessory nerve.
  - Phrenic nerve.[37]
  - Intercostals.
  - Partial contralateral plexus[23,32]: Used for C5–C6 avulsions.
  - Contralateral C7.[23]

Note: The more distal the recipient nerve the better, no useful recovery from anastomosing to donors proximal to the cords.
Complications include the following:
1. Damage to surrounding: Veins, arteries, trachea, esophagus, thoracic duct
2. Infection: Wound dehiscence, deep infection, abscess
3. Suture line disruption

50.12.7 Outcomes

In-continuity Brachial Plexus Outcomes

See ▶ Table 50.1.

Infraclavicular Stretch Outcomes

LSU medical center reports on surgical intervention of 1,019 traumatic BP lesions, 143 of which (28%) were infraclavicular stretch injuries. Outcomes were divided by division-cord and cord-nerve lesions (which are the majority of infraclavicular stretch injuries at 76%).[12]
Bottom line:
- **Favorable**: Lateral and posterior cords.
- **Unfavorable**: Medial cord and medial cord–ulnar nerve injuries were poor especially if excision and graft were needed.

Avulsion Outcomes

Avulsions treated with neurontization reveals up to 65 to 86% antigravity motor restoration at the level of the biceps and up to 20 to 43% at the level of finger flexion.[37,39,40] C7 hemicontralateral transfer has not shown adequate results when used independently.[23]

50.13 Extremities

50.13.1 Epidemiology

Upper extremity injury presenting the emergency department is associated with peripheral nerve injury about 1.7 to 2.5 of the time in children.[41] Radial nerve is the most commonly injured peripheral nerve of the extremities.[9,42]

- **Nerve injury associated with fractures**: Especially predominant in the upper extremities (80–90%).[41]
- **Direct penetrating or crush injury** can injure any regional peripheral nerve.
- **Compartment syndrome,** untreated for 12. hours, will likely yield permanent neurological dysfunction.[43]
- **Iatrogenic/injection injury**.

In adult polytrauma populations:

- **Humeral fractures** are associated with radial, ulnar, and median nerve injury (9.5, 3.8, 1.4%).[10] Although radial nerve injury is the most common peripheral nerve injured and is associated with humeral fracture,[42] supracondylar fractures may be more often associated with anterior interosseous nerve (AIN)/median nerve injury (from 10 to 15% of the time)[44] and a higher preponderance of ulnar injury depending on mechanism and fragment displacement (anterior).[45] Humeral neck fracture or shoulder dislocation has a greater correlation to axillary (16%), suprascapular (13%) over radial (10%).[46]
- **Forearm fractures** also results in greater ulnar nerve injury (2.4 %) versus median nerve (1.3%) injury.
- **Wrist fracture** most commonly associated with median nerve injury.[9]
- **Pelvic fracture** sciatic nerve injury rates (1.2–1.7%)[9] less commonly femoral nerve injury (0.16%).[9]
- **Femoral fracture** neck fracture associated with sciatic nerve injury (16%) midshaft associated with femoral nerve injury (0.16%).[9]
- **Elbow fractures** in children can be associated with nerve injury 5 to 19%.[45]
- **Distal lower extremity fractures** Peroneal nerve injury is the most common nerve injury associated with lower extremity trauma (2.2%) with femoral and tibial nerves being the least.[9]

50.13.2 Anatomy and Fractures Associated Nerve Injury

See **Appendix A.3** for nerve fracture association table.

50.14 Upper Extremity

50.14.1 Surgical Indications/ Outcomes

The majority of peripheral nerve injuries with closed fracture will improve spontaneously. About 82% of shoulder dislocation and humeral neck fractures had complete recovery at 4 months,[46] up to 96% of radial nerve recovered with humeral midshaft fractures.[47] About 90 to 100% of supracondylar fractures will exhibit complete spontaneous recovery, but may take up to 4 to 9 months.[48] Overall recovery rate for peripheral nerves of 85%, the extent of which is established by 18 months.[48] Most nerves need repair within 3 to 6 months[48]; however, radial nerve has a longer recovery time (6–9 months).[49] Distal denervation or no improvement on 3 to 4 month EMG (as compared with 6-week baseline) may support surgical exploration, functioning neuromas in continuity will likely improve from neurolysis alone, this sometimes will include clearance of boney callous formation from around the nerve.[47,50] Initial conservative management is considered to have more favorable outcomes when nerve injury is a "primary injury" (i.e., associated with the initial fracture),[50,51] whereas recommendations for iatrogenic injuries ("secondary injuries") associated with fracture reduction are less clear and often early exploration is indicated.[5,45]

Children often are observed over longer periods given their even greater chance of recovery (95%).[52] At this time, it is the fracture type that dictates exploration or not (complex or open fractures), and there is no clear consensus on early versus late exploration. Exploration of the nerve is recommended when open reduction is pursued.[5,42,45] More distal injury has better outcomes although outcomes can be nerve specific[49]:

- **High nerve regeneration potential:** Radial, musculocutaneous, and femoral.
- **Moderate nerve regeneration potential:** Median, ulnar, and tibial.
- **Poor nerve regeneration potential:** Peroneal.

See ▶ Table 50.2 for upper extremity outcomes.

Table 50.2 Upper extremity outcomes

Level of injury	Median			Radial			Ulnar		
	NTM 1 repair	NTM graft	ICL + NAP neurolysis	NTM 1 repair	NTM graft	ICL + NAP neurolysis	NTM 1 repair	NTM graft	ICL + NAP neurolysis
High	67%	67%	100%	80%	60%	93%	60%	100%	88%
Inter.	100%	67%	100%	100%	67%	100%	82%	57%	95%
Low	100%	71%	100%	(PIN) 100%	(PIN) 100%	(PIN) 100%	67%	100%	100%
Other	(AIN) N/A	(AIN) N/A	(AIN) 100%	(DF) 100%	(DF) 50%	(DF) 100%	N/A	N/A	N/A

Abbreviations: AIN, anterior interosseous nerve; DF, nerve to dorsal forearm; ICL, in-continuity lesion; NAP, nerve action potential; NTM, neurotmesis; PIN, posterior interosseus nerve.

Note: Values represent percentage of patients achieving recovery of strength grade 3 or better in a series of upper extremity injuries.[27]

50.15 Lower Extremity

Peripheral nerve injury in the lower extremity is more often associated with injection (for the proximal sciatic nerve), followed by fracture dislocation, contusion, compression (from motor vehicle collisions [MVC] most frequently gunshot wounds and in a delayed fashion with compartment syndrome or iatrogenic after fracture traction or reduction.[1,9,53] Sciatic nerve injury is associated with pelvic fracture approximately 1.2 to 1.7% of cases,[9,54] whereas femoral nerve is injured in less than 0.5% of the time with pelvic fractures[9] and possibly more proximally with iliopsoas hematoma.[55] The lumbosacral plexus courses over the posterior pelvic ring toward the sciatic notch. At this junction, the sciatic nerve can be injured in displaced pelvic fractures and crush injuries.[56] More often the sciatic nerve is injured beyond this point, where it lies adjacent to the ischial tuberosity. Here, posterior hip dislocations can injure the sciatic nerve 16% of the time.[57] The sciatic nerve is well protected in the thigh between the adductor magnus and biceps, and sciatic nerve laceration from femoral fracture here is rare.[56,58]

Distally, the peroneal nerve is much more susceptible to injury not only with fibular neck fracture, but also adduction knee injuries, and distal fibular or even tibial spiral fractures.[9] The peroneal nerve is the most common place where the sciatic component is injured and is found to be injured 2.2% of the time with fibular or tibial fractures.[59] The tibial nerve is more rarely injured as it courses protected between muscles for the majority of its course, found to be injured 0.5% of tibial or fibular fractures, and is more often injured in the lower extremity or ankle.[9]

50.15.1 Anatomical Considerations

Lumbar plexus: Involves nerve fibers from L2 to L5.

Mnemonic: "I Get Loud On Fridays": Iliohypogastric, Ilioinguinal, Genitofemoral, Lateral femoral cutaneous, Obturator, Femoral.

- **Femoral nerve**, exiting the pelvis deep to the inguinal ligament and is responsible for hip flexion and leg extension. Injury at this location is most common. Trauma is the most common cause of femoral nerve pathology.
- **Obturator nerve** exits via the obturator foramen, innervating the thigh adductors.
- **Sciatic nerve**, from both lumbar and sacral plexuses, passing through the greater sciatic foramen (inferior to the piriformis) innervating knee flexors and all muscles below the knee after dividing near popliteal fossa into the tibial and peroneal nerves.

Sacral plexus: other than its contribution to the sciatic nerve, the sacral plexus gives rise to

- **Gluteal nerves** (greater sciatic foramen) responsible for hip extension and abduction.
- **Pudendal nerves** (lesser sciatic foramen) to the pelvic floor.

50.15.2 Surgical Indications/ Outcomes

It is the fracture type that dictates open or closed reduction, no indication for immediate exploration with primary nerve palsy.

Table 50.3 Lower extremity outcomes

	Sciatic		Tibial			Common peroneal		
Level of injury	NTM 1 repair	ICL + NAP neurolysis	NTM 1 repair	NTM graft	ICL + NAP neurolysis	NTM 1 repair	NTM graft	ICL + NAP neurolysis
High	30–73%	69–95%	100%	55–94%	95%	84%	11–41%	82–93%
Intermediate	N/A	N/A	100%	64%	95%	N/A	15–31%	N/A
Low	78–95%	78–100%	N/A	64–100%	73%	N/A	57–76%	N/A

Abbreviations: ICL, in-continuity lesion; NAP, nerve action potential; NTM, neurotmesis.
Note: Values represent percentages of patients achieving recovery of strength grade 3 or better in a series of lower extremity injuries.[26,58,59]

Best lower extremity prognosis: Tibial nerve.
Worst lower extremity prognosis: Proximal peroneal division of sciatic nerve.

▶ Table 50.3 represents lower extremity outcomes.

50.16 Common Clinical Questions

1. How long after injury can wallerian degeneration be detected on neurophysiological testing?
2. How do second- and third-degree neuronal injury, using the Sunderland's classification, differ from each other?
3. A 13-year-old adolescent boy is evaluated in the emergency department after a high-speed motor vehicle collision and is found to have a fractured first rib on CXR and shoulder examination is limited. What is the most appropriate imaging modality to evaluate the neural elements?
4. What is the most commonly injured peripheral nerve and approximately what percentage will recover function with observation alone?
5. A 12-year-old boy has a type 1 Monteggia fracture and will be taken to the operating room for open reduction and internal fixation. He has no sensory deficit on examination, but gives poor effort with motor. What nerve(s) should be evaluated by neurosurgery intraoperatively?

50.17 Answers to Common Clinical Questions

1. 48 hours. Prior to this point, an absent response to proximal stimulus and an intact response to distal stimulus cannot differentiate conduction block from axonal disruption.
2. Both considered "axonotmesis" by Seddon, the important differentiating factor is disruption of the endoneurium in third-degree injury, conveying a more unpredictable neuronal recovery.
3. Bilateral brachial plexus MRI with axial cervical GRE sequences. CT myelography may more sensitive in detecting nerve root avulsion, however, MRI can delineate injury to the plexus and soft tissue as well as root avulsion and is the less invasive method.
4. The radial nerve is the most commonly injured nerve, especially with humeral shaft fracture and spontaneously recovers from 85 to 96% of the time. However, site of fracture is key with proximal humeral neck fractures more often disrupting axillary nerve and supracondylar fractures most commonly disrupting median nerve (or AIN).
5. Posterior interosseous nerve (PIN) is the most commonly injured nerve in Monteggia fracture (especially type 1) and would most often present without sensory deficit.

References

[1] Kline DG, Hudson AR. Nerve injuries. Operative Results for Major Nerve Injuries, Entrapments and Tumors. Philadelphia, PA: W.B. Saunders Company; 1995
[2] Tajima T, Imai H. Results of median nerve repair in children. Microsurgery. 1989; 10(2):145–146
[3] Frykman GK. Peripheral nerve injuries in children. Orthop Clin North Am. 1976; 7(3):701–716
[4] Zochodne DW. The challenges and beauty of peripheral nerve regrowth. J Peripher Nerv Syst. 2012; 17(1):1–18
[5] Hosalkar HS, Matzon JL, Chang B. Nerve palsies related to pediatric upper extremity fractures. Hand Clin. 2006; 22(1): 87–98
[6] Sulaiman W, Gordon T. Neurobiology of peripheral nerve injury, regeneration, and functional recovery: from bench top research to bedside application. Ochsner J. 2013; 13(1): 100–108
[7] Fox IK, Mackinnon SE. Adult peripheral nerve disorders: nerve entrapment, repair, transfer, and brachial plexus disorders. Plast Reconstr Surg. 2011; 127(5):105–118
[8] Sunderland S. A classification of peripheral nerve injuries producing loss of function. Brain. 1951; 74(4):491–516

[9] Noble J, Munro CA, Prasad VS, Midha R. Analysis of upper and lower extremity peripheral nerve injuries in a population of patients with multiple injuries. J Trauma. 1998; 45(1):116–122

[10] Lieberman AR. The axon reaction: a review of the principal features of perikaryal responses to axon injury. Int Rev Neurobiol. 1971; 14:49–124

[11] Dubuisson AS, Kline DG. Brachial plexus injury: a survey of 100 consecutive cases from a single service. Neurosurgery. 2002; 51(3):673–682, discussion 682–683

[12] Kim DH, Murovic JA, Tiel RL, Kline DG. Infraclavicular brachial plexus stretch injury. Neurosurg Focus. 2004; 16(5):E4

[13] Seddon HJ. Nerves Injuries Committee of the British Medical Research Council. In: Seddon HJ, ed. Peripheral nerve injuries. London: Her Majesty's Stationery Office, 1954. MRC Special Report Series, no. 282:10–11

[14] Gilbert A, Tassin JL. Réparation chirurgicale du plexus brachial dans la paralysie obstétricale. Chirurgie. 1984; 110 (1):70–75

[15] Blaauw G, Muhlig RS, Vredeveld JW. Management of brachial plexus injuries. Adv Tech Stand Neurosurg. 2008; 33:201–231

[16] Birchansky S, Altman N. Imaging the brachial plexus and peripheral nerves in infants and children. Semin Pediatr Neurol. 2000; 7(1):15–25

[17] Gilbert A, Pivato G, Kheiralla T. Long-term results of primary repair of brachial plexus lesions in children. Microsurgery. 2006; 26(4):334–342

[18] Dodds SD, Wolfe SW. Perinatal brachial plexus palsy. Curr Opin Pediatr. 2000; 12(1):40–47

[19] Varitimidis SE, Sotereanos DG. Partial nerve injuries in the upper extremity. Hand Clin. 2000; 16(1):141–149

[20] Kaufman Y, Cole P, Hollier L. Peripheral nerve injuries of the pediatric hand: issues in diagnosis and management. J Craniofac Surg. 2009; 20(4):1011–1015, 1011–1015

[21] Wolford LM, Stevao EL. Considerations in nerve repair. Proc Bayl Univ Med Cent. 2003; 16(2):152–156

[22] Dubuisson A, Kline DG. Indications for peripheral nerve and brachial plexus surgery. Neurol Clin. 1992; 10(4):935–951

[23] Spinner RJ, Kline DG. Surgery for peripheral nerve and brachial plexus injuries or other nerve lesions. Muscle Nerve. 2000; 23(5):680–695

[24] Murovic JA. Lower-extremity peripheral nerve injuries: a Louisiana State University Health Sciences Center literature review with comparison of the operative outcomes of 806 Louisiana State University Health Sciences Center sciatic, common peroneal, and tibial nerve lesions. Neurosurgery. 2009; 65 suppl 4:A18–A23

[25] Murovic JA. Upper-extremity peripheral nerve injuries: a Louisiana State University Health Sciences Center literature review with comparison of the operative outcomes of 1837 Louisiana State University Health Sciences Center median, radial, and ulnar nerve lesions. Neurosurgery. 2009; 65 suppl 4:A11–A17

[26] Witzel C, Rohde C, Brushart TM. Pathway sampling by regenerating peripheral axons. J Comp Neurol. 2005; 485(3): 183–190

[27] Tiel RL, Happel LT, Jr, Kline DG. Nerve action potential recording method and equipment. Neurosurgery. 1996; 39 (1):103–108, discussion 108–109

[28] Roganovic̕ Z, Pavlicevic̕ G. Difference in recovery potential of peripheral nerves after graft repairs. Neurosurgery. 2006; 59(3):621–633, discussion 621–633

[29] Nichols CM, Brenner MJ, Fox IK, et al. Effects of motor versus sensory nerve grafts on peripheral nerve regeneration. Exp Neurol. 2004; 190(2):347–355

[30] Siemionow M, Uygur S, Ozturk C, Siemionow K. Techniques and materials for enhancement of peripheral nerve regeneration: a literature review. Microsurgery. 2013; 33(4): 318–328

[31] Matz SO, Welliver PS, Welliver DI. Brachial plexus neuropraxia complicating a comminuted clavicle fracture in a college football player. Case report and review of the literature. Am J Sports Med. 1989; 17(4):581–583

[32] El-Gammal TA, El-Sayed A, Kotb MM, El Gammal. Surgical treatment of brachial plexus traction injuries in children, excluding obstetric palsy. Microsurgery. 2003; 23(1):14–17

[33] Midha R. Epidemiology of brachial plexus injuries in a multitrauma population. Neurosurgery. 1997; 40(6):1182–1188, discussion 1188–1189

[34] Michelow BJ, Clarke HM, Curtis CG, Zuker RM, Seifu Y, Andrews DF. The natural history of obstetrical brachial plexus palsy. Plast Reconstr Surg. 1994; 93(4):675–680, discussion 681

[35] Clarke HM, Curtis CG. An approach to obstetrical brachial plexus injuries. Hand Clin. 1995; 11(4):563–580, discussion 580–581

[36] Narakas AO, Hentz VR. Neurotization in brachial plexus injuries. Indication and results. Clin Orthop Relat Res. 1988 (237):43–56

[37] Samardzić M, Rasulić L, Grujicić D, Milicić B. Results of nerve transfers to the musculocutaneous and axillary nerves. Neurosurgery. 2000; 46(1):93–101, discussion 101–103

[38] Oberlin C, Teboul F, Severin S, Beaulieu JY. Transfer of the lateral cutaneous nerve of the forearm to the dorsal branch of the ulnar nerve, for providing sensation on the ulnar aspect of the hand. Plast Reconstr Surg. 2003; 112(5):1498–1500

[39] Liu Y, Lao J, Gao K, Gu Y, Zhao X. Functional outcome of nerve transfers for traumatic global brachial plexus avulsion. Injury. 2013; 44(5):655–660

[40] Midha R. Nerve transfers for severe brachial plexus injuries: a review. Neurosurg Focus. 2004; 16(5):E5

[41] Omer GE, Jr. Injuries to nerves of the upper extremity. J Bone Joint Surg Am. 1974; 56(8):1615–1624

[42] Niver GE, Ilyas AM. Management of radial nerve palsy following fractures of the humerus. Orthop Clin North Am. 2013; 44(3):419–424, x

[43] Rorabeck CH, Clarke KM. The pathophysiology of the anterior tibial compartment syndrome: an experimental investigation. J Trauma. 1978; 18(5):299–304

[44] Dormans JP, Squillante R, Sharf H. Acute neurovascular complications with supracondylar humerus fractures in children. J Hand Surg Am. 1995; 20(1):1–4

[45] Amillo S, Mora G. Surgical management of neural injuries associated with elbow fractures in children. J Pediatr Orthop. 1999; 19(5):573–577

[46] de Laat EA, Visser CP, Coene LN, Pahlplatz PV, Tavy DL. Nerve lesions in primary shoulder dislocations and humeral neck fractures. A prospective clinical and EMG study. J Bone Joint Surg Br. 1994; 76(3):381–383

[47] Pollock FH, Drake D, Bovill EG, Day L, Trafton PG. Treatment of radial neuropathy associated with fractures of the humerus. J Bone Joint Surg Am. 1981; 63(2):239–243

[48] Mohler LR, Hanel DP. Closed fractures complicated by peripheral nerve injury. J Am Acad Orthop Surg. 2006; 14(1): 32–37

[49] Roganović Z. Factors influencing the outcome of nerve repair. Vojnosanit Pregl. 1998; 55(2):119–131

[50] Böstman O, Bakalim G, Vainionpää S, Wilppula E, Pätiälä H, Rokkanen P. Radial palsy in shaft fracture of the humerus. Acta Orthop Scand. 1986; 57(4):316–319

[51] Ring D, Chin K, Jupiter JB. Radial nerve palsy associated with high-energy humeral shaft fractures. J Hand Surg Am. 2004; 29(1):144–147

[52] Mehlman CT, Strub WM, Roy DR, Wall EJ, Crawford AH. The effect of surgical timing on the perioperative complications of treatment of supracondylar humeral fractures in children. J Bone Joint Surg Am. 2001; 83-A(3):323–327

[53] Kim DH, Murovic JA, Tiel R, Kline DG. Management and outcomes in 353 surgically treated sciatic nerve lesions. J Neurosurg. 2004; 101(1):8–17

[54] Patterson FP, Morton KS. Neurologic complications of fractures and dislocations of the pelvis. Surg Gynecol Obstet. 1961; 112:702–706

[55] Kim DH, Kline DG. Surgical outcome for intra- and extrapelvic femoral nerve lesions. J Neurosurg. 1995; 83(5):783–790

[56] Johnson EW, Jr, Vittands IJ. Nerve injuries in fractures of the lower extremity. Minn Med. 1969; 52(4):627–633

[57] Morton KS. Traumatic dislocation of the hip: a follow up study. Can J Surg. 1959; 3:67–74

[58] Roganovic ́ Z. Missile-caused complete lesions of the peroneal nerve and peroneal division of the sciatic nerve: results of 157 repairs. Neurosurgery. 2005; 57(6):1201–1212, discussion 1201–1212

[59] Gurdjian ES, Smathers HM. Peripheral nerve injury in fractures and dislocations of long bones. J Neurosurg. 1945; 2:202–219

51 Management of Pediatric Head Trauma

Linda W. Xu, Gerald A. Grant

51.1 Introduction

Traumatic brain injuries (TBIs) in children lead to nearly 500,000 emergency room visits a year and over 2,000 deaths a year. The most common cause of injury in children of age 0 to 14 years are falls, followed by being struck by an object, motor vehicle accident, and assault. Trends for emergency department visits, hospitalizations, deaths, and mechanism are broken down by age and summarized in ▶ Table 51.1. While falls are the most common cause of TBI in children age 0 to 14 years, children age 15 to 19 years are more commonly injured from motor vehicle collisions (MVCs). Since MVCs are more likely to be fatal than other mechanisms, rates of fatal TBI are also highest in the 15- to 19-year age group. Patients age 0 to 14 years old have a 2 to 5% rate of death, but children age 15 to 19 years old have a 19% rate of death from TBI.[1]

Physical mechanisms of injury in traumatic brain injuries involve acceleration, deceleration, and rotational forces causing skull fractures, vascular injuries, direct impact to brain parenchyma, and axonal shear injury. Levels of injury in TBI can be loosely categorized into mild (Glasgow Coma Score ([*GCS*] *13–15*), moderate (*GCS 9–12*), and severe (*GCS ≤ 8*) based on GCS postresuscitation. Mild TBI is vastly more common than severe and often underreported as not all children with mild TBI are brought to medical attention.

51.2 Initial Emergency Room Evaluation

51.2.1 History

- Determine mechanism.
- Assess for seizures and loss-of-consciousness events.
- Current headache, stable, increasing or decreasing.
- Nausea or vomiting.
- Any history of bleeding disorders.

51.2.2 Physical

- Presence of scalp hematoma.
- Lacerations and abrasions on the scalp, assess whether full thickness.

Table 51.1 Summary of number of emergency department visits, hospitalizations, deaths, and mechanisms of injury for head trauma per year by age[1]

Age	ED visits	Hospitalizations	Deaths	Mechanism
0–4	251,546	15,239	998	5.1% MVC 64.2% Falls 0.1% Assault 21.4% Struck by object 9.1% Other
5–9	105,015	8,799	450	7.0% MVC 40.3% Falls 1.0% Assault 33.9% Struck by object 17.8% Other
10–14	117,387	11,098	726	5.6% MVC 36.5% Falls 9.7% Assault 29.5% Struck by object 18.8% Other
15–19	157,198	24,896	3,995	25.7% MVC 20.8% Falls 14.2% Assault 23.2% Struck by object 16.0% Other

Abbreviation: MVC, motor vehicle collision.

- Palpation for skull fractures.
- If fontanelle present, assess for bulging or firmness.
- Focal neurological symptoms.
- Evidence of basilar skull fractures (ecchymosis around eyes or ears, fluid drainage from the nares or ears).

51.2.3 Neuroimaging

- When to image?
  - Focal neurological findings.
  - Concern for skull fracture on examination.
  - Altered mental status.
  - Irritability.
  - Bulging fontanelle.
  - Persistent vomiting.
  - Seizure.
  - Prolonged loss of consciousness.
  - Concern for child abuse.[2,3,4]
- For patients with GCS 14 to 15 with mild head trauma, chance of clinically significant finding on computed tomography (CT) is 1%.[2,5]
  - Can consider observation without CT scan if very low risk.
  - In low-risk patients with normal mental status, no hematoma, no loss of consciousness, no skull fracture, and low-risk mechanism.
    - < 0.2% of patients < 2 years old have clinically significant findings on CT.
    - < 0.05% of patients > 2 years old have clinically significant findings on CT.[5]

51.3 Management of Mild TBI

Minor head trauma can be defined as an injury to the head in a patient that is awake, alert, and remains responsive throughout the event. In a **mild TBI**, the patient may be currently awake, alert, and responsive but have had a transient loss of consciousness (LOC), disorientation, or emesis and GCS 14 to 15 on presentation. In this population, 0.1 to 1% will require neurosurgical intervention.[3,5,6]

Roughly 5% of patients with mild TBI will have CT findings of either skull fracture or intracranial abnormality and can be classified as a **complicated mild TBI**.[5,6,7] Although this is a small population, there is some debate as to whether these patients have an eventually different functional outcome. Some adult studies show that those with complicated mild TBI have outcomes more similar to those with moderate head injuries (GCS 9–12) with deficits on neuropsychiatric testing and lower

GCS scores while other studies suggest that while there may be early differences (prolonged return to work), there are eventually no functional differences for those with complicated injuries than those with uncomplicated TBI.[7]

As 99% of patients with mild TBI do not require neurosurgical intervention, it is up for debate which of these patients should be admitted for monitoring in the hospital. In general, if there is any suspicion of injury that may lead to further decline, other medical issues that may make the patient unstable, or concern about supervision or mechanism of injury, patients should be admitted for observation. In general, patients who have mild TBI with no findings on initial CT have a low rate of delayed decline.[8,9] General criteria for admission for mild TBI may thus include the following:

- Intracranial injury on CT
- Depressed skull fracture
- Persistent vomiting
- Any concern for nonaccidental trauma

Concussion is a subset of mild TBI specifically defined as a low-velocity injury associated with a rapid onset of short-lived impairment in neurological function that resolves spontaneously. These symptoms are thought to be related to a functional disturbance rather than a structural disturbance. Common symptoms are as follows:

- Headache.
- Disorientation.
- Loss of consciousness.
- Amnesia.
- Irritability.
- Insomnia.
- Emotional lability.

Initial on-site evaluation for concussion should proceed as standard emergency care with evaluation of ABCs and precautions for any associated cervical spine injury. The patient needs to be evaluated by a medical provider and if one is not available on site, they should be taken for urgent referral. The patient should not be left unattended for the first hours after injury in case of neurological decline. If the concussion occurred in the setting of an athletic activity, the patient should not be allowed to return to play on the day of injury. Same day return to play can be associated with delayed onset of symptoms and higher rates of neuropsychological symptoms postinjury.[10]

There are several ways to grade concussions and recommendations for return to play, which are based on adult guidelines as summarized in

▶ Table 51.2. One concern about return to play stems from the risk of **second impact syndrome**. This phenomenon is seen when a second impact occurs while the first injury has not been resolved and triggers a synergistic response causing severe and devastating results. The most severe cases of second impact syndrome can appear as concussion symptoms initially, but is then followed by collapse, pupillary dilation, loss of eye movement, respiratory failure, and death.[11] This mechanism is thought to be related to loss of vascular autoregulation with rapid increase in intracranial pressure (ICP) and herniation, which can result in neurological deterioration in a matter of minutes. In a study of pediatric patients with GCS 13 to 15, up to 28% demonstrated impaired autoregulation following head trauma.[12] More

Table 51.2 Concussion grading and return-to-play guidelines.

	Grade I	Grade II	Grade III	Return to play (RTP)
Cantu guidelines	No LOC < 30 min amnesia	LOC < 5 min 30 min–24 h amnesia	LOC > 5 min > 24 h amnesia	Grade I: • 1st time—1 wk • 2nd time—2 wk • 3rd time—end season Grade II: • 1st time—1 wk • 2nd time—1 mo • 3rd time—end season Grade III: • 1st time—1 mo • 2nd time—end season
Colorado Medical Society Guidelines	Confusion	Confusion and amnesia	LOC	Grade I: • 1st time—15 min • 2nd time—1 wk Grade II: • 1st time—1 wk • 2nd time—2 wk with physician's approval Grade III: • 1st time—1–6 mo based on severity of LOC • 2nd time——6 mo–1 y with physician's approval
American Academy of Neurology Guidelines	No LOC and < 15 min confusion	No LOC and > 15 min confusion	LOC	As summarized in Colorado Medical Society Guidelines
4th International Conference on Concussion	No grading guidelines		Summary of how to progress through stepwise RTP • Must be asymptomatic for 24 h in each step • If any symptoms occur, drop back to previous step where patient was asymptomatic • At least 1 wk to progress through entire protocol • Absolutely no same day return to play if any concussion occurs	Stepwise RTP: • Stage 1: No activity—rest with goal of recovery • Stage 2: Light aerobic exercise—goal of increasing heart rate • Stage 3: Sport-specific exercise—training drills with no head impact • Stage 4: Noncontact training drills—complex training drills with resistive training • Stage 5: Full-contact practice—medical clearance to participate in normal training with goal of restoring functional skills • Stage 6: Return to play

Abbreviation: LOC, loss of consciousness.
Source: Data from from Cantu guidelines, Colorado Medical Society Guidelines, American Academy of Neurology, and the 4th International Conference on Concussion.[13,14,15]

detailed discussion of cerebral physiology and autoregulation can be found later in this chapter. Most physicians recommend a graduated return-to-play protocol if the patient is asymptomatic, with a drop down to previous activity level if the patient becomes symptomatic.[13,14,15] A general timeline is proposed in the adult concussion literature, but many choose to be more conservative with children when recommending timing of return to play, which may be left up to the prerogative of the individual physician.

In patients with a history of prior concussions, there may be long-term effects. In the most immediate period, **postconcussion syndrome** can develop in which the patient continues to have symptoms after the first week with headaches, dizziness, neuropsychiatric symptoms, or cognitive impairment.[15] About 10 to 15% of patients will develop prolonged symptoms after the initial period. Depression and other mental health problems can arise in this population as well. Sleep problems and anxiety can also be common and some will choose to treat these issues medically, but of note, if these symptoms are medically suppressed, the patient should not be considered at their baseline and should not be considered for return to play.[13]

After frequent and prolonged exposure to concussions, "punch drunk," dementia pugilistica, or **chronic traumatic encephalopathy (CTE)** has been well characterized and a real risk for those with repeated injuries. First characterized in 1928, those with multiple concussions later on in life developed mood and emotional lability, memory loss, tremor, and dysarthria. Autopsies at that time showed microhemorrhages replaced with gliosis or degenerative tissue.[16] In particular, there was destruction of the limbic system, atrophy of the cerebellum, and widespread neurofibrillary tangles. There does appear to be a correlation between the level of exposure to concussion (i.e., years playing in the NFL) and worse pathological findings on autopsy, although a direct link has not been proven.[10,17,18]

51.4 Management of Severe TBI and Polytrauma

Severe TBI is defined as GCS less than or equal to 8 and 39% of severe pediatric TBIs are associated with multiple other traumatic injuries.[19] Children with severe TBI have a 34% mortality rate, and only 16% survive with good outcomes or moderate disabilities.[20] These patients are best managed in a specialized pediatric trauma center.[21,22,23,24]

51.4.1 Cerebral Physiology

When a significant primary injury to the brain has occurred, the principles of management are to minimize the secondary insults to the brain. Pediatric patients seem to be even more vulnerable than their adult counterparts to subsequent diffuse cerebral edema and injury, possibly from higher cerebral blood volume and flow.[20,25,26]

While many principles of cerebral physiology in pediatrics are similar to adults, there are several factors that do change with age. In adults, the average cerebral blood flow is about 50 mL/100 g/min with more flow in the gray matter than white matter. It appears that this number is higher in young children age 2 to 4 years old and then decreases down to adult levels. Correspondingly, cerebral vascular resistance is also lowest in this young age group. Cerebral oxygen and glucose consumptions start lower at birth and then increase during childhood until they plateau at 3 to 9 years old and then decrease toward adult levels.[27,28]

As in adults, control of blood flow to the brain varies by metabolism, carbon dioxide levels, oxygen levels, blood viscosity, and autoregulation. Carbon dioxide levels can very rapidly regulate cerebral blood flow. There are studies in children under anesthesia that they are even more sensitive to these changes than adults are, with up to 14% change in blood flow velocity per 1 mm Hg change in end-tidal CO_2. Autoregulation is mostly controlled at the arteriole level and in adults, at mean arterial pressures (MAPs) between 60 and 160 mm Hg, cerebral blood flow is mostly constant as arterioles constrict or relax to maintain a stable amount of blood flow regardless of blood pressure changes. Outside of these levels, autoregulation is unable to compensate to maintain cerebral blood flow constant and the child can experience ischemia or hyperemia. Although some assume children can tolerate lower blood pressures than adults, studies actually show a similar range with best cerebral autoregulation with MAP above 60 mm Hg.[28]

After brain trauma, cerebral blood flow can become uncoupled from metabolism resulting in either ischemia or hyperemia. In the immediate hours after injury, ischemia is more common with damage from hypoperfusion for the first 12 hours. A second phase typically follows with hyperemia and increased ICP. The third phase is associated with vasospasm and ischemia which can again become problematic.[28]

Ischemia causes secondary injury with infarction, but hyperemia also causes secondary injury with increased chance of hemorrhage, diffuse brain swelling, and higher ICPs. It has been suggested that in young children that there is a greater concern for hyperemia compared with adults since baseline cerebral blood flow is higher. In mild pediatric head trauma, 17 to 28% have been found to have impaired autoregulation versus 42% in severe head injury.[12,28]

There is often a biphasic pattern of ICP elevation after severe head injury in children. After the initial injury and temporary ischemia, the release of inflammatory components from the primary cell injury can cause the first phase of dysregulation of cerebral blood flow, diffuse edema, and elevated ICP. A second phase often 3 to 7 days after initial injury when secondary injury cellular cascades again increase inflammatory cerebral markers can cause a second phase of elevated ICP.[28,29] Although cerebral blood flow and autoregulation are difficult to measure clinically, cerebral perfusion pressure (CPP) can often be used as a surrogate and guidelines for use are described later in this chapter.

Because of the principles of cerebral physiology after trauma in a child, it is critical to manage volume status, ICP, CPP, ventilation, and cerebral metabolism (seizures, sedation, paralysis) to minimize additional secondary brain injury.

51.4.2 Pediatric Blood Loss and Hypovolemia

In trauma, 39% of deaths can be attributed to exsanguination.[30] Children tend to have a higher oxygen consumption, higher cardiac output to blood volume ratio, and for the very young, the presence of fetal hemoglobin delivers less oxygen to tissue.[31] Despite having higher blood volume needs, children can mask hypovolemia and blood loss due to their physiological reserve. In fact, the blood pressure can remain normal with 25 to 30% total blood volume loss.[32] Hypotension can be difficult to recognize by those not familiar with pediatric patients as their baseline blood pressures can vary widely by age. By the time

hypotension or a drop in central venous pressure is noted, a patient can proceed rapidly to cardiovascular collapse. Hypotension in the setting of trauma is clearly associated with morbidity and mortality.[33,34]

Many are not familiar with baseline normal physiological ranges in pediatric patients. As a rough estimate for blood volume:

Normal systolic blood pressure $= 90 + 2 \times$ age
Hypotension $= 70 + 2 \times$ age
Blood volume $= 80$ mL/kg

In pediatric patients, less obvious signs of hypovolemia are particularly important such as:

- Decreased pulse pressure (< 20 mm Hg) and associated flattening in arterial line contour.
- Mottled skin.
- Drop in temperature.
- Lethargy.
- Metabolic acidosis.
- Decrease in palpable pulses.
- Decreased urine output.
- Increased capillary filling time.[32]

The pediatric guidelines for trauma suggest that access for pediatric resuscitation is critical. If two attempts at peripheral access have failed, the provider should move on to interosseus access.[35] Resuscitation should proceed in a graded fashion with the following protocol:

- Warm crystalloid boluses in 20 mg/kg units $\times$ 3.
- Type-specific or O-negative packed red blood cells (PRBCs) in 10 mg/kg boluses and locate source of bleeding as soon as possible.
- Monitor urine output to gauge success of resuscitation with goal urine output of greater than 2 mL/kg/h in infants and 1 to 1.5 mL/kg/h in older children.[36]

Head traumas can contribute significantly to blood loss as the scalp is especially vascular and open lacerations can lead to rapid exsanguination. Scalp hematomas can accumulate a significant amount of blood compared to the overall blood volume of a child. When assessing source of blood loss in a child, cranial injuries are not an insignificant potential source. Unlike adults though where internal bleeding in long bones and the abdominal cavities are typically the only spaces where exsanguination can occur internally, an infant with open sutures and the ability to expand their overall cranial volume can hide a significant amount of blood volume loss in the intracranial space.[37]

51.4.3 Coagulopathy

Coagulopathy can also particularly become a problem as platelets and coagulation factors are actively consumed during active blood loss and then subsequently become diluted as resuscitation begins. While whole blood has normal clotting factors, patients are frequently transfused with PRBC, transfusion of platelets or fresh frozen plasma (FFP) should be considered in addition to PRBC. Head injury patients are particularly prone to developing **disseminated intravascular coagulopathy (DIC)** as injured brain releases tissue thromboplastin.[37,38,39] DIC can be characterized by a precipitous drop in platelets, elevation in prothrombin time and partial thromboplastin time, drop in fibrinogen, and elevation in D-dimer. Up to 40% of pediatric patients with severe TBI will develop coagulopathy and this risk appears to correlate with severity of injury, increasing age, and intraparenchymal injuries.[39] Providers should therefore be especially vigilant in monitoring for coagulopathy when a head injury is suspected.

51.4.4 ICP Monitoring

Numerous studies have shown that high ICP is associated with poor outcome and aggressive treatment of elevated ICP can improve outcome. ICP monitoring provides a way to gauge current ICP and whether subsequent treatments are working to bring ICP to a normal range.

Generally, after resuscitation, ICP monitoring is indicated if the patient has GCS less than or equal to 8 and CT evidence of intracranial injury.[40] In one study, up to 86% of pediatric patients with GCS less than or equal to 8 had ICP greater than 20.[41] Patients without obvious CT findings of intracranial injury may also have elevated ICP and require an ICP monitor.

Note: In infants with severe head injury, an open fontanelle is not an adequate replacement for having a definitive ICP monitor in place.[42]

51.4.5 Treatment of Intracranial Hypertension

In studies of overall outcome, ICPs of greater than 40 mm Hg are highly associated with death and ICPs ranging from 20 to 40 with significant morbidity.[43,44,45] In general, the goals of ICP management are to keep ICPs below 20 mm Hg. However, some pediatric studies show that control of CPP may be more important than ICP in overall outcome. CPP is calculated as MAP minus ICP and studies in adults show better outcomes with CPP above 40 to 60.[46,47] In children, goal CPP tend to vary by age with higher CPP goals in older age groups than younger age groups with goals in the 40s to 50s in those ages 2 to 6 years and 50s to 60s in those ages 7 to 16 years.[48,49] Below the desired CPP goals the patient may experience cerebral ischemia and above the desired range the patient may experience hyperemia and subsequent elevation in ICP.[28,50,51] A biphasic increase in ICP has been reported in children after severe TBI, one immediately after injury, and one several days to a week after injury.[28,29,52]

In general, strategies for lowering ICP and maximizing CPP rely on the following methods:
- Cerebrospinal fluid (CSF) drainage.
- Sedation and neuromuscular blockade.
- Hyperosmolar therapy.
- Hyperventilation.
- Barbiturates.
- Temperature regulation.
- Surgical decompression.[42]

CSF Drainage

Ventriculostomy has been known to reduce ICP and in an adult study, CSF drainage to keep the ICP less than 15 showed a significant improvement in mortality down to 12% compared to 53% in medical management alone.[41,53]

In our practice, external ventricular drains (EVDs) are often placed in the emergency room or intensive care unit (ICU). We generally place EVDs on the right side unless contraindicated by large blood clots in the parenchyma or in the ventricle. The hair is shaved on the corresponding side in a generous area to allow for tunneling of the EVD catheter into a clean area of scalp. The entry point is generally at the mid-pupillary line about 1 cm anterior to the coronal suture. The EVD is passed to a premeasured length from available imaging (usually between 3 and 5 cm) until CSF returns. If there is a lower suspicion for a severe head injury and the GCS is 7 to 8, one may also place a superficial intraparenchymal strain gauge often called a "bolt." A bolt allows for ICP monitoring but does not have the ability to drain CSF to improve the elevations in ICP.

Hyperosmolar Therapy

The two most commonly used agents for hyperosmolar therapy are mannitol and 3% hypertonic saline infusion. Mannitol was first introduced in 1961 and is felt to work by both a rapid mechanism of decreased blood viscosity and thus decreasing blood vessel diameter and total intracranial blood volume, and a slower mechanism that acts directly by osmosis.[52,54,55,56,57] Mannitol can decrease ICP by about 10% with mean time for return to baseline being roughly 3 hours.[57] Mannitol is felt to have some risks for renal injury, having led to acute tubular necrosis and renal failure in early studies, however, at that time, patients were often kept hypovolemic while mannitol was administered. It is unclear if the renal toxicity would be significantly less if the patient is kept euvolemic during that time. However, it is also important to note that due to this quick and robust diuretic effect, volume status can be hard to manage in a very small child after mannitol administration. Mannitol is generally administered between 0.25 g/kg and 1 g/kg boluses with goal serum osmolarity of 320 mOsm/L.[42] We caution the use of mannitol in young children due to the risk for hypovolemia.

Three percent hypertonic saline has been used since the early 1900s with efficacy in lowering ICP and overall improved ICU courses when used in severe TBI. It has been studied in children with good results and no significant renal failure noted.[58,59,60,61] Some propose that with 3%, the Osm goal can be higher and that 0.1 to 1.0 mL/kg hour can be used with goal serum osmolarity up to 360 mOsm/L.[42,59]

Hyperventilation

The goal of hyperventilation is to reduce the serum pCO_2 and cause vasoconstriction and thus limit the total blood volume intracranially. Hypocapnia leads quickly to cerebral vasoconstriction, cerebral blood flow, cerebral blood volume, and can quickly change ICP. In children, as described above, they appear to be even more sensitive than adults to pCO_2 changes.[28] However, vasoconstriction also leads to risks of decreased cerebral perfusion.[62] Chronic hyperventilation can lead to a variety of problems including depleted bicarbonate supplies, causing the patient to become hyperresponsive to subsequent pCO_2 levels, left shift of the hemoglobin curve with decreased oxygen delivery, and increased brain ischemia.[63,64,65,66] Thus, hyperventilation is meant only for short-term use and only if ICP has been demonstrated to be high. There is no indication for prophylactic hyperventilation. As it is not a long-term mechanism for decreasing ICP,

hyperventilation is generally used only for brief periods in cases of herniation or acute deterioration to help while awaiting a more definitive method for lowering ICP. Hyperventilation goals can be to increase respiratory rate until $PaCO_2$ equals 30, less than 30 if used very aggressively. If planning for aggressive hyperventilation, one could consider monitoring for cerebral ischemia with brain tissue oxygen monitors or jugular venous oxygen monitors.[42]

Sedation

Sedation and paralysis are felt to reduce secondary injury after head trauma by reducing cerebral metabolism, minimizing patient agitation, and facilitating ventilation. There are number of agents that can be used for sedation which are often used in conjunction and thus difficult to study independently. The only sedative with strong evidence of correlation with lowering ICP more effectively than other agents is barbiturates which are discussed in the next section. Common sedatives used in pediatric trauma are summarized in ▶ Table 51.3. Opiates for pain management and benzodiazepines for sedation are commonly used for sedation to control ICP. Propofol is commonly used in neurosurgical patients as there is often a reduction in ICP from the agent itself, however, there have been concerns about propofol infusion syndrome, particularly in children. Therefore, long-term use is generally avoided.[67,68,69,70]

Neuromuscular blockade can decrease ICP by decreasing airway and thoracic pressures, decreasing shivering, posturing, and fighting the ventilator.[71] However, conversely it is also associated with pneumonia, cardiovascular side effects, increased ICU stay, myopathy, patient stress if not concomitantly sedated well, and inability to detect neurological changes.[42,72]

Barbiturates

Use of barbiturates was first described as a treatment for elevated ICP in the 1970s and have been correlated with improved outcomes.[73] It is thought that the mechanism of ICP reduction is threefold by suppressing overall metabolism, changing vascular tone, and eliminating free radicals with stabilization of neuronal membranes.[74,75] Generally pentobarbital and thiopental can both be used and there are no studies that directly compare the efficacy of either agent against each other. When initiating barbiturate coma, the patient should be

Table 51.3 Comparison of sedative agents frequently used in pediatrics for ICP management[67,68,69,70]

Agents	Pros	Cons	Use	Notes
Propofol	Rapid onset Rapid clearance Decreases cerebral metabolism and ICP Increases seizure threshold	Hypotension Pancreatitis Liver failure Propofol infusion syndrome	Induction: 1–2.5 mg/kg Maintenance: 1.5–4.5 mg/kg/h and titrate to sedation	Propofol infusion syndrome • First reported in children • Lactic acidosis • Cardiovascular collapse • At risk if using more than 4 mg/kg/h for > 48 h
Benzodiazepines	Less hypotension Raises seizure threshold Reduces cerebral metabolism and ICP	Slow wake up due to buildup of metabolites Withdrawal Delirium Respiratory depression Plateau with no increase in ICP control at high doses	Induction: 0.1 mg/kg Maintenance: 0.01–0.2 mg/kg/h	
Narcotics	Pain control Little effect on blood pressure	Could possibly increase ICP in high-dose boluses	Adjunct to other sedatives	
Dexmedetomidine	No respiratory depression Can be used in patients who are not intubated Decreases delirium	Hypotension Bradycardia Arrhythmia	Induction: 1 µg/kg Infusion: 0.42–1 µg/kg/h	

Abbreviation: ICP, intracranial pressure.

concomitantly on electroencephalogram (EEG) to titrate doses to maximal burst suppression to minimize cerebral metabolism. While you can check serum levels, studies have shown that serum levels don't predict well when a patient is truly burst suppressed. The drawback of barbiturate coma is that it often induces hemodynamic instability and requires concurrent use of cardiovascular drips to maintain adequate blood pressures and may be difficult to use in patients that are already hemodynamically unstable. In pediatric studies, use of barbiturates in patients without refractory intracranial hypertension may actually increase mortality due to hemodynamic problems, and thus it should never be used prophylactically or unless other methods of ICP control have failed.[76,77] When to stop a barbiturate coma can be up to the practitioner, but some suggest that ICP should be stable for at least 24 hours before trialing a barbiturate taper.

Pentobarbital:

Loading dose 10 mg/kg.

Maintenance 1 mg/kg/h with adjustments for burst suppression.[78]

Thiopental:

Loading dose 10 to 20 mg/kg.

Maintenance 3 to 5 mg/kg/h with adjustments for burst suppression.[79]

Temperature Regulation

Hyperthermia after a cerebral injury is thought to lead to increased metabolism, inflammation, excitotoxicity, and seizures. Thus, it was suggested that perhaps cooling a patient may improve neurological outcomes. A study in children in the 1970s showed 19/20 children survived with initial GCS of 4 after cooling, which is significantly better than historical controls.[80] There have been several adult studies more recently showing improved ICP and improved outcomes at 3 and 6 months from injury.[81,82,83] In one phase II trial in children, hypothermia did lower ICPs but were associated with some increase in arrhythmias and showed no definitive functional difference at 6 months from injury.[84] In general, all brain traumas should avoid hyperthermia and those with medically refractory ICP can be considered for a cooling protocol down to a temperature of 34 °C. During cooling it is important to monitor for coagulopathy, which can worsen existing bleeding, arrhythmias, and also to minimize shivering which can increase cerebral metabolism. Patients being cooled may need to be simultaneously paralyzed to minimize the effects of shivering. As cooling protocols limit examinations if the patient requires sedation and paralysis, and can worsen coagulopathy, it is also generally reserved for patients with refractory ICP to other methods of treatment.

Steroids

Steroids are used commonly in other neurosurgical pathologies like tumors and infections but in studies of steroid use in trauma, it has been correlated with increased infection rates but no corresponding improvement in outcomes.[85,86,87,88] Thus, there is *no indication for steroid use* in trauma.

Surgical Treatment

In general, if the patient has elevated ICP from a mass lesion, it is easy to make the decision to proceed with operative intervention to remove the mass lesion, whether it be a subdural, epidural, or intraparenchymal hematoma.

Epidural hematomas are classically associated with an immediate loss of consciousness with a lucid interval afterward, followed by headache, vomiting, and altered mental status. Often there are associated skull fractures and on CT the pattern of blood typically takes a lentiform shape and does not cross suture lines of the skull. Although previously it was felt that epidural hematomas are usually the result of arterial bleeding and thus can progress quickly and should all be surgically decompressed, more recent studies suggest that it is possible to manage patients who are neurologically intact with nonoperative treatment. In a study of 13 intact patients with epidural hematoma, all but one was successfully managed with nonoperative treatment and made a full recovery at follow-up after 4 months with follow-up CT scans showing complete resolution of bleed.[89] However, others argue nonoperative treatment can lead to prolonged hospitalization with continued issues with headache, nausea, and vomiting than a simple evacuation of an epidural.

Subdural hematomas typically result from shear injury to a cortical vein. In infants, it can be a result of shaken baby syndrome and nonaccidental trauma, which is addressed in a separate chapter. In general, patients with a subdural hemorrhage, evidence of brain compression, midline shift, and neurological deficit should be considered for evacuation. In an acute subdural, blood typically cannot be drained through burr holes and requires a full craniotomy, but chronic subdurals from distant trauma is often liquefied and can be successfully drained with just burr holes.

Less straightforward is deciding which patients require decompressive craniectomy. Goals for decompression are to reduce ICP, increase CPP, and prevent herniation. Decompressive craniectomy is efficacious in reducing ICP with a drop in ICP of 9 to 47 points at the time of durotomy.[45,90] However, as patients requiring decompressive craniectomy are also patients with very severe injuries, there is some question to whether this overall leads to desirable outcomes. There is some evidence that there are overall improved outcomes with craniectomy with better results in pediatric trauma patients than adults.[45,90,91] It is worth considering early in a child with refractory ICPs and a unilateral injury. In general, it is felt that patients should be considered if the patient meets the following criteria:[45,90,91,92]

1. Diffuse swelling on CT scan
2. Patient is within 48 hours of initial injury
3. No episodes of sustained ICP greater than 40 prior to surgery
4. GCS greater than 3 at some point after injury
5. Secondary deterioration after initial good clinical presentation
6. Evidence of herniation

Surgical technique for decompression can be a unilateral frontotemporalparietal decompression or bifrontal craniotomy. No studies directly compare these techniques but preference may depend on appearance on CT and whether there is more concern for unilateral or bilateral edema. Most surgeons also perform a duraplasty at the time of surgery. Generally, size of craniotomy is recommended to be as large as is safely possible as small craniectomy can cause sustained ICP problems and cerebral infarction at the borders of the craniectomy that undergo the most pressure to herniate outward.

Summary of treatment of elevated ICP (▶ Fig. 51.1).[42]

• *Tier 1:* Basic management of head trauma

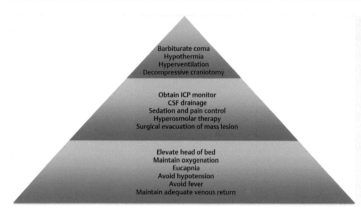

Fig. 51.1 Summary of treatment of elevated intracranial pressure. Tier 1: Basic management of head trauma. Tier 2: Suspected or confirmed ICP elevation. Tier 3: Refractory elevated ICP.

- *Tier 2:* Suspected or confirmed ICP elevation
- *Tier 3:* Refractory elevated ICP

51.4.6 Seizures

Posttraumatic seizures are common and can be classified as either early (within the first 7 days) or late (>7 days from injury). Seizures after initial injury can cause increased brain metabolism and ICP, leading to additional brain injury. In children, 20 to 39% of patients with severe TBI experience early posttraumatic seizures. Infants and children already have lower seizure threshold than adults and may have difficult to detect clinical seizures. Antiepileptics in severe TBI patients have been shown to decrease the percentage of patients that experience early seizures and has been associated with improved survival.[42,93,94]

Late posttraumatic seizures present in 7 to 12% of TBI patients and is not felt to be prevented by early use of prophylactic antiepileptics.[42] The risk of developing epilepsy is two times higher in the first 5 years after injury than those without head injury.[95] It can lead to further accidental injury and psychological changes, and these patients should generally be referred to a neurologist for long-term seizure management.

51.5 Surgical Pearls

- Head trauma is common in pediatrics with younger populations having more falls and older populations having more MVCs, leading to higher fatalities in older children.
- Mild TBI is defined as a patient with GCS greater than 13 on presentation and complicated mild TBI if the patient has an associated CT finding, who may functionally behave more like a patient with a moderate TBI. Only 1% will eventually need surgical intervention. Concussion is a functional disturbance in neurological dysfunction without any noted structural findings and is a subset of mild TBI.
- The principles of graded return to play indicate that the patient should return to activity through various stages starting with light activity to full activity, and drop back down to previous activity level if any symptoms are experienced. This is to minimize the occurrence of second impact syndrome which can be a fatal dysregulation of cerebral blood flow.
- Patient with multiple concussions or mild TBIs should be counseled on chronic traumatic encephalopathy (CTE) and implications later in life.
- Because of improved compensatory mechanisms in children to maintain heart rate and blood pressure, clinical signs of hypovolemia are more important to note early on rather than changes in vital signs.
- DIC is common in pediatrics and coagulation factors should be transfused in conjunction with PRBC.
- There is a basic tiered approach to elevated ICP management with baseline management of all head traumas, treatment methods for suspected or confirmed ICP elevation, and refractory ICP.
- CPP goals vary by age with goals of 40 to 50 in younger children and 50 to 60 in older children.
- Surgical decompression should be considered when there is a defined mass lesion.
- Surgery decompression should be considered early for diffuse brain edema if patient had an initially better neurological presentation and

had a subsequent decline due to herniation and surgical intervention can be offered quickly.

51.6 Common Clinical Questions

1. If ICP remains elevated after initiation of EVD placement and CSF drainage, 3% infusion, and sedation, what other steps can be taken at this point to lower ICP?
2. Are antiepileptic medications needed after head trauma? Do they reduce the chance of developing late posttraumatic seizures?
3. After a concussion, when should a child return to activities?
4. What is chronic traumatic encephalopathy?

51.7 Answers to Common Clinical Questions

1. If ICP is refractory to initial treatments, the next steps to consider are barbiturate coma and possibly hypothermia. If there is a mass lesion, surgical evacuation should be considered. If there is diffuse edema, overall clinical status should be considered and if appropriate for decompressive craniectomy, this step should be taken quickly. Hyperventilation can be used as a bridge therapy until another more definitive therapy can be initiated.
2. Antiepileptics should be considered for severe TBIs and has been shown to improve survival. It does not change the risk for late posttraumatic seizures.
3. After a concussion, the child should never return to play on the day of the event and should seek evaluation by a physician. Return to activities is based on a graded return to play where the child proceeds through graded steps of no activity, light activity, moderate activity, and full return to play with stop and drop back to previous activity level if the patient experiences any symptoms such as headache, nausea/vomiting, confusion, dizziness, dyscoordination, or mood changes. Recent recommendations are also encouraging return to school prior to return to play.
4. CTE is a condition after repeated head injuries where microhemorrhages are progressively replaced with degenerative tissue especially in the limbic system and cerebellum leading to permanent mood changes, memory loss,

tremor, and dysarthria. There is a direct correlation between exposure to concussions and severity of CTE.

References

[1] Faul MXL, Wald MM, Coronado VG. Traumatic brain injury in the United States: Emergency Department Visits, Hospitalizations and Deaths 2002–2006. Atlanta, GA: U.S. Department of Health and Human Services; 2010

[2] Osmond MH, Klassen TP, Wells GA, et al. Pediatric Emergency Research Canada (PERC) Head Injury Study Group. CATCH: a clinical decision rule for the use of computed tomography in children with minor head injury. CMAJ. 2010; 182(4): 341–348

[3] Schunk JE, Rodgerson JD, Woodward GA. The utility of head computed tomographic scanning in pediatric patients with normal neurologic examination in the emergency department. Pediatr Emerg Care. 1996; 12(3):160–165

[4] Stiell IG, Clement CM, Rowe BH, et al. Comparison of the Canadian CT Head Rule and the New Orleans Criteria in patients with minor head injury. JAMA. 2005; 294(12): 1511–1518

[5] Kuppermann N, Holmes JF, Dayan PS, et al. Pediatric Emergency Care Applied Research Network (PECARN). Identification of children at very low risk of clinically-important brain injuries after head trauma: a prospective cohort study. Lancet. 2009; 374(9696):1160–1170

[6] Dietrich AM, Bowman MJ, Ginn-Pease ME, Kosnik E, King DR. Pediatric head injuries: can clinical factors reliably predict an abnormality on computed tomography? Ann Emerg Med. 1993; 22(10):1535–1540

[7] Williams DH, Levin HS, Eisenberg HM. Mild head injury classification. Neurosurgery. 1990; 27(3):422–428

[8] Hamilton M, Mrazik M, Johnson DW. Incidence of delayed intracranial hemorrhage in children after uncomplicated minor head injuries. Pediatrics. 2010; 126(1):e33–e39

[9] Holmes JF, Borgialli DA, Nadel FM, et al. TBI Study Group for the Pediatric Emergency Care Applied Research Network. Do children with blunt head trauma and normal cranial computed tomography scan results require hospitalization for neurologic observation? Ann Emerg Med. 2011; 58(4): 315–322

[10] Guskiewicz KM, McCrea M, Marshall SW, et al. Cumulative effects associated with recurrent concussion in collegiate football players: the NCAA Concussion Study. JAMA. 2003; 290(19):2549–2555

[11] Saunders RL, Harbaugh RE. The second impact in catastrophic contact-sports head trauma. JAMA. 1984; 252 (4):538–539

[12] Jünger EC, Newell DW, Grant GA, et al. Cerebral autoregulation following minor head injury. J Neurosurg. 1997; 86(3):425–432

[13] Giza CC, Kutcher JS, Ashwal S, et al. Summary of evidence-based guideline update: evaluation and management of concussion in sports: report of the Guideline Development Subcommittee of the American Academy of Neurology. Neurology. 2013; 80(24):2250–2257

[14] McCrory P, Meeuwisse WH, Aubry M, et al. Consensus statement on concussion in sport: the 4th International Conference on Concussion in Sport held in Zurich, November 2012. J Am Coll Surg 216(5):e55–e71

[15] Cantu RC. Head injuries in sport. Br J Sports Med. 1996; 30 (4):289–296

[16] Corsellis JA, Bruton CJ, Taylor DC, Falconer MA. [Localized dysplasia of the cerebral cortex based on tissue examinations which were obtained during neurosurgical interventions in epileptics]. Psychiatr Neurol Med Psychol Beih. 1973; 17–18: 43–53

[17] McKee AC, Stern RA, Nowinski CJ, et al. The spectrum of disease in chronic traumatic encephalopathy. Brain. 2013; 136(pt 1):43–64

[18] Lehman EJ, Hein MJ, Baron SL, Gersic CM. Neurodegenerative causes of death among retired National Football League players. Neurology. 2012; 79(19):1970–1974

[19] Chiaretti A, De Benedictis R, Della Corte F, et al. The impact of initial management on the outcome of children with severe head injury. Childs Nerv Syst. 2002; 18(1–2):54–60

[20] Levin HS, Aldrich EF, Saydjari C, et al. Severe head injury in children: experience of the Traumatic Coma Data Bank. Neurosurgery. 1992; 31(3):435–443, discussion 443–444

[21] Hall JR. Impact of traumatic subarachnoid hemorrhage on outcome in nonpenetrating head injury. Part II: relationship to clinical course and outcome variables during acute hospitalization. J Trauma. 1997; 42(6):1196–1197

[22] Hulka F, Mullins RJ, Mann NC, et al. Influence of a statewide trauma system on pediatric hospitalization and outcome. J Trauma. 1997; 42(3):514–519

[23] Johnson DL, Krishnamurthy S. Send severely head-injured children to a pediatric trauma center. Pediatr Neurosurg. 1996; 25(6):309–314

[24] Potoka DA, Schall LC, Gardner MJ, Stafford PW, Peitzman AB, Ford HR. Impact of pediatric trauma centers on mortality in a statewide system. J Trauma. 2000; 49(2):237–245

[25] Tepas JJ, III, DiScala C, Ramenofsky ML, Barlow B. Mortality and head injury: the pediatric perspective. J Pediatr Surg. 1990; 25(1):92–95, discussion 96

[26] Lang DA, Teasdale GM, Macpherson P, Lawrence A. Diffuse brain swelling after head injury: more often malignant in adults than children? J Neurosurg. 1994; 80(4):675–680

[27] Chiron C, Raynaud C, Mazière B, et al. Changes in regional cerebral blood flow during brain maturation in children and adolescents. J Nucl Med. 1992; 33(5):696–703

[28] Udomphorn Y, Armstead WM, Vavilala MS. Cerebral blood flow and autoregulation after pediatric traumatic brain injury. Pediatr Neurol. 2008; 38(4):225–234

[29] Dardiotis E, Karanikas V, Paterakis KN, Fountas K, Hadjigeorgiou GM. Traumatic Brain Injury and Inflammation: Emerging Role of Innate and Adaptive Immunity. In: Agrawal A, ed. Brain Injury–Pathogenesis, Monitoring, Recovery and Management. Rijeka: InTech; 2012:23–38

[30] Sauaia A, Moore FA, Moore EE, et al. Epidemiology of trauma deaths: a reassessment. J Trauma. 1995; 38(2):185–193

[31] Barcelona SL, Thompson AA, Coté CJ. Intraoperative pediatric blood transfusion therapy: a review of common issues. Part I: hematologic and physiologic differences from adults; metabolic and infectious risks. Paediatr Anaesth. 2005; 15 (9):716–726

[32] McFadyen JG, Ramaiah R, Bhananker SM. Initial assessment and management of pediatric trauma patients. Int J Crit Illn Inj Sci. 2012; 2(3):121–127

[33] Pigula FA, Wald SL, Shackford SR, Vane DW. The effect of hypotension and hypoxia on children with severe head injuries. J Pediatr Surg. 1993; 28(3):310–314, discussion 315–316

[34] Kokoska ER, Smith GS, Pittman T, Weber TR. Early hypotension worsens neurological outcome in pediatric patients with moderately severe head trauma. J Pediatr Surg. 1998; 33(2):333–338

[35] McNamara RM, Spivey WH, Unger HD, Malone DR. Emergency applications of intraosseous infusion. J Emerg Med. 1987; 5(2):97–101

[36] American College of Surgeons. ATLS: Advanced Trauma Life Support for Doctors. 8th ed. Chicago, IL: American College of Surgeons; 2008

[37] Barcelona SL, Thompson AA, Coté CJ. Intraoperative pediatric blood transfusion therapy: a review of common issues. Part II: transfusion therapy, special considerations, and reduction of allogenic blood transfusions. Paediatr Anaesth. 2005; 15 (10):814–830

[38] Hymel KP, Abshire TC, Luckey DW, Jenny C. Coagulopathy in pediatric abusive head trauma. Pediatrics. 1997; 99(3):371–375

[39] Talving P, Lustenberger T, Lam L, et al. Coagulopathy after isolated severe traumatic brain injury in children. J Trauma. 2011; 71(5):1205–1210

[40] Narayan RK, Kishore PR, Becker DP, et al. Intracranial pressure: to monitor or not to monitor? A review of our experience with severe head injury. J Neurosurg. 1982; 56 (5):650–659

[41] Shapiro K, Marmarou A. Clinical applications of the pressure-volume index in treatment of pediatric head injuries. J Neurosurg. 1982; 56(6):819–825

[42] Adelson PD, Bratton SL, Carney NA, et al. American Association for Surgery of Trauma, Child Neurology Society, International Society for Pediatric Neurosurgery, International Trauma Anesthesia and Critical Care Society, Society of Critical Care Medicine, World Federation of Pediatric Intensive and Critical Care Societies. Guidelines for the acute medical management of severe traumatic brain injury in infants, children, and adolescents. Chapter 4. Resuscitation of blood pressure and oxygenation and prehospital brain-specific therapies for the severe pediatric traumatic brain injury patient. Pediatr Crit Care Med. 2003; 4 suppl 3:S12–S18

[43] Pfenninger J, Kaiser G, Lütschg J, Sutter M. Treatment and outcome of the severely head injured child. Intensive Care Med. 1983; 9(1):13–16

[44] Esparza J, M-Portillo J, Sarabia M, Yuste JA, Roger R, Lamas E. Outcome in children with severe head injuries. Childs Nerv Syst. 1985; 1(2):109–114

[45] Cho DY, Wang YC, Chi CS. Decompressive craniotomy for acute shaken/impact baby syndrome. Pediatr Neurosurg. 1995; 23(4):192–198

[46] Robertson CS, Valadka AB, Hannay HJ, et al. Prevention of secondary ischemic insults after severe head injury. Crit Care Med. 1999; 27(10):2086–2095

[47] Changaris DG, McGraw CP, Richardson JD, Garretson HD, Arpin EJ, Shields CB. Correlation of cerebral perfusion pressure and Glasgow Coma Scale to outcome. J Trauma. 1987; 27(9):1007–1013

[48] Chambers IR, Jones PA, Lo TY, et al. Critical thresholds of intracranial pressure and cerebral perfusion pressure related to age in paediatric head injury. J Neurol Neurosurg Psychiatry. 2006; 77(2):234–240

[49] Chambers IR, Stobbart L, Jones PA, et al. Age-related differences in intracranial pressure and cerebral perfusion pressure in the first 6 hours of monitoring after children's head injury: association with outcome. Childs Nerv Syst. 2005; 21(3):195–199

[50] Downard C, Hulka F, Mullins RJ, et al. Relationship of cerebral perfusion pressure and survival in pediatric brain-injured patients. J Trauma. 2000; 49(4):654–658, discussion 658–659

[51] Elias-Jones AC, Punt JA, Turnbull AE, Jaspan T. Management and outcome of severe head injuries in the Trent region 1985–90. Arch Dis Child. 1992; 67(12):1430–1435

[52] Bouma GJ, Muizelaar JP. Cerebral blood flow, cerebral blood volume, and cerebrovascular reactivity after severe head injury. J Neurotrauma. 1992; 9 suppl 1:S333–S348

[53] Ghajar JB. Significant lateralisation of supratentorial ICP after blunt head trauma. Acta Neurochir (Wien). 1993; 120(1–2): 98–99

[54] Wise BL, Chater N. Effect of mannitol on cerebrospinal fluid pressure. The actions of hypertonic mannitol solutions and of urea compared. Arch Neurol. 1961; 4:200–202

[55] Muizelaar JP, Wei EP, Kontos HA, Becker DP. Mannitol causes compensatory cerebral vasoconstriction and vasodilation in response to blood viscosity changes. J Neurosurg. 1983; 59 (5):822–828

[56] Muizelaar JP, Lutz HA, III, Becker DP. Effect of mannitol on ICP and CBF and correlation with pressure autoregulation in severely head-injured patients. J Neurosurg. 1984; 61(4): 700–706

[57] James HE. Methodology for the control of intracranial pressure with hypertonic mannitol. Acta Neurochir (Wien). 1980; 51(3–4):161–172

[58] Fisher B, Thomas D, Peterson B. Hypertonic saline lowers raised intracranial pressure in children after head trauma. J Neurosurg Anesthesiol. 1992; 4(1):4–10

[59] Khanna S, Davis D, Peterson B, et al. Use of hypertonic saline in the treatment of severe refractory posttraumatic intracranial hypertension in pediatric traumatic brain injury. Crit Care Med. 2000; 28(4):1144–1151

[60] Peterson B, Khanna S, Fisher B, Marshall L. Prolonged hypernatremia controls elevated intracranial pressure in head-injured pediatric patients. Crit Care Med. 2000; 28(4): 1136–1143

[61] Simma B, Burger R, Falk M, Sacher P, Fanconi S. A prospective, randomized, and controlled study of fluid management in children with severe head injury: lactated Ringer's solution versus hypertonic saline. Crit Care Med. 1998; 26(7):1265–1270

[62] Muizelaar JP, van der Poel HG, Li ZC, Kontos HA, Levasseur JE. Pial arteriolar vessel diameter and CO2 reactivity during prolonged hyperventilation in the rabbit. J Neurosurg. 1988; 69(6):923–927

[63] Muizelaar JP, Marmarou A, Ward JD, et al. Adverse effects of prolonged hyperventilation in patients with severe head injury: a randomized clinical trial. J Neurosurg. 1991; 75(5): 731–739

[64] Schneider GH, von Helden A, Lanksch WR, Unterberg A. Continuous monitoring of jugular bulb oxygen saturation in comatose patients—therapeutic implications. Acta Neurochir (Wien). 1995; 134(1–2):71–75

[65] von Helden A, Schneider GH, Unterberg A, Lanksch WR. Monitoring of jugular venous oxygen saturation in comatose patients with subarachnoid haemorrhage and intracerebral haematomas. Acta Neurochir Suppl (Wien). 1993; 59:102–106

[66] Kiening KL, Härtl R, Unterberg AW, Schneider GH, Bardt T, Lanksch WR. Brain tissue pO2-monitoring in comatose patients: implications for therapy. Neurol Res. 1997; 19(3): 233–240

[67] Spitzfaden AC, Jimenez DF, Tobias JD. Propofol for sedation and control of intracranial pressure in children. Pediatr Neurosurg. 1999; 31(4):194–200

[68] Farling PA, Johnston JR, Coppel DL. Propofol infusion for sedation of patients with head injury in intensive care. A preliminary report. Anaesthesia. 1989; 44(3):222–226

[69] Bray RJ. Propofol infusion syndrome in children. Paediatr Anaesth. 1998; 8(6):491–499

[70] Flower O, Hellings S. Sedation in traumatic brain injury. Emerg Med Int. 2012; 2012:637171

[71] Vernon DD, Witte MK. Effect of neuromuscular blockade on oxygen consumption and energy expenditure in sedated, mechanically ventilated children. Crit Care Med. 2000; 28(5): 1569–1571

[72] Hsiang JK, Chesnut RM, Crisp CB, Klauber MR, Blunt BA, Marshall LF. Early, routine paralysis for intracranial pressure control in severe head injury: is it necessary? Crit Care Med. 1994; 22(9):1471–1476

[73] Bruce DA, Raphaely RC, Goldberg AI, et al. Pathophysiology, treatment and outcome following severe head injury in children. Childs Brain. 1979; 5(3):174–191

[74] Piatt JH, Jr, Schiff SJ. High dose barbiturate therapy in neurosurgery and intensive care. Neurosurgery. 1984; 15(3): 427–444

[75] Cruz J. Adverse effects of pentobarbital on cerebral venous oxygenation of comatose patients with acute traumatic brain swelling: relationship to outcome. J Neurosurg. 1996; 85(5): 758–761

[76] Kasoff SS, Lansen TA, Holder D, Filippo JS. Aggressive physiologic monitoring of pediatric head trauma patients with elevated intracranial pressure. Pediatr Neurosci. 1988; 14(5):241–249

[77] Pittman T, Bucholz R, Williams D. Efficacy of barbiturates in the treatment of resistant intracranial hypertension in severely head-injured children. Pediatr Neurosci. 1989; 15 (1):13–17

[78] Eisenberg HM, Frankowski RF, Contant CF, Marshall LF, Walker MD. High-dose barbiturate control of elevated intracranial pressure in patients with severe head injury. J Neurosurg. 1988; 69(1):15–23

[79] Nordby HK, Nesbakken R. The effect of high dose barbiturate decompression after severe head injury. A controlled clinical trial. Acta Neurochir (Wien). 1984; 72(3–4):157–166

[80] Gruszkiewicz J, Doron Y, Peyser E. Recovery from severe craniocerebral injury with brain stem lesions in childhood. Surg Neurol. 1973; 1(4):197–201

[81] Shiozaki T, Sugimoto H, Taneda M, et al. Effect of mild hypothermia on uncontrollable intracranial hypertension after severe head injury. J Neurosurg. 1993; 79(3):363–368

[82] Marion DW, Penrod LE, Kelsey SF, et al. Treatment of traumatic brain injury with moderate hypothermia. N Engl J Med. 1997; 336(8):540–546

[83] Clifton GL, Allen S, Barrodale P, et al. A phase II study of moderate hypothermia in severe brain injury. J Neurotrauma. 1993; 10(3):263–271, discussion 273

[84] Adelson PD, Ragheb J, Kanev P, et al. Phase II clinical trial of moderate hypothermia after severe traumatic brain injury in children. Neurosurgery. 2005; 56(4):740–754, discussion 740–754

[85] Fanconi S, Klöti J, Meuli M, Zaugg H, Zachmann M. Dexamethasone therapy and endogenous cortisol production in severe pediatric head injury. Intensive Care Med. 1988; 14 (2):163–166

[86] Cooper PR, Moody S, Clark WK, et al. Dexamethasone and severe head injury. A prospective double-blind study. J Neurosurg. 1979; 51(3):307–316

[87] Klöti J, Fanconi S, Zachmann M, Zaugg H. Dexamethasone therapy and cortisol excretion in severe pediatric head injury. Childs Nerv Syst. 1987; 3(2):103–105

[88] James HE, Madauss WC, Tibbs PA, McCloskey JJ, Bean JR. The effect of high dose dexamethasone in children with severe closed head injury. A preliminary report. Acta Neurochir (Wien). 1979; 45(3–4):225–236

[89] Balmer B, Boltshauser E, Altermatt S, Gobet R. Conservative management of significant epidural haematomas in children. Childs Nerv Syst. 2006; 22(4):363–367

[90] Taylor A, Butt W, Rosenfeld J, et al. A randomized trial of very early decompressive craniectomy in children with traumatic brain injury and sustained intracranial hypertension. Childs Nerv Syst. 2001; 17(3):154–162

[91] Polin RS, Shaffrey ME, Bogaev CA, et al. Decompressive bifrontal craniectomy in the treatment of severe refractory posttraumatic cerebral edema. Neurosurgery. 1997; 41(1):84–92, discussion 92–94

[92] Guerra WK, Gaab MR, Dietz H, Mueller JU, Piek J, Fritsch MJ. Surgical decompression for traumatic brain swelling: indications and results. J Neurosurg. 1999; 90(2):187–196

[93] Lewis RJ, Yee L, Inkelis SH, Gilmore D. Clinical predictors of post-traumatic seizures in children with head trauma. Ann Emerg Med. 1993; 22(7):1114–1118

[94] Tilford JM, Simpson PM, Yeh TS, et al. Variation in therapy and outcome for pediatric head trauma patients. Crit Care Med. 2001; 29(5):1056–1061

[95] Annegers JF, Grabow JD, Groover RV, Laws ER, Jr, Elveback LR, Kurland LT. Seizures after head trauma: a population study. Neurology. 1980; 30(7 pt 1):683–689

52 Abusive Head Trauma

Mark S. Dias

52.1 Definitions and Nomenclature

Abusive head trauma reflects a combination of injuries to an infant, most commonly less than 24 months of age, resulting from child abuse. The injuries were originally described by Guthkelch in 1972 and Caffey in 1974; the term shaken baby syndrome was adopted in 1984 to emphasize the contribution of shaking as a mechanistic injury. In 1987, Duhaime and colleagues first described impact injuries in a significant proportion of cases and suggested the term shaken impact syndrome.[1] Multiple studies have described both shaking as well as impact; the literature confirms both that (1) shaking can cause brain injury, subdural hematoma (SDH), retinal hemorrhage (RH), and even death, and (2) evidence of impact injuries may be lacking even when impact has occurred. Therefore, the term abusive head trauma (AHT) has been more recently proposed by many, including the American Academy of Pediatrics,[2] to account for the contributions of shaking, impact, and other injury mechanisms. *The term abusive head trauma should be used rather than shaken baby syndrome since, in any particular case, the injury mechanism(s) are not known with absolute certainty.*

AHT produces a constellation of injuries, not all of which need to be present to make the diagnosis. AHT is an important type of childhood head trauma, the proper and accurate recognition of which is vital both for the protection of the child from harm and the caregiver from wrongful prosecution. The principal injuries include the following:

- *Subdural hematoma:* SDHs are present, on average, in 80% of cases of AHT. They may be hyperdense, isodense, hypodense, or of mixed density. Mixed-density SDH are more common in AHT than in accidental injuries; some of these likely reflect multiple episodes of injury although more recent studies suggest that some may occur after a single trauma and may reflect an admixture of clotted and unclotted blood, cerebrospinal fluid (CSF), and serum.[3] Some, but not all, studies have suggested a preponderance of interhemispheric and tentorial SDH in AHT.[4]
- *Primary brain injury:* Brain injuries can include superficial or deep contusions and cortical lacerations, deeper white matter injuries, and hypoxic-ischemic injuries. Contusions are mostly superficial and are visible as hyperdense punctate hemorrhages on computed tomography (CT). In contrast, ischemic-anoxic injuries are hypodense on CT scans, and hyperintense on T2- and fluid-attenuated inversion recovery (FLAIR)-weighted magnetic resonance imaging (MRI) sequences; diffusion and apparent diffusion coefficient (ADC) MRI sequences establish these as ischemic-anoxic in nature. A particular pattern involves a reversal of the densities of the hemispheres compared with either the deep gray nuclei or the cerebellum (*reversal sign*). At the extreme, the entire hemisphere is hypodense ("big black brain").
- *Retinal hemorrhages:* RHs are seen, on average, in 80% of cases of AHT.[5] The number and location may vary widely. Not all RHs are diagnostic of AHT; RHs are increasingly specific for AHT when they are (1) more numerous in number, (2) extend beyond the posterior pole (the perimacular region) to the edges (ora serrata) of the retina, (3) involve multiple retinal layers (preretinal, intraretinal, and subretinal), and (4) include retinoschisis or macular folds. Retinoschisis is the retinal finding that is most specific to AHT and represents a physical tearing within the layers of the retina producing a hemorrhagic cavity within the neural retina. As of this writing only five cases of traumatic retinoschisis have been reported outside of the setting of AHT (these include cases of crush injuries to the head, high-speed vehicular trauma, and fall from great height). RHs are present in only 3 to 5% of accidentally injured children and, when present, they are usually few, limited to the posterior pole and intraretinal in location. Other conditions that may produce RH are covered in an excellent reference by Levin.[5]
- *Signs of cranial impact injury:* Impact injuries are reported in about one-quarter to one-half of cases of AHT, and skull fractures in about one-quarter.[6,7,8] Evidence of impact may include both physical signs such as soft tissue swelling, bruising, lacerations or abrasions, and radiographic evidence such as soft tissue swelling or skull fractures.

- *Spine injuries:* Spine and spinal cord injuries have previously been thought to be rare in AHT. However, more recent studies, using more modern autopsy techniques that do not cut across the cervicomedullary junction, have increasingly demonstrated evidence of ligamentous or bony cervical spine injuries, as well as injuries to the spinal cord and upper cervical roots and ganglia, in up to 78% of cases on MRI scans[9] and 70% of fatal cases at autopsy.[10] Posterior ligamentous and bony injuries are more common than are vertebral body fractures. Spinal SDH may also be present, particularly in cases having posterior fossa SDH; thoracolumbar SDH likely reflect dropdown of blood from the cranium to the most dependent portion of the spine.
- *Other injuries:* The presence of other, noncranial traumatic injuries is important to document and needs to be considered in the holistic evaluation of AHT. Bruises, burns, or patterned marks on the skin should be sought, particularly on padded surfaces and torso, and particularly among nonambulatory infants. Rib fractures are present in approximately one-third of cases; although any part of the rib may be fractured, many studies demonstrate that posterior rib fractures, where the rib abuts the vertebral transverse process, is the most common location. Long bone fractures are present in about one-quarter of cases; classic metaphyseal lesions (CMLs), also known as corner fractures, of the limb metaphases are particularly suggestive of abuse. Liver, spleen, pancreatic, or bowel injuries reflect coexisting occult abdominal trauma.

52.2 Clinical Presentation

Children with AHT are young; 80 to 90% are under 12 months of age at diagnosis.[11] The type, severity, and extent of injuries are typically inconsistent with either the story provided or the developmental age of the child (e.g., a fall from height in an infant < 4 months of age who can't roll, or multiple bruises in a child who is not yet cruising). Often the story changes as time goes on as additional injuries are discovered that the alleged perpetrator can't explain. The most common presentations include the following, virtually always while alone with a single adult, and without an adequate explanation:

- Sudden and unexplained screaming, crying, or extreme irritability.

- Sudden lethargy or alteration in level of consciousness.
- Eyes rolling back in head.
- Apnea or disordered breathing.
- Seizures.
- Loss of motor tone or limpness.
- Emesis.

The presence of coma, disordered breathing or apnea, significant RHs or retinoschisis, and multiple seizures over the first 72 hours that are difficult to control are all significant indicia of AHT.

The history is a vital part of the evaluation for AHT. It should be obtained from both parents and/ or any witnesses to the events independently using open-ended questions, and the entire conversation should be recorded in the medical record immediately after the interview, being as accurate and complete as possible. Questions will obviously be dependent on the situation, but important questions to record include What exactly happened? Where and how was the baby positioned at the time? Where were you when it happened? What exactly did the baby do? If an accidental trauma was described, how exactly did it happen? If the baby fell, how far, off of what, on what surface did they land, did they hit anything else on the way down? Who else was in the room with, or in proximity to you? What were you doing with the baby at the time? What did you do in response to the changes in the baby? How did the baby react to that? Did you perform cardiopulmonary resuscitation (CPR) (including chest compressions)? Were you injured (e.g., if the story involves an adult falling with the baby)? Who else cares for the baby and at what times? When did each person last care for the baby? Have you witnessed any other injuries prior to the day this happened?

It is also vital to carefully document an injury time line as completely and accurately as possible. When was the baby last seen by another adult acting normally? When did they last eat and how much (head injured babies will not eat much)? Have they been unusually fussy or irritable lately (perhaps suggesting a prior injury)? Have there been any recent seizures or abnormal motor movements? Radiological interpretation can also provide clues as to when an injury occurred; for example, studies suggest that (1) a hypodense component of an acute SDH most commonly appears within 3 to 12 days after AHT and (2) parenchymal hypodensities appear commonly within 1 to 3 hours.[4,9] One must be careful about correlating the clinical and imaging findings to establish a time frame during which the abuse might have occurred.

52.3 Differential Diagnosis of AHT

The history and physical findings in combination usually suggest the possibility of AHT. However, it is important to keep an open mind and contemplate other potential causes of the injuries. The differential diagnosis of AHT includes a large number of other diseases,[5,6,12,13] only a few of which are discussed in detail here. Obviously whether to consider any of these depends on the circumstances of the injury, the clinical findings, and the results of ancillary tests.

Differentiating AHT from accidental injury is the most frequent dilemma. However, multiple studies of accidental injuries in children confirm the following:

- The overwhelming majority of household and/or short falls are benign. Significant brain injury, prolonged coma, disordered breathing and/or apnea, multiple seizures, and radiographic evidence of ischemic-anoxic brain injury are extraordinarily uncommon in short falls (< 4 ft). The risk of dying from a short fall is, at greatest, approximately 0.25%.[14] When they do occur, coma and/or death are most frequently due to large and expanding extra-axial mass lesions.[15]
- SDH is statistically much less frequent in accidental trauma than in AHT (where it averages 80%). Moreover, when it occurs in the setting of accidental injury, SDH is usually small, focal, and underlying a site of impact injury. In contrast, AHT more commonly produces diffuse, bilateral, panhemispheric, interhemispheric, and/or tentorial SDH.
- Intracranial injuries from short falls more commonly include scant, focal cortical subarachnoid hemorrhage and/or tiny superficial cortical contusions that are almost always associated with a skull fracture and/or soft tissue scalp swelling; hypodensities and deeper white matter injuries are rare.
- Epidural hematomas occur more commonly in association with *accidental* injuries and, in young children, may not be associated with a skull fracture; on occasion they may be associated with a small number of RH as well.

Birth trauma is another consideration. Birth trauma is a known cause of RH in 40% of newborns.[5] However, most resolve within days of birth, and all reported cases have resolved by 4 postnatal weeks. Similarly, recent studies have demonstrated that birth-related SDH are common in asymptomatic infants (8–46%).[16,17,18] They are more common in vaginal and assisted deliveries. Most are located in the occipital and infratentorial locations, and virtually all are gone by 4 weeks postnatal. Rebleeding has only been described in one asymptomatic case.[17] Birth trauma should not be a cause for acute deterioration in an infant more than 4 weeks' postnatal. Although rebleeding into a chronic birth-related SDH has been proposed as a potential cause for acute deterioration weeks or months later, there is not a single reported case to support this theory.

An underlying coagulopathy should be excluded. Many institutions perform only a complete blood count (CBC) with platelet counts and a prothrombin time (PT), partial thromboplastin time (PTT), and international normalized ratio (INR); others recommend more sophisticated testing to include fibrinogen and fibrin split products (to evaluate for disseminated intravascular coagulopathy [DIC]), von Willebrand's factor, and factors VIII, IX, and XIII.[19] Hemorrhagic disease of the newborn should be considered in the infant up to 6 months of age with a greatly prolonged PT, particularly in a child who is breast-fed, has significant diarrhea, has been on prolonged antibiotics, or has had neonatal hepatitis/biliary atresia, and whose PT corrects readily with the administration of vitamin K. A significant coagulopathy other than DIC should prompt a hematology consult for further evaluation.

Vascular malformations and aneurysms are rare causes of intracranial hemorrhage in infancy, and are usually readily distinguished by the location of the hemorrhage as subarachnoid or intraparenchymal rather than subdural. Although RH may occur in the setting of aneurysmal intracranial hemorrhage in adults (Terson's syndrome), these are extraordinarily rare in childhood if they occur at all, and are readily distinguished from RH associated with AHT. A brain MRI, magnetic resonance angiography (MRA), and magnetic resonance venography (MRV) will usually exclude these conditions.

Intracranial infections are rarely confused with AHT. Neither meningitis nor viral encephalitis are associated with SD or severe RH. Fevers, nuchal rigidity, and an elevated white blood cell (WBC), erythrocyte sedimentation rate (ESR), and C-reactive protein (CRP) are usually present. Postmeningitic subdural hygromas can develop (especially after pneumococcal and *Haemophilus influenzae* meningitis), but acute SDH does not occur. Subdural empyema is usually readily distinguished from SDH based on the history, laboratory tests, and neuroimaging; a contrast-enhanced CT or MRI will disclose leptomeningeal enhancement.

Genetic, metabolic, and other conditions that can mimic AHT in infants may include the following:

- *Glutaric aciduria (GA):* Produces episodic neurological decline with extensor motor movements, hyper- or hypotonia, and seizures; choreoathetoid movements develop later in life. Neuroimaging demonstrates enlarged extra-axial CSF spaces, temporal fossa arachnoid cysts, and, later, characteristic putaminal hyperintensities.[20] A routine newborn metabolic screen (mandated in most states) virtually excludes GA.
- *Menkes' kinky-hair disease:* X-linked recessive disorder characterized by short, friable, and twisted hair (pili torti); poor growth; severe and early neurological deterioration; characteristic skeletal deformities (wormian skull bones, metaphyseal defects); and characteristic facies. Neuroimaging demonstrates atrophy, enlarged extra-axial CSF spaces with tortuous cerebral vessels, and SDHs or effusions.
- *Ehlers–Danlos syndrome:* A disorder characterized by hypermobile joints, hyperelastic skin, dystrophic scarring particularly around the flexor creases of joints, and poor healing of skin wounds. Approximately 30% of affected individuals also have a qualitative functional platelet disorder. A family history may reveal ruptured cerebral or thoracic aortic aneurysms in other family members. SDHs can rarely be present.
- *Arachnoid cysts:* Temporal fossa cysts may be associated with SDH or hygroma either spontaneously or in response to trauma; RHs are extraordinarily rare and if present are intraretinal and limited to the posterior pole.
- *Benign extra-axial collections of infancy (BECI):* BECI is characterized by macrocrania with progressive cranial enlargement over the first 12 to 18 months of life; neuroimaging demonstrates an accumulation of CSF in the subarachnoid spaces, associated with mild ventricular enlargement in 40%. A family history of macrocephaly is present in 40% of families. The infants are asymptomatic and develop normally. The fluid is subarachnoid in location;

therefore, the fluid is isointense to CSF on CT and all MRI sequences, it does not compress the sulci (in fact, the sulci are typically widened giving the erroneous picture of brain atrophy), and the cortical bridging blood vessels cross the space to the overlying arachnoid. In contrast, a subdural hematoma or hygroma is not entirely isointense to CSF and causes compression of both the sulci and the bridging vessels. An associated SDH may occur in approximately 2 to 3% of cases of BECI.[21,22] In virtually every case, the infant is asymptomatic and the BECI and SDH are is discovered during an evaluation for macrocephaly; there is no associated brain injury or other evidence of trauma and RH have been described in only one case.[23]

52.4 Work-up of AHT

In addition to a thorough history and physical examination, the following studies that should be considered (depending on the circumstances) include the following:

- A complete coagulation profile as described above.
- Brain MRI, MRA, and MRV, as well as a cervical spine MRI. A complete spine MRI should be considered as spinal SDH in the thoracic or lumbar regions may be missed.
- A retinal examination by a pediatric or retinal ophthalmologist who is experienced in interpreting RH.
- A complete skeletal survey.
- Liver function tests, amylase, urinalysis, and/or abdominal CT if abdominal trauma is suspected.
- Consultation with a geneticist if an underlying metabolic or genetic condition is suspected.
- A child abuse pediatrician should always be consulted if available.
- If a reasonable suspicion of abuse is present, all health care providers are *mandated to report suspected abuse to legal agencies* (usually a state Department of Children and Youth).

52.5 Treatment

The medical and surgical treatment of AHT is largely identical to the treatment of any severe traumatic brain injury and includes the following:

- Intubation for the child with Glasgow Coma Score (GCS) less than 8 for airway control.
- Seizure prophylaxis is particularly important given both the frequency with which seizures

occur in AHT and the difficulty in controlling them. Prophylaxis with phenobarbital, phenytoin, or levetiracetam should be instituted at the onset; a second agent may be necessary if seizures continue despite maximal doses of a single agent. Seizures usually subside after the first 3 to 4 days.

- Standard intracranial pressure (ICP) management using osmotic diuretics and/or hypertonic saline and external ventricular drainage as primary measures.
- Surgical management is rarely needed. SDH are usually small and nonoperative; larger acute SDH should be evacuated. Chronic SDH may be treated with either repeated aspirations (usually through the anterior fontanelle), a subdural drain, or a subdural-peritoneal shunt if necessary.
- Consideration may be given to decompressive craniotomy if ICP cannot be controlled and/or there is significant shift on neuroimaging studies.

52.6 Outcome

Outcome from AHT is poorer than for other types of traumatic brain injury.

- Mortality averages 20 to 25%.
- Half of survivors will suffer significant neurological deficits such as spasticity, seizures, blindness (from RH and/or cortical injury), and focal neurological deficits.
- As many as 80% will suffer measurable cognitive and/or behavioral deficits.
- Neuroimaging studies often demonstrate multifocal encephalomalacia or global brain atrophy, evidence of cortical laminar necrosis (tram-track hyperdensities that follow the gyral surfaces), *ex vacuo* ventricular enlargement, and widened subarachnoid spaces.
- Rebleeding into chronic SDH occurs in about 15%, but is virtually always asymptomatic and usually discovered incidentally on routine follow-up neuroimaging studies.[9] It does not, in itself, indicate repeated abuse.

52.7 Other Considerations

- Medical information gathering is critical to the successful evaluation and prosecution of AHT. The evaluation of AHT should be left to physicians who are experienced in its evaluation and knowledgeable about the differential diagnosis.
- It is no longer acceptable to naively equate SDH and RH with AHT without careful consideration of alternate diagnoses. A thorough history and work-up looking both for associated injuries and evidence of other medical conditions is important.
- Chart documentation is extremely important from a medicolegal standpoint. Avoid the use of the word shaken baby syndrome as the mechanism(s) are unknown in individual cases and this generates unnecessary confusion. Stick to the facts, avoiding inflammatory or judgmental statements about the alleged perpetrator and/or family, particularly concerning social or demographic issues.
- Don't jump to conclusions. Avoid making overly dogmatic statements about causation—one way or another—before the history has been fully obtained and all of the medical information is available.
- Do not testify in court as an expert witness without first knowing all of the clinical information and the pertinent literature on AHT. It is easy for the uninformed clinician to derail a medicolegal investigation with ill-considered or incorrect remarks in the courtroom.

References

[1] Duhaime AC. Closed head injury without fractures. In: Albright AL, Pollack I, Adelson D, eds. Principles and Practice of Pediatric Neurosurgery. New York, NY: Thieme; 1999: 799–811

[2] Christian CW, Block R, Committee on Child Abuse and Neglect, American Academy of Pediatrics. Abusive head trauma in infants and children. Pediatrics. 2009; 123(5): 1409–1411

[3] Vinchon M, Noizet O, Defoort-Dhellemmes S, Soto-Ares G, Dhellemmes P. Infantile subdural hematomas due to traffic accidents. Pediatr Neurosurg. 2002; 37(5):245–253

[4] Dias MS, Backstrom J, Falk M, Li V. Serial radiography in the infant shaken impact syndrome. Pediatr Neurosurg. 1998; 29 (2):77–85

[5] Levin AV. Retinal haemorrhages and child abuse. In: David TJ, ed. Recent Advances in Paediatrics. Edinburgh, UK: Churchill Livingstone; 2000;18:151–219

[6] Minns RA, Brown JK. Neurological perspectives of non-accidental head injury and whiplash/shaken baby syndrome: an overview. In: Minns RA, Brown JK, eds. Shaking and other Non-Accidental Head Injuries in Children. London, UK: Cambridge University Press; 2005:1–105

[7] Starling SP, Patel S, Burke BL, Sirotnak AP, Stronks S, Rosquist P. Analysis of perpetrator admissions to inflicted traumatic brain injury in children. Arch Pediatr Adolesc Med. 2004; 158 (5):454–458

[8] Vinchon M, de Foort-Dhellemmes S, Desurmont M, Delestret I. Confessed abuse versus witnessed accidents in infants: comparison of clinical, radiological, and ophthalmological data in corroborated cases. Childs Nerv Syst. 2010; 26(5):637–645

[9] Bradford R, Choudhary AK, Dias MS. Serial neuroimaging in infants with abusive head trauma: timing abusive injuries. J Neurosurg Pediatr. 2013; 12(2):110–119

[10] Brennan LK, Rubin D, Christian CW, Duhaime A-C, Mirchandani HG, Rorke-Adams LB. Neck injuries in young pediatric homicide victims. J Neurosurg Pediatr. 2009; 3(3):232–239

[11] Kesler H, Dias MS, Shaffer M, Rottmund C, Cappos K, Thomas NJ. Demographics of abusive head trauma in the Commonwealth of Pennsylvania. J Neurosurg Pediatr. 2008; 1 (5):351–356

[12] Greeley CS. Conditions confused with head trauma. In: Jenny C, ed. Child Abuse and Neglect: Diagnosis, Treatment, and Evidence. St. Louis, MO: Elsevier; 2011:441–450

[13] Reece RM. Differential diagnosis of inflicted childhood neurotrauma. In: Reece RM, Nicholson CE, eds. Inflicted Childhood Neurotrauma. Elk Grove, IL: American Academy of Pediatrics; 2003

[14] Alexander RC, Levitt CJ, Smith WL. Abusive head trauma. In: Reece RM, Ludwig S, eds. Child Abuse. Medical Diagnosis and Management. Philadelphia, PA: Lippincott Williams and Wilkins; 2001:47–80

[15] Hall JR, Reyes HM, Horvat M, Meller JL, Stein R. The mortality of childhood falls. J Trauma. 1989; 29(9):1273–1275

[16] Looney CB, Smith JK, Merck LH, et al. Intracranial hemorrhage in asymptomatic neonates: prevalence on MR images and relationship to obstetric and neonatal risk factors. Radiology. 2007; 242(2):535–541

[17] Rooks VJ, Eaton JP, Ruess L, Petermann GW, Keck-Wherley J, Pedersen RC. Prevalence and evolution of intracranial hemorrhage in asymptomatic term infants. AJNR Am J Neuroradiol. 2008; 29(6):1082–1089

[18] Whitby EH, Griffiths PD, Rutter S, et al. Frequency and natural history of subdural haemorrhages in babies and relation to obstetric factors. Lancet. 2004; 363(9412):846–851

[19] Thomas AE. The bleeding child; is it NAI? Arch Dis Child. 2004; 89(12):1163–1167

[20] Strauss KA, Puffenberger EG, Robinson DL, Morton DH. Type I glutaric aciduria, part 1: natural history of 77 patients. Am J Med Genet C Semin Med Genet. 2003; 121C(1):38–52

[21] Greiner MV, Richards TJ, Care MM, Leach JL. Prevalence of subdural collections in children with macrocrania. AJNR Am J Neuroradiol. 2013; 34(12):2373–2378

[22] McKeag H, Christian CW, Rubin D, Daymont C, Pollock AN, Wood J. Subdural hemorrhage in pediatric patients with enlargement of the subarachnoid spaces. J Neurosurg Pediatr. 2013; 11(4):438–444

[23] Piatt JH, Jr. A pitfall in the diagnosis of child abuse: external hydrocephalus, subdural hematoma, and retinal hemorrhages. Neurosurg Focus. 1999; 7(4):e4

Section X

Infections

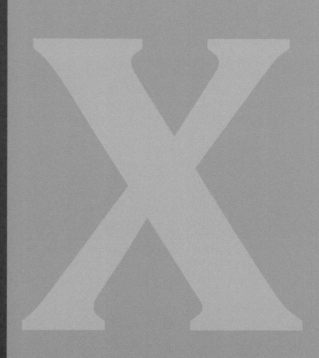

53 Evaluation and Management of Pediatric Intracranial Infections

Jonathan R. Ellenbogen, Richard P.D. Cooke, Conor L. Mallucci

53.1 Introduction

Central nervous system (CNS) infections in the pediatric population are life-threatening diseases in which early recognition and appropriate treatment may prevent long-term brain injury or death. The causal agents are different in the pediatric population when compared to the adult population, and so are the presenting symptoms. It is therefore important to know and understand the clinical presentations of these conditions in children in order to evaluate and manage these conditions appropriately. This chapter will focus on epidural and brain abscesses, subdural empyema, bacterial and viral meningitis, and encephalitis. Tuberculous, fungal, and parasitic infections of the CNS will be discussed in a different chapter.

53.2 Bacterial Meningitis

53.2.1 Background

Meningitis is the most common CNS infection and can be classified according to causative agent, for example, viral or bacterial, or on the basis of the duration of symptoms, that is, acute, subacute, or chronic. Subacute meningitis is defined as the one that ongoing for more than 1 week. Chronic meningitis occurs if the symptoms have been ongoing for a month or longer.

Bacterial meningitis usually arises via hematogenous spread from mucosal surfaces. Other modes of transmission include contiguous spread from an infected mastoid/middle ear or paranasal sinus, rupture of a parenchymal abscess, transmission from dysraphic lesions, and penetrating trauma.

In neonates (< 28 days old) the most common causative organisms are likely to be acquired around the time of birth from the maternal genital and gastrointestinal tract, and are *Streptococcus agalactiae* (group B *Streptococcus*), *Escherichia coli*, *Streptococcus pneumoniae*, and *Listeria monocytogenes*.[1] *L monocytogenes* meningitis is rare (~ 5% of neonatal meningitis) with most cases occurring in the first week of life in predominantly premature infants, and are related to maternal infection. The neonatal case fatality rate is around 10 to 12.4%.[2] The risk factors for neonatal meningitis include antenatal chorioamnionitis, premature rupture of membranes, less than 37 weeks' gestation, and having a previous newborn with early-onset disease.[3]

In children over the age of 3 months the most common pathogens arise from the upper respiratory tract and include *Neisseria meningitidis* (meningococcus), *S. pneumoniae* (pneumococcus), and *Haemophilus influenzae* type b (Hib). The case fatality rate in this group varies between 1.9 and 11%.[2] *N. meningitidis* infection leading to meningococcal disease is the leading infectious cause of death in early childhood (case fatality rate ~ 10%) and can be fatal within hours of the first symptoms appearing. The highest incidence occurs among children aged under 2 years; another period of increased risk occurs in adolescence and early adulthood. The disease is more frequent in winter months and is associated with smoking, crowding, and recent viral respiratory illness. It most commonly presents as bacterial meningitis (15%) or septicemia (25%), or as a combination of the two syndromes (60%).[2] Rarely the disease presents as pneumonia, arthritis, osteomyelitis, pericarditis, endophthalmitis, or conjunctivitis.

The epidemiology of pediatric bacterial meningitis has changed dramatically following the introduction of routine vaccination. Hib was the main cause of bacterial meningitis in children under 5 years old before the introduction of the Hib conjugate vaccine in 1992. It is now the third most common causative organism after *N. meningitidis* and *S. pneumoniae*. Similar results have been found since the introduction of the meningococcal C (MenC) conjugate vaccine in 1999 against serogroup C meningococcus, and the pneumococcal conjugate vaccine in 2006 against pneumococcal disease. Serogroup B meningococcus is now the most common cause of bacterial meningitis (and septicemia) in children and young people aged 3 months or older. A vaccine is available but not in routine use.

53.2.2 Evaluation

Most children with meningitis present with a temperature over 38 °C or fever (90%), vomiting (70%), and headache (3–58%). Respiratory symptoms are not an uncommon finding. Under one-third of children present having had a seizure (13–30%), with shock being a less common finding at presentation (8–17%). Over two-thirds of children with meningitis experience impaired consciousness (60–87%), with around 10% presenting with coma. Most are "irritable" or "agitated." Between 62 and 75% will report neck stiffness or some back rigidity.[2] Brudzinski's sign can be elicited in approximately two-thirds of children and Kernig's sign is present in approximately half of children. Approximately 80% of children will have one of these signs; neck stiffness, Kernig's sign, or Brudzinski's sign.[2]

Children under 2 years old present similarly but two-thirds will present with poor feeding and the prevalence of seizures ranges from 22 to 55.2%.[2] Approximately half present with a bulging fontanelle.

In neonates, fever and irritability is common (79%), however, the classical symptoms of nuchal rigidity and bulging fontanelle are not usually evident (17% and 13%, respectively). A quarter of neonates present with lethargy and 17% with seizures. Nonspecific gastrointestinal symptoms (anorexia and/or vomiting, diarrhea, and abdominal distension) are more frequent (50, 29, and 17%, respectively) than respiratory symptoms (respiratory distress [17%] and apnea [13%]).[2]

Clinical features vary with age. Although fever is a common nonspecific symptom, it is more often absent in neonates. Babies are less likely to have symptoms and signs of meningism, extremity pain or hemorrhagic rash, whereas older children and young people are more likely to have meningism, confusion/altered mental state, hemorrhagic rash, or extremity pain. The majority of children and young people with meningococcal disease will develop a hemorrhagic rash during their illness, but this may be primarily absent, and may initially be blanching or macular in nature.

Bacterial and viral causes of meningitis cannot be differentiated reliably based on clinical features alone. However, children with viral meningitis are less likely to have shock, decreased level of consciousness, or seizures than are those with bacterial meningitis. Symptoms and signs that are considered typical of meningeal irritation (headache, neck stiffness, or photophobia) occur in a minority of children and young people before hospital admission, but they are more likely to occur in older children and young people. Herpes simplex encephalitis should be considered as an alternative diagnosis.

53.2.3 Investigations

Laboratory Tests

The diagnosis of meningitis is established upon the clinical history, physical examination, and laboratory investigations. The definitive test for meningitis is a lumbar puncture, measuring the opening pressure, with laboratory examination of the cerebrospinal fluid (CSF). Although performance of a lumbar puncture is contraindicated if the following are present, this should not delay commencement of appropriate antibiotic treatment:

- Signs suggesting raised intracranial pressure (ICP).
  - Reduced or fluctuating level of consciousness (Glasgow Coma Score [GCS] < 9 or a drop of ≥ 3).
  - Relative bradycardia and hypertension.
  - Focal neurological signs.
  - Abnormal posture or posturing.
  - Unequal, dilated, or poorly responsive pupils.
  - Papilloedema.
  - Abnormal "doll's eye" movements.
- Shock.
- Extensive or spreading purpura.
- After seizures until stabilized.
- Coagulation abnormalities.
  - Coagulation results outside the normal range.
  - Platelet count below 100×10^9/L.
  - Receiving anticoagulant therapy.
- Local superficial infection at the lumbar puncture site.
- Respiratory insufficiency (lumbar puncture is considered to have a high risk of precipitating respiratory failure in the presence of respiratory insufficiency).

CSF examination should include white blood cell count and examination, total protein and glucose concentrations, Gram stain and microbiological culture. A corresponding laboratory-determined blood glucose concentration should be measured. In bacterial meningitis one might expect to find raised protein, low glucose levels, and raised white blood cells with neutrophilic predominance. The normal values for CSF differ between laboratories but approximate values are as below:
- Appearance to the naked eye: clear and colorless.
- Total protein concentration: 0.15 to 0.45 g/L.
- Glucose concentration: 2.78 to 4.44 millimole/L (~ 60% of the plasma value).
- Cell count (per microliter): 0 to 5 white blood cells (WBCs) (0–20 in neonates), no RBCs.

(If RBCs are present and the blood WBC count is within the normal range, more than one WBC per 500–1000 CSF RBCs can be expected in a child or young person with meningitis and should not be ignored).

The normal CSF opening pressure should be in the range of 10 to 100 mm H_2O in less than 8 year olds and between 60 and 200 mm H_2O in greater than 8 year olds. CSF opening pressures above 250 mm H_2O indicates raised ICP.

If a child has an unexplained petechial rash and fever, that is, suspected meningitis, then the following should also be performed:
- Full blood count.
- C-reactive protein (CRP).
- Coagulation screen.
- Blood cultures.
- Advanced molecular testing (including polymerase chain reaction [PCR]).
- Blood glucose.
- Blood gas.

The finding of a high CRP (> 99 mg/L) is specific but not sensitive for meningococcal disease in children with fever and a rash. A low CRP does not exclude meningococcal disease. Be aware that the CRP may be normal and the WBC count normal or low even in severe meningococcal disease. Serum CRP levels of more than 20 mg/L and procalcitonin of more than 0.5 ng/mL have greater than 83% sensitivity for differentiating bacterial meningitis from aseptic meningitis.[2]

Imaging

In children and young people with a reduced or fluctuating level of consciousness (GCS < 9 or a drop of ≥ 3) or with focal neurological signs, perform a computed tomography (CT) scan to rule out alternative intracranial pathology. Patients should be clinically stable before scanning takes place, but this should not delay appropriate treatment. Imaging is not performed to make a diagnosis of meningitis, but it can be used to look for its complications and sequelae including hydrocephalus, abscess, empyema, and raised ICP. CT alone is unreliable for identifying raised ICP, therefore clinical assessment should also be used to decide whether it is safe to perform a lumbar puncture.

In meningitis, a CT scan is often normal. Mild ventriculomegaly and enlargement of the subarachnoid spaces are early abnormalities. Contrast-enhanced T1-weighted magnetic resonance imaging (MRI) is the imaging modality of choice, looking for enhancement of the leptomeninges over the cerebral convexities, although this can be difficult as normal meninges enhance. Contrast-enhanced fluid-attenuated inversion recovery (FLAIR) imaging increases the specificity over contrast-enhanced T1-weighted images for this.[3]

53.2.4 Management

Clinical progress should be monitored via frequent vital sign measurements of respiratory rate, heart rate, blood pressure, conscious level (GCS/APVU), temperature, perfusion (capillary refill time), and oxygen saturations. It is important to ensure that appropriate investigation and management of metabolic disturbances, seizures, raised ICP, respiratory support, and fluid balance is undertaken.

Medical/Antimicrobial

Treat with an intravenous third-generation cephalosporin (e.g., ceftriaxone) immediately if the CRP and/or WBC count (especially neutrophil count) is raised, as this indicates an increased risk of having meningococcal disease.

There is not enough evidence in children to show that CSF WBC, protein, or glucose values have sufficient diagnostic accuracy to confirm or exclude bacterial meningitis as compared to viral or "aseptic" meningitis. Therefore, in cases of suspected bacterial meningitis start antibiotic treatment—start before CSF result available if there is a delay in obtaining CSF—if the CSF WBC count is abnormal:
- In neonates, at least 20 cells/µL (be aware that even if fewer than 20 cells/µL, bacterial meningitis should still be considered if other symptoms and signs are present).
- In older children and young people more than 5 cells/µL or more than 1 neutrophil/µL, regardless of other CSF variables.

The empirical antibiotic protocols of choice are[2] as below:
- Children older than 3 months—intravenous ceftriaxone for at least 10 days.
- Children younger than 3 months—intravenous cefotaxime plus either amoxicillin or ampicillin for at least 14 days.
- Suspected meningococcal disease—intravenous ceftriaxone for 7 days.
- Children and young people who have recently travelled outside the United Kingdom or have had prolonged or multiple exposure to

antibiotics (within the past 3 months and who may have penicillin-resistant pneumococcus)—vancomycin in addition to the above antibiotics.

- In children younger than 3 months, ceftriaxone may be used as an alternative to cefotaxime (with or without ampicillin or amoxicillin), but be aware that ceftriaxone should not be used in premature babies or in babies with jaundice, hypoalbuminemia, or acidosis as it may exacerbate hyperbilirubinemia.

Below are the antibiotic protocols, which should be employed for confirmed bacterial meningitis unless directed otherwise by the results of antibiotic sensitivities.[2]

Children and young people older than or equal to 3 months.

- *H. influenzae* type b meningitis—intravenous ceftriaxone for 14 days.
- *S. pneumoniae* meningitis—intravenous ceftriaxone for 14 days.

Children younger than 3 months.

- Group B streptococcal meningitis—intravenous cefotaxime at least 14 days.
- *L. monocytogenes* meningitis—intravenous amoxicillin or ampicillin for 21 days, plus gentamicin for at least the first 7 days.
- Gram-negative bacilli meningitis—intravenous cefotaxime for at least 21 days.

In children with bacterial meningitis from high-income settings, there is no evidence from meta-analyses that corticosteroids reduce mortality or short-term neurological sequelae, but there is evidence that adjunctive corticosteroids reduce the risk of severe hearing loss and long-term neurological sequelae following bacterial meningitis. Give dexamethasone (0.15 mg/kg to a maximum dose of 10 mg, four times daily for 4 days) for suspected or confirmed bacterial meningitis as soon as possible, that is, at the same time as the initial dose of antibiotic (may not have CSF results available) if lumbar puncture reveals any of the following:

- Frankly purulent CSF.
- CSF WBC count greater than 1,000/μL.
- Raised CSF WBC count with protein concentration greater than 1 g/L.
- Bacteria on Gram stain.

There is no evidence to support the use of corticosteroids in children younger than 3 months with bacterial meningitis.

Neurosurgical

Neurosurgical intervention is only required in the event of raised ICP which is not managed by medical means. In the majority of these cases, external ventricular drain (EVD) placement allows drainage of CSF and can act as a conduit for intrathecal antibiotic administration.

Burr hole and subdural washouts are sometimes required for persistent subdural effusions in the context of ongoing raised CRP and poor clinical response to antibiotics alone (▶ Fig. 53.1). Neurosurgical intervention may be required to deal with complications of meningitis which are discussed later.

53.2.5 Prognosis

If meningitis is not efficiently and adequately treated, it can spread via the leptomeningeal sheaths of the penetrating cortical vessels in the perivascular spaces resulting in cerebritis and brain abscess formation. Spread of infection to the ependymal surface results in ventriculitis and aqueductal ependymitis causing hydrocephalus.

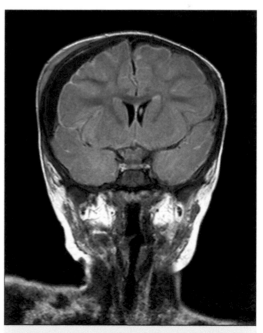

Fig. 53.1 Coronal T1 MRI of a 16-month old boy, presenting with meningitis secondary to chicken pox infection, demonstrating a right-sided subdural empyema. Patient was surgically treated via burr hole drainage isolating *Streptococcus pyogenes*.

Ventriculitis occurs in 30% of patients and can be as high as 92% in neonates.[3] Necrosis in vessel walls can result in arterial or venous thrombosis, and overall cerebral infarctions are seen in up to 30% of neonates.[3] Neonatal meningitis is a common recognized cause of hydrocephalus requiring ventriculoperitoneal (VP) shunt placement.

Meningitis can result in significant long-term sequelae including those of hearing loss, orthopedic complications (damage to bones and joints), skin complications (including scarring from necrosis), psychosocial problems, neurological and developmental problems, and renal failure. These need to be fully appreciated, investigated, and managed prior to discharge and in follow-up.

Group B *Streptococcus* appears to have the worst outcomes, with an average of 29% of survivors developing moderate or severe disabilities. An average of 22% of *S. pneumoniae* survivors develop moderate or severe disabilities and approximately 5% develop hearing deficits require cochlear implants. An average of 19% of *E. coli* sufferers develop moderate or severe disabilities. Nine percent of *N. meningitidis* survivors develop severe or moderate disabilities and approximately 0.5% develop hearing deficits require cochlear implants. *H. influenzae* has the least damaging long-term effects, with only 1% of survivors developing severe or moderate disabilities and 3.2% requiring cochlear implants.[2]

53.3 Viral Meningitis

53.3.1 Background

Viral meningitis is relatively common although probably underreported. It occurs at any age but most commonly in young children. A study of 12,000 children in Finland reported the annual incidence of presumed viral meningitis to be 219 per 100,000 in infants younger than 1 year and 27.8 per 100,000 overall in children younger than 14.[4]

The most common cause of viral meningitis is the enteroviruses. Mumps virus infection was the commonest cause prior to the introduction of the mumps, measles, and rubella (MMR) vaccination, as 15% of patients with mumps develop meningitis.[5]

53.3.2 Evaluation

As described previously, it is difficult to distinguish viral meningitis from bacterial meningitis as both are characterized by acute onset of fever and irritability. There are considerable benefits in making this distinction swiftly, in terms of both reducing antibiotic usage and hospital bed occupancy and reassuring parents. Rapid PCR is available to enable prompt diagnosis. Children with viral meningitis frequently report nausea, vomiting, headache, and neck stiffness, while more children with bacterial meningitis present with the more serious symptoms of fever, seizures, lethargic or comatose state, toxic or moribund state, bulging fontanelle, Brudzinski's sign, and Kernig's sign. Photophobia is not a predictor of meningitis type.

Untreated patients with bacterial meningitis show progressive deterioration whereas spontaneous recovery is usual in viral cases. Suspected encephalitis warrants empirical antiviral treatment as discussed below, while viral meningitis does not. History and examination can yield clues as to viral causes. The viral causes are the same as those that cause viral encephalitis. It is important to elicit in the history recent illness contacts, foreign travel, and rodents/tick exposure, HIV risk factors/immunocompetence, immunization status (specifically MMR/mumps), and if appropriate, sexual history. In addition, during examination, evidence of a rash, lymphadenopathy, pharyngitis, and parotid swelling should be sought.

53.3.3 Investigations

Laboratory Tests

Investigation is the same as that required for suspected bacterial meningitis. CSF analysis is required via a lumbar puncture, unless it is contraindicated. A blood glucose concentration is essential and should be collected immediately before lumbar puncture. Although characteristically associated with a mononuclear pleocytosis, neutrophils may predominate initially in viral meningitis (▶ Table 53.1).[5] In a study of 138 children with aseptic meningitis, 57% had a CSF polymorphonuclear predominance that persisted beyond 24 hours.[6]

As discussed previously serum CRP concentration and peripheral blood white cell count can be helpful markers but do not reliably discriminate diagnoses.

CSF viral analysis using PCR is the initial investigation of choice. Other tests can be performed specific to the likely causative agent. If enterovirus is suspected, then culture and PCR of throat swabs and stool samples should be performed. If herpes simplex virus (HSV) or varicella-zoster virus (VZV) is suspected, then HSV type-specific serum

Table 53.1 Typical CSF findings in bacterial and viral meningitis

Meningitis cause	WCC (cells/mm^3/10^6 cells/L)	Predominant cell	CSF: serum glucose (normal ≥ 0.5)	Protein (normal 0.2–0.4)
Viral	50–1,000	Mononuclear (may be neutrophilic early in course)	>0.5	0.4–0.8
Bacterial	100–5,000	Neutrophilic (mononuclear after antibiotics)	<0.5	0.5–2

Source: Adapted from Logan and MacMahon.[5]

Table 53.2 Causes of viral encephalitis

Sporadic causes of viral encephalitis		Travel-related causes of encephalitis	
Herpes viruses	Herpes simplex virus types 1 and 2	The Americas	West Nile
	Varicella-zoster virus		La Crosse
	Epstein–Barr virus		St Louis
	Cytomegalovirus		Dengue
	Human herpes virus 6 and 7		Rabies
Enteroviruses	Coxsackieviruses	Europe/Middle East	Tick-borne encephalitis
	Echoviruses		West Nile
	Parechovirus	Africa	West Nile
	Poliovirus		Rift Valley fever virus
Paramyxoviruses	Measles virus		Crimean–Congo hemorrhagic fever
	Mumps virus		Dengue
Other (rarer causes)	Flu viruses		Rabies
	Adenovirus	Asia	Japanese encephalitis
	Parvovirus		West Nile
	Lymphocytic choriomeningitis virus		Dengue
	Rubella virus		Murray Valley encephalitis
			Rabies
			Nipah
		Australasia	Murray Valley encephalitis
			Japanese encephalitis

Source: Adapted from Thompson et al.[7]

serology, together with PCR, culture, immunofluorescence, electron microscopy, and Tzanck's smear of skin lesion samples/scraping should be performed. In suspected mumps meningitis serum serology should be performed together with PCR of throat swabs, urine samples, blood and oral fluid. If Epstein–Barr virus (EBV) is suspected, then EBV-specific serology, viral capsule antigen IgM and IgG, and Epstein–Barr nuclear antigen IgG tests should be performed together with CSF PCR and the Monospot test.[5]

Imaging

As discussed previously, viral meningitis in itself is not associated with abnormalities on imaging.

53.3.4 Pathogens

Enteroviruses

The Enterovirus groups (▶ Table 53.2) are small nonenveloped RNA viruses of the picornavirus family and are the commonest cause of viral meningitis. Infections with these ubiquitous viruses are mostly asymptomatic, but they have a tendency to be neuroinvasive giving rise to neurological manifestations ranging from aseptic meningitis to meningoencephalitis and paralytic poliomyelitis. Focal neurological signs or seizures are rare, except in neonates who are mostly at risk of developing meningoencephalitis and severe systemic complications such as myocarditis or necrotizing enterocolitis, which are associated with substantial mortality.[8] Coxsackie B viruses and echoviruses account for most cases of enterovirus meningitis.[5] Infection may be accompanied by mucocutaneous manifestations including localized vesicles such as in hand, foot, and mouth disease (enterovirus 71); herpangina (coxsackie virus A); and generalized maculopapular rash (echovirus 9).[8] Infants and young children with no immunity are most susceptible to enteroviruses, and the incidence decreases with age. Infection is seasonal in temperate climates, the highest in summer and autumn, but high all year round in tropical and subtropical climates.[5,8]

Herpes Simplex Viruses (HSV2, HSV1)

HSV is the second most common cause of viral meningitis in adolescents. The rate of childhood infection with HSV1 has declined with a fall in seropositivity rates among 10- to 14-year olds from 34 (1986–1987) to 24% (1994–1995).[9] It is important to understand that HSV meningitis and encephalitis are discrete entities in the immunocompetent host, rather than part of a continuous spectrum. HSV meningitis is a self-limiting condition in patients with normal immunity, whereas HSV encephalitis is a life-threatening medical emergency warranting emergent antiviral treatment. See "Encephalitis" section.

Constitutional symptoms of primary herpes infection may occur, with malaise and clinical features of genital HSV infection. One-third of cases with primary HSV-2 meningitis are complicated by sacral radiculomyelitis (manifesting as urinary retention, constipation, paraesthesias, and motor weakness).[5]

Mumps

The most common neurological manifestation of mumps virus infection is meningitis, which is two to five times more common in male than female patients.[8] Mumps meningitis can precede or follow the parotid swelling, and 50% of cases occur in the absence of parotitis. It is a recognized cause of hydrocephalus.

53.3.5 Management

Treatment is mostly supportive and includes analgesics, antipyretics, antiemetics, maintenance of fluid balance, and prevention and treatment of complications. There are no specific treatment recommendations for enterovirus or VZV meningitis beyond the usual treatment for zoster, and management is conservative.

Immunoglobulin replacement has a role in patients with hypogammaglobulinemia, who are prone to severe and chronic enteroviral disease.

53.3.6 Prognosis

Enterovirus and mumps meningitis in most cases is self-limiting and carries a good prognosis, although it can progress to meningoencephalitis resulting in a sudden deterioration in mental status or seizures as discussed later. HSV2 meningitis causes neurological complications more often than most other viral meningitis: around one-third of all patients in one study developed complications; however, virtually all of these had resolved after 6 months.[7] There is some evidence that in children with meningitis under 1 year of age, subtle neurodevelopmental problems such as language may later be detected.[7] A UK study of children with meningitis in the first year of life found that 42% of children with echovirus meningitis had mild or moderate neurological disability by the age of 5 years.[10]

53.4 Encephalitis

53.4.1 Background

Encephalitis is an uncommon but potentially devastating diffuse inflammatory process of the brain parenchyma caused by a variety of infective pathogens (with viruses being the commonest) or inflammatory/immune pathologies (▶ Table 53.2). The annual rate of encephalitis in children in the United Kingdom is 2.8/100,000, with the highest incidence in infants under 1 year of age, 8.7/100,000. There is no sex preponderance (2.9 in boys vs. 2.8/100,000 in girls). Although a prospective multicenter study found the overall incidence to be higher at around 10.5/100,000 child-years, with an incidence of 18.4/100,000 child-years in children younger than 1 year.[11]

Variations in the geographical distribution of disease and their vectors exist, but globally the commonest viruses are HSV (22%), followed by varicella (21%), adenovirus (4%), mumps virus, and arbovirus (e.g., Japanese encephalitis virus and West Nile virus) spread via the hematogenous route across the blood–brain barrier.[3,7] Others in the United Kingdom include cytomegalovirus (CMV), EBV, measles virus, and enterovirus. Spread to the CNS via peripheral nerves occurs in HSV1 and polio virus. Parasites and fungi are rare causes of encephalitis, and usually affect only immuno-compromised patients.

53.4.2 Evaluation

Symptoms are generally nonspecific, which makes diagnosis difficult, but it is usually associated with prodromal acute febrile "flu-like" illness followed by relatively acute onset of severe headaches, nausea, vomiting, and altered consciousness. Symptoms can include seizures, meningism, and focal neurological deficit. Diagnosis can therefore be confused with that of bacterial meningitis. Presentation may be subtle with personality/behavioral or language/speech disturbances prior to becoming frankly encephalopathic, or may be more subacute in immunocompromised individuals.

An understanding of the pathogenesis of encephalitis can help with appropriate diagnoses and treatment as most present as a result of a mixture of direct viral cytopathology and a parainfectious or postinfectious inflammatory or immune-mediated response.

History is important in etiology, as with viral meningitis. Vaccination, travel history, and social history (HIV) is important, as is a history of a rash (chickenpox [VZV], slapped cheek syndrome (parvovirus), hand, foot, and mouth disease (enterovirus), and roseola (human herpesvirus 6 [HHV-6]). Parotitis, abdominal pain (pancreatitis), or testicular pain (orchitis) may be present in those with mumps.[7]

Important examination findings include signs of meningism (bulging fontanelle in a young infant, and nuchal rigidity or positive Kernig's sign in older children) but these may not always be present. It is important to assess the conscious level and monitor for signs of raised ICP, as well as identifying subtle seizures.

53.4.3 Investigations

Laboratory Tests

The following are recommended to be performed routinely[7]:
- Full blood count and film—which may show lymphocytosis.
- Urea and electrolytes.
- Liver function tests—raised hepatic enzymes may be seen in EBV & CMV.
- Raised amylase in mumps.
- Capillary glucose, laboratory blood glucose.
- Blood gas (arterial or capillary or venous).
- Lactate.
- Urinalysis (dipstick) for ketones, glucose, protein, nitrites, and leucocytes.
- Plasma ammonia (taken from a venous or arterial sample).
- Blood culture—may identify bacteria or fungi.
- Approximately 1 to 2 mL plasma to be separated, frozen, and saved for later analysis if required.
- Approximately 1 to 2 mL of plain serum to be saved for later analysis if required.
- Approximately 10 mL of urine to be saved.

Culture, PCR, or immunofluorescence techniques may be able to identify respiratory viruses, measles, enteroviruses, *Chlamydophila pneumoniae* and *Mycoplasma pneumoniae* from a throat swab. Using a nasopharyngeal aspirate, respiratory viruses (influenza A, parainfluenza, adenoviruses, and respiratory syncytial virus [RSV]) can be identified using PCR, antigen detection, or culture. Stool samples may reveal infection with enteroviruses or measles viruses, and urine samples may reveal infection with mumps virus, through PCR or culture. If vesicles are present, a viral swab should be taken from the vesicle for detection of VZV or HSV by immunofluorescence or PCR. Urine can be cultured for CMV, mumps, or measles virus. Serum and CSF IgM antibodies or a rising IgG concentration may allow identification of infection with HSV, VZV, CMV, EBV, RSV, adenovirus, influenza A and B virus, parainfluenza and enteroviruses, rotavirus, *M. pneumoniae*, and arboviruses.[7]

A lumbar puncture should be performed in all cases of suspected encephalitis unless contraindications exist (see "Bacterial meningitis" section). CSF should be sent for the following investigations:

- Microscopy, culture, and sensitivity analysis.
- PCR for HSV types 1 and 2 and VZV (HHV-6 and HHV-7, CMV, EBV, enteroviruses, respiratory viruses, HIV, and *C. pneumonia*).
- Glucose, lactate, and oligoclonal bands (with paired serum sample).

CSF examination may reveal a mononuclear pleocytosis and moderately elevated protein level, or the CSF red blood cell count may be raised in hemorrhagic encephalitis. The presence of eosinophils suggests infection with helminths, but is also seen with toxoplasma infection, *Rickettsia rickettsii*, and infection with *M. pneumoniae*. A decreased CSF glucose concentration suggests a bacterial, fungal, or protozoal etiology, but may occur in viral encephalitis. Although up to 10% of patients with viral encephalitis will have a completely normal CSF, at least initially, and therefore a second lumbar puncture should be considered if clinical evidence of encephalitis continues.[7]

Occasionally pathological diagnosis may have to be made via tissue/brain biopsy, but this is not always feasible. Despite use of a wide range of investigations, the etiology of encephalitis remains unknown in approximately one-third of cases.[7] Therefore, a diagnosis of encephalitis is made in most patients who have an appropriate history and clinical presentation together with markers of brain inflammation (CSF pleocytosis and/or inflammatory changes on brain MRI).

53.4.4 Pathogens
Herpes Simplex Virus 1

HSV is the commonest cause of sporadic encephalitis. HSV1 is the commonest cause of herpes encephalitis in children over the age of 6 months.[3] About 30% of all cases of HSV1 infection occur in patients younger than 20 years. As a consequence of the increasing incidence of genital herpes, clinical cases of HSV encephalitis in the United Kingdom are set to increase.[5] The virus penetrates the oral and nasal mucosa and remains dormant in the trigeminal ganglion, after initial infection. After reactivation (70% of all cases of HSV encephalitis already have antibodies present) the virus spreads along the branches of the trigeminal nerve in the anterior and middle cranial fossa.[7] It is not understood why the virus reactivates, but two mutations in children that result in impaired interferon-production and a predisposition to herpes encephalitis have been identified.[7] The disease begins in the anterior and medial parts of the temporal lobes, spreads to the insular cortex, inferior parts of the frontal lobes, and the cingulate gyri. Bilateral involvement is common. Basal nuclei are usually spared. In those that survive multifocal encephalomalacia, cortical gyriform calcification and ventriculomegaly are seen.

53.4.5 Varicella Virus

Varicella-zoster infection is common in childhood and results in chickenpox, but fewer than 0.1% have CNS complications. Symptoms usually develop within 10 days of the onset of skin rash and include headache, vomiting, dysarthria, hemiparesis, and signs of raised ICP. Varicella infection results in a significant vasculitis causing infarcts of the basal ganglia resulting in focal neurological deficit, which can be sometimes delayed to between 1 and 4 months following the initial skin rash.

Measles Virus

Measles involves the CNS as either acute postinfectious encephalitis, progressive infectious encephalitis, or as subacute sclerosing panencephalitis (SSPE). Acute postinfectious encephalitis is an autoimmune process with perivascular inflammation, which causes hemorrhage and demyelination resulting in acute hemorrhagic leukoencephalitis. Progressive infectious encephalitis is associated with impaired cell immunity resulting in progressive neurological deterioration with seizures and altered mental state. SSPE is caused by reactivation of the measles virus after many years of latency. This results in behavioral change, mental deterioration, ataxia, myoclonus, and visual disturbance. Followed eventually by severe dementia, quadriparesis, and autoimmune instability. Most patients die within 1 to 3 years after the onset of the disease.

Rasmussen's Encephalitis

First described by Rasmussen in 1958, this chronic localized encephalitis is one of the common causes of intractable epilepsy in childhood. Affected children usually present between the ages of 2 and 14 years with the mean age of 7 years. Symptoms include hemiparesis, dysphasia, hemianopia, and mental deterioration together with progressive refractory seizures. Surgical resection of the affected hemisphere is the only effective treatment. It is thought to be due to a slow viral infection like EBV or CMV, or an autoimmune cause.

Acute Demyelinating Encephalomyelitis

This autoimmune postinfectious encephalitis, with or without myelitis results in demyelination. It occurs after a vaccination or late in the course of a viral infection. Symptoms occur a few days to a few weeks after a viral event. Presentation is with seizures, ataxia, and altered mental state. Most cases are self-limiting, with most patients making a complete recovery although between 10 and 30% have some permanent neurological deficit. The disease can relapse rarely with the chances of a second attack greater in patients who are more than 10 years of age at initial presentation. A hemorrhagic variant is described in which involved brain undergoes hemorrhagic necrosis. The prognosis is poor with most patients dying days to weeks after onset.

Imaging

MRI demonstrates inflammation of the white matter, and occasionally meninges, with neuronal loss. Some viruses have predilection to involve certain brain areas. Diffusion-weighted imaging (DWI) shows abnormalities earlier and more extensively than the standard T2-weighted imaging. In HSV1, hemorrhage can occasionally be seen and enhancement occurs in the subacute phase involving the cortex and overlying meninges. In varicella infection, lesions are often seen in the gray–white junction, cerebral cortex, basal ganglia, and in the cerebellum. Angiography can demonstrate associated vasculitis demonstrating narrowing of the distal internal carotid artery (ICA) and proximal anterior and middle cerebral arteries. In acute postinfectious measles, encephalitis MRI demonstrates T2 hyperintensity in the thalami, basal ganglia, and cortex.

In SSPE, there is diffuse atrophy with multifocal areas of T2 hyperintensity in periventricular and subcortical white matter. There is not usually contrast enhancement. There is typical asymmetric involvement of the temporal and parietal lobes. The basal ganglia are involved in 20 to 35% of cases and the brainstem is involved late in the disease. In Rasmussen's encephalitis, initial imaging is often normal. Subsequent imaging demonstrates areas of T2 signal especially in the frontal and temporal lobes. Atrophy of the involved regions and subcortical white matter involvement is seen later. Basal ganglia involvement is seen in about 65% of cases.[3]

In acute demyelinating encephalomyelitis (ADEM), involved areas show low attenuation on CT and increased T2/FLAIR signal with bilateral asymmetric involvement. DWI shows increased water diffusion. Periventricular white matter and deep cerebral nuclei involvement is seen in 50% of cases. The brainstem, cerebellum, and spinal cord are involved in about 30 to 50% of cases. Spinal imaging should be obtained that shows contrast enhancement in the subacute stages and evidence of swelling and increased T2 signal within the cord.[3]

53.4.6 Management

Children are often inpatients for several weeks due to prolonged courses of intravenous treatments often coupled with lengthy recovery and rehabilitation. Some children will need management in an intensive care setting.

Medical/Antimicrobial

At the time of clinical presentation, the pathogen is uncertain and therefore broad-spectrum intravenous antimicrobials and antiviral treatment, acyclovir, should be initiated pending the results of diagnostic studies. Suitable broad-spectrum antimicrobials include a third-generation cephalosporin such as ceftriaxone, to cover *S. pneumoniae*, *H. influenzae*, and *N. meningitidis* infections in addition to ampicillin or amoxicillin to cover *L. monocytogenes* (although listeriosis in immunocompetent children is very unusual). Despite treatment with acyclovir, two-thirds of patients with HSV encephalitis are left with significant neurological impairment.[7] However, high-dose acyclovir (60 mg/kg/day intravenously) given for 21 days for HSV encephalitis in neonates has been shown to reduce the rates of relapse and improve neurological outcome.[12] In adults and children older than 12 years, the current recommended treatment regime is intravenous acyclovir 10 mg/kg every 8 hours (i.e., 30 mg/kg/day) for 21 days. The British National Formulary for children states that children aged 3 months to 12 years should receive intravenous acyclovir 500 mg/m^2 every 8 hours. Rates of relapse of herpes encephalitis have been reported to be as high as 26% but do not occur if treatment is given for longer than 14 days and at doses greater than or equal to 30 mg/kg/day.[7] A negative CSF PCR result at the end of treatment is associated with a better outcome and antiviral therapy should be continued in the context of a positive PCR.[7]

Steroids are the mainstay of treatment for children with ADEM and are usually given as first-line treatment to children with an antibody-mediated encephalitis. Treatment with intravenous immunoglobulin, plasma exchange, and other immunosuppressants, including cyclophosphamide and azathioprine have been used.[7]

Neurosurgical

Neurosurgical input may be required to confirm the diagnosis via biopsy of affected brain tissue, where the diagnosis is equivocal or difficult. The area of brain to biopsy is guided by the MRI characteristics of involvement. Care should be taken to avoid eloquent areas as much as possible. Biopsy may be undertaken using a frame-based or frameless stereotactic method.

In rare cases of viral encephalitis causing brain shift and threat to life due to herniation decompressive craniectomy has been described as an effective treatment to improve outcome.[13]

53.4.7 Prognosis

Studies on long-term outcome are limited although the literature suggests morbidity rates of up to 67% in children with HSV encephalitis, with seizures and developmental delay being most common.[7] A Swedish retrospective study between 2000 and 2004, of 93 children admitted with acute encephalitis found that 60% of patients had sequelae at discharge from hospital.[14] In 24% of cases, symptoms included cognitive impairment, motor impairment, ataxia, dysphasia, or epilepsy. Although relatively small numbers of all children with RSV encephalitis made a full recovery, however, 66% of children with enterovirus encephalitis had ataxia, fatigue, and personality change and 60% of children with VZV encephalitis had ataxia.

Memory impairment was present in both cases of HSV encephalitis, and of the two children with EBV encephalitis one suffered from anxiety and one with ataxia, cognitive problems, and epilepsy.[14]

In this study, predictors of adverse outcomes were focal neurology at the time of presentation, with 84% having symptoms at discharge, and encephalopathy, CSF pleocytosis, and positive neuroimaging finding. Seizures or age at presentation were not predictive of symptoms at discharge.[14] Other studies have suggested that predictors of poor outcome include a GCS of less than 6 and disease present for more than 4 days prior to starting treatment.[7]

53.5 Brain Abscess, Subdural Empyema, and Extradural Empyema

53.5.1 Background

Brain abscess and subdural empyemas are relatively uncommon but serious infections. In the United Kingdom, over a 10-year period between 1999 and 2009, 121 children presented with brain abscesses to four large pediatric neurosurgical centers.[15]

Brain abscesses arise as localized areas of cerebritis that evolve through four stages of evolution into a collection of intraparenchymal purulent material: early cerebritis (3–5 days), late cerebritis (5–14 days), early capsule formation, and late capsule formation (weeks to months) (▶ Table 53.3). The infection most commonly is a complication of bacterial meningitis but can result via direct spread from contiguous sites such as sinusitis or mastoiditis (▶ Fig. 53.2), through hematogenous seeding, for example, in congenital heart disease, or via direct inoculation as occurs with penetrating injury from trauma, or surgery. Neurological deficit arises as a consequence of mass effect/

Table 53.3 MRI appearances during evolution of parenchymal abscesses

Abscess evolution	Appearance on T1	Appearance on T2	Contrast appearance
Early cerebritis	Heterogeneous hyperintensity	Heterogeneous hyperintensity	Patchy enhancement
Late cerebritis	Hyperintense rim Hypointense cavity	Hypointense rim Hyperintense cavity	Intense wall enhancement
Early capsular	Hyperintense rim Hypointense cavity	Hypointense rim Hyperintense cavity	Intense wall enhancement
Late capsular	Isointense capsule	Hypointense capsule	Smooth and intense enhancement

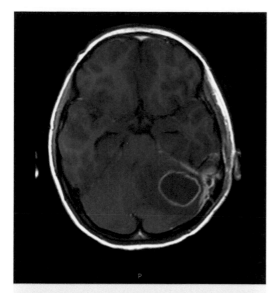

Fig. 53.2 Axial contrast-enhanced T1 MRI of a 10-year old girl presenting with mastoiditis, demonstrating a left cerebellar abscess. Patient was surgically treated via burr hole drainage under electromagnetic image guidance and *S. intermedius* was isolated. This patient went on to develop venous sinus thrombosis and secondary hydrocephalus requiring insertion of a ventriculoperitoneal shunt.

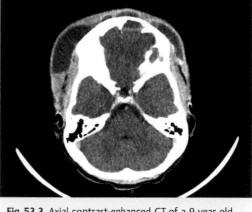

Fig. 53.3 Axial contrast-enhanced CT of a 9-year old girl, presenting generally unwell with frontal sinusitis, demonstrating Pott's puffy tumor and a frontal extradural abscess. Patient was surgically treated via a craniotomy and drainage isolating *S. constellatus*.

Epidural abscesses are almost always secondary to or associated with other infections such as a mastoiditis, sinusitis, or osteomyelitis of the skull. As the abscess expands, it strips the dura from the skull due to the pressure of the expanding inflammatory mass. As a result of its relatively slow-growing nature, symptoms are often insidious and, depending on its location, focal neurological signs may develop due to the pressure effect of continued expansion.

compression of adjacent structures, direct destruction, or infarction secondary to vasculitis. The location tends to vary with age; cerebellar abscesses are more common in younger children and temporal lobe abscesses in older children.[16] Deep abscess location, particularly in the parieto-occipital lobes, has a higher propensity to rupture into the ventricular system causing ventriculitis, which is a life-threatening event, associated with poor outcome. This can occur as the collagen abscess capsule is thicker and better developed on the cortical side than the ventricular side, probably due to the increased vascularity on the cortical side.[3]

Subdural empyema is a rare and life-threatening complication of sinusitis in children. It may also occur following meningitis in 2% of infants, penetrating head injury, cranial osteomyelitis, or via hematogenous spread. Pott's puffy tumor is a non-neoplastic complication of acute sinusitis characterized by osteomyelitis of the frontal bone and subperiosteal abscess formation and thus forehead swelling, hence the name. This infection can spread intracranially causing epidural abscess, subdural empyema, and brain abscess, and can

be associated with cortical vein thrombosis (▶ Fig. 53.3). Sinusitis occurs in 5 to 10% of all respiratory tract infection in children, and only in a minority of cases, there is an intracranial spread with involvement of the subdural or extradural compartment, via bone erosion or more commonly by indirect hematogenous spread.[17] The frontal sinus is the most common culprit followed by the ethmoid, sphenoid, and maxillary sinuses. The overall reported incidence of subdural empyema is between 10 and 41% of all localized intracranial infective processes, with a decreasing mortality rate from 42% in the 1950s to 12% in the 1990s.[18] The supratentorial compartment is more commonly affected (90–95% of cases) with a reported incidence of infratentorial subdural empyema in children of 0.6 to 1.9%.[18] Aggressive management of these cases with craniotomy evacuation of the subdural or extradural collection, endoscopic or antral washout of the sinuses, and parenteral antibiotic therapy has led to a decrease mortality rate, although delayed diagnosis and recurrent collections still appear to be problems and contributing factors in its morbidity or mortality.[18]

53.5.2 Evaluation

A recent UK study demonstrated the male:female ratio to be 1:1 but with a bimodal age presentation distribution, with peaks at younger than 2 and 11 years, boys presenting older than girls (median 11 vs. 8 years).[15,19,20] The commonest underlying medical conditions predisposing patients to these infections include congenital heart disease and immunodeficiency. The commonest preceding infection is sinusitis in approximately a third or more of patients.[15,20] The commonest symptoms at presentation are nonspecific but headache and abnormal focal neurology and/or altered consciousness are often present, and seizures occur in up to 30%.[18] The classic triad of headache, fever, and focal neurological findings is highly suggestive of intracranial abscess formation, although the percentage of children presenting with this triad in the literature varies between 13 and 70%.[15,20] Brain abscess should be a strong consideration in a child who presents with new onset of acute headaches or first-time seizures, especially when focal neurological signs are present. In the neonate, a brain abscess is a potential cause of irritability, a bulging fontanelle, and a rapid increase in head circumference[16] (▶ Fig. 53.4).

53.5.3 Investigations

Laboratory Tests

Analysis of blood inflammatory markers such as white cell count and CRP should be undertaken, as should blood cultures. Obtaining CSF via a lumbar puncture in the presence of a brain abscess may be life threatening due to a risk of herniation. If CSF is obtained, there may be a mild mononuclear pleocytosis, slight elevation of protein, and a normal concentration of glucose; however, the culture tends to be sterile unless the abscess has ruptured into the ventricular system.[16]

Samples of pus taken intraoperatively should be sent for microscopy, culture, and sensitivity. The use of further molecular diagnostic techniques, such as PCR and 16/18 s rDNA testing, is often useful in increasing the diagnostic yield from pus samples.

Imaging

MRI is the cerebral imaging choice as it allows prompt confirmation of the clinical diagnosis,

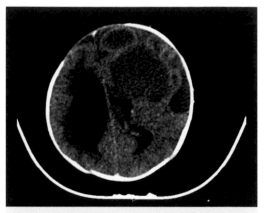

Fig. 53.4 Axial CT scan of a 3-month old girl infant, presenting with symptoms of sepsis and macrocephaly, demonstrating a left frontal loculated intracerebral abscess. Patient was surgically treated via transfontanelle drainage isolating *S. pneumoniae*. In subdural empyema, the presentation may be prolonged and insidious with nonspecific symptoms such as malaise, fever, rhinorrhea, and cough. The interval of time between the onset of first symptoms (rhinorrhea, cellulitis, feeling unwell, pyrexia) and the development of symptoms indicative of intracranial infection has been reported to be between 2 and 6 weeks.[18] These nonspecific symptoms can be easily overlooked by the family physician, leading to the delayed diagnosis often seen, but this period of time offers a therapeutic window in which aggressive treatment of sinus infection may prevent the formation of subdural empyema.

abscess location, and number.[16] It has been shown to have a sensitivity of up to 100%.[15]

Brain abscess in infants and newborns tend to be located in the periventricular white matter as opposed to the subcortical white matter seen in adults. Subdural empyemas are usually shaped in a crescent and occur along the cerebral convexities in approximately 50% of cases and along the falx in 20% of cases. On CT, they appear as extra-axial fluid collections that are isointense or slightly hyperintense to CSF. On T1-weighted MRI, they show mild hyperintense signal when compared to CSF, and on T2-weighted imaging, they are isointense or hyperintense. There is restricted diffusion on DWI and apparent diffusion coefficient (ADC) imaging, which is useful to distinguish them from hygromas or chronic hematomas. There is marked rim enhancement, on contrast administration, caused by inflammatory changes of the limiting membrane caused by hypervascularity and fibrosis. Surrounding parenchyma may have abnormal signal due to cerebritis and ischemia secondary to venous thrombosis.

DWI and MR spectroscopy can aid in the differentiation of a brain abscess from tumor. Brain abscesses show peaks of aliphatic amino acids like alanine, succinate, acetate, leucine, isoleucine, and valine,[3] whereas tumors generally show increased choline with reduced N-acetylaspartate on MR spectroscopy. Pus in abscesses has restricted diffusion and appears hyperintense on DWI.[21] Serial scanning should be used for follow-up to compare abscess size over time to aid treatment protocols and ensure resolution. Contrast enhancement should not be used as a guide to treatment response as it may persist, presumably due to fibrosis, following treatment completion.

Susceptibility-weighted imaging (SWI) MRI exploits the magnetic susceptibility differences between different tissues and is exquisitely sensitive to blood, iron, and calcification. SWI may be helpful in the recognition of infective emboli associated with systemic sepsis[22] (▶ Fig. 53.5).

If an MRI cannot be obtained, a CT scan with intravenous contrast should be performed, or in the neonate, bedside cranial ultrasonography is an alternative.

53.5.4 Pathogens

Historically subdural empyema was a disease of infancy associated with meningitis and caused by *H. influenzae* type b. The incidence of which has dropped dramatically since the introduction of national vaccination programs.

The most common pathogens are streptococci attributed to over 50% of cases, with the commonest

belonging to the *Streptococcus milleri* group (*Streptococcus intermedius*, *Streptococcus anginosus*, and *Streptococcus constellatus*).[15,20] These are normal flora in the mouth and gastrointestinal (GI) tract. Other organisms include *Haemophilus* sp, *Enterobacter*, *Citrobacter*, and *Pseudomonas* (▶ Table 53.4). Children with penetrating trauma

Table 53.4 Common causative organisms of brain abscess in children, organized by predisposing factors

Predisposing factor	Causative organism(s)
Neonate	*Proteus* spp *Citrobacter* spp *Enterobacter* spp
Immunocompromised	*Nocardia* spp Fungi *Mycobacterium tuberculosis*
Congenital heart disease	*Streptococcus viridans* Microaerophilic streptococci *Haemophilus* spp
Middle ear infection	Streptococci (aerobic and anaerobic) Enterobacteriaceae *Pseudomonas* spp
Sinusitis	Streptococci (aerobic and anaerobic) *Staphylococcus aureus* Enterobacteriaceae
Oral cavity infection	Mixed anaerobic flora Streptococci (aerobic and anaerobic) *S. aureus* Enterobacteriaceae
Posttraumatic	*S. aureus* *Streptococcus* spp Enterobacteriaceae

Source: Adapted from Sheehan et al.[16]

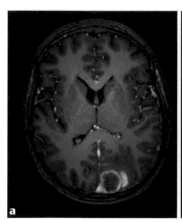
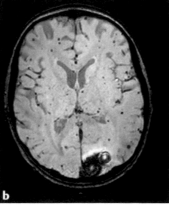

Fig. 53.5 (a) Axial contrast-enhanced T1 MRI of a 9-year old boy, presenting with systemic sepsis requiring extracorporeal membrane oxygenation with a pleural empyema and osteomyelitis, demonstrating a left occipital abscess. (b) Susceptibility-weighted imaging MRI of the same patient demonstrating microemboli not identified on the standard T1 with contrast MRI.

or postneurosurgery are more likely have *Staphylococcus aureus* infections. Very few abscesses are caused by anaerobic bacteria. Fungal and amoebic abscess are very rare and generally in immunocompromised hosts. Multiple pathogens have been found in up to 25% of cases. In those cases where a pathogen is not identified from samples taken intraoperatively, it is important to culture material from different sites that include blood, phlegm, urine and stool cultures, and CSF as this can often lead to positive results.

53.5.5 Management

Medical/Antimicrobial

The importance of obtaining a sample for culture cannot be overemphasized but empirical treatment should be commenced as soon as possible.
- Ceftriaxone/cefotaxime plus metronidazole as initial treatment.
- If meningitis or cyanotic congenital heart disease is present, then ceftriaxone alone may be sufficient.
- In penetrating trauma/postneurosurgery, treatment should cover *S. aureus*, but there are insufficient data to support whether flucloxacillin or a carbapenem should be used or whether ceftriaxone is sufficient.
- Meropenem is the first-line choice in the severely ill or immunocompromised.
- Vancomycin should be added if the patient is methicillin-resistant *S. aureus* (MRSA)-colonized or is from a high-prevalence area.

The optimal duration of treatment is not known but the consensus is that brain abscesses should be treated with a total of 6 weeks of antibiotics, of which at least 1 to 2 weeks should be intravenous, guided by improvement in clinical condition, MRI findings, and blood inflammatory markers.[15,16,23] Oral step-down antibiotics would include amoxicillin/clavulanate, although alternatives such as clindamycin or rifampicin may be suitable, and treatment should be guided by culture results.[15,23] Some studies have suggested shorter courses can be advocated but at present, there is limited data to support this.

Seizure Prophylaxis

There are no studies to guide the prophylactic use of antiepileptic therapy in children with brain abscesses. Some practitioners favor short-term prophylactic use of antiepileptic drugs in all children with a brain abscess, others commence antiepileptic therapy only in patients whose presentation includes a seizure. If anticonvulsants are started, be mindful of the possible pharmacological interactions between antibiotics and anticonvulsants in calculating dosages.

Neurosurgical

Cerebral Abscess

Consideration of treating cerebritis, small solitary abscesses (< 2 cm in diameter), or those in which the causative agent has been identified by antimicrobials alone is possible,[16] although thought should be given to surgical drainage. Surgical drainage is required if there is (1) deteriorating neurological deficit or consciousness, (2) marked mass effect on imaging, (3) failure of antibiotic treatment, (4) need to obtain organism samples for culture.

Surgical drainage can often be performed using frameless stereotactic burr hole aspiration (CT, MRI, or ultrasound based), or via neuroendoscopy, without the need for a craniotomy. The use of intraoperative ultrasonography can further help to ensure abscess evacuation. The majority of children only require a single aspiration.[16,24] If there is a progressive neurological deterioration, or nonresolution or growth of the abscess despite adequate and appropriate antimicrobial therapy, then repeat aspiration or craniotomy should be performed. Craniotomy allows more complete evacuation and debridement of the infected parenchyma together with the abscess wall, but its size should be as small as possible. Intracranial foreign bodies associated with abscesses, such as shunt tubing or deep brain electrodes, should be removed.

Surgical complications associated with burr hole aspiration or craniotomy include hemorrhage, CSF leakage, seizure, stroke, and risk to life. It is important when planning a needle trajectory for aspiration that in addition to avoiding eloquent areas does not penetrate the ventricle due to the risk of seeding the infection.

Subdural Empyema

This is a neurosurgical emergency that commonly requires emergency craniotomy. Craniotomy and evacuation of the pus collection followed by intravenous antibiotic treatment is the standard neurosurgical treatment in most neurosurgical centers.

It has been reported that wide craniotomy with pus washout and deloculation of the collection, if saeptae are present, allows better control of raised ICP and reduced incidence of reaccumulation.[18,25] If sinus disease is the causative insult, then consideration of a sinus washout by the otolaryngology team during the same operating sitting should be made. Attempts should not be made to remove formed adherent pus from the arachnoid due to risk of damaging underlying parenchyma (▶ Fig. 53.6).

The empyema may recollect at the site of the original craniotomy or a de novo focus of infection may form in a different location. The reaccumulation rate requiring reoperation has been reported to vary between 18 and 33%.[18,26] Therefore, postoperative imaging is an essential tool in the early detection of possible recollections.

Subdural empyema may present with associated lesion such as an intra-axial abscess, extradural collection, bone infection, soft tissue infection, meningitis, or hydrocephalus. The incidence of these associated lesions varies with the location and the severity of the subdural infection, but the treating team must be mindful to monitor for these.

Epidural Abscess

Treatment consists of appropriate antibiotic therapy combined with neurosurgical drainage with thorough irrigation, either through burr holes, craniotomy, or craniectomy. In epidural abscesses, consideration should be made to removal of infected bone especially if it is sequestered or previously devascularized by surgery or trauma. In suppuration complicating craniofacial reconstruction where bone loss would create irreparable defects, the bone may be replaced, and prolonged antibiotic administration planned. This may be successful in preserving bone fragments until they are revascularized or resorbed.

53.5.6 Prognosis

Although relatively rare in children, intracranial suppuration is associated with significant morbidity and mortality. The potential long-term sequelae depend on abscess location and cortical involvement but can include among others seizures, hemiparesis, cognitive deficits, and cranial nerve dysfunction. Approximately a third of children will not return to their predisease state, having focal neurological deficits, and approximately 6% will die.[15,20] Predisposing factors to a poorer outcome include age younger than 5 years and a GCS less than or equal to 8 at admission.[15] It is therefore essential that early diagnosis combined with the prompt initiation of empirical antimicrobial therapy and neurosurgical intervention are instigated to try and minimize long-term sequelae.

53.6 Common Clinical Questions

1. In neonates what are the common causative organisms of bacterial meningitis and from where are they generally acquired?
2. What are the contraindications to performing a lumbar puncture?
3. What are the commonest global causes of viral encephalitis?
4. What are the four stages of brain abscesses evolution?
5. What are the indications for surgical drainage of brain abscesses?

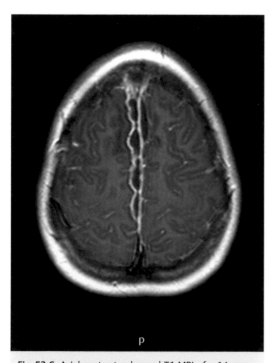

Fig. 53.6 Axial contrast-enhanced T1 MRI of a 14-year old adolescent girl, presenting with 2 weeks of headache and partially treated frontal sinusitis resulting in meningitis, demonstrating a parafalcine subdural empyema. Patient was surgically treated via a bifrontal craniotomy and drainage isolating *Streptococcus* species.

53.7 Answers to Common Clinical Questions

1. In neonates (< 28 days old), the most common causative organisms are likely to be acquired around the time of birth from the maternal genital and GI tract, and are *S. agalactiae* (Group B *Streptococcus*), *E. coli*, *S. pneumoniae*, and *L. monocytogenes*.

2. Performance of a lumbar puncture is contraindicated if the following signs are present:
   - Signs suggesting raised ICP:
     - Reduced or fluctuating level of consciousness (GCS < 9 or a drop of ≥ 3)
     - Relative bradycardia and hypertension
     - Focal neurological signs
     - Abnormal posture or posturing
     - Unequal, dilated, or poorly responsive pupils
     - Papilloedema
     - Abnormal "doll's eye" movements
   - Shock
   - Extensive or spreading purpura
   - After seizures until stabilized
   - Coagulation abnormalities:
     - Coagulation results outside the normal range
     - Platelet count below $100 \times 109/L$
     - Receiving anticoagulant therapy
   - Local superficial infection at the lumbar puncture site.
   - Respiratory insufficiency (lumbar puncture is considered to have a high risk of precipitating respiratory failure in the presence of respiratory insufficiency).

3. Globally the commonest causes of viral encephalitis are herpes simplex virus (22%), followed by varicella (21%), adenovirus (4%), and mumps virus.

4. The four stages of evolution of brain abscesses are early cerebritis (3–5 days), late cerebritis (5–14 days), early capsule formation, and late capsule formation (weeks to months).

5. Surgical drainage is required if there is:
   - Deteriorating neurological deficit or consciousness.
   - Marked mass effect on imaging.
   - Failure of antibiotic treatment.
   - Need to obtain organism samples for culture.

References

[1] Brouwer MC, Tunkel AR, van de Beek D. Epidemiology, diagnosis, and antimicrobial treatment of acute bacterial meningitis. Clin Microbiol Rev. 2010; 23(3):467–492

[2] National Collaborating Centre for Women's and Children's Health. Bacterial Meningitis and Meningococcal Septicaemia in Children. London, UK: RCOG Press; 2010

[3] Parmar H, Ibrahim M. Pediatric intracranial infections. Neuroimaging Clin N Am. 2012; 22(4):707–725

[4] Rantakallio P, Leskinen M, von Wendt L. Incidence and prognosis of central nervous system infections in a birth cohort of 12,000 children. Scand J Infect Dis. 1986; 18(4):287–294

[5] Logan SA, MacMahon E. Viral meningitis. BMJ. 2008; 336 (7634):36–40

[6] Negrini B, Kelleher KJ, Wald ER. Cerebrospinal fluid findings in aseptic versus bacterial meningitis. Pediatrics. 2000; 105 (2):316–319

[7] Thompson C, Kneen R, Riordan A, Kelly D, Pollard AJ. Encephalitis in children. Arch Dis Child. 2012; 97(2):150–161

[8] Chadwick DR. Viral meningitis. Br Med Bull. 2006; 75–76:1–14

[9] Vyse AJ, Gay NJ, Slomka MJ, et al. The burden of infection with HSV-1 and HSV-2 in England and Wales: implications for the changing epidemiology of genital herpes. Sex Transm Infect. 2000; 76(3):183–187

[10] Bedford H, de Louvois J, Halket S, Peckham C, Hurley R, Harvey D. Meningitis in infancy in England and Wales: follow up at age 5 years. BMJ. 2001; 323(7312):533–536

[11] Koskiniemi M, Korppi M, Mustonen K, et al. Epidemiology of encephalitis in children. A prospective multicentre study. Eur J Pediatr. 1997; 156(7):541–545

[12] Kimberlin DW, Lin CY, Jacobs RF, et al. National Institute of Allergy and Infectious Diseases Collaborative Antiviral Study Group. Safety and efficacy of high-dose intravenous acyclovir in the management of neonatal herpes simplex virus infections. Pediatrics. 2001; 108(2):230–238

[13] Pérez-Bovet J, Garcia-Armengol R, Buxó-Pujolràs M, et al. Decompressive craniectomy for encephalitis with brain herniation: case report and review of the literature. Acta Neurochir (Wien). 2012; 154(9):1717–1724

[14] Fowler A, Stödberg T, Eriksson M, Wickström R. Childhood encephalitis in Sweden: etiology, clinical presentation and outcome. Eur J Paediatr Neurol. 2008; 12(6):484–490

[15] Felsenstein S, Williams B, Shingadia D, et al. Clinical and microbiologic features guiding treatment recommendations for brain abscesses in children. Pediatr Infect Dis J. 2013; 32 (2):129–135

[16] Sheehan JP, Jane JA, Ray DK, Goodkin HP. Brain abscess in children. Neurosurg Focus. 2008; 24(6):E6

[17] Waseem M, Khan S, Bomann S. Subdural empyema complicating sinusitis. J Emerg Med. 2008; 35(3):277–281

[18] Osman Farah J, Kandasamy J, May P, Buxton N, Mallucci C. Subdural empyema secondary to sinus infection in children. Childs Nerv Syst. 2009; 25(2):199–205

[19] Wong TT, Lee LS, Wang HS, et al. Brain abscesses in children— a cooperative study of 83 cases. Childs Nerv Syst. 1989; 5(1):19–24

[20] Leotta N, Chaseling R, Duncan G, Isaacs D. Intracranial suppuration. J Paediatr Child Health. 2005; 41(9–10):508–512

[21] Nickerson JP, Richner B, Santy K, et al. Neuroimaging of pediatric intracranial infection–part 1: techniques and bacterial infections. J Neuroimaging. 2012; 22(2): e42–e51

[22] Lai PH, Chang HC, Chuang TC, et al. Susceptibility-weighted imaging in patients with pyogenic brain abscesses at 1.5T: characteristics of the abscess capsule. AJNR Am J Neuroradiol. 2012; 33(5):910–914

[23] Infection in Neurosurgery Working Party of the British Society for Antimicrobial Chemotherapy. The rational use of antibiotics in the treatment of brain abscess. Br J Neurosurg. 2000; 14(6):525–530

[24] Goodkin HP, Harper MB, Pomeroy SL. Intracerebral abscess in children: historical trends at Children's Hospital Boston. Pediatrics. 2004; 113(6):1765–1770

[25] Hendaus MA, Corporation HM. Subdural empyema in children. Glob J Health Sci. 2013; 5(6):54–59

[26] Glickstein JS, Chandra RK, Thompson JW. Intracranial complications of pediatric sinusitis. Otolaryngol Head Neck Surg. 2006; 134(5):733–736

54 Evaluation and Management of Pediatric Spinal Infections

Lydia J. Liang, Mari L. Groves

54.1 Introduction

Spinal infections have been recognized throughout history.[1] Regional variability in socioeconomic changes and endemic microbial flora has led to differences in the epidemiology of spinal infections worldwide. While advances in medical technology have enhanced the ease of detection and options for definitive treatment of these infections, they have also promoted the development of spinal infections by increasing the number of patients on iatrogenic immunosuppression and incidence of iatrogenic infections. Infections of the spine are relatively rare, yet often present with variable, nonspecific symptoms, requiring a high index of suspicion from clinicians. Spinal infections in the pediatric population are generally less common and less completely characterized than those in adults.[1,2]

From a neurosurgical perspective, spinal infections can be broadly divided into three categories by location—(1) infections of the spinal cord; (2) infections of the nerve roots and meninges; and (3) infections of the spinal axis, including the vertebrae, disks, and epidural space. Infections of the spinal axis can be further subdivided into spontaneous pyogenic infections, iatrogenic infections, and granulomatous infections caused by mycobacterium, fungi, unusual bacteria, and parasites. This chapter will focus on infections of the spinal cord and spinal axis. The severity of spinal infections relates to the number of structures involved, vertebral level of involvement, presence or absence of neurological symptoms, delay in diagnosis, virulence of the organisms involved, and immunological status of the host.

Risk factors for children and adults include intravenous (IV) drug abuse, AIDS, and chronic conditions such as diabetes. Medical interventions such as immunosuppression, chronic indwelling catheters for venous access, or chemotherapy also increase the risk for spinal infections.

The vertebral end plate is the most commonly reported focus of vertebral infection, followed by the disk space itself, epidural abscess formation, and paraspinal abscess formation.[3]

Spinal axis infections:

- Average delay in diagnosis is 3 months, average recovery period is 12 months.[3]

- Pyogenic spinal infections (PSIs)—neutrophil predominant:
  - More frequent in males (55–75%).[3]
  - Annual incidence now estimated at between 5 and 10 cases per million[1] (17–19).
  - Diskitis—infection of the intervertebral disk.[4,5,6]
    - Affects children of all ages, but its prevalence is highest in children younger than 5 years, and adolescents.[7,8]
    - Lumbosacral (78%) > thoracic > cervical disease.[3,9]
  - Pyogenic vertebral osteomyelitis (PVO) (▶ Fig. 54.1)—infection of the vertebral body/pyogenic spondylodiskitis—infection of the vertebral body and adjacent disk.[10]
    - Affects older children past the age of 8 years, incidence peaks in adolescence and again in later adult years.
    - About 2 to 7% of all cases of osteomyelitis involve the spine.
    - In persons younger than 20 years, the incidence is 0.3 per 100,000, but rises sharply in late adulthood to 6.5 per 100,000.
  - Spinal epidural abscess (SEA) (▶ Fig. 54.1) purulent collection between the bone and dura mater:[11,12]
    - Majority of cases of SEA in children are individual case reports. Overall incidence of SEA ranges from 2 to 20 per 100,000.
    - Less common than cranial epidural abscesses. Commonly secondary to pyogenic or tubercular diskitis and osteomyelitis.
    - More common in girls than in boys.
- Granulomatous spinal infections:
  - Tuberculosis (TB) of the spine (Pott's disease; tuberculosis spondylodiskitis [TS])—caused by *Mycobacterium Tuberculosis*.
    - More common in developing world with higher rates of TB.
    - Spinal TB occurs in 1 to 3% of people infected with TB.
    - Predilection for anterior vertebral body involvement of the thoracolumbar spine, although posterior vertebral body can be involved.
    - Axial skeleton accounts for about 60% of all cases of TB osteomyelitis.[13]

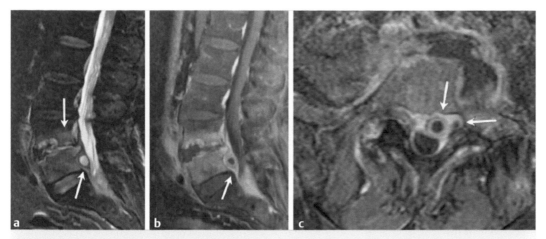

Fig. 54.1 (a) Sagittal fat-suppressed T2-weighted imaging demonstrating vertebral osteomyelitis at the L4–L5 level, seen as poorly defined zones with high signal in the marrow of the vertebral bodies (*arrows*) and corresponding gadolinium contrast enhancement on (b) sagittal and (c) axial fat-suppressed T1-weighted imaging (*arrows*). Abnormal high signal on T2-weighted imaging is seen involving the L4–L5 disk as well as irregularities at the end plates of the adjacent vertebral bodies. The infection extends posteriorly to involve the epidural soft tissues, and there is an epidural abscess at the L5 level (*arrow* in b). (Reproduced with permission from Differential Diagnosis in Neuroimaging: Spine, 2017. Meyers, Steven. Fig. 1.193)

○ Up to 10% of patients have multiple involved levels with intervening normal "skip" regions. Unlike in adult patients, children rarely present with paraplegia.

○ Neurological loss observed in 10 to 60% of patients.[2,14]

- Brucellosis:

○ Most common zoonosis in humans. About 20 to 25% of systemic brucellosis cases involve children. In children, transmission occurs from infected animals to humans via consumption of raw milk or milk products.

○ Cutaneous, hematological, and respiratory complications are most common in children.

○ May be present focally or diffusely.[2]

• Iatrogenic infections:

- Rates of surgical site infections (SSIs) following pediatric spine surgery range from 3.7 to 8.5%.[15,16]

- Reported risk factors include inappropriate timing of antibiotics, previous spine surgery, complex medical comorbidities, age, more than 10 vertebrae fused, increase intraoperative blood loss, obesity, infection prophylaxis with clindamycin, and prolonged intraoperative hypothermia.[17,18,19] Skin preparation before surgery, wound irrigation before closure, nutritional status, and preoperative antibiotic administration have also been hypothesized as major factors influencing infection.

- Financial costs range from $26,977 to $961,722 secondary to hospital readmissions and repeat surgeries.[20]

• Intramedury spinal cord abscess (ISCA)—suppurative infection of the central nervous system (CNS) similar to pyogenic brain abscesses[21]:

- Isolated infection of the spinal cord is uncommon overall, with only 96 cases published between 1830 and 2011,[22] yet over 40% of ISCA presents in patients younger than 20 years, with 25 to 27% of patients younger than 10 years.[23,24]

- Male predilection—60 to 70% of cases occur in men.[23,24]

- Most frequently found in the thoracic region (32%) > cervical (17%) > lumbar (12%).

- About 69% of all abscesses involved some portion of the thoracic cord.[23]

- Causative organisms include *Schistosoma* (particularly common children), *Candida* infection, *Aspergillus*, and nocardiosis.[14]

- Predisposing conditions include congenital heart disease, disorders of the immune system, underlying spinal cord tumors, and dermal sinuses, which may give rise to intraspinal abscesses outside and inside the cord.[14]

- Higher incidence in IV drug users.[25]

Infective organisms can be carried to the spine by direct inoculation through surgical manipulation or a penetrating injury, by local spread from continuous structures, or hematogenously from a distant site of infection.[1,3] Infections tend to be localized in a single region (i.e., vertebral body, disk, and epidural space), but may involve multiple regions concurrently. For pyogenic and nonpyogenic infections that spread hematogenously from a primary source of infection other than the spine, a proposed mechanism of spread begins with bacteria lodging in the capillary loop or postcapillary venous channels in the end plate. The infection can extend anteriorly to create a paravertebral abscess, longitudinally along the spinal axis to cause diskitis, or posteriorly to cause myelitis or an epidural abscess. In most cases, infection of the vertebral body is limited by the cartilage-capped end plates. As the infection progresses, suppurative inflammation and tissue necrosis eventually result in end plate erosions and infection of the vertebral body. The bone softens and may collapse under the body's weight, leading to deformity or kyphosis. Neurological deficits are caused by direct extension of the infection to the neural elements, or secondary compression from pathological fracture as a result of bone softening.[3]

Tuberculous infections, on the other hand, typically feature a slow inflammatory response initiated by bacteria, with the formation of a tuberculous granuloma in the vertebral end plate.[26] It caseates centrally and forms an abscess, which may extend in any direction. The abscess grows "cold" and large and may compress adjacent structures, extend into the spinal canal, or develop into a sinus.[2,27] Pathological fracture of the vertebral body following the development of a fibrous ankylosis most commonly in the thoracic spine may eventually result in angular kyphosis and compromise of the spinal canal by sequestration of vertebra and disk or by dislocation of one spinal segment.[28]

54.2 Anatomy

The vertebral body is composed of a central zone and a peripheral zone, with an epiphyseal ring surrounding the outer rim of the vertebral body surface. It is slightly raised, externally overlapping the outer surface of the vertebral body, and internally slopes to meet the peripheral zone of the bony end plate. The bony end plate is separated from the intervertebral disk by a central cartilaginous end plate, which consists of hyaline cartilage. The annulus fibrosis of the intervertebral disk is firmly adherent to the epiphyseal ring, where the central portion is less firmly attached[29,30] (▶ Fig. 54.2).

At the level of each vertebra, the vertebral artery, intercostal artery, or lumbar arteries provide nutrient vessels that enter the vertebral body, form anastomoses at each level, and join with a posterior nutrient and venous network. Vascular loops and channels formed by these anastomoses in the bony end plate supply nutrients to the intervertebral disk via diffusion through the cartilaginous end plate, as the disk is avascular even in infants.[28,31,32] These loops are more prominent in children than adults, and diminish with age. In children younger than 8 years, this vasculature extends beyond the ossification center into the surrounding cartilage directly in close proximity to the border of the intervertebral disk.[33,34] This provides a more direct route of infectious spread

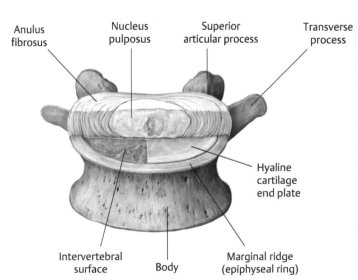

Anulus fibrosus · Nucleus pulposus · Superior articular process · Transverse process · Hyaline cartilage end plate · Intervertebral surface · Body · Marginal ridge (epiphyseal ring)

Fig. 54.2 Structure of intervertebral disk. Anterosuperior view with the anterior half of the disk and the right half of the end plate removed. The intervertebral disk consists of an external fibrous ring (annulus fibrosus) and a gelatinous core (nucleus pulposus). (Reproduced with permission from Thieme. Atlas of Anatomy, 2nd ed. Chapter 1 Bones, Ligaments & Joints, Fig 1.18.)

to the intervertebral disk and may explain the distinctly higher incidence of diskitis in children compared to adults. Notably, a high proportion of cultures in diskitis are negative.[28]

The extensive venous drainage of the spine provides an opportunity for retrograde spread of infection. The external and internal venous plexuses run the length of the spine, and communicate with venous systems throughout the body, including the pelvic, prostatic, sacral, pulmonary, caval, thoracoabdominal, scalp, skull, and facial venous systems (▶ Fig. 54.3 and ▶ Fig. 54.4).[26,30]

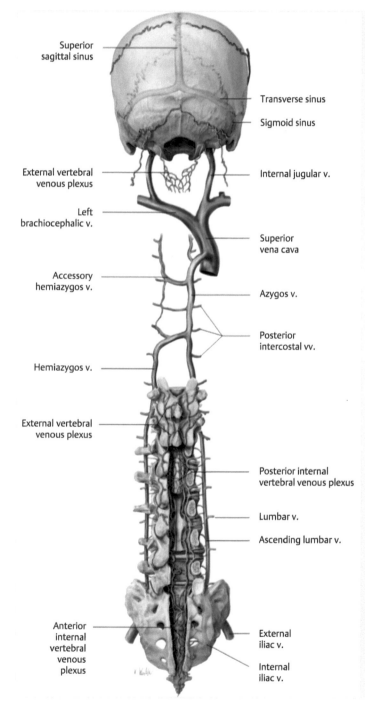

Fig. 54.3 Veins of the back. Vertebral venous plexus, posterior view with vertebral canal windowed in the lumbar and sacral spine. (Reproduced with permission from Thieme. Atlas of Anatomy, 2nd ed. Fig. 4.2 B.)

Superior sagittal sinus

Transverse sinus

Sigmoid sinus

External vertebral venous plexus

Internal jugular v.

Left brachiocephalic v.

Superior vena cava

Accessory hemiazygos v.

Azygos v.

Posterior intercostal vv.

Hemiazygos v.

External vertebral venous plexus

Posterior internal vertebral venous plexus

Lumbar v.

Ascending lumbar v.

Anterior internal vertebral venous plexus

External iliac v.

Internal iliac v.

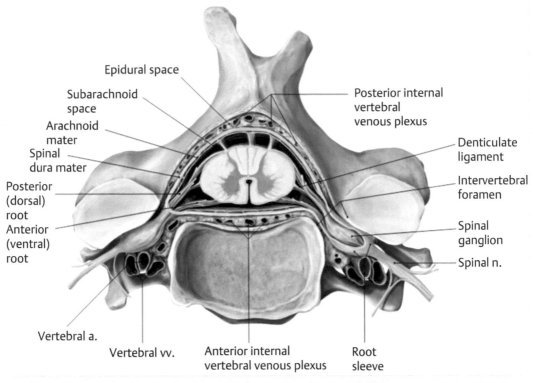

Fig. 54.4 Spinal cord in situ: transverse section. Spinal cord at level of C4 vertebra. (Reproduced with permission from Thieme. Atlas of Anatomy, 2nd ed. Fig. 2.20.)

54.3 Examination

54.3.1 History and Physical Examination

The history of patients with spinal infection is relatively nondiagnostic. One series found 85% of patients presented with pain.[9] Pain occurs primarily in the infected area with changes in position, ambulation, and other forms of activity, and may be referred to the abdomen, hips, or genitals. The intensity of the pain varies from mild to extreme. Particularly sharp or lancinating pain and the presence of a rapidly progressing neurological deficit implicates SEA over PVO or diskitis.[35] Young children or toddlers may present with a limp or refusal to walk, and may hold their spine erect to minimize pain. The pediatric assessment can be difficult because young children in pain are often agitated, fearful, and marginally cooperative, and they may not be able to relate the character or localization of their pain clearly. A useful diagnostic examination in children involves requesting the patient to pick up an object from the floor. The child will generally be unwilling to flex the spine and instead will squat to lower the body.[2] In older children and young athletes, the prevalence of back pain increases (24–36%) and back pain from diskitis or osteomyelitis may be mistaken for a sports injury.[36]

Constitutional symptoms include anorexia, malaise, night sweats, intermittent fever, and weight loss, but patients only rarely appear systemically ill. Other symptoms include dysphagia or neck stiffness. Temperature elevation, if present, usually is minimal, and more suggestive of spondylodiskitis over diskitis. Tenderness to palpation over the affected level is the most common physical sign. Sustained paraspinal spasm, torticollis, bizarre posturing, severe stiffness of the hamstring, and generalized weakness may be present also and are indicative of the acute process. A history of an immune-suppressing disease or a recent infection, or both, is common. A history of epidural catheters for regional anesthesia and spinal instrumentation strongly suggest SEA. Spinal deformity and paralysis are serious, late complications of the disease.[2,3,14,28]

Because of the depth of the spine, abscess formation is difficult to identify, unless it points superficially. Children with tuberculosis disease of the spine often present with large paraspinal abscesses (62%). A paraspinal abscess commonly presents as a swelling in the groin below the inguinal because of extension along the psoas muscle. Straight leg raising examination usually is not helpful because it may be negative or may elicit back or rarely leg pain.[37]

Neurological findings rarely are radicular and more frequently involve multiple nerve groups. Deficits such as weakness, numbness, or incontinence suggest a compressive lesion, epidural empyema, or intradural infection, over diskitis. ISCAs almost always involve motor (83–94%) or sensory (60–78%) deficits, and roughly half (51–56%) of patients will have loss of sphincter control at the time of diagnosis.[21,22,25] Central cord syndrome has been reported in two-thirds of patients with paralysis from cord compression, and anterior cord syndrome was found in one-third. Neurological symptoms are most frequent with infections in the cervical and thoracic areas and are least common with infections in the thoracolumbar region. The development of neurological signs should suggest the possibility of neural compression from abscess formation, bone collapse, or direct neural infection. Severe kyphosis from bony collapse develops in a significant proportion of children with tuberculosis of the spine (3%). When neurological symptoms appear, they may progress rapidly unless active decompression or drainage is undertaken.

Overall, a high index of clinical suspicion for spinal infection in any child presenting with back pain and nonspecific constitutional symptoms expedites the diagnosis and prevents the neurological morbidity that may accompany diagnostic delays. This suspicion increases for patients presenting with worsening nonmechanical back pain (e.g., worse at night, not relieved with rest) in immunocompromised patients, patients with travel history to endemic areas, and other risk factors that also apply to adults mentioned previously.

54.3.2 Laboratory

The goals of the laboratory work-up are to identify and isolate the causative organism to guide therapy and monitor the course of treatment. The standard work-up includes a complete blood count (CBC) with differential, measurement of the erythrocyte sedimentation rate (ESR), and C-reactive protein (CRP), and blood cultures, ideally taken during the initial febrile phase of the illness before antibiotics have been administered. Temporarily withholding antibiotics may be considered in patients who are not declining clinically, if antibiotic therapy has already been initiated and blood cultures are unrevealing.[38]

Blood culture is positive in approximately 50% of spinal infections.[2,3] The most common organism causing PSI is *Staphylococcus aureus*.[27] *S. aureus* with other gram-positive organisms such as *Staphylococcus epidermidis*, *Streptococcus viridans*, *Streptococcus pneumoniae*, *Streptococcus faecalis*, *Propionibacterium*, and diphtheroids account for the vast majority of PSIs. Gram-negative organisms causing PSIs are less frequent and may be associated with gastrointestinal or genitourinary sources of infection. Organisms responsible for ISCA include *Staphylococcus*, *Streptococcus*, *Actinomyces*, *Proteus mirabilis*, *Pneumococcus*, *Listeria monocytogenes*, *Haemophilus*, and *Escherichia coli*. These may arise from contiguous spread from a dermal sinus tract, postoperatively, or secondary to odontogenic bacteremia.[22]

If the blood cultures are negative, an image-guided or open biopsy may be indicated in patients who do not respond to empirical therapy and who are not in need of immediate surgical debridement (see **Biopsy** section below). In diagnosing tuberculosis disease of the spine, the Mantoux (tuberculin skin) test is nearly always positive secondary to BCG immunization which is widely conducted in the developing world. Definitive diagnosis only follows positive culture of a biopsy, but acid-fast bacilli culture may take 6 to 8 weeks. Advances in polymerase chain reaction (PCR) techniques specific for *Mycobacterium* DNA have hastened diagnosis.[2,28] Positive serology is helpful for diagnosing brucellosis (sensitivity is 65–95%), but the specificity is low because of the presence of antibodies in the bloodstream in regions of endemic flora.

The ESR and CRP are used to identify and clinically monitor the treatment spinal infections. They are not diagnostic tests and only indicate an inflammatory process. The ESR and CRP levels are normal to mildly elevated in diskitis, elevated in 71 to 97% of children with vertebral osteomyelitis,[3] and uniformly increased in SEA.[35] Both the ESR and CRP are elevated after surgery, but the CRP level tends to peak within the first 2 postoperative days and then declines rapidly to normal within 14 days given no postoperative infection, compared to the ESR which may be elevated for up to 4 weeks after surgery with no postoperative infection. The CRP level thus serves as a more sensitive marker for early detection of postoperative spine infections when compared with ESR, and can also be used to monitor the antibiotic treatment of an infection in the same way.[3]

Leukocytosis is not especially helpful in diagnosing spinal infection. White blood cell counts may decrease in infants. High white blood cell counts may indicate areas of infection other than the spine. CD4 counts are not helpful in determining the presence of infection in HIV patients but can help in determining the location and course of infection. Patients with CD4 count greater than 200/mL tend to have spinal infections that respond to antibiotics. Patients with CD4 counts less than 200/mL are more susceptible to osteoarticular and soft tissue infections.

54.3.3 Radiology

Imaging techniques are used to confirm the clinical impression.[3] Plain radiographs of the involved area are the most common initial study in patients with spinal infection. Radiographic findings, which appear 2 weeks to 3 months after the onset of the infection, include disk space narrowing, vertebral end plate irregularity or loss of the normal contour of the end plate, loss of normal lordosis in the cervical or lumbar spine, defects in the subchondral portion of the end plate, and hypertrophic (sclerotic) bone formation in pyogenic and nonpyogenic infections. Occasionally, paravertebral soft tissue masses may be noted with involvement of nearby areas of the spine. Late radiographic findings may include vertebral collapse, segmental kyphosis, and bony ankylosis, particularly in late tuberculosis infections. The sequence of events may range from 2 to 8 weeks for early findings to more than 2 years for later findings. The only definable abnormality on plain radiographs and computed tomography (CT) scans related specifically to early tuberculosis is fine calcification in the paravertebral soft tissue space. In brucellosis, the vertebral body is characteristically spared, without deformity.

CT identifies paravertebral soft tissue swelling and abscesses much more readily and can monitor changes in the size of the spinal canal. CT also offers a more detailed demonstration of the nature of destruction of the bone, end plate, disk, and soft tissue densities. Postmyelogram CT more clearly defines compression of the neural elements by abscess or bone impingement and helps determine whether the infection extends to the neural structures themselves.

Magnetic resonance imaging (MRI) is the gold standard for diagnosing infectious disorders of the spine in the pediatric age group.[14,39,40] MRI distinguishes infected from normal tissues, but does not differentiate between pyogenic and nonpyogenic infections and cannot eliminate the need for diagnostic biopsy. MRI may be difficult to attain in children without sedation. It is often performed in emergencies because of the often aspecific clinical presentation that may raise the suspicion of spinal cord compression. Intravenous administration of contrast (i.e., gadolinium) greatly enhances the identification and delineation of spinal infection. Spinal infections in the vertebral bodies and disks demonstrate decreased signal intensity on T1-weighted images, representing subchondral fibrosis and bone sclerosis. In T2-weighted images, the signal intensity is increased in the vertebral disk, representing tissue edema, and markedly decreased in the vertebral body. The granulation tissue associated with diskitis and vertebral osteomyelitis often resembles an abscess on MRI, appearing as areas of increased uptake. Intramedullary infections demonstrate hyperintensity on T2-weighted images, irregular ring enhancement, cord expansion, and restricted diffusion.[25,41]

The imaging of ISCAs follows the same progression as brain abscesses. MRI reveals early and late myelitis. Early myelitis appears as hyperintense on T2-weighted and proton density-weighted sequences. T1-weighted sequences show isointense to hypointense signal changes with a widened spinal cord. Late myelitis, about 7 days after the initial presentation, corresponds to the pathological stage of capsular formation, with more clearly defined marginal enhancement on contrast-enhanced T1-weighted images, while T2-weighted hyperintense signal changes become less diffuse.[22,42] MRI is not a reliable method of documenting resolution of spinal infections. Clinical findings, such as decreased pain and improved neurological function, seem to be better indicators than improvement seen on MRI.

Radionuclide studies are relatively effective in identifying spinal infection. These techniques include technetium-99 m (99 m Tc) bone scan, gallium-67 (67 Ga) scan, and indium-111-labeled leukocyte (111 In WBC) scan. In infection, diffuse activity is seen on the blood pool images of the 99 m Tc bone scan, and becomes focal on delayed views. This marked reactivity may persist for months. The 67 Ga scan is a good adjunct to bone scanning for the detection of osteomyelitis and it may be useful to document clinical improvement because it changes rapidly with the resolution of the acute active infection.[26] The 111 In WBC scan is useful in detecting abscesses and differentiating between noninfectious lesions, but it does not differentiate between acute and chronic infections.[28]

54.3.4 Biopsy

Invasive procedures for diagnosis are recommended only for failure of conservative management or for immunocompromised or immunosuppressed patients. If an invasive procedure is required, image-guided biopsy typically offers the least morbid option for directly obtaining a tissue sample. Time, host resistance, bacterial virulence, prior antibiotic exposure, and culture of the proper anatomical part all are factors in successful isolation of the offending organism. An exception is diskitis in children younger than 6 years, which may be viral in origin. Needle biopsy is rarely performed in these cases, and these patients may be the only group in whom careful monitoring without antibiotics is reasonable. An open surgical biopsy has a higher yield for the confirmation of a positive bacterial culture and is obligated if image-guided aspiration fails to grow an organism and the patient does not respond to medical management.

54.4 Nonsurgical Management

Identification of a causative organism through blood cultures or biopsy allows appropriate antibiotic therapy in concordance with consideration of surgical management. Treatment goals are aimed at resolving the infection, eliminating pain, and preventing the development of more serious infection or neurological compromise. CRP profiles are useful to monitor the activity of most infections, especially pyogenic infections. Serial MRI is not recommended to guide duration of antibiotic therapy, because improvements in the appearance on MRI tend to lag significantly behind clinical improvement.

Recommendations vary considerably for childhood diskitis. Nonoperative therapy, consisting of analgesia and immobilization for pain control, can resolve diskitis in almost all pediatric cases and is particularly appropriate for immunocompetent patients.[2,3,28] In the past, no difference in the outcome was reported in children who receive bed rest or antibiotic therapy. A course of antibiotics is now recommended for initial treatment, because prolonged or recurrent symptoms can occur in children not receiving antibiotics.[28] The standard course is 7 to 10 days of intravenous antibiotics with a follow-up period of 2 to 3 days of oral antibiotics that can be extended up to 6 weeks based on clinical findings. Patients should be followed up for at least 12 to 18 months and reassessed if symptoms recur or ESR and CRP fail to return to normal.

For osteomyelitis, long-term antimicrobial therapy with immobilization is the optimal treatment.[18] The recommended course is 6 weeks of appropriate intravenous antibiotic therapy with possibility of extension to 8 to 12 weeks, depending on the clinical and laboratory findings.[43]

In SEA acquired postoperatively, *Staphylococcus* species resistant to methicillin are seen (methicillin-resistant *S. aureus* [MRSA]), whereas community-acquired infections are most commonly broadly sensitive to methicillin (methicillin-sensitive *S. aureus* [MSSA]). However, surgical intervention is almost always indicated once a SEA is diagnosed.

Treatment for tuberculosis disease of the spine (TS) is medical only if TS is diagnosed early, the neurological examination is intact, and there is no bony destruction. A common regimen consists of rifampin, isoniazid, ethambutol, and pyrazinamide for 2 months, followed by rifampin and isoniazid for a variable period of 7 to 9 additional months. This has a success rate of 93% in neurologically intact patients.[3,28] Whether or not to immobilize patients is controversial, given the risks of bed rest balanced against the concern for vertebral collapse. Brucellosis requires at least two antibiotics (tetracycline, doxycycline, or rifampin) over 6 weeks.

54.5 Surgical Indications

Surgical treatment is indicated when there is clinically significant instability of the spine, neurological deterioration, or severe infection, including septicemia or persistent infection after nonoperative treatment (day). Sampling of infectious tissue to provide diagnostic cultures can also be performed during surgery. For a diagnosed spinal epidural abscess and other frank abscesses on imaging, surgical intervention is virtually always indicated due to the possibility of sudden and irreversible neurological decline despite antibiotic treatments.[2,14] Prompt surgery is also indicated for all intramedullary spinal cord abscesses.

For tuberculosis disease of the spine, reports have demonstrated up to 94% improvement when surgery is performed as early as possible, followed by chemotherapy. Long-term results from surgery with postoperative chemotherapy are superior to nonoperative management in terms of spinal stability and alignment, with less angular kyphosis. The involvement of multiple vertebrae significantly increases the risk of kyphosis and collapse and may prompt surgical intervention in the absence of neurological symptoms. Children have a greater potential to develop kyphosis with growth over time.[2] Indications for surgery in TS parallel those for pyogenic infections—neurological compromise that may be arrested, progressive or severe kyphosis or angulation, severe pain associated with kyphosis or collapse, evidence of progression of disease while the patient on optimized medical therapy, and a diagnosis in doubt.[2]

Situations in which surgical intervention might not be appropriate include: (1) the presence of a very small amount of fluid in the epidural space (particularly if it extends over multiple levels) and no evidence of neurological impairment, (2) the presence of complete neurological deficit for longer than 3 days, (3) profound and overwhelming comorbidity adversely affecting the likelihood that the patient will survive an operation, and (4) refusal of the patient to consent to operative intervention.[2]

54.6 Surgical Technique

For pyogenic infections, surgical goals include the evacuation of free pus from the epidural space, the sampling of infectious tissue to provide diagnostic cultures, and the maintenance and protection of spinal stability. For granulomatous infections, surgical goals include the decompression of neural elements, stabilization of columnar spinal stability, and correction of any kyphosis that may be present.[26,28]

In a patient with an epidural abscess, surgical goals can most often be accomplished with a decompressive laminectomy over the length of the abscess.[28,37] The purulent collection is almost uniformly posterior in all reported pediatric cases of SEA, but even when the collection is anterior, a laminectomy will often suffice to provide drainage and allow the sampling of material for diagnostic culture. An initial strategy of alternating hemila-

minotomies for multilevel abscesses allows vigorous irrigation of the epidural space while still retaining the posterior tension band to prevent later spinal instability. Posterior instrumentation and fusion provides spinal stability during the postoperative healing process.

Surgical approaches for tuberculosis disease of the spine have been debated in the medical literature. Limited surgery consists of laminectomy, which is the preferred procedure when the primary problem is a dorsal epidural collection of granulation material without kyphosis. Laminectomy is insufficient when the patient has significant vertebral body disease because of the potential for delayed kyphosis and the inability to address any ventral spinal cord compression that may be present. Posterior instrumented fusion can meaningfully augment stabilization but can do little to correct kyphosis.[26]

When vertebral body involvement has produced wedging and kyphosis, a more radical operation for TS involves an anterior approach with complete resection of infected and compromised vertebral bodies and secondary reconstruction with a bone graft (the Hong Kong procedure).[44,45] Radical surgery in TS is superior to nonsurgical management in terms of long-term spinal stability and alignment with less angular kyphosis. Recent reports have emphasized the addition of anterior stabilizing instrumentation for better outcomes, although posterior instrumentation is equally effective.[2,28] Vertebrectomy is associated with better long-term correction of kyphosis and angulation compared to laminectomy. Posterior instrumented fusion can be done at same time or in a staged manner 1 to 2 weeks after the initial surgical debridement in order to allow for an interval of IV antibiotics.[26] Single-stage anterior–posterior reconstruction is viable when sufficient debridement and stabilization can be achieved. More extensive surgery appears to be more effective in correcting the degree of deformity in children, but only a very limited experience in young children has been reported to date.[2]

Best practice guidelines on minimizing surgical site infections in high-risk pediatric spinal surgery were compiled by consensus and include preoperative, perioperative, and postoperative recommendations. Preoperative recommendations include a chlorhexidine skin wash at home the night before surgery, urine cultures, a Patient Education sheet, and a nutritional assessment. Perioperative guidance includes clipping over shaving if removing hair, IV cefazolin and prophylaxis for gram-negative bacilli, limited OR access, intraoperative wound irrigation, and vancomycin powder applied in bone grafts and to surgical sites. Postoperatively, impervious dressings are preferred, and dressing changes should be minimized to the extent possible.[46]

Treatment of postoperative spinal infections, including acute postoperative infections, consists of initial drainage and debridement with primary closure done in layers over a drain. Repeat irrigation and debridement of the wound with cultures and layered closure over drains is done at 48-hour intervals until the wound is without necrotic tissue, and cultures and Gram stain are negative. Well-fixed implants, assessed during debridement, should be left in place and removed only when the fusion is solid or when fixation is lost as infection can be treated around instrumentation. Bone graft pieces that are loose should be removed at the time of debridement. Recalcitrant wounds may require negative pressure wound therapy, V–Y flaps, or free flaps when bone or implants are exposed.[3]

To minimize spinal infections after placement of epidural catheters, tunneling the catheter before exiting the skin may help in reducing the risk of infection. The use of 0.5% chlorhexidine in 80% ethanol rather than 10% povidone–iodine for decontamination of the skin before insertion of an epidural catheter has been promoted by some as a method of preventing catheter infections in a pediatric population.[1]

Surgery for intramedullary spinal cord abscesses should be prompt, and include laminectomies at the involved levels, intradural exploration, midline myelotomy, and irrigation and drainage of the abscess cavity.

54.7 Complications

In patients with diskitis and associated vertebral osteomyelitis, laminectomy alone is associated with a high rate of clinical deterioration. For an established disk space infection at L4–L5, the blood vessels are usually adherent to the spine, which can make surgical treatment challenging due to risk of blood vessel injury. Any spinal surgery may be complicated with surgical site infections following the operation.[20]

54.8 Postoperative Care

Appropriate antibiotic therapy is required after surgical treatment. Selective antibiotics based on

biopsy results should be used according to the specific disease entity. For most pyogenic infections, 4 to 6 weeks of antibiotics are recommended, whereas fungal, granulomatous, and especially mycobacterial infections require longer periods of postoperative antibiotic treatment. Relapse often occurs when the course of antibiotics is discontinued before 6 weeks and/or the sedimentation rate and CRP levels are abnormal.

External immobilization is mandatory following debridement and grafting. Halo (vest, cast, or pelvic) immobilization for an average of 3 months is used after cervical and cervicothoracic procedures until the spine is clinically judged to have united. Removable or nonremovable thoracolumbar immobilization is used after thoracic and thoracolumbar procedures until the grafts have completely healed (9–12 months). Lumbosacropelvic immobilization is used after low lumbar procedures and should be from the hip to the knee of at least one leg for 6 to 8 weeks, followed by thoracolumbosacral immobilization until the graft has healed and the infection has resolved. Mobilization is started gradually and continued for 6 to 8 weeks, and the patient should be carefully watched for increasing kyphosis or other signs of disease activity.[3]

54.9 Outcomes

Even if an absolute diagnosis is not made, most spinal infections resolve symptomatically and radiographically within 9 to 24 months of onset when recognized early and treated appropriately.[47] Recurrence of infection and periods of decreased immune response are always possible, as are delayed complications of kyphosis, paralysis, and myelopathy. These risks are greatest during the period when the infection is controlled but the bone is still soft, when the healing process has not advanced to the point where solid bone has formed around the infected tissue.[3]

• In patients with diskitis and osteomyelitis, many authors report a favorable prognosis after antibiotic treatment with restoration of disk space height. Children with persistent radiological changes were found to be more prone to backache.[48] However, the amount of disk space restoration is variable. In one series of 16 children with contiguous diskitis and osteomyelitis, Song et al found that after antibiotic treatment, the disk space was partially restored 2 to 3 months after the initial visit in some patients but then became progressively narrower.[48] No patients achieved full restoration of disk space.

- In virtually all series of SEA, the best predictor of neurological outcome is the patient's preoperative neurological condition.[2]
- For intramedullary spinal cord abscesses, prognosis is inversely related to the acuity of onset of symptoms and directly related to the use of antibiotics in conjunction with prompt surgical drainage. Mortality among patients treated nonoperatively is 100%, whereas surgically treated patients improve or have a complete recovery in approximately 78% of cases.[22] Death is most frequently due to the presence of multiple CNS abscesses.

54.10 Surgical Pearls

- Surgical intervention for tuberculous osteomyelitis may be either via laminectomy with antibiotics and bracing or via anterior vertebrectomy and reconstruction. The two approaches do not differ in efficacy for local disease control, but vertebrectomy is associated with a reduced rate of complications related to kyphosis and angulation.
- For every spine biopsy, send tissue for appropriate cultures and pathological study. Uncommon infections such as tuberculosis and fungal infections will often be identified first by microscopic evaluation.

54.11 Common Clinical Questions

1. What are the surgical indications for a laminectomy over a more radical surgery for dealing with spinal infection?
2. How do you minimize the surgical site infections following high-risk pediatric spinal surgery?
3. What is the standard treatment for childhood diskitis sand osteomyelitis, and surgical site infections?

54.12 Answers to Common Clinical Questions

1. Laminectomy remains the preferred procedure when the primary problem for most surgical decompression and biopsy. However, if there is significant mobility of the spine with significant vertebral body disease, instrumented fusion with possible corpectomy is necessary given the potential for delayed kyphosis and the inability to address any significant ventral disease.

2. (a) Preoperative recommendations include a chlorhexidine skin wash at home the night before surgery, urine cultures, a Patient Education sheet, and a nutritional assessment. (b) Perioperative guidance includes clipping over shaving if removing hair, IV cefazolin and prophylaxis for gram-negative bacilli, limited OR access, intraoperative wound irrigation, and vancomycin powder applied in bone grafts and to surgical sites. (c) Postoperatively, impervious dressings are preferred, and dressing changes should be minimized to the extent possible.[46]

3. (a) Child diskitis: 7 to 10 days of IV antibiotics followed by up to 6 weeks of PO antibiotics based on imaging. Patients should be followed for up to 12 to 18 months and reassessed if symptoms recur or ESR/CRP fail to return to normal. (b) Osteomyelitis and spinal epidural abscess: 6 weeks of targeted IV antibiotic therapy with extension to 8 to 12 weeks depending on clinical and laboratory findings. (c) Surgical site infections: 4 to 6 weeks of targeted antibiotic therapy with possible maintenance on oral antibiotic therapy depending on clinical and laboratory findings.

References

[1] Vollmer DG, Tandon N. Infections of the spine. In: Winn HR, ed. Youmans Neurological Surgery. 6th ed. Philadelphia, PA: Saunders; 2011

[2] Blount JP, Naftel RP, Ditty BJ, Conklin MJ. Infections of the spinal axis. In: Albright AL, Pollack IF, Adelson PD, eds. Principles and Practice of Pediatric Neurosurgery. New York, NY: Thieme; 2015: 1065–1073

[3] Camillo FX. Infections of the spine. In: Canale ST, Beaty JH, eds. Campbell s Operative Orthopaedics. 12th ed. Philadelphia, PA: Elsevier; 2013

[4] Chandrasenan J, Klezl Z, Bommireddy R, Calthorpe D. Spondylodiscitis in children: a retrospective series. J Bone Joint Surg Br. 2011; 93(8):1122–1125

[5] Early SD, Kay RM, Tolo VT. Childhood diskitis. J Am Acad Orthop Surg. 2003; 11(6):413–420

[6] Fernandez M, Carrol CL, Baker CJ. Discitis and vertebral osteomyelitis in children: an 18-year review. Pediatrics. 2000; 105(6):1299–1304

[7] Brown R, Hussain M, McHugh K, Novelli V, Jones D. Discitis in young children. J Bone Joint Surg Br. 2001; 83(1):106–111

[8] Cushing AH. Diskitis in children. Clin Infect Dis. 1993; 17(1): 1–6

[9] Dormans JP, Moroz L. Infection and tumors of the spine in children. J Bone Joint Surg Am. 2007; 89 suppl 1:79–97

[10] Eismont FJ, Bohlman HH, Soni PL, Goldberg VM, Freehafer AA. Vertebral osteomyelitis in infants. J Bone Joint Surg Br. 1982; 64(1):32–35

[11] Boody BS, Jenkins TJ, Maslak J, Hsu WK, Patel AA. Vertebral osteomyelitis and spinal epidural abscess: an evidence-based review. J Spinal Disord Tech. 2015; 28(6):E316–E327

[12] Hawkins M, Bolton M. Pediatric spinal epidural abscess: a 9-year institutional review and review of the literature. Pediatrics. 2013; 132(6):e1680–e1685

[13] Khoo LT, Mikawa K, Fessler RG. A surgical revisitation of Pott distemper of the spine. Spine J. 2003; 3(2):130–145

[14] Rossi A. Pediatric spinal infection and inflammation. Neuroimaging Clin N Am. 2015; 25(2):173–191

[15] Glotzbecker MP, Riedel MD, Vitale MG, et al. What's the evidence? Systematic literature review of risk factors and preventive strategies for surgical site infection following pediatric spine surgery. J Pediatr Orthop. 2013; 33(5):479–487

[16] Smith J, Bhatia NN. Postoperative spinal infections. In: Herkowitz H, Garfin SR, Eismont FJ, Bell GR, Balderston RA, eds. Rothman-Simeone: The Spine. 6th ed. Philadelphia, PA: Elsevier; 2011

[17] Fei Q, Li J, Lin J, et al. Risk factors for surgical site infection following spinal surgery: a meta-analysis. World Neurosurg. 2016; 95:507–515

[18] Glotzbecker MP, Vitale MG, Shea KG, Flynn JM, POSNA committee on the Quality, Safety, Value Initiative (QSVI). Surgeon practices regarding infection prevention for pediatric spinal surgery. J Pediatr Orthop. 2013; 33(7):694–699

[19] Meng F, Cao J, Meng X. Risk factors for surgical site infection following pediatric spinal deformity surgery: a systematic review and meta-analysis. Childs Nerv Syst. 2015; 31(4):521–527

[20] Glotzbecker MP, Garg S, Akbarnia BA, Vitale M, Hillaire TS, Joshi A. Surgeon practices regarding infection prevention for growth friendly spinal procedures. J Child Orthop. 2014; 8(3):245–250

[21] Chan CT, Gold WL. Intramedullary abscess of the spinal cord in the antibiotic era: clinical features, microbial etiologies, trends in pathogenesis, and outcomes. Clin Infect Dis. 1998; 27(3):619–626

[22] Javahery RJ, Levi AD. Spinal intradural infections. In: Herkowitz H, Garfin SR, Eismont FJ, Bell GR, Balderston RA, eds. Rothman-Simeone: The Spine. 6th ed. Philadelphia, PA: Elsevier; 2011

[23] Bartels RH, Gonera EG, van der Spek JA, Thijssen HO, Mullaart RA, Gabreëls FJ. Intramedullary spinal cord abscess. A case report. Spine. 1995; 20(10):1199–1204

[24] Menezes AH, Graf CJ, Perret GE. Spinal cord abscess: a review. Surg Neurol. 1977; 8(6):461–467

[25] Baruah D, Chandra T, Bajaj M, et al. A simplified algorithm for diagnosis of spinal cord lesions. Curr Probl Diagn Radiol 2015;44(3):256–266

[26] Tay BK, Deckey J, Hu SS. Spinal infections. J Am Acad Orthop Surg. 2002; 10(3):188–197

[27] Yoon YK, Jo YM, Kwon HH, et al. Differential diagnosis between tuberculous spondylodiscitis and pyogenic spontaneous spondylodiscitis: a multicenter descriptive and comparative study. Spine J. 2015; 15(8):1764–1771

[28] Day GA, McPhee IB. Spine Infections: an algorithmic approach. In: Slipman C, Derby R, Simeone F, Mayer T, eds.

[29] Dar G, Masharawi Y, Peleg S, et al. The epiphyseal ring: a long forgotten anatomical structure with significant physiological function. Spine. 2011; 36(11):850–856

[30] Wiley AM, Trueta J. The vascular anatomy of the spine and its relationship to pyogenic vertebral osteomyelitis. J Bone Joint Surg Br. 1959; 41-B:796–809

[31] Coventry MB. Anatomy of the intervertebral disk. Clin Orthop Relat Res. 1969; 67(67):9–15

[32] Whalen JL, Parke WW, Mazur JM, Stauffer ES. The intrinsic vasculature of developing vertebral end plates and its nutritive significance to the intervertebral discs. J Pediatr Orthop. 1985; 5(4):403–410

[33] Ferguson WR. Some observations on the circulation in foetal and infant spines. J Bone Joint Surg Am. 1950; 32-A(3):640–648

[34] Ho PS, Yu SW, Sether LA, Wagner M, Ho KC, Haughton VM. Progressive and regressive changes in the nucleus pulposus. Part I. The neonate. Radiology. 1988; 169(1):87–91

[35] Auletta JJ, John CC. Spinal epidural abscesses in children: a 15-year experience and review of the literature. Clin Infect Dis. 2001; 32(1):9–16

[36] Haus BM, Micheli LJ. Back pain in the pediatric and adolescent athlete. Clin Sports Med. 2012; 31(3):423–440

[37] Rigamonti D, Liem L, Sampath P, et al. Spinal epidural abscess: contemporary trends in etiology, evaluation, and management. Surg Neurol. 1999; 52(2):189–196, discussion 197

[38] Cottle L, Riordan T. Infectious spondylodiscitis. J Infect. 2008; 56(6):401–412

[39] Chahoud J, Kanafani Z, Kanj SS. Surgical site infections following spine surgery: eliminating the controversies in the diagnosis. Front Med (Lausanne). 2014; 1:7

[40] Sze G, Bravo S, Baierl P, Shimkin PM. Developing spinal column: gadolinium-enhanced MR imaging. Radiology. 1991; 180(2):497–502

[41] Crema MD, Pradel C, Marra MD, Arrivé L, Tubiana JM. Intramedullary spinal cord abscess complicating thoracic spondylodiscitis caused by Bacteroides fragilis. Skeletal Radiol. 2007; 36(7):681–683

[42] Roh JE, Lee SY, Cha SH, Cho BS, Jeon MH, Kang MH. Sequential magnetic resonance imaging finding of intramedullary spinal cord abscess including diffusion weighted image: a case report. Korean J Radiol. 2011; 12(2):241–246

[43] Concia E, Prandini N, Massari L, et al. Osteomyelitis: clinical update for practical guidelines. Nucl Med Commun. 2006; 27(8):645–660

[44] Nussbaum ES, Rockswold GL, Bergman TA, Erickson DL, Seljeskog EL. Spinal tuberculosis: a diagnostic and management challenge. J Neurosurg. 1995; 83(2):243–247

[45] Obaid-ur-Rahman, Ahmad S, Hussain T. Anterior surgical interventions in spinal tuberculosis. J Coll Physicians Surg Pak. 2009; 19(8):500–505

[46] Vitale MG, Riedel MD, Glotzbecker MP, et al. Building consensus: development of a Best Practice Guideline (BPG) for surgical site infection (SSI) prevention in high-risk pediatric spine surgery. J Pediatr Orthop. 2013; 33(5):471–478

[47] Martin RJ, Yuan HA. Neurosurgical care of spinal epidural, subdural, and intramedullary abscesses and arachnoiditis. Orthop Clin North Am. 1996; 27(1):125–136

[48] Song KS, Ogden JA, Ganey T, Guidera KJ. Contiguous discitis and osteomyelitis in children. J Pediatr Orthop. 1997; 17(4):470–477

Interventional Spine: An Algorithmic Approach. Philadelphia, PA: Elsevier; 2008:401–415

55 Surgical Considerations in Tuberculosis, Fungal, and Parasitic Infections of CNS in Children

Chandrashekhar Deopujari, Dattatraya Muzumdar, Sonal Jain

55.1 Introduction

Tuberculosis (TB) is a chronic granulomatous disease caused by acid-fast bacilli, in the *Mycobacterium tuberculosis* complex. It has a propensity to affect multiple organs and is potentially life threatening. It is still regarded as a leading cause of death worldwide due to a single infectious agent. The incidence of TB is on decline in developing as well as industrialized countries, but the emergence of multidrug-resistant form of tuberculosis is of concern since it has worsened morbidity and mortality. Children who are persistently exposed to individuals with tuberculosis are usually at high risk of contracting the dreaded illness. Low immunity, malnutrition, and overcrowding are the principal contributing factors. Central nervous system (CNS) TB is a devastating manifestation of the infection, accounting for about 10% of all cases of TB especially TB meningitis.[1] The occurrence of vasculitis, arachnoiditis, direct parenchymal injury, and raised intracranial pressure (ICP) is responsible for the poor outcome.[1,2] Delay in diagnosis is another significant cause for mortality in underdeveloped countries. Involvement of the spine, also known as Pott's disease accounts for 1 to 2% of the world spinal deformity. It can result in complications, such as arachnoiditis, intramedullary tuberculoma, and spinal cord compression from epidural abscess. There are no specific international guidelines for the diagnosis and treatment of CNS tuberculosis and the treatment is largely institution specific. There are no studies, which demonstrate the superiority of an individual treatment protocol over another.

55.2 Pathogenesis

Mycobacterium TB commonly causes CNS tuberculosis, although in immunocompromised patients other species may be involved. Following initial pulmonary infection, the tuberculous bacteria may enter the systemic circulation and subsequently reach the CNS, which is rich in oxygen establishing in the meninges, subpial or subependymal region of the brain, or the spinal cord. It is known as the Rich focus, which may rupture into the subarachnoid space or ventricular system leading to meningitis. Alternatively, the meninges can be involved due to rupture of a tuberculoma into a vessel in the subarachnoid space, or rupture of miliary tubercles in miliary TB. It can rarely be involved following contiguous spread of infection from the adjacent bone.

The classic feature of tuberculous CNS disease is the formation of dense, gelatinous, inflammatory exudate along the basal surface of the cerebrum. In advanced cases, it may involve the leptomeninges over the cerebral convexities, and extend into the ventricular system, can cause ependymitis and choroid plexitis.[1,2]

Cell-mediated immune response is usually seen. The parenchymal tuberculous focus can develop into tuberculoma or brain abscess if the immunity is low.

The tuberculous affliction of the CNS manifests in a variety of clinical syndromes.

55.3 Tuberculous Meningitis

Tuberculous meningitis (TBM) in developing countries is more common among infants and children. The basal exudates can cause obstruction to cerebrospinal fluid (CSF) flow, causing hydrocephalus. It can also result in obliterative vasculitis due to occlusion of blood vessels at the base of the brain.[3,4] Tuberculous meningitis is characterized by basal exudates, which cause abnormal meningeal enhancement, hydrocephalus, and cerebral infarction. This triad is specific for the diagnosis of TBM.

The complications of meningitis include hyponatremia, hydrocephalus, vasculitis, cranial nerve involvement, and associated multiple tuberculomas.[3]

55.3.1 Hyponatremia

Hyponatremia is common in TBM and is independently associated with worse outcome. In conjunction with raised ICP, it may contribute to poor outcome through worsening cerebral edema, and its surveillance and prevention are of paramount importance. It manifests as either syndrome of inappropriate antidiuretic hormone secretion (SIADH) or cerebral salt-wasting syndrome (CSW).[3] It usually results due to hypothalamic injury or inflammation.

55.3.2 Hydrocephalus

Hydrocephalus is a sequelae or complication of tubercular meningitis.[1,2,3,4] The inflammatory basal exudates cause obstruction to the CSF flow resulting in a communicating type of hydrocephalus in about 80% of the cases. Noncommunicating or obstructive hydrocephalus can occur either because of obstruction of fourth ventricular outlet foramina by the basal exudates, or when there is obstruction of the aqueduct either due to a strangulation of the brainstem by exudates or by a subependymal tuberculoma. Trapped or loculated ventricle is also seen due to entrapment of a part of a ventricle by ependymitis. Sometimes, there is a combination of noncommunicating (obstructive) and communicating (defective absorption) hydrocephalus, which may be difficult to treat. It is found to be a cause of failure of endoscopic third ventriculostomy. About 50% of patients with TBM have chest X-rays suggesting active or previous pulmonary tuberculosis; 10% have miliary disease, which strongly suggests CNS involvement.[4,5]

55.3.3 Vasculitis

The inflammatory basal predominantly involving the circle of Willis. The adventitial and media are affected initially and later the lumen of the vessel. It causes reactive subendothelial cellular proliferation leading to complete occlusion and thrombus formation. Middle cerebral and lenticulostriate arteries are the most common vessels involved.

55.3.4 Cranial Nerve Involvement

Cranial nerve involvement in TBM is variable and is seen in 17 to 70% of patients. It primarily occurs due to ischemia of the nerve or entrapment of the nerve in basal exudates causing neuritis or perineuritis or there may be a tuberculoma on the nerve within the subarachnoid course. The proximal portion of the nerve at root entry zone is usually affected. The brainstem nucleus of the nerve in proximity can be affected. Permanent loss of function can ensue in late stages due to fibrosis.[1,2,3,4,5,6]

55.3.5 Tuberculous Encephalitis and Encephalopathy

Tuberculous encephalitis results from parenchymal inflammation adjacent to the meninges. It shows edema, perivascular infiltration, and a microglial reaction, known as border zone reaction. Tuberculous encephalopathy is a delayed type IV hypersensitivity reaction caused by tuberculous protein. It is a fulminant immunological mechanism resulting in extensive damage to the white matter and perivascular demyelination. Infants and young children with pulmonary TB are commonly affected. There is a high incidence of mortality despite antituberculous medication.[5,6]

55.3.6 Tuberculomas

Tuberculomas are among the most common intracranial mass lesions.[7,8,9] They can occur at any age. They can be solitary or multiple and can occur anywhere in the brain parenchyma.[10,11,12] In children, they predominate in the infratentorial compartment.[10] Tuberculomas arise when tubercles in the parenchyma of brain enlarge without rupturing into the subarachnoid space. They usually occur in the absence of TBM, but may occur with meningitis because of the extension of CSF infection into the adjacent parenchyma via cortical veins or Virchow–Robin spaces. Presence of tuberculomas at the corticomedullary junction suggests the hematogenous spread of infection, because there is narrowing of the arterioles at the gray/white matter junction. Initially, tuberculomas show typical noncaseating granulomatous reaction, which is predominantly lymphocytic and subsequently develops a central area of caseating necrosis. The central area of necrosis is initially solid and later may liquefy. Miliary tuberculomas are usually associated with meningitis and most of these patients have a primary pulmonary focus of infection. They are usually less than 2 to 5 mm in size. The occurrence of intramedullary tuberculoma is rare.[13,14,15]

55.3.7 Tuberculous Brain Abscess

Tuberculous brain abscess is rare.[16,17,18,19,20,21] It can be solitary or multiple. It is an encapsulated collection of pus with abundant viable tubercle bacilli without classic tubercular granuloma formation. The wall is thicker than pyogenic abscess. They can mimic ontogenic–pyogenic abscess.[18] It can occur from parenchymal tuberculous granulomas or via the spread of tuberculous foci in the meninges to the brain. According to the Whitener criteria for tuberculous abscess, it should reveal macroscopic evidence of abscess formation within the brain parenchyma, and, on histological confirmation, the abscess wall should be composed of vascular granulation tissue containing acute and chronic inflammatory cells and tubercle bacilli.[19,20]

55.3.8 Calvarial Tuberculosis

Calvarial tuberculosis is rare, even in areas where tuberculosis is endemic because of paucity of lymphatics in the calvarial bone.[21,22] It occurs secondary to hematogenous spread from the primary focus such as pulmonary, cervical or hilar lymphadenitis, renal or systemic tuberculosis. Less commonly it can arise from tuberculous mastoiditis or spinal tuberculosis. The outer table is usually the first to be destroyed, though eventually both tables can be affected. It could occur as small, circumscribed punched out defect in the bone with granulation tissue covering both internal and external aspect with little tendency for osteitis to spread in the bone or periosteum surrounding the defect or widespread destruction of the inner table with abundant extradural granulation tissue in the form of pachymeningitis externa.[23,24] In circumscribed and sclerotic type, there is marked thickening of the bone because of lack of blood supply to the diseased bone. Younger population is at higher risk to develop calvarial tuberculosis and it is rare in infancy. The most common sites of involvement are frontal and parietal bones, both the bones have large amount of cancellous bone.[25,26,27] They commonly present as scalp swelling, discharging sinus, and pain, rarely patient may present with seizure or motor deficit. Plain X-ray of the skull can be helpful. Areas of rarefaction are seen early in the disease, which develop into punched out defects with a central sequestrum later on.[28] Both osteolytic and osteoblastic areas may be seen. Rarely, sclerosis may be seen and indicates secondary infection. CT scan of the brain is helpful in assessing the extent of bone destruction, scalp swelling, and degree of intracranial involvement (▶ Fig. 55.1).[27] Combination of surgical excision and antitubercular therapy are the preferred treatment. With early diagnosis and a combination of surgical and medical management, all cases of calvarial tuberculosis are potentially curable. Surgery is indicated to establish the diagnosis, to remove thick extradural granulation tissue and necrotic bone, and in patients with sinus discharge, intracranial extensions, and large collections of caseating material causing mass effect.[21,22,23,24,25,26,27,28]

55.3.9 Spinal Tuberculosis

TB spondylitis, also called as Pott's disease, was first described by Percival Pott in 1779. Tuberculous spondylodiskitis is an important cause of spinal infection in developing countries. Early diagnosis and prompt treatment are essential to avoid morbidity. It constitutes 2 to 4% of all cases of osteomyelitis. The lumbar spine is the most commonly affected region, followed by the thoracic and cervical spine and, rarely, the sacrum. The thoracolumbar junction is a common site involved in tuberculous spondylitis. It results from hematogenous spread, both arterial and venous; direct contamination; and direct spread from adjoining abscess. The arteries at the anterior aspect of the vertebra possess the richest supply, accounting for the initial infective focus in the anterior subchondral bone. The Batson paravertebral venous plexus of valveless veins provides a potential route of retrograde spread from abdominal veins. Direct contamination of the spine may occur after surgery or after spinal canal puncture, although the incidence is low. It could manifest as solitary vertebral body involvement, multifocal skip lesions, pure

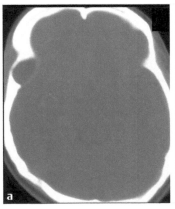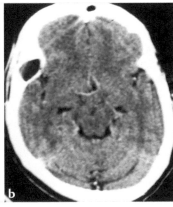

Fig. 55.1 **(a)** Axial CT bone window showing right greater wing of sphenoid bone erosion. **(b)** Axial contrast CT showing hypodense poorly enhancing granulation tissue in the right greater wing of sphenoid bone.

posterior element involvement. Spinal meningitis, arachnoiditis, or myelitis may ensue. Epidural abscess may occur.

55.3.10 Clinical Profile, Imaging, and Diagnosis

The most common signs include fever, headache, vomiting, and an altered sensorium. Neck rigidity and cranial nerve palsies are commonly seen.[1,6] Variable degrees of encephalitis, hydrocephalus, and infarction are responsible for altered sensorium in tubercular meningitis.

Focal deficits may occur in the forms of mild to total weakness of the limbs or varying degrees of cranial nerve palsy. The cranial nerves are involved via arachnoiditis, and motor weakness is usually secondary to infarctions of the subcortical white matter. Among the cranial nerves, the abducens and oculomotor nerves are frequently involved. Motor deficits are measured by the Barthel index, which are categorized by activities of daily living. Patients with tuberculomas usually present with headache, seizures, focal neurological deficit, and features of raised intracranial tension. Infratentorial tuberculomas may present with brainstem syndromes, cerebellar symptoms, and multiple cranial nerve palsies.[10] Hydrocephalus has been described as a marker of visual impairment. Tuberculous abscesses have an acute clinical presentation and a rapid deteriorating course than tuberculomas, with symptoms of fever, headache, and focal neurological signs. The clinical symptoms of spinal TB in children are often insidious and include back pain, fever, paraparesis, sensory disturbance, and bowel and bladder dysfunction. About 3% of children with spinal TB develop severe kyphosis greater than 60 degrees. The risk factors for the development of severe kyphotic deformity are the following: being younger than 10 years of age, involvement of three or more vertebral bodies, and thoracic spine localization. Severe kyphosis results in spinal cord compression over the apex of the deformity and cardiopulmonary dysfunction from restrictive lung disease and is cosmetically unacceptable.

On clinical suspicion of tubercular meningitis, CSF examination is the initial modality of investigation.[3] The diagnosis of tubercular meningitis is based on definite and probable criteria. Definitive diagnosis of tuberculous meningitis depends on the detection of the tubercle bacilli in the CSF, either by smear examination or by bacterial culture.[5,6,7] The predominance of CSF lymphocytosis is highly suggestive of tubercular meningitis, which is reported to be greater than 50% in 80 to 83% of patients. Low levels of CSF glucose and elevated levels of protein are also seen. The polymerase chain reaction (PCR) constitutes a rapid method of detecting the M. tuberculosis genome in CSF, and allows for a rapid and specific diagnosis of tuberculous meningitis.[6] The identification of bacilli is difficult since cultures take a long time for processing and the bacilli may disappear rapidly from CSF after treatment has been instituted.[6] Acid-fast bacilli in the context of centrifuged CSF may be evident in 20 to 90% of cases. However, the small sample volume, low bacillary load, and presence of PCR inhibitors in samples may account for low sensitivity. The yield of positive mycobacterial cultures from CSF in tubercular meningitis varies from 19 to 70%.[5,6,7,8] The diagnostic utility of skin testing being positive for CNS tuberculosis varies from 10 to 20% to 50%.

Molecularly based techniques include commercially available nucleic acid amplification (NAA) methods and other PCR-based methods, antibody detection, antigen detection, or chemical assays such as adenosine deaminase (ADA) and tuberculostearic acid measurements.[29] Commercial nucleic acid amplification (NAA) assays for the diagnosis of TBM are 56% sensitive and 98% specific and the diagnostic yield of NAA increases when large volumes of CSF are processed. The sensitivity of CSF microscopy and culture falls rapidly after the start of treatment, whereas mycobacterial DNA may remain detectable within the CSF until 1 month after the start of treatment. The measured sensitivities and specificities of ADA in the CSF range from 44 to 100% and 71 to 100%, respectively. Standardized cutoffs of ADA values for the diagnosis of TBM have not been established, and the values used in various studies ranged from greater than 5 to greater than 15 IU/L. It is helpful in predicting poor neurological outcomes among pediatric TBM cases.[30,31] A raised ADA activity in the CSF of patients with CNS TB lacks specificity. CSF ADA activity is not recommended as a routine diagnostic test for CNS tuberculosis. Tuberculostearic acid has good sensitivity, but requirement of expensive equipment has limited its clinical use.[31]

The imaging findings are summarized in ▶ Table 55.1.

Contrast-enhanced computed tomography (CT) is the investigation of choice since it is easily available and can be quickly performed to establish diagnosis. CT scan can depict the presence of

Table 55.1 Imaging features

MR imaging	Tuberculous meningitis	Tuberculoma	Cysticercosis	Fungal granuloma	Hydatid cyst
T1 WI	Hyperintense	Hypointense	Hypointense with hyperintense dot within cyst	Variable, low to intermediate to isointense	Hypointense
T2 WI	Nonspecific	Hypointense	Hyperintense	Hypointense	Hypointense
Contrast	Basal enhancement	Homogenous/ring enhancement with central hypointensity	Present	Peripherally enhancing	Nil
Magnetic transfer	Hyperintense	-	-	-	-
Diffusion WI	Restriction (infarction)	-	-	-	-

Abbreviations: MR, magnetic resonance; WI, weighted.

hydrocephalus, infarcts, and basal exudates.[32] The presence of periventricular lucency in isolation can suggest ischemia but along with a rounded third ventricle is suggestive of interstitial edema and raised ICP syndrome. In some series, normal results are reported in up to 5% of cases. Hydrocephalus is a frequent accompaniment of tuberculous meningitis with an incidence varying between 50 and 80%. CT cannot predict the level of CSF block in TBM because both types of hydrocephalus can present with panventricular dilation.[32] The presence of basal enhancement, hydrocephalus, tuberculoma, and infarction were more common in TBM than in children with pyogenic meningitis. They reported that basal enhancement, tuberculomas, or both were 100% specific and 89% sensitive for the diagnosis of TBM. Andronikou and colleagues suggested nine criteria for the diagnosis of TBM on CT. Przybojewski and colleagues evaluated these nine criteria and showed high specificity for all the criteria, and 100% specificity for four individual criteria.[32] It has been shown that sensitivity has been improved when more than one criterion was present. Presence of hyperdensity on precontrast scans in the basal cisterns might be the specific sign of TBM in children. The reported incidence of infarcts on CT varies from 20.5 to 38%.

Magnetic resonance imaging (MRI) has been shown to be superior to CT in evaluating patients with suspected meningitis and its associated complications.[33,34,35] Noncontrast MRI shows little or no evidence of meningitis in early stages of the disease. Contrast-enhanced MRI shows abnormal meningeal enhancement in the basal cisterns, and sylvian fissures (▶ Fig. 55.2). The cerebral convexities show enhancement in severe and late-stage

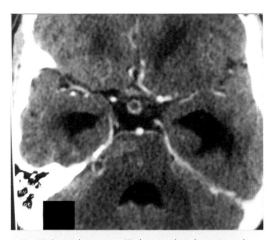

Fig. 55.2 Axial contrast CT showing basal meningeal inflammation with dilated ventricles and periventricular ooze suggestive of meningitis with hydrocephalus.

TBM. Tentorial and cerebellar meningeal involvement is less common. There could be minimal or absent meningeal enhancement in immunocompromised patients although some reports show no significant difference. The newer sequences of MR imaging along with qualitative and quantitative information of CSF flow and dynamics is helpful to differentiate between types of hydrocephalus and postoperative evaluation in patients with third ventriculostomy. However, the flow around fourth ventricle may not be easily appreciated. MR ventriculography has been used to evaluate CSF flow dynamics and in patients with hydrocephalus. MRI depicts hemorrhagic transformation of infarcts better. Multiple infarcts in the anterior circulation territory favored tuberculous etiology.

MR angiogram reveals small segmental narrowing, uniform narrowing of large segments, irregular beaded appearance of vessels, or complete occlusion with contrast-enhanced MRI being more sensitive to detect smaller vessels. The infarcts mostly involve thalamus, basal ganglia, and internal capsule regions. Diffusion-weighted MR imaging helps in early detection of infarction and in delineating the extent of infarction.

Magnetic transfer (MT) MRI is considered superior to conventional MRI for showing abnormal meninges.[36] It also helps in differentiating tuberculous meningitis from other causes of meningitis. The abnormal meninges appearing hyperintense on precontrast T1-weighted (T1W) MT images is considered to strongly suggest tuberculous meningitis. Also, the MT ratio (MTR) is significantly different from brain parenchyma and inflamed meninges, because the inflammatory exudate in TBM is composed of cellular infiltrate, degenerated

and partially caseated fibrin, tubercles, and, less commonly, bacilli.

Radiograph/CT pneumoencephalography or contrast-enhanced cisternography done via lumbar puncture may help in differentiating communicating and noncommunicating hydrocephalus, if MRI is not available.[32,33,34,35,36]

Imaging findings of tuberculoma depends on whether it is noncaseating or caseating with solid or liquid center. A solid noncaseating tuberculoma is isodense or slightly hypodense to the surrounding brain parenchyma on CT and hypointense on both T1W and T2W images on MRI. It shows homogeneous enhancement on contrast administration (▶ Fig. 55.3 and ▶ Fig. 55.4). The cellular components of the noncaseating tuberculomas appear brighter on MT T1W imaging differentiating it from metastases, lymphomas, and other infective granulomas.[32,33,34,35,36] The target sign, a central calcification or nidus surrounded by ring

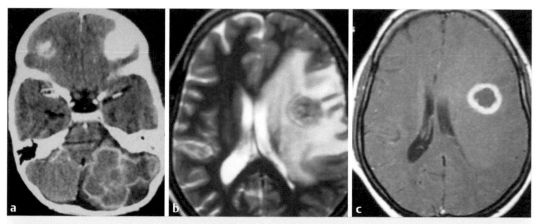

Fig. 55.3 (a) Axial contrast CT showing ring-enhancing conglomerate lesions in the left cerebellum. (b) Axial T2 image showing hypointense solid lesion with perifocal edema in the left frontoparietal brain. (c) Axial contrast image showing hypointense thick irregularly ring-enhancing lesion in the left frontoparietal brain.

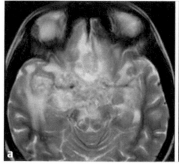
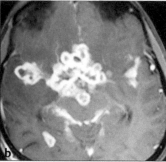

Fig. 55.4 (a) Axial T2 image showing hypointense solid conglomerate lesions in the suprasellar and bilateral sylvian fissures. There is severe perifocal edema. (b) Axial contrast image showing the peripheral enhancing solid lesions depicting crenated margins.

enhancement on postcontrast images, is considered pathognomonic of tuberculoma. Solid caseating granulomas with T2 hypointense center can be confused with lymphoma and fungal and cysticercus granulomas. These lesions appear hypointense on T1 W MT images surrounded with a hyperintense rim. En plaque tuberculomas are hyperdense on noncontrast CT scans, isointense to brain on T1 W MRI, and isointense to hypointense on T2 W images with homogeneous postcontrast enhancement. Tuberculomas can mimic neurocysticercosis, fungal granulomas, and tumors like lymphomas, glioma, and metastases. Newer imaging techniques, like diffusion imaging, MR spectroscopy (MRS), and MT imaging may help in differentiating these conditions.[33,34,35,36]

MRS is specific for the diagnosis of tuberculoma, which show large cellular component appearing bright on MT imaging and with a choline peak on spectroscopy. Dynamic contrast enhancement (DCE) MRI has been used by to correlate the relative cerebral blood volume values with the cellular and necrotic components of tuberculomas and also with the expression of various immunohistochemical markers. Serial diffusion tensor imaging (DTI) has been used to evaluate brain tuberculomas and may be of value in assessing the therapeutic response of tuberculomas that are treated only with specific antituberculous drugs. Fluorodeoxyglucose positron emission tomography can be helpful in differentiating an atypical tuberculoma from other neoplastic and nonneoplastic CNS lesions. It can also be used in the follow-up of tuberculomas.

Imaging findings of tuberculous brain abscess are usually nonspecific. They present as large, frequently multiloculated, ring-enhancing lesions with perilesional edema and mass effect (▶ Fig. 55.5). Diffusion-weighted imaging shows restricted diffusion with low apparent diffusion coefficient (ADC) values because of the presence of inflammatory cells in the pus. MRS helps in differentiating tuberculous abscess from those of pyogenic and fungal causes.[33,34,35] MRS shows lipid, lactate, and phosphoserine without evidence of cytosolic amino acids, in contrast with pyogenic abscess. MT imaging can differentiate tuberculous from pyogenic abscesses. The rim of tuberculous abscesses shows lower MTR values compared with pyogenic abscesses.[36]

55.3.11 Spinal Tuberculosis

MRI is currently the imaging modality of choice, given its superior ability in the detection of soft

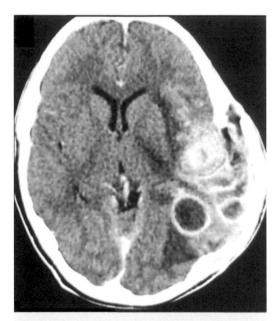

Fig. 55.5 Axial contrast CT image showing conglomerate of multiple ring-enhancing lesions in the left posterior temporal brain.

tissue and bone marrow changes even in patients with normal radiographs.[34,35] MRI of the entire spine should be performed to exclude multilevel involvement and skip lesions. Bone marrow edema is an early sign of infection that is seen as areas of hypointensity on T1 W images, and hyperintense areas on T2 W, short tau inversion recovery (STIR), and proton density fat-suppressed sequences (▶ Fig. 55.6). T1 W images are the most sensitive in detecting marrow edema. A contrast-enhanced T1 W sequence with fat suppression provides valuable additional information and is highly recommended. Vertebral end plate erosion is seen as loss of the normal T1-hypointense line on sagittal MR images. Diskal enhancement patterns include homogeneous disk enhancement, patchy nonconfluent areas of disk enhancement, and varying areas of peripheral disk enhancement, most often being T1 hypointense, T2-heterogeneously hyperintense, and epidural masses, which are slightly T1 hypointense and T2 hyperintense. Compression or displacement of the spinal cord should be looked for in the presence of epidural masses, which may show craniocaudal migration. Spinal cord involvement in the form of infarction and syringomyelia may occur as a complication of arachnoiditis. Tuberculous pus formation may occur between the dura and the leptomeninges and may appear

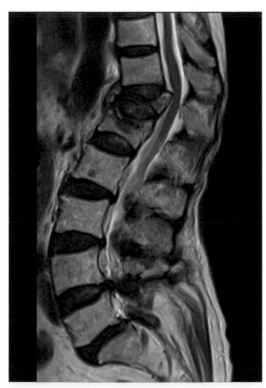

Fig. 55.6 Axial T2 image of the dorsolumbar spine showing destruction and collapse of D12–L1 vertebra resulting in kyphosis and spinal cord compression.

loculated. It appears hyperintense on T2 W and isointense to hypointense on T1 W images. The dural granulomas appear hypointense to isointense on T2 W and isointense on T1 W images. Rim enhancement can be seen on postcontrast images. Epidural TB lesions generally appear to be isointense to the spinal cord on T1 W images and have mixed intensity on T2 W images. In postcontrast images, uniform enhancement can be seen if the TB inflammatory process is phlegmonous, whereas peripheral enhancement is seen if true epidural abscess formation or caseation has developed. Epidural tuberculous abscess may occur as primary lesions or may be seen in association with arachnoiditis, myelitis, spondylitis, and intramedullary, and dural tuberculomas.

55.3.12 Treatment

The primary line of treatment for tuberculous meningitis is medical therapy with antituberculous multidrug chemotherapy.[1,4,5,6,7,8,9,31] The primary drugs include rifampicin (10 mg/kg), isoniazid (5 mg/kg), ethambutol (20 mg/kg) or streptomycin (20 mg/kg), and pyrazinamide (25 mg/kg) for 3 months followed with isoniazid and rifampicin daily for the next 6 months and continued with isoniazid and ethambutol for 15 months. The therapy is prolonged and is continued for 2 years.[1,4,5,6,7,8,9] In certain situations like relapse, therapy can be continued for 1 more year. Steroids can be added if the patient has pronounced meningitis and appears sick. All patients with TBM may receive adjunctive corticosteroids regardless of disease severity at presentation.[4,5,6,7,8,9,31] Adults (> 14 years) should be administered dexamethasone 0.4 mg/kg/24 h with a tapering course over 6 to 8 weeks. Children can be given prednisolone 4 mg/kg/24 h (or equivalent dose dexamethasone: 0.6 mg/kg/24 h) for 4 weeks, followed by a tapering course over 4 weeks. It has been shown to significantly improve survival rate. They are withheld if the patient has also manifested with lung tuberculosis. Patients with multidrug-resistant tuberculosis are administered second and third line of antituberculous drugs including kanamycin or ethionamide. The liver and renal functions are closely monitored during the course of therapy. Visual charting is performed to detect abnormality with color vision.

The therapy for children with TB meningitis includes controlled ventilation maintaining normal oxygenation and $paCO_2$ concentrations.[1,3,6] Intravascular volume should be maintained at all times with blood and fluids, maintaining normal hematocrit and electrolyte concentration. Fluid restriction is not recommended. Hypotonic fluids should be avoided to prevent hyponatremia. The head of the bed may be elevated to reduce intracranial venous pressure as long as normal central venous pressures are maintained by adequate volume replacement.

55.3.13 Hyponatremia

The mainstay of treatment for SIADH has been based on fluid restriction unless patients are severely symptomatic, in which case hypertonic saline is used. Diuretics and urea have been used. Demeclocycline has been used in chronic SIADH. The treatment of CSW revolves around fluid and Na replacement because these patients develop hyponatremia in the setting of volume depletion.[37] Fludrocortisone or hypertonic saline has yielded good results. Correction of chronic hyponatremia should be performed very slowly (< 0.5 mM/h) or rapid correction risks the development of central pontine myelinolysis.[1,3]

55.3.14 Hydrocephalus

The hydrocephalus is graded as mild if the third ventricle or temporal horns were dilated (> 2 mm), as moderate if rounding of the frontal horns occurred, and as severe if periventricular lucency was present on imaging. Patients with symptomatic hydrocephalus or radiologically worsening hydrocephalus benefit from CSF diversion procedures. The Palur grading system (Vellore grading system) was based on the presence or absence of neurological deficits and level of sensorium (▶ Table 55.2).[38] The grading system is useful to grade the patients in retrospective studies, but it has some degree of subjectivity in assessing sensorium. Therefore, the modified Vellore grading system is used which includes the Glasgow Coma Scale (▶ Table 55.3). The latter grading system is reproducible across different levels of clinical expertise and across different disciplines of health care workers and is, therefore, a more reliable system. However, both grading systems correlate well with outcome and prognostication.

Medical management with tapering doses of steroids and decongestants including acetazolamide (100 mg/kg) and frusemide (1 mg/kg) can be tried for a few days or a week in patients in grades I and II.[38] Grades II and III patients should be monitored closely during this period to detect any worsening or lack of improvement and a shunt should be promptly offered in case of failure of medical management. In good grade patients, prolonging medical therapy could be harmful and may lead to irreversible brain damage. Grade IV patients should undergo external ventricular drainage and shunt should be inserted if they show neurological improvement.[39,40]

Ventricular tap is sometimes indicated as an emergency measure to assess and reduce the CSF pressure and stabilize the neurological condition. It can also yield ventricular CSF for examination. Serial ventricular tap every 6 to 8 hours can be done till definitive CSF diversion procedure is contemplated. The initial choice of surgical procedure is ventriculoperitoneal shunt. Bhagwati et al have observed that reduction in ICP and size of the ventricles is helpful to improve periventricular perfusion and enhance drug delivery to the tissues in a more effective manner.[41] The complications of shunt surgery include shunt infection and shunt blockade requiring one or multiple revisions. Poor general condition of patient and high CSF protein and cellular content were responsible for frequent shunt blockages. Agarwal et al reported shunt-related complications in 11 (30%) children and three of 37 children had to undergo multiple shunt revisions. Palur et al reported that 26 of 114 (22.8%) patients had to undergo one or more shunt revisions, one patient requiring more than three revisions.[38] Sil and Chatterjee reported a shunt infection rate of 15.6% and revision rate of 43.8% in their series of 37 children who underwent shunt surgery for TBM with hydrocephalus.[42] Multiple revisions were done in 18.7% of patients.

Endoscopic third ventriculostomy is an option for patients who have completed at least 4 weeks of antituberculous therapy.[43] It is technically demanding and should be performed by a surgeon who is skilled in endoscopic procedures.[44,45,46,47,48] It is difficult to recognize anatomical landmarks since the floor of the third ventricle is frequently thick and the subarachnoid space is also likely to

Table 55.2 Palur's grading for TB meningitis–induced hydrocephalus

	Description
I. 1.	Headache, vomiting, fever, and/or neck stiffness
2.	No neurological deficit
3.	Normal sensorium
II 1.	Normal sensorium
2.	Neurological deficit present
III 1.	In altered sensorium but easily arousable
2.	Dense neurological deficit may or may not be present
IV 1.	Deeply comatose
2.	Decerebrate or decorticate posturing

Abbreviation: TB, tuberculosis.

Table 55.3 Modified Vellore Grading Scale for TB meningitis–induced hydrocephalus

Grade	Variables
I	GCS 15 Headache, vomiting, fever ± neck stiffness. No neurological deficit
II	GCS 15 Neurological deficit present
III	GCS 9–14 Neurological deficit may or may not be present
IV	GCS 3–8 Neurological deficit may or may not be present

Abbreviations: TB, tuberculosis; GCS, Glasgow Coma Scale.

be obliterated by exudates in early stages of the disease.[47,48] The basilar artery and its branches are at enhanced risk of injury. The tubercles and granulation tissue on the thick floor of third ventricle bleed when touched and obscure the endoscopic field. Patients with longer duration of symptoms and ATT were more likely to benefit from the ETV.[47]

With the advent of effective antitberculous chemotherapy and steroids, the indication for surgery is rare.[1,6,31] The role of routine adjunctive corticosteroids for all patients with tuberculomas without meningitis is controversial. They may be helpful in those patients whose symptoms are not controlled, or are worsening, on anti-tuberculosis therapy. Intrathecal hyaluronidase has been tried in children with communicating hydrocephalus but does not offer any particular advantage over shunt insertion in terms of regression of specific neurological deficit or overall functional improvement.[49] Surgical excision of tuberculomas or tuberculous abscess is performed only when there is a rapid clinical deterioration following optimal medical therapy.[49,50,51,52] Intraventricular tuberculous abscess threatening to develop acute obstructive hydrocephalus or formation of a subdural empyema may necessitate a craniotomy. Biposy correlation may be warranted to establish diagnosis in cases of coinfection with HIV contributing to differential diagnosis.

55.3.15 Outcome and Prognostication

The factors contribute to this poor outcome include cerebrovascular involvement with resultant cerebral ischemia, abscess formation, hydrocephalus and raised ICP, direct parenchymal injury, hyponatremia, seizures, and delayed diagnosis. The grade at presentation is the best and most consistent predictor of outcome following shunt surgery in patients with TBM. The presence of infarcts in the basal ganglia and internal capsule are also likely to indicate a poor outcome following shunting.[1,3,6,38,41,42]

The outcome of TBM with hydrocephalus is finally dependent on the response of the disease to antituberculous therapy.[38,41,49,50,51,52] It is understandable that in patients with drug-resistant TB either multidrug-resistant TB (MDR-TB) or extensively drug-resistant TB (XDR-TB), the outcome is likely to be poor. There are, however, no studies, which have reported on the outcome following

surgery for drug-resistant TBM. Home-based treatment of childhood neurotuberculosis is feasible in selected patients under close supervision in areas where there is high incidence of tuberculosis coupled with HIV infection resulting in severe bed shortages in secondary and tertiary hospitals.[53]

55.3.16 Pott's Disease

The early TB spondylitis without spinal cord compression or neurological deficits can be treated conservatively with chemotherapy. However, surgery is recommended for patients with spinal cord compression or neurological compromise, significant spinal deformity, persistent severe axial pain, or disease progression on maximal medical therapy.[54] Steroids may be helpful in patients who are deteriorating on antituberculous therapy.

Various surgical approaches have been reported in the treatment of TB spondylitis in the pediatric age group.[55,56] Short- and long-term clinical outcomes were similar when radical surgery was compared with debridement alone, but the correction of kyphosis and deformity was better in children undergoing radical surgery with anterior reconstruction than in patients undergoing debridement alone. In addition, radical surgery seems to decrease the length of drug therapy because clinical and radiographic outcomes were similar for chemotherapeutic regimens prescribed for 6, 9, or 18 months when combined with radical surgery.[54,55,56] In children, the skeletal immaturity of young children should be recognized minimizing the number of fused segments, especially in the thoracic spine, to avoid complications such as iatrogenic short trunk, crankshaft deformity, and pulmonary hypoplasia from restricted growth of the rib cage. Moreover, younger patients exhibit a more progressive form of TB, with increased risk of extrapulmonary disease and progressive vertebral body collapse placing them at a higher risk for disabling complications than adults.

The surgical technique of choice for spinal TB has been a matter of continuous debate.[56] Posterior-only operations in spinal TB traditionally have had unfavorable outcomes because they were usually limited to laminectomy with or without fusion, whereas the unaddressed spinal cord compression was located anteriorly.[55,56] Modern techniques, such as vertebral column resection via a posterior approach, allow circumferential decompression of the spinal cord, correction of acute segmental deformity, and resection of the infectious focus.[56]

55.3.17 Fungal Diseases of Central Nervous System

Intracranial fungal infections are reported but intracranial fungal masses requiring neurosurgical intervention are uncommon.[57,58,59,60] They are rare in children.[61] However, in the recent years it has seen an upsurge due to HIV infections, increased use of immunosuppressants, increased incidence of diabetes mellitus and prolonged survival in organ transplants, and patients undergoing cancer adjuvant therapy.[62,63,64,65,66,67,68,69] There is relative paucity of literature on this subject and hence the management of intracranial fungal masses is not standardized.[62,63,64] The mainstay of fungal infections, however, is still antifungal therapy. It is still unclear whether the role of surgery involves a biopsy, partial or radical excision and its relation to the long-term outcome.

55.3.18 Pathogenesis

Fungi are ubiquitous organisms. They are often nonpathogenic or result in a self-limited illness in otherwise healthy humans. Fungi that grow as yeast include *Candida* and *Cryptococcus*, whereas *Aspergillus* and *mucormycosis* grow with branching hyphae. *Coccidioidomycosis* is an example of a dimorphic fungus. Fungi that grow as yeasts spread hematogenously, entering the meningeal microcirculation owing to their small size, resulting in seeding of the subarachnoid space and meningitis. Although parenchymal disease is less common with yeast organisms, both *Candida* and *Cryptococcus* may manifest as primarily parenchymal abnormalities with the formation of granulomas or abscesses. The hyphal forms of fungal pathogens often cause parenchymal disease, because the larger morphology precludes access to the meningeal microcirculation. The larger cerebral vessels may also become involved, resulting in vasculitis with thrombosis and mycotic aneurysm formation.

The commonest fungus that produces intracranial fungal masses (IFM) is the *Aspergillus* species.[57,58,59,60] *Aspergillus flavus* is generally implicated as the causative organism in patients who are immunocompetent, whereas *Aspergillus fumigatus* is more frequently reported in immunocompromised individuals. The other fungi causing IFMs include *Cryptococcus*, mucormycosis, *Candida*, *Cladosporium*, and dematiaceous fungi. Inhaled fungal spores, which travel to the lung parenchyma, are most often removed by an immunocompetent immune system. They can also occur related to indwelling catheters, fungal disease in other organs, or trauma, with the infection subsequently being eliminated by a combination of the host's reticuloendothelial, cellular, and humoral defense system. Direct penetration of the blood–brain barrier through hematogenous route, in immunocompromised or rarely immunocompetent patient may result in meningitis or cerebritis. It may also result following setting of neurosurgical procedures or secondary to adjacent sinus disease. Fungal aneurysms are caused usually by *Aspergillus* or mucormycosis.[62,63,64] The angioinvasive nature of these organisms leads to the digestion of the elastic lamina of the vessels by the production of the enzyme elastase.

The commonest focus of infection for intracranial fungal masses is the paranasal sinuses (PNSs) and the mastoid sinuses, rarely lungs and heart especially in the presence of artificial heart valves.[62,63,64,65,66,67,68,69] In some patients with IFM, however, no obvious systemic source for the fungal infection is discernible.[62] Rarely, fungal infection may follow direct inoculation of the brain during intracranial or transsphenoidal surgery or following trauma. Sharma et al reported two patients who developed IFMs following intracranial surgery.[70] IFM include, HIV infection organ transplantation, cancer chemotherapy, prolonged steroid therapy, autoimmune disorders such as systemic lupus erythematosus and tuberculosis.

Fungal infections can lead to meningitis, meningoencephalitis, vasculitis, abscess formation, and granuloma formation.[57,58,59,60,61,62] Most reported studies have identified *Cryptococcus*, *Aspergillus*, and *Candida* species as the most common organisms in fungal infections of the CNS.[62,63,64,65,66,67,68,69] However, granuloma formation has been reported to be most common with *Aspergillus*.

55.3.19 Prevalence and Clinical Profile

Intracranial fungal masses can be seen in any age group, but most patients are in the third, fourth, and fifth decades of life.[57,58,59,60,61,62] They have been reported even in neonates, infants, and young children. Intracranial fungal masses in immunocompetent patients have been predominantly reported from Indian subcontinent, Middle east, Africa, and California in the United States. The hot, dry climate coupled with a high content of *Aspergillus* spores in the atmosphere may be a probable cause. Nearly 50% of patients with IFMs have no overt predisposing illness or evidence of immunosuppression. There might be a subclinical impairment of cell-mediated immunity. There has been an increase in the number of invasive fungal infections in recent times. The incidence was 5.1% in 1992, 6.6% in 1996, and 10.4% in 2005. The cumulative prevalence of IFMs in transplant recipients varied between 0.5 and 1%.[57,58,63,64,65,66,67,68,69] It has been observed that IFMs would constitute about 1 per 1,000 neurosurgical procedures performed at major neurosurgical centers accounting for their rarity.

The clinical presentation can be indolent and vary from a few days to several months or even years.[64] The clinical presentation is not specific but can be divided into the following five distinct types depending on the nature of the disease:[64]

- Involvement of the cranial nerves I to VI with orbital and nasal symptoms. These symptoms/signs are common in patients with fungal infections that originate in the PNS and spread to the intracranial compartment by the contiguous route.
- Focal neurological deficits due to involvement of any part of the neuraxis.
- "Stroke-like" presentation with sudden onset of hemiparesis reported in 6 to 10% of patients. Fungal aneurysms can present with subarachnoid hemorrhage.
- Raised ICP, seizures, and altered sensorium. The altered sensorium can result from raised ICP, ischemia due to the vasculitis associated with the concomitant fungal meningitis and fungal meningoencephalitis.
- Fever is an infrequent symptom, seen in only 10 to 31% of patients.

55.3.20 Imaging and Diagnosis

CT scans can show paranasal sinusitis, small areas of bony destruction, and absence of separation of periosteum from the medial orbital wall. Jinkins et al described five cases with varying radiological findings, including large tumor-like enhancing granulomatous masses within the brain tissue, nodular meningeal granuloma, paranasal sinusitis, orbital masses with brain destruction, infections with vasculitis, and aneurysm formation. The differential diagnosis of a similar mass in isolation included an abscess, tuberculoma, meningioma, and glioma (depending on location).

The characteristic MRI appearances for various fungal granulomas have been described and have shown some variability among organisms. For example, cryptococcoma appears to have low T2-weighted signal intensity, contrasting with the surrounding hyperintense cerebral edema (▶ Fig. 55.7). Aspergillomas, however, have intermediate signal intensity for the granuloma, surrounded by perilesional edema on T2-weighted images (▶ Fig. 55.8). Gupta et al who reported an intracranial aspergilloma that simulated a meningioma by demonstrating isointense T1 signal to the brain parenchyma and isointense T2 signal to the white matter.[71]

Parenchymal involvement of CNS fungal disease may result in granuloma formation, cerebritis, and/or abscess formation. Imaging findings of cerebritis are nonspecific but typically include increased T2/fluid-attenuated inversion recovery (FLAIR) signal abnormality associated with a variable amount of enhancement. The common locations involved are the frontal lobes, anterior cranial fossa without frontal lobe involvement, and followed by middle cranial fossa, sellar and temporal regions.

Fungal abscesses often multiple and near the gray–white matter junction related to the hematologic distribution of fungal organisms. Fungal

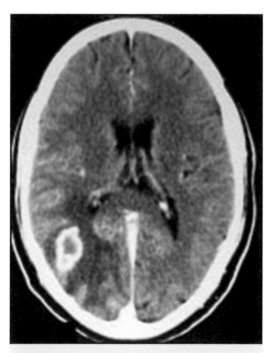

Fig. 55.7 Axial contrast CT image showing the hypodense center with peripherally enhancing lesion in the right parietal brain. There is perifocal edema.

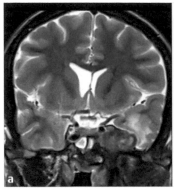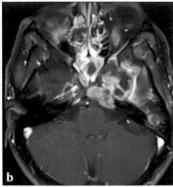

Fig. 55.8 (a) Coronal T2-weighted MR image showing the hypointense left cavernous sinus lesion characteristic of *Aspergillus*. (b) Axial T1-weighted contrast MR image showing the heterogenous enhancement.

abscesses may also involve the deep gray matter nuclei involvement of the deep gray matter nuclei. Bacterial abscesses are more often single and spare the basal ganglia. The imaging appearance of an intracranial fungal abscess is similar to a pyogenic abscess typically demonstrating a ring-enhancing lesion with a hypointense T2 rim, which may show restricted diffusion. Immunocompromised patients may have a variable imaging appearance, as shown by Enzmann and colleagues, who studied 15 immunocompromised patients with CNS infections and concluded that six of eight patients afflicted with *Aspergillus* had minimal to no enhancement on imaging with intravenous contrast.[72] MRS demonstrated identification of multiple signals between 3.6 and 3.6 ppm and may confer further specificity to the diagnosis.

Fungal infections that affect immunocompetent hosts include *Cryptococcus neoformans*, *Coccidioides immitis*, *Histoplasma capsulatum*, and *Blastomyces dermatitidis*, whereas *Aspergillus* and *Candida* are most often seen in immunocompromised hosts.

Aspergillus is among the most commonly isolated organism from fungal brain abscesses. *Aspergillus* abscesses may be surrounded by low signal intensity on T2-weighted and gradient-echo images. The hypointense T2 signal rim has been attributed to small amount of hemorrhage with hemosiderin-laden macrophages and a dense population of hyphae at the abscess rim. Peripherally restricted diffusion may be present. Another striking feature of *Aspergillus* is the tendency for the organism to invade blood vessels. In the retrospective analysis by Nadkarni and Goel,[63] 3 of 10 patients were found to have autopsy-proven evidence of intracranial vascular invasion with secondary thrombosis. Vascular invasion is facilitated by the release of the enzyme elastase, which facilitates intramural vascular invasion. Secondary complications of vascular invasion include vasculitis, infarction, rarely mycotic aneurysms, and intracranial hemorrhage. Imaging findings of hemorrhage are common in association with *Aspergillus* infection.

55.3.21 Treatment

Surgical treatment is required in the following situations: (1) stereotactic biopsy as a means to establish diagnosis and identification of organism; (2) surgical excision, to remove or reduce the mass effect; and (3) external ventricular drain to treat sequelae such as hydrocephalus and conversion to ventricular shunt placement, if necessary. In addition, intracavitary administration of amphotericin B has been advised.[65,66,67,68,69] Stereotactic drainage of aspergillosis brain abscesses with long-term survival has been reported by Goodman et al.[73]

Stereotactic procedures might yield a good outcome in selected patients, but whenever feasible, safe radical excision of the IFM along with normal nervous tissue around it should be done. Medical therapy with antifungal agents is required for prolonged periods following surgery in patients with IFM.[57,58,59,60,61,62,63,64,65,66,67,68,69] Surgical extirpation of the paranasal sinus disease by functional endoscopic sinus surgery (FESS) should be performed whenever it is associated with intracranial fungal masses.[64,74,75,76,77,78,79,80,81,82,83,84] Fungal aneurysms should be treated with clipping or endovascular treatment after sufficient duration of antifungal therapy.[85] However, the ultimate outcome may not be always gratifying.[86]

The treatment of cryptococcal meningitis is essentially chemotherapy.[87] A 4-week regimen is advocated for patients who have no underlying disease or immunosuppressive therapy and early recognition of meningitis without concomitant neurological sequelae. After 4 weeks of therapy, the CSF India Ink preparation should be negative and CSF cryptococcal antigen titers b1: 8 at 4 weeks. Patients who do not meet the above criteria should receive at least 6 weeks of therapy and long-term maintenance treatment should be considered for patients with the AIDS.

55.3.22 Outcome

In spite of advances in the management of fungal CNS infections, there is a uniformly high mortality and morbidity reported in almost all series of patients with IFMs. The mortality rates range from around 40% in immunocompetent patients to 92% in transplant recipients. The newer drugs and more aggressive surgical procedures have not significantly improved the mortality and morbidity rates of patients with intracranial fungal masses.[70,74,75,76,77] However, earlier diagnosis has reduced the mortality rate. The cause of delay in treatment could be multifold. In India, most patients are treated with antituberculous therapy on empirical basis. Amphotericin B is notorious for causing renal and liver failure and has other serious side effects. Other contributing factors were presence of extensive paranasal sinus involvement, postoperative meningoencephalitis, and ventriculitis. Sometimes, the diagnosis is revealed only at postmortem.[67] Rhinocerebral mucormycosis has a high mortality associated with it. In immunocompetent patients, the survival is 75% but it decreases to 60% in patients with diabetes mellitus and to only 20% in those with other systemic disorders.[69] The outcome is better in immunocompetent patients than those who are immunocompromised. The rhinocerebral form of the disease has a better survival than those with the primary intracranial form. The main cause of mortality and morbidity is vasculitis and stroke. It can occur even distant to the site of lesion.

55.3.23 Conclusions

A high index of suspicion should be present in cases of immunocompromised patients with intracranial mass lesions. Diabetic patients with intracranial and rhinocerebral mass lesions should be treated and evaluated early for fungal etiology. Early diagnosis, aggressive surgical procedures, and antibiotic therapy for CNS fungal infections may reduce morbidity and mortality. The presence of intracranial fungal granulomas in immunocompromised patients is associated with significant morbidity and mortality. Control of the underlying condition determines the outcome.

55.3.24 Neurocysticercosis

Cysticercosis is caused by the larval form (cysticercus) of the cestode *Taenia solium* or the pork tapeworm.[88] Man is an accidental intermediate host who becomes infected by consuming eggs in the gravid proglottids of the adult tapeworm shed in the stools of a carrier of the worm. The larvae of *T. solium* lodge selectively in certain organs of the body such as the subcutaneous tissues, eyes, muscles, and the brain.

Neurocysticercosis (NCC) is the commonest parasitic infestation of the brain and it is estimated that nearly 50 million people worldwide suffer from this disease.[89] Approximately, 50,000 individuals with NCC die each year due to the disease.[90] Seizures or epilepsy is the commonest manifestation of NCC affecting nearly 80% of patients.[91]

55.3.25 Clinicopathogenesis of NCC

Cysticercus cysts reach the parenchyma of the brain through the hematogenous route. Once they are lodged in the brain, the larvae undergo degeneration and pass through four stages namely (i) vesicular, (ii) colloidal, (iii) granular–nodular, and (iv) calcific stages.[91] Degeneration of the larvae in large numbers can lead to severe edema and raised ICP causing headache, vomiting, altered sensorium known as "cysticercotic encephalitis," which is seen in some children and adolescents. It carries high risk of morbidity and can even be fatal.

Solitary cysticercus granuloma (SCG) is the commonest cause of focal seizures in Indian patients.[91] The seizures are usually complex partial seizures of short duration, rarely status epilepticus (1.7%).[92] It can be associated with hippocampal sclerosis responsible for mesial temporal lobe epilepsy. It can cause obstructive hydrocephalus by blocking the circulation of CSF. Papilledema has been reported in 2.3 to 6.6% of children, less common than in adults.[92] The cysts, which reside dormant in the subarachnoid spaces at the base of the brain or the sylvian fissures, are termed as "racemose cysticercus cyst." They can cause infarcts of the brainstem and the basal ganglia. Focal deficits were seen in 4% of children,[92] as compared to 16% of adults.[93]

Extraparenchymal cysts are rare in children.[94] They may be found in the ventricular and subarachnoid spaces presenting as chronic meningitis, basilar arachnoiditis, or obstructive hydrocephalus. Ophthalmic cysticercosis may lodge in subretinal space, vitreous humor, anterior chamber, or conjunctiva. They may cause sudden blindness, ocular palsy, or visual diminution.

NCC rarely affects the spinal cord. Intramedullary cysticercus granulomas are occasionally known to cause paraparesis.[95]

55.3.26 Diagnosis of NCC

CT scan and MRI of the brain and spinal cord reveal the primary diagnosis. On CT scan, lesions are single and less than 20 mm in size—termed as single small enhancing computed tomographic lesion (SSECTL).[96] Some children may have multiple lesions; disseminated NCC with numerous cysts may give the so-called "starry-sky" appearance, which is typical of NCC (▶ Fig. 55.9). Vesicular cysts are nonenhancing with no perifocal edema while colloidal cyst have ring enhancement with scolex appearing as bright high-density eccentric nodule. Calcified cysts are small and generally without any edema. In extraparenchymal NCC, CT may show hydrocephalus, enhancement of tentorium and

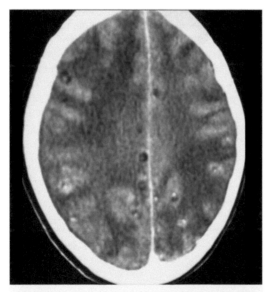

Fig. 55.9 Axial CT image showing multiple disk lesions with central scolex in bilateral cerebral hemispheres suggestive of disseminated cysticercosis.

basal cisterns due to arachnoiditis, and occasionally infarcts.[97] On MRI, visualization of the cysts is better, isointense to white matter and bright on T2-weighted images, scolex being seen well with proton-density sequences. Calcified lesions appear hypointense on all MRI sequences and may at times be missed. 3DCISS is more sensitive in diagnosis of intraventricular cysts. High ADC is seen in core of cysticercus cyst than tubercular abscess.[97]

Serological tests include enzyme-linked immunosorbent assay (ELISA), which is 50% sensitivity and 65% specificity in the CSF. Most of the laboratory tests are usually noncontributory.[94]

The differential diagnosis includes tuberculoma, microabscess, low-grade neoplasm, metastasis, toxoplasmosis, and fungal infection.

55.3.27 Surgery for NCC

The primary treatment of NCC is medical therapy and primarily consists of symptomatic treatment including analgesics, anticonvulsants, and steroids.[90,94] Cysticidal drugs (praziquantel and albendazole) are known to destroy live larval cysts whether in the parenchyma, ventricles, or the subarachnoid spaces and possibly hasten the resolution of granulomas. Albendazole is preferred over praziquantel for its lower cost and side effects. A dose of 15 mg/kg body weight in two divided doses for 15 days is the most commonly used regime. The bioavailability of albendazole increases with coadministration of steroids and is not affected by phenytoin and carbamazepine, which is affected with praziquantel.[94] Patients with cysticercotic encephalitis may have a fatal outcome if treated with cysticidal drugs due to the increase in edema around the degenerating cysts.[90]

The primary indication for surgery in NCC is as follows:

- Extraparenchymal NCC: Intraventricular cysts, hydrocephalus due to racemose cysts, hydrocephalus due to ependymitis caused by NCC.
- Spinal cysticercosis: Intramedullary, extramedullary.

In addition to above, surgery may be required for a large parenchymal colloidal or subarachnoid cyst causing mass effect, confirm diagnosis in atypical cysticercus granuloma, and surgery for intractable epilepsy.[90,94,98]

55.3.28 Surgery for Intraventricular Cysts

Patients with intraventricular cysts usually present with persistent or intermittent features of raised ICP. A CT or MRI shows the cyst, which has similar density to CSF and occasionally a scolex is seen as a hyperintense dot within the cyst (▶ Fig. 55.10). 3DCISS or FLAIR MR sequences may confirm the diagnosis. The commonest location of the cyst is in the fourth ventricle followed by the lateral and third ventricles. An inflamed cyst will enhance on contrast administration and be densely adherent to the surrounding ependyma and choroid plexus.

Medical therapy for intraventricular cyst may take several days or weeks to act and clinical deterioration might occur during that period. Sudden death with intra–third ventricular cysts has been reported.[99,100,101] The minimally invasive endoscopic excision of the cyst is the procedure of choice since it avoids a large craniotomy and reduces the manipulation of the brain. However, the surgeon should have adequate experience in endoscopic surgery, which will help minimize complications and inadequate excision. A rigid scope is sufficient for use in the lateral and third ventricular cysts, but a flexible scope is better for posterior third ventricle and aqueductal cysts. The excision of lateral and third ventricular cysts can be combined with other procedures such as septostomy to create a communication between both the lateral ventricles and a third ventriculostomy to relieve hydrocephalus due to an obstruction in the region of the aqueduct.[102] Endoscopic surgery for fourth ventricle cyst is more demanding, which can be approached through the precoronal burr hole using rigid scope. The cyst can be excised through the aqueduct. It is paramount that the entire scope assembly with the cyst should be delivered through the burr hole. A flexible endoscope is needed for cysts presenting at the foramen of Magendie. Dense adhesions in this region might preclude safe excision of the cyst and the procedure may need to be abandoned. In such a situation, a shunt would be needed to treat the hydrocephalus and medical therapy with albendazole and praziquantel is required.[103] Inadvertent rupture of intraventricular cyst during excision has rarely lead to an untoward incident. It does not cause dissemination of the disease or anaphylactic reaction. Madrazo et al devised a pipette to perform an atraumatic removal of the cysts.[104] In patients who have multiple cysts, oral albendazole (15 mg/kg body weight in two daily divided doses) for 2 weeks is administered. A course of steroids (prednisolone or dexamethasone) can be given for the first 5 to 7 days of albendazole therapy. The hydrocephalus usually resolves in about 70% of patients. A shunt is necessary in cases where there is ependymitis following degeneration of cysts within the ventricles or subarachnoid spaces. Repeated shunt revisions may be required since the CSF may have high protein or cell content and even due to obstruction of the shunt by small cysts or inflammatory exudates. Shunts have also been known to be the cause of migration of fourth ventricular cysts into the third or lateral ventricles due to a siphon effect.[90,94,102,103] A standard shunt system is suitable for use in patients with hydrocephalus due to NCC. Long-term steroid therapy with daily oral prednisone at a dose of 50 mg three times a week for up to 2 years has been shown to reduce the rate of shunt dysfunction from 60 to 13%.[90,102,103] However, prophylaxis for tuberculosis with isoniazid is recommended as prolonged steroid therapy, can predispose a patient to tuberculous infection.[104]

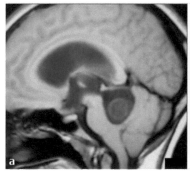
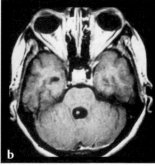

Fig. 55.10 (a) Sagittal T1-weighted MR image showing a cyst in the fourth ventricle, hypointense center with a smooth peripheral margin. **(b)** Axial T1-weighted MR image showing the fourth ventricular cyst with a scolex in the center.

55.3.29 Surgery for Parenchymal and Racemose Cysts

They present with signs of acute to subacute raised ICP and focal neurological deficits. They are usually in the colloidal stage of evolution. Diffusion-weighted sequences may be needed to distinguish these lesions from epidermoid cysts.

Surgery might be required on an emergent basis to reverse the deficits and reduce the raised ICP.[90, 94,98] Craniotomy and excision of cyst leads to good outcome. Cysts are usually delivered easily. However, if the cyst wall is densely adherent to the neurovascular structures in the vicinity, they can be subtotally excised. The cysts might present in suprasellar cisterns, cerebellopontine cisterns causing pressure effect on the adjacent critical structures.

A typical solitary cysticercus granuloma presenting with seizures does not require surgery. In 7% of patients, the granuloma can enlarge and can have atypical radiology and mimic tuberculoma or an abscess.[90] In such situation, stereotactic excision or biopsy may be needed especially in eloquent areas of brain. If there is a high index of suspicion, then serum should be tested for cysticercus antibodies and if found positive, then either symptomatic therapy or treatment with albendazole will avoid a surgical exploration.

NCC can cause intractable epilepsy due to an epileptogenic scar around a cortical cysticercus lesion such as a granuloma or mesial temporal sclerosis (MTS) associated with NCC.[94,105] It can cause MTS by various mechanisms such as kindling, seizures, and due to inflammation spreading from an adjacent degenerating cysticercus cyst. These patients should undergo presurgical evaluation for epilepsy surgery and dealt with accordingly.

55.3.30 Spinal Cysticercosis

Intramedullary and extramedullary cysticercal cysts in the spinal cord are rare (▶ Fig. 55.11). They need to be excised in case of spinal cord compression or if the diagnosis is uncertain. If there is no spinal cord compression and there is evidence of cysticercal infection from a positive enzyme-linked immunotransfer blot (EITB) for cysticercal antibodies in the serum, medical therapy can be

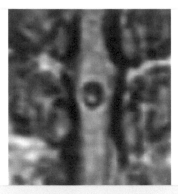

Fig. 55.11 Coronal T1 contrast MR image showing the thoracic intramedullary large hypointense cyst with a scolex in the center.

administered using steroid therapy alone for a maximum of 2 weeks or albendazole with steroid therapy for 2 weeks.[90,94,95]

55.3.31 Complications and Prevention

The major complications for endoscopic surgery include intraventricular hemorrhage, forniceal damage, CSF leak, seizures, and meningitis.[99,102, 103,104] These complications occur in fewer than 5% of patients. Patients with intraventricular cysts, large parenchymal cysts, large racemose cysts causing mass effect, and for biopsy or excision of atypical SCG have an excellent outcome. About 75% of patients with NCC who underwent surgery had improved at a follow-up of 3 years. Shunt surgery for hydrocephalus caused by cysticercotic meningitis is complicated by frequent shunt revisions for blockages or infection in as many as 68% of patients and carries a mortality of 50% on long-term follow-up.[90,94,98,100] Mortality is high in patients with basal racemose cysticercosis.

The possible strategies to control cysticercosis include health education emphasizing the need for hygienic practices such as hand washing after defecation and before eating, mass chemotherapy for taeniasis and vaccination of pigs.[89,90,94]

55.3.32 Conclusions

NCC is primarily treated with medical therapy. Surgery is required in patients with NCC include large parenchymal cysts, spinal cord cysts, atypical SCG, and surgery for intractable epilepsy. Endoscopic surgery is the procedure of choice for excision of intraventricular cysticercal cysts as it is minimally invasive. Shunt surgery is needed for hydrocephalus associated with cysticercotic meningitis. Hydrocephalus has a poor outcome with the need for multiple shunt revisions and a high morbidity and mortality.

55.3.33 Hydatid Disease

Cerebral involvement by hydatid disease occurs in 1 to 4% of patients infected with the parasite.[106,107] The majority are males, belonging to younger age group. They usually reach considerable size before the patient becomes symptomatic. The common signs and symptoms are usually attributable to raised ICP. In children, they present with increasing head size. This is probably because of the slow growth and expansion of these cysts within the cranial cavity. Posterior fossa cysts obstruct the CSF pathways, causing hydrocephalus. Other symptoms such as hemiparesis, seizures, visual field defects, and gait disturbances may vary with the cyst location.[108,109] Intracranial hydatid cyst may also be classified as primary or secondary.

The primary cysts are formed as a result of direct infestation of the larvae in the brain without demonstrable involvement of other organs. In primary multiple cysts, each cyst has a separate pericyst with brood capsule scolices and these originate from multiple larvae affecting brain after crossing the gastrointestinal tract, liver, lungs, and right side of heart without affecting them. The primary cysts are fertile as they contain scolices and brood capsules, hence rupture of primary cyst can result in recurrence. The secondary multiple cysts results from spontaneous, traumatic, or surgical rupture of the primary intracranial hydatid cyst and they lack brood capsule and scolices. The secondary intracranial hydatid cysts are therefore infertile and the resultant risk of recurrence after their rupture is negligible. Primary multiple cysts are uncommon and isolated case reports of primary multiple hydatid cysts have appeared in the literature.[109]

CT/MRI reveals a well-defined, smooth, thin-walled, spherical homogenous cystic lesions. The intensity of the cystic contents is similar to that of CSF. On unenhanced CT scans, the cyst wall is iso-dense or hyperdense to brain tissue (▶ Fig. 55.12). The cyst wall has low intensity on both T1- and T2-weighted images (▶ Fig. 55.13). Usually, no enhancement of the walls is noted in simple cysts. Based on the presence or absence of pericystic edema and contrast enhancement, hydatid cysts are classified into simple (noncomplicated) cysts with no edema or contrast enhancement,

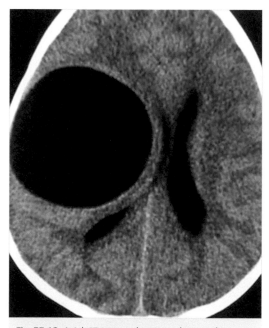

Fig. 55.12 Axial CT image showing a large right frontoparietal cyst with smooth margins.

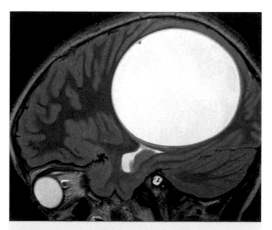

Fig. 55.13 Sagittal T2-weighted MR image showing hyperintense cyst with smooth margins in the posterior parietal brain causing mass effect. There is no perifocal edema.

and infected or complicated cysts with edema and contrast enhancement.[107,108,109] The growing cyst produces a compressed layer of host tissue surrounding it, called the pericyst. The compressed cerebral parenchyma (the pericyst) shows increased vascularity and reactive gliosis.

The differential diagnosis of cerebral cystic hydatidosis includes abscess, cystic tumor, arachnoid cyst, glioependymal cyst, and porencephalic cyst.[106,107,108,109] Brain abscess and cystic tumor usually have significant rim enhancement, surrounding edema, and mural nodules. Other cystic lesions are not spherical in shape and are not surrounded entirely by brain parenchyma.

Multiple cerebral hydatid cysts are rather rare and result from spontaneous, traumatic, or surgical rupture of a solitary primary cyst or as a consequence of a cyst rupture elsewhere and embolization of hydatids to the brain.[109,110] Only three cases of multiple primary hydatid cysts of the brain have been described.[109,110]

Rupture of hydatid cysts can occur in three ways: contained, communicating, and direct.[107,108,109,110,111] Contained rupture occurs when only the endocyst ruptures and the cyst contents are confined within host-derived pericyst.

Complicated hydatid cysts may further be classified according to the status of the germinal membranes. Intact complicated hydatid cysts have well-preserved germinal membranes while ruptured-complicated hydatid cysts have intact pericysts with ruptured, free-floating membranes. Intact complicated cysts need to be excised along with the pericyst, especially when multiple in number, owing to the absence of any plane of dissection. Ruptured-complicated but contained hydatid cysts are analogous to brain abscesses with floating hyaline membranes, acting as foreign bodies within purulent material. Surgery remains the treatment of choice, with intact cyst removal without spillage of fluid being the main prognostic factor.[112,113,114,115,116,117] Care should be exercised to prevent cyst migration while managing intraventricular small cysts. Irrigation with scolicidal agents like 1% cetrimide and 10% formalin is not recommended as prophylaxis.[111,112] Antihelminthics such as albendazole (oral 10 mg/kg for 3 months) should be administered, including during the perioperative period.

55.3.34 Conclusion

Intracranial hydatid cysts can occur as primary solitary cysts, in both the supra- and infratentorial compartments. Both these locations may also have multiple primary hydatid cysts. Cyst wall enhancement is a rare finding, but can be present at times. Gravity can be put to use in removing these cysts, supplementing the Dowling technique. Infected hydatid cysts that have ruptured in contained manner behave just like a brain abscess containing a foreign body and can be tackled in the same fashion.

References

[1] Vadivelu S, Effendi S, Starke JR, Luerssen TG, Jea A. A review of the neurological and neurosurgical implications of tuberculosis in children. Clin Pediatr (Phila). 2013; 52(12): 1135–1143

[2] Be NA, Kim KS, Bishai WR, Jain SK. Pathogenesis of central nervous system tuberculosis. Curr Mol Med. 2009; 9(2): 94–99

[3] Figaji AA, Sandler SI, Fieggen AG, Le Roux PD, Peter JC, Argent AC. Continuous monitoring and intervention for cerebral ischemia in tuberculous meningitis. Pediatr Crit Care Med. 2008; 9(4):e25–e30

[4] Bhagwati SN, Singhal BS. Raised intracranial pressure as a mode of presentation in tuberculous meningitis. Neurol India. 1970; 18(2):116–119

[5] Dastur HM. Diagnosis and neurosurgical treatment of tuberculous disease of the CNS. Neurosurg Rev. 1983; 6(3): 111–117

[6] Waecker NJ. Tuberculous meningitis in children. Curr Treat Options Neurol. 2002; 4(3):249–257

[7] Dastur HM. A tuberculoma review with some personal experiences. I. Brain. Neurol India. 1972; 20(3):111–126

[8] Bhagwati SN, Parulekar GD. Management of intracranial tuberculoma in children. Childs Nerv Syst. 1986; 2(1):32–34

[9] Dastur HM. A tuberculoma review with some personal experiences. II. Spinal cord and its coverings. Neurol India. 1972; 20(3):127–131

[10] Parihar V, Yadav YR, Sharma D. Giant extra-axial posterior fossa tuberculoma in a three-year-old child. Neurol India. 2009; 57(2):218–220

[11] van Toorn R, Schoeman JF, Donald PR. Brainstem tuberculoma presenting as eight-and-a-half syndrome. Eur J Paediatr Neurol. 2006; 10(1):41–44

[12] Jain R, Kumar R. Suprasellar tuberculoma presenting with diabetes insipidus and hypothyroidism—a case report. Neurol India. 2001; 49(3):314–316

[13] Chitre PS, Tullu MS, Sawant HV, Ghildiyal RG. Co-occurrence of intracerebral tuberculoma with lumbar intramedullary tuberculoma. J Child Neurol. 2009; 24(5):606–609

[14] Dastur HM, Shah MD. Intramedullary tuberculoma of the spinal cord. Indian Pediatr. 1968; 5(10):468–471

[15] Kumar R, Kasliwal MK, Srivastava R, Sharma BS. Tuberculoma presenting as an intradural extramedullary lesion. Pediatr Neurosurg. 2007; 43(6):541–543

[16] Andronikou S, Greyling PJ. Devastating yet treatable complication of tuberculous meningitis: the resistant TB abscess. Childs Nerv Syst. 2009; 25(9):1105–1106, discussion 1107, 1109–1110

[17] Abraham R, Kumar S, Scott JX, Agarwal I. Tuberculous brain abscess in a child with tetralogy of Fallot. Neurol India. 2009; 57(2):217–218

[18] Muzumdar D, Balasubramaniam S, Melkundi S. Tuberculous temporal brain abscess mimicking otogenic pyogenic abscess. Pediatr Neurosurg. 2009; 45(3):220–224

[19] Chakraborti S, Mahadevan A, Govindan A, et al. Clinicopathological study of tuberculous brain abscess. Pathol Res Pract. 2009; 205(12):815–822

[20] Kumar R, Pandey CK, Bose N, Sahay S. Tuberculous brain abscess: clinical presentation, pathophysiology and treatment (in children). Childs Nerv Syst. 2002; 18(3–4): 118–123

[21] Diyora B, Kumar R, Modgi R, Sharma A. Calvarial tuberculosis: a report of eleven patients. Neurol India. 2009; 57(5):607–612

[22] Ramdurg SR, Gupta DK, Suri A, Sharma BS, Mahapatra AK. Calvarial tuberculosis: uncommon manifestation of common disease—a series of 21 cases. Br J Neurosurg. 2010; 24(5):572–577

[23] Jadhav RN, Palande DA. Calvarial tuberculosis. Neurosurgery. 1999; 45(6):1345–1349, discussion 1349–1350

[24] Gupta PK, Kolluri VR, Chandramouli BA, Venkataramana NK, Das BS. Calvarial tuberculosis: a report of two cases. Neurosurgery. 1989; 25(5):830–833

[25] Singh G, Kumar S, Singh DP, Verma V, Mohammad A. A rare case of primary tuberculous osteomyelitis of skull vault. Indian J Tuberc. 2014; 61(1):79–83

[26] García-García C, Ibarra V, Azcona-Gutiérrez JM, Oteo JA. Calvarial tuberculosis with parenchymal involvement. Travel Med Infect Dis. 2013; 11(5):329–331

[27] Dawar P, Gupta DK, Sharma BS, Jyakumar A, Gamanagatti S. Extensive calvarial tuberculosis presenting as exophytic ulcerated growth on scalp in an infant: an interesting case report with review of literature. Childs Nerv Syst. 2013; 29 (7):1215–1218

[28] Raut AA, Nagar AM, Muzumdar D, et al. Imaging features of calvarial tuberculosis: a study of 42 cases. AJNR Am J Neuroradiol. 2004; 25(3):409–414

[29] Figaji AA, Fieggen AG. The neurosurgical and acute care management of tuberculous meningitis: evidence and current practice. Tuberculosis (Edinb). 2010; 90(6):393–400

[30] Schoeman J, Wait J, Burger M, et al. Long-term follow up of childhood tuberculous meningitis. Dev Med Child Neurol. 2002; 44(8):522–526

[31] Ramzan A, Nayil K, Asimi R, Wani A, Makhdoomi R, Jain A. Childhood tubercular meningitis: an institutional experience and analysis of predictors of outcome. Pediatr Neurol. 2013; 48(1):30–35

[32] Przybojewski S, Andronikou S, Wilmshurst J. Objective CT criteria to determine the presence of abnormal basal enhancement in children with suspected tuberculous meningitis. Pediatr Radiol. 2006; 36(7):687–696

[33] Pienaar M, Andronikou S, van Toorn R. MRI to demonstrate diagnostic features and complications of TBM not seen with CT. Childs Nerv Syst. 2009; 25(8):941–947

[34] Chatterjee S, Saini J, Kesavadas C, Arvinda HR, Jolappara M, Gupta AK. Differentiation of tubercular infection and metastasis presenting as ring enhancing lesion by diffusion and perfusion magnetic resonance imaging. J Neuroradiol. 2010; 37(3):167–171

[35] Andronikou S, van Toorn R, Boerhout E. MR imaging of the posterior hypophysis in children with tuberculous meningitis. Eur Radiol. 2009; 19(9):2249–2254

[36] Gupta R. Magnetization transfer MR imaging in central nervous system infections. Indian J Radiol Imaging. 2002; 12:51–58

[37] Nagotkar L, Shanbag P, Dasarwar N. Cerebral salt wasting syndrome following neurosurgical intervention in tuberculous meningitis. Indian Pediatr. 2008; 45(7):598–601

[38] Palur R, Rajshekhar V, Chandy MJ, Joseph T, Abraham J. Shunt surgery for hydrocephalus in tuberculous meningitis: a long-term follow-up study. J Neurosurg. 1991; 74(1): 64–69

[39] Lamprecht D, Schoeman J, Donald P, Hartzenberg H. Ventriculoperitoneal shunting in childhood tuberculous meningitis. Br J Neurosurg. 2001; 15(2):119–125

[40] Peng J, Deng X, He F, et al. Role of ventriculoperitoneal shunt surgery in grade IV tubercular meningitis with hydrocephalus. Childs Nerv Syst. 2012; 28(2):209–215

[41] Bhagwati SN. Ventriculoatrial shunt in tuberculous meningitis with hydrocephalus. J Neurosurg. 1971; 35(3): 309–313

[42] Sil K, Chatterjee S. Shunting in tuberculous meningitis: a neurosurgeon's nightmare. Childs Nerv Syst. 2008; 24(9): 1029–1032

[43] Husain M, Jha DK, Rastogi M, Husain N, Gupta RK. Role of neuroendoscopy in the management of patients with tuberculous meningitis hydrocephalus. Neurosurg Rev. 2005; 28(4):278–283

[44] Chugh A, Husain M, Gupta RK, Ojha BK, Chandra A, Rastogi M. Surgical outcome of tuberculous meningitis hydrocephalus treated by endoscopic third ventriculostomy: prognostic factors and postoperative neuroimaging for functional assessment of ventriculostomy. J Neurosurg Pediatr. 2009; 3(5):371–377

[45] Siomin V, Constantini S. Endoscopic third ventriculostomy in tuberculous meningitis. Childs Nerv Syst. 2003; 19(5–6): 269

[46] Figaji AA, Fieggen AG, Peter JC. Endoscopic third ventriculostomy in tuberculous meningitis. Childs Nerv Syst. 2003; 19(4):217–225

[47] Figaji AA, Fieggen AG. Endoscopic challenges and applications in tuberculous meningitis. World Neurosurg. 2013; 79 suppl 2:S24.e9–24.e14

[48] Bhagwati S, Mehta N, Shah S. Use of endoscopic third ventriculostomy in hydrocephalus of tubercular origin. Childs Nerv Syst. 2010; 26(12):1675–1682

[49] Bhagwati SN, George K. Use of intrathecal hyaluronidase in the management of tuberculous meningitis with hydrocephalus. Childs Nerv Syst. 1986; 2(1):20–25

[50] Kumar R, Prakash M, Jha S. Paradoxical response to chemotherapy in neurotuberculosis. Pediatr Neurosurg. 2006; 42(4):214–222

[51] Perez-Alvarez F, Serra C, Mayol L, Liarte A. Unusual central nervous system tuberculosis debut in children: stroke. Childs Nerv Syst. 2008; 24(5):539–540

[52] Poonnoose SI, Rajshekhar V. Rate of resolution of histologically verified intracranial tuberculomas. Neurosurgery. 2003; 53(4):873–878, discussion 878–879

[53] Schoeman J, Malan G, van Toorn R, Springer P, Parker F, Booysen J. Home-based treatment of childhood neurotuberculosis. J Trop Pediatr. 2009; 55(3):149–154

[54] Jain AK, Sreenivasan R, Mukunth R, Dhammi IK. Tubercular spondylitis in children. Indian J Orthop. 2014; 48(2): 136–144

[55] Hu J, Li D, Kang Y, et al. Active thoracic and lumbar spinal tuberculosis in children with kyphotic deformity treated by one-stage posterior instrumentation combined anterior debridement: preliminary study. Eur J Orthop Surg Traumatol. 2014; 24 suppl 1:S221–S229

[56] Varatharajah S, Charles YP, Buy X, Walter A, Steib JP. Update on the surgical management of Pott's disease. Orthop Traumatol Surg Res. 2014; 100(2):229–235

[57] Mathur M, Johnson CE, Sze G. Fungal infections of the central nervous system. Neuroimaging Clin N Am. 2012; 22 (4):609–632

[58] Riddell J, IV, Shuman EK. Epidemiology of central nervous system infection. Neuroimaging Clin N Am. 2012; 22(4): 543–556

[59] Deshpande DH, Desai AP, Dastur HM. Aspergillosis of the central nervous system. A clinical and mycopathological study of 9 cases. Neurol India. 1975; 23(4):167–175

[60] Sharma RR, Lad SD, Desai AP, Lynch PG. Surgical management of fungal infections of the nervous system. In: Schmidek HH, ed. Schmidek and Sweet Operative Neurosurgical Techniques: Indications, Methods and Results. 4 th ed. Philadelphia, PA: WB Saunders Company; 2000:1726–1755

[61] Cuccia V, Galarza M, Monges J. Cerebral aspergillosis in children. Report of three cases. Pediatr Neurosurg. 2000; 33(1):43–48

[62] Nadkarni TD, Desai KI, Muzumdar D, Goel A, Shenoy A. Ischaemic complications after surgical resection of intracranial aspergilloma. J Clin Neurosci. 2003; 10(4):500–502

[63] Nadkarni T, Goel A. Aspergilloma of the brain: an overview. J Postgrad Med. 2005; 51 suppl 1:S37–S41

[64] Rajshekhar V. Surgical management of intracranial fungal masses. Neurol India. 2007; 55(3):267–273

[65] Shamim MS, Siddiqui AA, Enam SA, Shah AA, Jooma R, Anwar S. Craniocerebral aspergillosis in immunocompetent hosts: surgical perspective. Neurol India. 2007; 55(3): 274–281

[66] Raman Sharma R. Fungal infections of the nervous system: current perspective and controversies in management. Int J Surg. 2010; 8(8):591–601

[67] Mehta VS, Bhatia R, Mohapatra LN, Banerji AK. Intracranial mycotic infection in non-immunosuppressed individuals. J Indian Med Assoc. 1985; 83(6):185–188

[68] Sethi PK, Khanna L, Batra A, et al. Central nervous system fungal infections: observations from a large tertiary hospital in northern India. Clin Neurol Neurosurg. 2012; 114(9): 1232–1237

[69] Agarwal R, Kalita J, Marak RS, Misra UK. Spectrum of fungal infection in a neurology tertiary care center in India. Neurol Sci. 2012; 33(6):1305–1310

[70] Sharma BS, Khosla VK, Kak VK, et al. Intracranial fungal granuloma. Surg Neurol. 1997; 47(5):489–497

[71] Gupta R, Singh AK, Bishnu P, Malhotra V. Intracranial Aspergillus granuloma simulating meningioma on MR imaging. J Comput Assist Tomogr. 1990; 14(3):467–469

[72] Enzmann DR, Brant-Zawadzki M, Britt RH. CT of central nervous system infections in immunocompromised patients. AJR Am J Roentgenol. 1980; 135(2):263–267

[73] Goodman ML, Coffey RJ. Stereotactic drainage of Aspergillus brain abscess with long-term survival: case report and review. Neurosurgery. 1989; 24(1):96–99

[74] Young RF, Gade G, Grinnell V. Surgical treatment for fungal infections in the central nervous system. J Neurosurg. 1985; 63(3):371–381

[75] Dubey A, Patwardhan RV, Sampth S, Santosh V, Kolluri S, Nanda A. Intracranial fungal granuloma: analysis of 40 patients and review of the literature. Surg Neurol. 2005; 63 (3):254–260, discussion 260

[76] Siddiqui AA, Shah AA, Bashir SH. Craniocerebral aspergillosis of sinonasal origin in immunocompetent patients: clinical spectrum and outcome in 25 cases. Neurosurgery. 2004; 55(3):602–611, discussion 611–613

[77] Jamjoom AB, al-Hedaithy SA, Jamjoom ZA, et al. Intracranial mycotic infections in neurosurgical practice. Acta Neurochir (Wien). 1995; 137(1–2):78–84

[78] Jinkins JR, Siqueira E, Al-Kawi MZ. Cranial manifestations of aspergillosis. Neuroradiology. 1987; 29(2):181–185

[79] Jiang PF, Yu HM, Zhou BL, et al. The role of an Ommaya reservoir in the management of children with cryptococcal meningitis. Clin Neurol Neurosurg. 2010; 112(2):157–159

[80] Patiroglu T, Unal E, Yikilmaz A, Koker MY, Ozturk MK. Atypical presentation of chronic granulomatous disease in an adolescent boy with frontal lobe located Aspergillus abscess mimicking intracranial tumor. Childs Nerv Syst. 2010; 26(2):149–154

[81] Vlaardingerbroek H, van der Flier M, Borgstein JA, Lequin MH, van der Sluis IM. Fatal Aspergillus rhinosinusitis during induction chemotherapy in a child with acute lymphoblastic leukemia. J Pediatr Hematol Oncol. 2009; 31(5):367–369

[82] Giacchino M, Chiapello N, Riva C, et al. Intracranial aspergillosis in children successfully treated with antifungal therapy and surgical intervention. Pediatr Infect Dis J. 2006; 25(4):379–381

[83] Liu JK, Schaefer SD, Moscatello AL, Couldwell WT. Neurosurgical implications of allergic fungal sinusitis. J Neurosurg. 2004; 100(5):883–890

[84] Panda NK, Balaji P, Chakrabarti A, Sharma SC, Reddy CE. Paranasal sinus aspergillosis: its categorization to develop a treatment protocol. Mycoses. 2004; 47(7):277–283

[85] Loeys BL, Van Coster RN, Defreyne LR, Leroy JG. Fungal intracranial aneurysm in a child with familial chronic mucocutaneous candidiasis. Eur J Pediatr. 1999; 158(8):650–652

[86] Hurst RW, Judkins A, Bolger W, Chu A, Loevner LA. Mycotic aneurysm and cerebral infarction resulting from fungal sinusitis: imaging and pathologic correlation. AJNR Am J Neuroradiol. 2001; 22(5):858–863

[87] Chan KH, Mann KS, Yue CP. Neurosurgical aspects of cerebral cryptococcosis. Neurosurgery. 1989; 25(1):44–47, discussion 47–48

[88] Escobar A. The pathology of neurocysticercosis. In: Palacios E, Rodriguez Carabajal I, Taveras J, eds. Cysticercosis of the Central Nervous System. Illinois: Charles C. Thomas; 1983:27–54

[89] Eddi C, Nari A, Amanfu W. Taenia solium cysticercosis/ taeniosis: potential linkage with FAO activities; FAO support possibilities. Acta Trop. 2003; 87(1):145–148

[90] Rajshekhar V. Surgical management of neurocysticercosis. Int J Surg. 2010; 8(2):100–104

[91] Rajshekhar V, Raghava MV, Prabhakaran V, Oommen A, Muliyil J. Active epilepsy as an index of burden of neurocysticercosis in Vellore district, India. Neurology. 2006; 67(12):2135–2139

[92] Singhi P, Ray M, Singhi S, Khandelwal N. Clinical spectrum of 500 children with neurocysticercosis and response to albendazole therapy. J Child Neurol. 2000; 15(4):207–213

[93] Del Brutto OH, Santibañez R, Noboa CA, Aguirre R, Díaz E, Alarcón TA. Epilepsy due to neurocysticercosis: analysis of 203 patients. Neurology. 1992; 42(2):389–392

[94] Singhi P, Singhi S. Neurocysticercosis in children. Indian J Pediatr. 2009; 76(5):537–545

[95] Garg RK, Nag D. Intramedullary spinal cysticercosis: response to albendazole: case reports and review of literature. Spinal Cord. 1998; 36(1):67–70

[96] Misra S, Verma R, Lekhra OP, Misra NK. CT observations in partial seizures. Neurol India. 1994; 42:24–27

[97] Singhi PD, Baranwal AK. Single small enhancing computed tomographic lesion in Indian children—I: evolution of current concepts. J Trop Pediatr. 2001; 47(4):204–207

[98] Colli BO, Martelli N, Assirati JA, Jr, Machado HR, de Vergueiro Forjaz S. Results of surgical treatment of neurocysticercosis in 69 cases. J Neurosurg. 1986; 65(3): 309–315

[99] Bergsneider M, Nieto JH. Endoscopic management of intraventricular cysticer-cosis. In: Singh G, Prabhakar S, eds. Taenia Solium Cysticercosis: from Basic to Clinical Sscience. Oxon, UK: CABI Publishing; 2002:399–410

[100] Apuzzo MLJ, Dobkin WR, Zee CS, Chan JC, Giannotta SL, Weiss MH. Surgical considerations in treatment of intraventricular cysticercosis. An analysis of 45 cases. J Neurosurg. 1984; 60(2):400–407

[101] Couldwell WT, Chandrasoma P, Apuzzo ML, Zee CS. Third ventricular cysticercal cyst mimicking a colloid cyst: case report. Neurosurgery. 1995; 37(6):1200–1203

[102] Bergsneider M. Endoscopic removal of cysticercal cysts within the fourth ventricle. Technical note. J Neurosurg. 1999; 91(2):340–345

[103] Bergsneider M, Holly LT, Lee JH, King WA, Frazee JG. Endoscopic management of cysticercal cysts within the lateral and third ventricles. Neurosurg Focus. 1999; 6(4):e7

[104] Madrazo I, García-Rentería JA, Sandoval M, López Vega FJ. Intraventricular cysticercosis. Neurosurgery. 1983; 12(2): 148–152

[105] Singla M, Singh P, Kaushal S, Bansal R, Singh G. Hippocampal sclerosis in association with neurocysticercosis. Epileptic Disord. 2007; 9(3):292–299

[106] Erşahin Y, Mutluer S, Güzelbağ E. Intracranial hydatid cysts in children. Neurosurgery. 1993; 33(2):219–224, discussion 224–225

[107] Gupta S, Desai K, Goel A. Intracranial hydatid cyst: a report of five cases and review of literature. Neurol India. 1999; 47 (3):214–217

[108] Khaldi M, Mohamed S, Kallel J, Khouja N. Brain hydatidosis: report on 117 cases. Childs Nerv Syst. 2000; 16(10–11): 765–769

[109] Joseph BV, Haran RP, Chandy MJ. Surgery for multiple intracranial hydatid cysts. Neurol India. 2003; 51(2):295–296

[110] Onal C, Erguvan-Onal R, Yakinci C, Karayol A, Atambay M, Daldal N. Can the requirement of a diversion procedure be predicted after an uncomplicated intracranial hydatid cyst surgery? Pediatr Neurosurg. 2006; 42(6):383–386

[111] Ciurea AV, Fountas KN, Coman TC, et al. Long-term surgical outcome in patients with intracranial hydatid cyst. Acta Neurochir (Wien). 2006; 148(4):421–426

[112] Izci Y, Tüzün Y, Seçer HI, Gönül E. Cerebral hydatid cysts: technique and pitfalls of surgical management. Neurosurg Focus. 2008; 24(6):E15

[113] Dagtekin A, Koseoglu A, Kara E, et al. Unusual location of hydatid cysts in pediatric patients. Pediatr Neurosurg. 2009; 45(5):379–383

[114] Turgut M. Intracranial extradural hydatid cysts: review of the literature. Acta Neurochir (Wien). 2010; 152(10):1805–1806

[115] Altas M, Serarslan Y, Davran R, Evirgen O, Aras M, Yilmaz N. The Dowling-Orlando technique in a giant primary cerebral hydatid cyst: a case report. Neurol Neurochir Pol. 2010; 44 (3):304–307

[116] Duishanbai S, Jiafu D, Guo H, et al. Intracranial hydatid cyst in children: report of 30 cases. Childs Nerv Syst. 2010; 26 (6):821–827

[117] Mohindra S, Savardekar A, Gupta R, Tripathi M, Rane S. Varied types of intracranial hydatid cysts: radiological features and management techniques. Acta Neurochir (Wien). 2012; 154(1):165–172

481

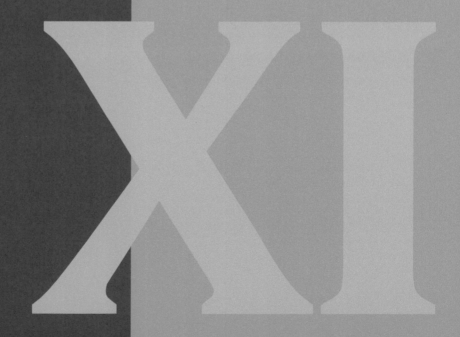

Section XI

Operating Room Basics

56 Neuronavigation in Pediatric Neurosurgery

Ulrich-Wilhelm N. Thomale

56.1 Introduction

Among other recent advances in Pediatric neurosurgery, neuronavigation is one of the relevant ones. This technique has made surgical procedures shorter with smaller approaches, more effective and thus safer. Although for neuronavigation, only a very few prospective randomized trials were performed to proof its efficacy, this technique became routine use in all neurosurgical fields over the past decades. In the development of its broad application, boundaries of surgical indications have partially been crossed by navigation techniques since the precise planning and execution of surgery especially of deep seated became better accessible. In the following chapter, we would like to define different techniques of neuronavigation and go through the wide range of indications as used in pediatric neurosurgery.

56.2 Terminology

56.2.1 Definition

Navigation is the process of determining, establishing, and maintaining a course or trajectory to a target location.[1]

Neuronavigation is technically a neurosurgical computer-assisted guiding system in which an anatomical image dataset is registered in its spatial orientation to the related patients' anatomy using virtual coordinates defined in an invisible reference system.

56.2.2 Related Terminology

Computer-assisted surgery is a broader definition for surgical planning and performance systems, in which computer data processing is used to assist specific steps before or within the surgical procedure. Neuronavigation is one possible computer-assisted technique.

In **frameless stereotaxy**, unlike frame-based stereotaxy, where the mechanical frame is used as coordinate system fixed toward the patients' head and visualized in an image dataset, the frame is replaced by a virtual coordinate system defined by an optical (camera) or magnetic (electromagnetic source) reference system.

Image guidance defines any surgical procedure guided by imaging or image data, which may also include intraoperative imaging techniques (ultrasound, computed tomography [CT], magnetic resonance imaging [MRI]) besides navigation.

56.3 Technique

56.3.1 Systems

Optical Navigation

A camera is used to register any spatial orientation of two to three markers defining the geometry of a reference frame,[2,3,4,5,6] which is rigidly attached to the fixed patient positioning system (e.g., pin clamp) and instruments in order to localize their spatial relation to the patients' anatomy in correlation to the image dataset (mean system accuracy: 0.22 mm).[7] In infants with open fontanelles in which rigid pin fixation is not possible, indirect fixation of the patient to the table as well as reference frame attachment to the table can overcome this problem (▶ Fig. 56.1a). As an alternative, the reference frame may directly be attached to the bone structures overcoming the need for head fixation or pinless fixation systems are used.[8,9,10] Children with closed fontanelle until the age of, for example, 10 years should be fixated with a four-pin pediatric clamp system (▶ Fig. 56.1b). Free line of sight from the camera toward the surgical site including the reference frame and all navigated instruments are warranted during surgery (▶ Fig. 56.2).

Active Reference Marker System

Markers are giving active infrared signals toward the camera system to detect their spatial localization. Electric supply is needed with batteries or cables integrated or attached to the reference frame or instruments.

Passive Reference System

Infrared signals are emitted by the camera reflected by passive markers attached to the reference frame or instruments to detect their spatial position. No cable or batteries are needed.

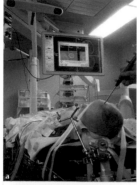
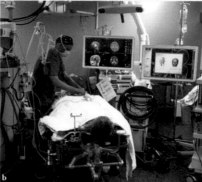
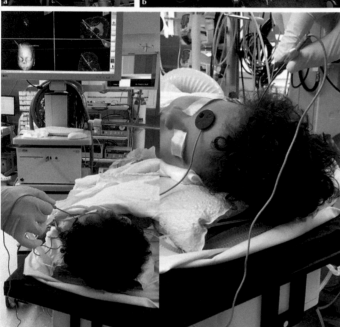
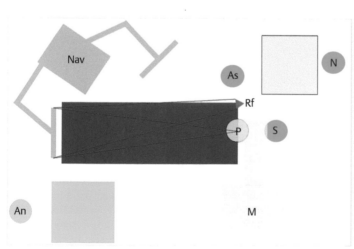

Fig. 56.1 Age- and system-dependent positioning. **(a)** Infant positioning for optical navigation system on a vacuum mattress secured with tape toward the table. Reference frame is attached to the table. **(b)** Child positioning for optical navigation (closed fontanelle with age up to 10 years) four-pin fixation clamp with the reference frame attached to the clamp. **(c)** Positioning for electromagnetic navigation without head fixation attaching the reference localizer to the forehead (electromagnetic source: box on left).

Fig. 56.2 Schematic arrangement of the OR components during microscopic navigation using an optical system. An, anesthetist; As, assistance; M, microscope; N, nurse; Nav, optical navigation system; P, patient; Rf, reference frame; S, surgeon.

56.3.2 Electromagnetic Navigation

An electromagnetic source is building a magnetic field in which active magnetic sensors either rigidly attached to the patient may localize the registered anatomy (reference localizer) or integrated within navigated instruments which can be spatially detected and visualized in the image dataset in relation to the patient's anatomy (mean system precision: 0.99–2.24 mm).[7,11] The system is easier to handle during surgery since no rigid fixation of the head is needed (advantageous for infants, ▶ Fig. 56.1c).[12,13,14,15] Line of sight is not an issue during surgery, however, any magnetic material within the positioning table or surgical instruments brought into the electromagnetic field may negatively influence the system-related accuracy.

56.3.3 Workflow

- Image data acquisition.
- Virtual planning: definition of regions of interests, targets and trajectories, definition of landmarks and registration points.
- Registration of the image data in correlation to the related patient's anatomy.
- Tracking and navigation of the surgical procedure.

Imaging

Volume dataset of CT (thin-sliced sections, may be reconstructed from spiral CT scan), MRI contrast enhanced, (MP-Rage, 3D-FFE, T1 sequence with high anatomical resolution), may be fused to thin sliced T2 sequences which can be reconstructed along virtual planes and along any defined trajectories.

Registration

Marker Registration

May be performed with visible markers attached to the patients' anatomy and defined within the image dataset (skin—fiducials, bone—screw markers) or by anatomical landmarks which are clearly identified on the patient's anatomy and within the images (e.g., nasion, epicanthus, lateral orbital rim, tragus, etc.). Fiducial skin marker ($n \geq 6$) registration reveals a mean precision of 1 to 1.9 mm.[16,17] Screw marker registration was described to be more precise than skin fiducials

(1.35 vs. 1.85 mm),[18] however, with the necessity of further intervention for its placement.

Surface Registration

Surface registration is achieved with multiple point acquisition along the most characteristic anatomical structures (facial mask) and widest possible regions which is then correlated to the 3D surface reconstruction of the volume dataset. This is nowadays routinely used and may be acquired with a laser scanner (mean precision: 1.8–3 mm)[16,17] or an active touch-sensitive pointer, which is advantageous for including haired skin regions in the registration in parietal and occipital approaches.

Tracking and Navigation

Patient position and attachment of any reference localizer (optical or electromagnetical) must be carefully planned to establish good registration quality and to avoid interference during surgery and navigation. Intraoperative tracking and navigation includes pointer-based techniques to identify the preplanned entry point on the patient's anatomy and trajectory toward the respective target. Registered surgical instruments may be included in the navigation process such as catheter stylets,[13,19,20] forceps,[21,22,23] or endoscopes[8,24,25,26,27] tracked with their geometric information and tip position.

Microscope integration into navigation includes tracking of the focus level and viewing direction visualized in the image dataset of the navigation.[28,29] Augmented reality may be integrated by contour guidance displaying any targets or regions of interest in the microscopic field of view. This has the advantage that navigation can be performed parallel to microsurgical intervention without interruption by pointer integration.

56.3.4 Multimodal Image Integration in Navigation

Functional imaging, metabolic imaging, and angiography might be integrated in the visualization of the image dataset and fused to high-resolution image data guiding surgical-related information. Avoiding morbidity close to eloquent areas might better be avoided by visualizing them in the image data.[30,31,32] Integrating diffusion tensor imaging (DTI) tractography into the navigation has high value for surgical planning but must be interpreted carefully during surgery due to the brain shift and changes by tumor compression.[33] Angiography integration may help to localize feeder entry into a nidus of arteriovenous malformations (AVMs) or intraoperative visualization of aneurysm-related anatomy.[34,35,36] Metabolic imaging is relevant for targeted biopsies for metabolic active tumor parts and to correlate image information with histological evaluation (▶ Fig. 56.3).[37,38,39,40]

56.3.5 Intraoperative Imaging and Navigation

Intraoperative imaging together with navigation may be conducted together with preoperative imaging data and later updating the surgical modified anatomy. It may also be used for combining registration by using the intraoperative image dataset of the patient. That might be achieved when the image source is directly linked to the navigation system.

Ultrasound Navigation

Ultrasound navigation is an easy and cost-effective tool for gaining an image update with reasonable time effort. Navigation systems are available with direct integration of the ultrasound probe as navigated tool. Ultrasound image interpretation may require experience by the user which is more likely established in pediatric neurosurgery.[41,42,43,44,45]

Intraoperative MRI may be of relevance in pediatric brain tumor surgery in extensive mass lesions or low-grade tumor entities. The need for high investments and the time-consuming efforts does restrict its use in big medical centers and for selected cases. Updating the surgical-related spatial changes (brain shift) over time and identifying tumor remnants is possible with high image quality. Low-field MRI machines are more often integrated in the operating room (OR), while high-field 3Tesla machines are often used in a dual OR concepts for parallel diagnostic use during long surgeries.[46,47,48,49,50,51]

Intraoperative CT is less relevant for pediatric neurosurgery in order to avoid radiation exposure.[52,53,54,55] Spinal instrumentation, however, is a relevant indication in which 3D C-arm imaging combined with navigation may effectively be used for proper pedicle screw placement.[56]

56.4 Indications

56.4.1 Ventricular Catheter Placement

Guided placement of ventricular catheters has shown to be beneficial for more accurate placement

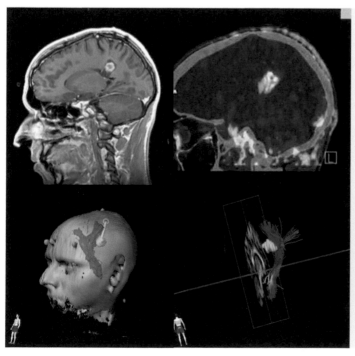

Fig. 56.3 Multimodal image integration in a postcentral paracallosal lesion with nodular FET–PET hotspot and visualization of the pyramidal tract anterior to the lesion, selecting a postcentral approach.

and longer survival of the functioning catheters.[13,57] Neuronavigation was introduced as an effective guiding tool. Indications were described for slit ventricle syndrome, narrow and displaced ventricles in shunt surgery, reservoirs for intrathecal chemotherapy, and external ventricular drains for traumatic brain injury. Frameless stereotactic systems,[19,58,59] electromagnetic navigation,[13,20,57,60,61] ultrasound-guided navigation,[41] and navigated endoscopic systems[62] are used. These introduce high technical and time-consuming efforts for a relative short surgical intervention, which are justified especially for applying accuracy in lifelong implants.

Recently, a simple navigation system based on guiding tool assisted by smartphone technology was introduced in order to reduce the time effort and to apply accuracy of ventricular placement in a high number of patients, which has significantly reduced incorrect catheter placement within a prospective randomized trial.[63,64]

56.4.2 Endoscopy

Combining neuronavigation together with endoscopy is reasonable and useful since endoscopy often uses small openings and the freedom of action is limited by this entry. Thus, the point of entry as well as the trajectories must be well defined in preoperative planning as well as intraoperative application by navigation. Brain shift during intraventricular surgery may be a relevant problem in navigated endoscopy necessitating constant verification of the endoscope's view and position depicted in the navigation system. This problem may be reduced by establishing continuous irrigation with balanced in and outflow to void collapse of the paraventricular structures. Navigated endoscopy is used for several indications.

Ventricular Endoscopy

For endoscopic third ventriculostomy (ETV), navigation has been discussed to be useful.[26,65] In enlarged ventricles, navigation may not be necessary and the entry point can accurately be measured in the sagittal image with a trajectory from the floor of the third ventricle through the foramen of Monro toward the skull surface in relation to the nasion and 2 cm lateral to the midline.[66] In narrow ventricles, navigation is reasonable to enter the lateral ventricle safely.[67,68,69]

Ventricular cysts are heterogeneous and fenestration toward regular cerebrospinal fluid (CSF)

spaces is most often the surgical aim. The entry point must be individually defined in each patient and the trajectory should enable free working space at the target of fenestration. Indications for arachnoid cysts of different locations,[70,71,72,73,74] for septum pellucidum cysts,[75,76] intraventricular cysts,[25] and Dandy–Walker–like malformations[77,78] are described.

Multiloculated hydrocephalus (MLHC) is a complex situation after ventriculitis during neonatal period. Anatomical distortion causing lack of anatomical landmarks and multiple compartments are presented often with active volume changes. Navigation is necessary to apply an individual and effective plan for surgical therapy in order to simplify the most often necessary shunt system with minimal amount of catheter placements.[24,79,80] Repeated navigated endoscopy procedures are often necessary in early active state of MLHC.

Isolated ventricles alone are the simpler form of MLHC and must be treated with fenestration foramen of Monro plasty,[81] septostomy, or stent placement especially in isolated forth ventricle[82,83] by navigated endoscopic guidance.

Ventricular tumors have also an individual appearance and are often initially diagnosed or treated by navigated endoscopy. Endoscopic resection is possible if they are small or well accessible.[84,85,86] Cystic tumor compartments might need fenestration or stent placement.[87,88]

Endoscopic biopsy is also relevant in pineal region tumors especially challenging when combined with ETV.[89] Single burr hole entry points may well be planned with navigated techniques.[90]

Skull Base Surgery

Endoscopy was introduced for accessing skull base lesions transnasally or transorally.[91,92,93] In smaller children, this techniques might be limited or be less standardized since pneumatization develops at later stage.[94,95] Navigation is especially helpful in approaching either very small lesions or extensive destructing lesions when the regular anatomy is destroyed either by endoscopic means ore microsurgical technique.[93,96,97,98,99,100,101] Additionally, X-ray exposure can be reduced while penetrating the skull base. Not only tumor surgery, but also CSF leaks due to trauma or malformations may well be treated.[102,103] The clivus and craniocervical junction may also be approached by navigated endoscopic-assisted techniques.[104,105,106]

Endoscopic Assistance for Intraparenchymal Lesions

Deep-seated intraparenchymal lesions may be approached with navigated endoscopic assistance directly or with the help of port devices.[86,107] Pineal region tumors were described to be approached transtentorially by navigated endoscopic assistance.[108] Similarly, hippocampal depth electrodes have been placed.[109]

56.4.3 Navigated Microsurgery

Since early times of neuronavigation, *cavernomas* were the classical indication for navigated microsurgical resection.[36,110,111,112,113,114] This was associated with a more comfortable and safer surgery in children.[115]

Most of the supratentorial located *tumors* in pediatric cohort are deep seated tumors in which neuronavigation is helpful. Hemispheric, intraventricular, thalamic, and hypothalamic tumors are approached by the help of neuronavigation on a routine basis in most countries.[116,117,118,119,120] By the means of neuronavigation, deep seated tumors can be precisely targeted and by using augmented reality contour overlays in the miscroscope, the extension of the tumor can better be estimated at different microscopic magnifications to aim for more extensive resection.[120] Especially, for intraventricular tumors, navigated placement of tubular retraction devices are developed.[121,122] In surgical resection of tumors close to eloquent areas, the combination of neuronavigation and brain mapping[123] or transcranial magnetic stimulation is used.[124] For infratentorial lesions, intrinsic cerebellar hemispheric tumors and often brainstem tumors are operated by guidance of neuronavigation.[125,126,127] This also holds true for extensive skull base[128] or orbitocranial tumors.[129,130]

Intraoperative imaging might further enhance the grade surgical resection by intraoperative imaging using ultrasound[42,44,131] or MRI[46,132,133,134] in extensive tumor lesions or deep-seated low-grade lesions with similar appearance characteristics like brain tissue.

56.4.4 Frameless Stereotaxy

For navigation, different frameless stereotactic systems are available which have the major advantage that preoperative imaging can be used saving significant time of anesthesia, and that no stereotactic frame needs to be attached to the children's head which represents difficulties in all younger children. However, the accuracy of frameless stereotactic systems are described to be lower.[135] Using these systems, lesions should exceed diameters of 10 to15 cm depending on their depth location.[21,135,136] Diagnostic yield and complication rates were described to be similar in frame-based compared to frameless techniques.[137,138] Indications are generally biopsies,[22,136,139,140] catheter placement, for example, for cyst aspiration or stent placements,[4,141,142] or the placement of depth electrodes for seizure monitoring as stereo EEG.[15]

56.4.5 Epilepsy Surgery

Neuronavigation is widely used in epilepsy surgery for different reasons.[143,144,145] Resection of epileptogenic hamartomas[85,146] is regularly navigated procedures similar to other heterotopic[147] or focal epileptogenic lesions.[148,149] The placement of intraoperative electrodes for seizure mapping being either grid electrodes or depth electrodes can accurately be placed by navigation.[15,150,151,152] The correlation of monitoring results by defining epileptogenic regions as targets can intraoperatively well identified by navigation.[28,153,154,155] Complex epilepsy surgeries such as insular surgery[156,157] hemispherotomies[158] and callosotomies[159] can additionally be guided by neuronavigation.

56.4.6 Spine

Spinal instrumentation in scoliosis surgery[160,161] or craniocervical junction reconstruction[105,162] was described to be guided by neuronavigational techniques alone and/or together with intraoperative imaging.[56,163] In addition, spinal tumors or neurenteric cysts were approached with navigated techniques.[54,164,165]

56.5 Common Clinical Questions

1. How do you practically gain maximal accuracy by fiducial marker or surface registration?
2. Is it obligatory to have an optical parallel to an electromagnetic navigation system?
3. What are the possible solutions for navigating suboccipital approaches in prone positioning?
4. What are the limitations of stenting the sylvian aqueduct in an isolated fourth ventricle?

56.6 Answers to Common Clinical Questions

1. For skin fiducial marker registration, the following essentials are necessary to acknowledge during registration. First, at least six fiducials must be placed. Second, the fiducials must be placed so that they can be reached by the pointer in the respective position. Third, the area of fiducial placement should be as wide as possible including tight skin areas over the forehead, temporal region, and the mastoid. For surface matching, active sensitive touch pointers might have the disadvantage to take longer for multiple surface point acquisition, but the great advantage over the laser pointer is that hairy skin and the entire face mask can be included in the registration. To combine landmark registration together with surface registration gives highest accuracy and best practicability.

2. Electromagnetic navigation system is an easy and fast usage system but includes most often the disadvantage that multimodal image datasets and individual instruments cannot as easily be included in the navigation procedure. That makes it a decent navigation system for simple tasks such as ventricular catheter placement. Those can also be established by optic navigation systems with only low amount of additional efforts. Optical navigation system should cover the entire range of indications needed in navigated neurosurgery.

3. For optical navigation systems, registration in prone positioning might be painful. However, it is well possible when the camera is positioned on the side of the patient focusing on the area in front of the face below the table. Surface registration can then be performed by touch pointer registration including landmarks, multiple points on the facial mask, and the wide range of hairy skin in parietal and occipital regions. After registration, the camera might be moved back at the foot of the table for free line of sight during surgery.

4. Stenting the sylvan aqueduct is generally indicated only in isolated fourth ventricle and in cases with short aqueductal stenosis. To avoid any injury to the midbrain while approaching the stent, the direction of the sylvian aqueduct defines the trajectory toward the skull surface which determines the entry point at relative close proximity to the midline (1.5–2 cm).

Under endoscopic vision and with great care to the deviating structures around the foramen of Monro, the catheter is then approached through the aqueduct into the fourth ventricle. In cases where the roof of the fourth ventricle is already deviated supratentorially, the catheter might be advanced through a double layer membrane at this location under navigated endoscopic guidance.

References

[1] Franz MO, Mallot HA. Biometic robot navigation. Robot Auton Syst. 2000; 30:133–153

[2] Tirakotai W, Riegel T, Sure U, Bozinov O, Hellwig D, Bertalanffy H. Clinical application of neuro-navigation in a series of single burr-hole procedures. Zentralbl Neurochir. 2004; 65(2):57–64

[3] Tuominen J, Yrjänä SK, Katisko JP, Heikkilä J, Koivukangas J. Intraoperative imaging in a comprehensive neuronavigation environment for minimally invasive brain tumour surgery. Acta Neurochir Suppl (Wien). 2003; 85:115–120

[4] Vitaz TW, Hushek SG, Shields CB, Moriarty TM. Interventional MRI-guided frameless stereotaxy in pediatric patients. Stereotact Funct Neurosurg. 2002; 79(3–4):182–190

[5] Vougioukas VI, Hubbe U, Hochmuth A, Gellrich NC, van Velthoven V. Perspectives and limitations of image-guided neurosurgery in pediatric patients. Childs Nerv Syst. 2003; 19(12):783–791

[6] Wagner W, Gaab MR, Schroeder HW, Sehl U, Tschiltschke W. Experiences with cranial neuronavigation in pediatric neurosurgery. Pediatr Neurosurg. 1999; 31(5):231–236

[7] Kral F, Puschban EJ, Riechelmann H, Freysinger W. Comparison of optical and electromagnetic tracking for navigated lateral skull base surgery. Int J Med Robot. 2013; 9 (2):247–252

[8] Mangano FT, Limbrick DD, Jr, Leonard JR, Park TS, Smyth MD. Simultaneous image-guided and endoscopic navigation without rigid cranial fixation: application in infants: technical case report. Neurosurgery. 2006; 58(4) suppl 2: ONS-E377; discussion E377

[9] Reavey-Cantwell JF, Bova FJ, Pincus DW. Frameless, pinless stereotactic neurosurgery in children. J Neurosurg. 2006; 104(6) suppl:392–395

[10] Sadda P, Azimi E, Jallo G, Doswell J, Kazanzides P. Surgical navigation with a head-mounted tracking system and display. Stud Health Technol Inform. 2013; 184:363–369

[11] Barszcz S, Roszkowski M, Daszkiewicz P, Jurkiewicz E, Maryniak A. Accuracy of intraoperative registration during electromagnetic neuronavigation in intracranial procedures performed in children. Neurol Neurochir Pol. 2007; 41(2): 122–127

[12] Choi KY, Seo BR, Kim JH, Kim SH, Kim TS, Lee JK. The usefulness of electromagnetic neuronavigation in the pediatric neuroendoscopic surgery. J Korean Neurosurg Soc. 2013; 53(3):161–166

[13] Hayhurst C, Beems T, Jenkinson MD, et al. Effect of electromagnetic-navigated shunt placement on failure rates: a prospective multicenter study. J Neurosurg. 2010; 113(6):1273–1278

[14] McMillen JL, Vonau M, Wood MJ. Pinless frameless electromagnetic image-guided neuroendoscopy in children. Childs Nerv Syst. 2010; 26(7):871–878

[15] Wray CD, Kraemer DL, Yang T, et al. Freehand placement of depth electrodes using electromagnetic frameless stereotactic guidance. J Neurosurg Pediatr. 2011; 8(5):464–467

[16] Schicho K, Figl M, Seemann R, et al. Comparison of laser surface scanning and fiducial marker-based registration in frameless stereotaxy. Technical note. J Neurosurg. 2007; 106 (4):704–709

[17] Schlaier J, Warnat J, Brawanski A. Registration accuracy and practicability of laser-directed surface matching. Comput Aided Surg. 2002; 7(5):284–290

[18] Thomp, son EM, Anderson GJ, Roberts CM, Hunt MA, Selden NR. Skull-fixated fiducial markers improve accuracy in staged frameless stereotactic epilepsy surgery in children. J Neurosurg Pediatr. 2011; 7(1):116–119

[19] Gil Z, Siomin V, Beni-Adani L, Sira B, Constantini S. Ventricular catheter placement in children with hydrocephalus and small ventricles: the use of a frameless neuronavigation system. Childs Nerv Syst. 2002; 18(1–2):26–29

[20] Hermann EJ, Capelle HH, Tschan CA, Krauss JK. Electromagnetic-guided neuronavigation for safe placement of intraventricular catheters in pediatric neurosurgery. J Neurosurg Pediatr. 2012; 10(4):327–333

[21] Gralla J, Nimsky C, Buchfelder M, Fahlbusch R, Ganslandt O. Frameless stereotactic brain biopsy procedures using the Stealth Station: indications, accuracy and results. Zentralbl Neurochir. 2003; 64(4):166–170

[22] Grunert P, Espinosa J, Busert C, et al. Stereotactic biopsies guided by an optical navigation system: technique and clinical experience. Minim Invasive Neurosurg. 2002; 45(1):11–15

[23] Owen CM, Linskey ME. Frame-based stereotaxy in a frameless era: current capabilities, relative role, and the positive- and negative predictive values of blood through the needle. J Neurooncol. 2009; 93(1):139–149

[24] Schulz M, Bohner G, Knaus H, Haberl H, Thomale UW. Navigated endoscopic surgery for multiloculated hydrocephalus in children. J Neurosurg Pediatr. 2010; 5(5):434–442

[25] Schroeder HW, Wagner W, Tschiltschke W, Gaab MR. Frameless neuronavigation in intracranial endoscopic neurosurgery. J Neurosurg. 2001; 94(1):72–79

[26] Rohde V, Behm T, Ludwig H, Wachter D. The role of neuronavigation in intracranial endoscopic procedures. Neurosurg Rev. 2012; 35(3):351–358

[27] Coelho G, Kondageski C, Vaz-Guimarães Filho F, et al. Frameless image-guided neuroendoscopy training in real simulators. Minim Invasive Neurosurg. 2011; 54(3):115–118

[28] Cho DY, Lee WY, Lee HC, Chen CC, Tso M. Application of neuronavigator coupled with an operative microscope and electrocorticography in epilepsy surgery. Surg Neurol. 2005; 64(5):411–417, discussion 417–418

[29] Ganslandt O, Behari S, Gralla J, Fahlbusch R, Nimsky C. Neuronavigation: concept, techniques and applications. Neurol India. 2002; 50(3):244–255

[30] Zhu FP, Wu JS, Song YY, et al. Clinical application of motor pathway mapping using diffusion tensor imaging tractography and intraoperative direct subcortical stimulation in cerebral glioma surgery: a prospective cohort study. Neurosurgery. 2012; 71(6):1170–1183, discussion 1183–1184

[31] Qiu TM, Zhang Y, Wu JS, et al. Virtual reality presurgical planning for cerebral gliomas adjacent to motor pathways in an integrated 3-D stereoscopic visualization of structural MRI and DTI tractography. Acta Neurochir (Wien). 2010; 152(11):1847–1857

[32] Roessler K, Donat M, Lanzenberger R, et al. Evaluation of preoperative high magnetic field motor functional MRI (3 Tesla) in glioma patients by navigated electrocortical stimulation and postoperative outcome. J Neurol Neurosurg Psychiatry. 2005; 76(8):1152–1157

[33] Kinoshita M, Yamada K, Hashimoto N, et al. Fiber-tracking does not accurately estimate size of fiber bundle in pathological condition: initial neurosurgical experience using neuronavigation and subcortical white matter stimulation. Neuroimage. 2005; 25(2):424–429

[34] Akdemir H, Oktem S, Menkü A, Tucer B, Tuğcu B, Günaldi O. Image-guided microneurosurgical management of small arteriovenous malformation: role of neuronavigation and intraoperative Doppler sonography. Minim Invasive Neurosurg. 2007; 50(3):163–169

[35] Coenen VA, Dammert S, Reinges MH, Mull M, Gilsbach JM, Rohde V. Image-guided microneurosurgical management of small cerebral arteriovenous malformations: the value of navigated computed tomographic angiography. Neuroradiology. 2005; 47(1):66–72

[36] Rohde V, Spangenberg P, Mayfrank L, Reinges M, Gilsbach JM, Coenen VA. Advanced neuronavigation in skull base tumors and vascular lesions. Minim Invasive Neurosurg. 2005; 48(1):13–18

[37] Pirotte B, Goldman S, Van Bogaert P, et al. Integration of [11C] methionine-positron emission tomographic and magnetic resonance imaging for image-guided surgical resection of infiltrative low-grade brain tumors in children. Neurosurgery. 2005; 57 suppl 1:128–139, discussion 128–139

[38] Pirotte B, Goldman S, Massager N, et al. Combined use of 18F-fluorodeoxyglucose and 11C-methionine in 45 positron emission tomography-guided stereotactic brain biopsies. J Neurosurg. 2004; 101(3):476–483

[39] Messing-Jünger AM, Floeth FW, Pauleit D, et al. Multimodal target point assessment for stereotactic biopsy in children with diffuse bithalamic astrocytomas. Childs Nerv Syst. 2002; 18(8):445–449

[40] Floeth FW, Pauleit D, Wittsack HJ, et al. Multimodal metabolic imaging of cerebral gliomas: positron emission tomography with [18F]fluoroethyl-L-tyrosine and magnetic resonance spectroscopy. J Neurosurg. 2005; 102(2):318–327

[41] Heussinger N, Eyüpoglu IY, Ganslandt O, Finzel S, Trollmann R, Jüngert J. Ultrasound-guided neuronavigation improves safety of ventricular catheter insertion in preterm infants. Brain Dev. 2013; 35(10):905–911

[42] Roth J, Biyani N, Beni-Adani L, Constantini S. Real-time neuronavigation with high-quality 3D ultrasound SonoWand in pediatric neurosurgery. Pediatr Neurosurg. 2007; 43(3):185–191

[43] Rygh OM, Cappelen J, Selbekk T, Lindseth F, Hernes TA, Unsgaard G. Endoscopy guided by an intraoperative 3D ultrasound-based neuronavigation system. Minim Invasive Neurosurg. 2006; 49(1):1–9

[44] Ulrich NH, Burkhardt JK, Serra C, Bernays RL, Bozinov O. Resection of pediatric intracerebral tumors with the aid of intraoperative real-time 3-D ultrasound. Childs Nerv Syst. 2012; 28(1):101–109

[45] Woydt M, Krone A, Soerensen N, Roosen K. Ultrasound-guided neuronavigation of deep-seated cavernous haemangiomas: clinical results and navigation techniques. Br J Neurosurg. 2001; 15(6):485–495

[46] Vitaz TW, Hushek S, Shields CB, Moriarty T. Intraoperative MRI for pediatric tumor management. Acta Neurochir Suppl (Wien). 2003; 85:73–78

[47] Samdani A, Jallo GI. Intraoperative MRI: technology, systems, and application to pediatric brain tumors. Surg Technol Int. 2007; 16:236–243

[48] Kremer P, Tronnier V, Steiner HH, et al. Intraoperative MRI for interventional neurosurgical procedures and tumor resection control in children. Childs Nerv Syst. 2006; 22(7): 674–678

[49] Kaya S, Deniz S, Duz B, Daneyemez M, Gonul E. Use of an ultra-low field intraoperative MRI system for pediatric brain tumor cases: initial experience with 'PoleStar N20'. Turk Neurosurg. 2012; 22(2):218–225

[50] Jankovski A, Francotte F, Vaz G, et al. Intraoperative magnetic resonance imaging at 3-T using a dual independent operating room-magnetic resonance imaging suite: development, feasibility, safety, and preliminary experience. Neurosurgery. 2008; 63(3):412–424, discussion 424–426

[51] Avula S, Mallucci CL, Pizer B, Garlick D, Crooks D, Abernethy LJ. Intraoperative 3-Tesla MRI in the management of paediatric cranial tumours–initial experience. Pediatr Radiol. 2012; 42(2):158–167

[52] Acosta FL, Jr, Quinones-Hinojosa A, Gadkary CA, et al. Frameless stereotactic image-guided C1-C2 transarticular screw fixation for atlantoaxial instability: review of 20 patients. J Spinal Disord Tech. 2005; 18(5):385–391

[53] Ersahin M, Karaaslan N, Gurbuz MS, et al. The safety and diagnostic value of frame-based and CT-guided stereotactic brain biopsy technique. Turk Neurosurg. 2011; 21(4):582–590

[54] Rajasekaran S, Kamath V, Shetty AP. Intraoperative Iso-C three-dimensional navigation in excision of spinal osteoid osteomas. Spine. 2008; 33(1):E25–E29

[55] Reig AS, Stevenson CB, Tulipan NB. CT-based, fiducial-free frameless stereotaxy for difficult ventriculoperitoneal shunt insertion: experience in 26 consecutive patients. Stereotact Funct Neurosurg. 2010; 88(2):75–80

[56] Hott JS, Papadopoulos SM, Theodore N, Dickman CA, Sonntag VK. Intraoperative Iso-C C-arm navigation in cervical spinal surgery: review of the first 52 cases. Spine. 2004; 29(24):2856–2860

[57] Levitt MR, O'Neill BR, Ishak GE, et al. Image-guided cerebrospinal fluid shunting in children: catheter accuracy and shunt survival. J Neurosurg Pediatr. 2012; 10(2):112–117

[58] Azeem SS, Origitano TC. Ventricular catheter placement with a frameless neuronavigational system: a 1-year experience. Neurosurgery. 2007; 60(4) suppl 2:243–247, discussion 247–248

[59] Stieglitz LH, Giordano M, Samii M, Luedemann WO. A new tool for frameless stereotactic placement of ventricular catheters. Neurosurgery. 2010; 67(3) suppl operative: ons131–ons135, discussion ons135

[60] Aufdenblatten CA, Altermatt S. Intraventricular catheter placement by electromagnetic navigation safely applied in a paediatric major head injury patient. Childs Nerv Syst. 2008; 24(9):1047–1050

[61] Clark S, Sangra M, Hayhurst C, et al. The use of noninvasive electromagnetic neuronavigation for slit ventricle syndrome and complex hydrocephalus in a pediatric population. J Neurosurg Pediatr. 2008; 2(6):430–434

[62] Turner MS, Nguyen HS, Payner TD, Cohen-Gadol AA. A novel method for stereotactic, endoscope-assisted transtentorial placement of a shunt catheter into symptomatic posterior fossa cysts. J Neurosurg Pediatr. 2011; 8(1):15–21

[63] Thomale UW, Knitter T, Schaumann A, et al. Smartphone-assisted guide for the placement of ventricular catheters. Childs Nerv Syst. 2013; 29(1):131–139

[64] Thomale UW, Schaumann A, Stockhammer F, et al. GAVCA study: randomized, multicenter trial to evaluate the quality of ventricular catheter placement with a mobile health assisted guidance technique. Neurosurgery 2017 (e-pub ahead of print). doi:10.1093/neuros/nyx420

[65] Broggi G, Dones I, Ferroli P, Franzini A, Servello D, Duca S. Image guided neuroendoscopy for third ventriculostomy. Acta Neurochir (Wien). 2000; 142(8):893–898, discussion 898–899

[66] Knaus H, Abbushi A, Hoffmann KT, Schwarz K, Haberl H, Thomale UW. Measurements of burr-hole localization for endoscopic procedures in the third ventricle in children. Childs Nerv Syst. 2009; 25(3):293–299

[67] Di Rocco C, Cinalli G, Massimi L, Spennato P, Cianciulli E, Tamburrini G. Endoscopic third ventriculostomy in the treatment of hydrocephalus in pediatric patients. Adv Tech Stand Neurosurg. 2006; 31:119–219

[68] Erşahin Y, Arslan D. Complications of endoscopic third ventriculostomy. Childs Nerv Syst. 2008; 24(8):943–948

[69] Naftel RP, Tubbs RS, Reed GT, Wellons JC, III. Small ventricular access prior to rigid neuroendoscopy. J Neurosurg Pediatr. 2010; 6(4):325–328

[70] Di Rocco F, Yoshino M, Oi S. Neuroendoscopic transventricular ventriculocystostomy in treatment for intracranial cysts. J Neurosurg. 2005; 103 suppl 1:54–60

[71] Greenfield JP, Souweidane MM. Endoscopic management of intracranial cysts. Neurosurg Focus. 2005; 19(6):E7

[72] Karabatsou K, Hayhurst C, Buxton N, O'Brien DF, Mallucci CL. Endoscopic management of arachnoid cysts: an advancing technique. J Neurosurg. 2007; 106 suppl 6:455–462

[73] Spacca B, Kandasamy J, Mallucci CL, Genitori L. Endoscopic treatment of middle fossa arachnoid cysts: a series of 40 patients treated endoscopically in two centres. Childs Nerv Syst. 2010; 26(2):163–172

[74] Van Beijnum J, Hanlo PW, Han KS, Ludo Van der Pol W, Verdaasdonk RM, Van Nieuwenhuizen O. Navigated laser-assisted endoscopic fenestration of a suprasellar arachnoid cyst in a 2-year-old child with bobble-head doll syndrome. Case report. J Neurosurg. 2006; 104 suppl 5:348–351

[75] Meng H, Feng H, Le F, Lu JY. Neuroendoscopic management of symptomatic septum pellucidum cysts. Neurosurgery. 2006; 59(2):278–283, discussion 278–283

[76] Borha A, Ponte KF, Emery E. Cavum septum pellucidum cyst in children: a case-based update. Childs Nerv Syst. 2012; 28 (6):813–819

[77] Weinzierl MR, Coenen VA, Korinth MC, Gilsbach JM, Rohde V. Endoscopic transtentorial ventriculocystostomy and cystoventriculoperitoneal shunt in a neonate with Dandy-Walker malformation and associated aqueductal obstruction. Pediatr Neurosurg. 2005; 41(5):272–277

[78] Sikorski CW, Curry DJ. Endoscopic, single-catheter treatment of Dandy-Walker syndrome hydrocephalus: technical case report and review of treatment options. Pediatr Neurosurg. 2005; 41(5):264–268

[79] Paraskevopoulos D, Biyani N, Constantini S, Beni-Adani L. Combined intraoperative magnetic resonance imaging and navigated neuroendoscopy in children with multicompartmental hydrocephalus and complex cysts: a feasibility study. J Neurosurg Pediatr. 2011; 8(3):279–288

[80] Tabakow P, Czyz M, Jarmundowicz W, Zub W. Neuroendoscopy combined with intraoperative low-field magnetic imaging for treatment of multiloculated

hydrocephalus in a 7-month-old infant: technical case report. Minim Invasive Neurosurg. 2011; 54(3):138–141

[81] Oi S, Enchev Y. Neuroendoscopic foraminal plasty of foramen of Monro. Childs Nerv Syst. 2008; 24(8):933–942

[82] Hamada H, Hayashi N, Kurimoto M, Endo S. Endoscopic aqueductal stenting via the fourth ventricle under navigating system guidance: technical note. Neurosurgery. 2005; 56 suppl 1:E206–, discussion E206

[83] Schulz M, Goelz L, Spors B, Haberl H, Thomale UW. Endoscopic treatment of isolated fourth ventricle: clinical and radiological outcome. Neurosurgery. 2012; 70(4):847–858, discussion 858–859

[84] Hopf NJ, Grunert P, Darabi K, Busert C, Bettag M. Frameless neuronavigation applied to endoscopic neurosurgery. Minim Invasive Neurosurg. 1999; 42(4):187–193

[85] Ng YT, Rekate HL, Prenger EC, et al. Endoscopic resection of hypothalamic hamartomas for refractory symptomatic epilepsy. Neurology. 2008; 70(17):1543–1548

[86] Di X. Multiple brain tumor nodule resections under direct visualization of a neuronavigated endoscope. Minim Invasive Neurosurg. 2007; 50(4):227–232

[87] Tirakotai W, Hellwig D, Bertalanffy H, Riegel T. The role of neuroendoscopy in the management of solid or solid-cystic intra- and periventricular tumours. Childs Nerv Syst. 2007; 23(6):653–658

[88] Pettorini BL, Tamburrini G, Massimi L, Caldarelli M, Di Rocco C. Endoscopic transventricular positioning of intracystic catheter for treatment of craniopharyngioma. Technical note. J Neurosurg Pediatr. 2009; 4(3):245–248

[89] Souweidane MM, Krieger MD, Weiner HL, Finlay JL. Surgical management of primary central nervous system germ cell tumors: proceedings from the Second International Symposium on Central Nervous System Germ Cell Tumors. J Neurosurg Pediatr. 2010; 6(2):125–130

[90] Knaus H, Matthias S, Koch A, Thomale UW. Single burr hole endoscopic biopsy with third ventriculostomy-measurements and computer-assisted planning. Childs Nerv Syst. 2011; 27(8):1233–1241

[91] Al-Mefty O, Kadri PA, Hasan DM, Isolan GR, Pravdenkova S. Anterior clivectomy: surgical technique and clinical applications. J Neurosurg. 2008; 109(5):783–793

[92] Di Rocco F, Oi S, Samii A, et al. Neuronavigational endoscopic endonasal sellar and parasellar surgery using a 2-mm-diameter lens rigid-rod endoscope: a cadaver study. Neurosurgery. 2007; 60(4) suppl 2:394–400, discussion 400

[93] Kaptain GJ, Vincent DA, Sheehan JP, Laws ER, Jr. Transsphenoidal approaches for the extracapsular resection of midline suprasellar and anterior cranial base lesions. Neurosurgery. 2001; 49(1):94–100, discussion 100–101

[94] van Lindert EJ, Ingels K, Mylanus E, Grotenhuis JA. Variations of endonasal anatomy: relevance for the endoscopic endonasal transsphenoidal approach. Acta Neurochir (Wien). 2010; 152(6):1015–1020

[95] Tsioulos K, Del Pero MM, Philpott C. Pneumatisation of turbinates and paranasal sinuses in children: case report. J Laryngol Otol. 2013; 127(4):419–422

[96] Alotaibi N, Hanss J, Benoudiba F, Bobin S, Racy E. Endoscopic removal of large orbito-ethmoidal osteoma in pediatric patient: Case report. Int J Surg Case Rep. 2013; 4(12):1067–1070

[97] Jagannathan J, Prevedello DM, Ayer VS, Dumont AS, Jane JA, Jr, Laws ER. Computer-assisted frameless stereotaxy in transsphenoidal surgery at a single institution: review of 176 cases. Neurosurg Focus. 2006; 20(2):E9

[98] Jo KW, Shin HJ, Nam DH, et al. Efficacy of endoport-guided endoscopic resection for deep-seated brain lesions. Neurosurg Rev. 2011; 34(4):457–463

[99] Joshi SM, Hewitt RJ, Storr HL, et al. Cushing's disease in children and adolescents: 20 years of experience in a single neurosurgical center. Neurosurgery. 2005; 57(2):281–285, discussion 281–285

[100] Fei Z, Zhang X, Jiang XF, Liu WP, Wang XL, Xie L. Removal of large benign cephalonasal tumours by transbasal surgery combined with endonasal endoscopic sinus surgery and neuronavigation. J Craniomaxillofac Surg. 2007; 35(1):30–34

[101] Kanaan IN. Minimally invasive approach to management of pituitary adenomas. Minim Invasive Neurosurg. 2005; 48 (3):169–174

[102] Ibrahim AA, Magdy EA, Eid M. Endoscopic endonasal multilayer repair of traumatic ethmoidal roof cerebrospinal fluid rhinorrhea in children. Int J Pediatr Otorhinolaryngol. 2012; 76(4):523–529

[103] Qiao L, Xue T, Zha DJ, et al. Determining leak locations during transnasal endoscopic repair of cerebrospinal fluid rhinorrhea. Auris Nasus Larynx. 2011; 38(3):335–339

[104] Dasenbrock HH, Clarke MJ, Bydon A, et al. Endoscopic image-guided transcervical odontoidectomy: outcomes of 15 patients with basilar invagination. Neurosurgery. 2012; 70(2):351–359, discussion 359–360

[105] Visocchi M, Doglietto F, Della Pepa GM, et al. Endoscope-assisted microsurgical transoral approach to the anterior craniovertebral junction compressive pathologies. Eur Spine J. 2011; 20(9):1518–1525

[106] Visocchi M, Della Pepa GM, Doglietto F, Esposito G, La Rocca G, Massimi L. Video-assisted microsurgical transoral approach to the craniovertebral junction: personal experience in childhood. Childs Nerv Syst. 2011; 27(5):825–831

[107] Almenawer SA, Crevier L, Murty N, Kassam A, Reddy K. Minimal access to deep intracranial lesions using a serial dilatation technique: case-series and review of brain tubular retractor systems. Neurosurg Rev. 2013; 36(2):321–329, discussion 329–330

[108] Shirane R, Kumabe T, Yoshida Y, et al. Surgical treatment of posterior fossa tumors via the occipital transtentorial approach: evaluation of operative safety and results in 14 patients with anterosuperior cerebellar tumors. J Neurosurg. 2001; 94(6):927–935

[109] Bahuleyan B, Omodon M, Robinson S, Cohen AR. Frameless stereotactic endoscope-assisted transoccipital hippocampal depth electrode placement: cadaveric demonstration of a new approach. Childs Nerv Syst. 2011; 27(8):1317–1320

[110] Conrad M, Schonauer C, Morel Ch, Pelissou-Guyotat I, Deruty R. Computer-assisted resection of supra-tentorial cavernous malformation. Minim Invasive Neurosurg. 2002; 45(2):87–90

[111] Enchev YP, Popov RV, Romansky KV, Marinov MB, Bussarsky VA. Neuronavigated surgery of intracranial cavernomas—enthusiasm for high technologies or a gold standard? Folia Med (Plovdiv). 2008; 50(2):11–17

[112] Gralla J, Ganslandt O, Kober H, Buchfelder M, Fahlbusch R, Nimsky C. Image-guided removal of supratentorial cavernomas in critical brain areas: application of neuronavigation and intraoperative magnetic resonance imaging. Minim Invasive Neurosurg. 2003; 46(2):72–77

[113] Winkler D, Lindner D, Trantakis C, et al. Cavernous malformations—navigational supported surgery. Minim Invasive Neurosurg. 2004; 47(1):24–28

[114] Wurm G, Fellner FA. Implementation of T2*-weighted MR for multimodal image guidance in cerebral cavernomas. Neuroimage. 2004; 22(2):841–846

[115] Winkler D, Lindner D, Strauss G, Richter A, Schober R, Meixensberger J. Surgery of cavernous malformations with and without navigational support—a comparative study. Minim Invasive Neurosurg. 2006; 49(1):15–19

[116] Baroncini M, Vinchon M, Minéo JF, Pichon F, Francke JP, Dhellemmes P. Surgical resection of thalamic tumors in children: approaches and clinical results. Childs Nerv Syst. 2007; 23(7):753–760

[117] Esposito V, Paolini S, Morace R, et al. Intraoperative localization of subcortical brain lesions. Acta Neurochir (Wien). 2008; 150(6):537–542, discussion 543

[118] Fronda C, Miller D, Kappus C, Bertalanffy H, Sure U. The benefit of image guidance for the contralateral interhemispheric approach to the lateral ventricle. Clin Neurol Neurosurg. 2008; 110(6):580–586

[119] Ren H, Chen X, Sun G, et al. Resection of subependymal giant cell astrocytoma guided by intraoperative magnetic resonance imaging and neuronavigation. Childs Nerv Syst. 2013;29(7):1113–1121

[120] Spalice A, Ruggieri M, Grosso S, et al. Dysembryoplastic neuroepithelial tumors: a prospective clinicopathologic and outcome study of 13 children. Pediatr Neurol. 2010; 43(6): 395–402

[121] Recinos PF, Raza SM, Jallo GI, Recinos VR. Use of a minimally invasive tubular retraction system for deep-seated tumors in pediatric patients. J Neurosurg Pediatr. 2011; 7(5):516–521

[122] Jo KI, Chung SB, Jo KW, Kong DS, Seol HJ, Shin HJ. Microsurgical resection of deep-seated lesions using transparent tubular retractor: pediatric case series. Childs Nerv Syst. 2011; 27(11):1989–1994

[123] Gupta N, Berger MS. Brain mapping for hemispheric tumors in children. Pediatr Neurosurg. 2003; 38(6):302–306

[124] Coburger J, Musahl C, Henkes H, et al. Comparison of navigated transcranial magnetic stimulation and functional magnetic resonance imaging for preoperative mapping in rolandic tumor surgery. Neurosurg Rev. 2013; 36(1):65–75, discussion 75–76

[125] Lunsford LD, Khan AA, Niranjan A, Kano H, Flickinger JC, Kondziolka D. Stereotactic radiosurgery for symptomatic solitary cerebral cavernous malformations considered high risk for resection. J Neurosurg. 2010; 113(1):23–29

[126] Ng WH, Mukhida K, Rutka JT. Image guidance and neuromonitoring in neurosurgery. Childs Nerv Syst. 2010; 26(4):491–502

[127] Pirotte BJ, Lubansu A, Massager N, et al. Clinical impact of integrating positron emission tomography during surgery in 85 children with brain tumors. J Neurosurg Pediatr. 2010; 5(5):486–499

[128] Venkataramana NK, Anantheswar YN. Pediatric anterior skull base tumors: our experience and review of literature. J Pediatr Neurosci. 2010; 5(1):1–11

[129] Gao D, Fei Z, Jiang X, et al. The microsurgical treatment of cranio-orbital tumors assisted by intraoperative electrophysiologic monitoring and neuronavigation. Clin Neurol Neurosurg. 2012; 114(7):891–896

[130] Siomin V, Spektor S, Beni-Adani L, Constantini S. Application of the orbito-cranial approach in pediatric neurosurgery. Childs Nerv Syst. 2001; 17(10):612–617

[131] Kanno H, Ozawa Y, Sakata K, et al. Intraoperative power Doppler ultrasonography with a contrast-enhancing agent for intracranial tumors. J Neurosurg. 2005; 102(2): 295–301

[132] Levy R, Cox RG, Hader WJ, Myles T, Sutherland GR, Hamilton MG. Application of intraoperative high-field magnetic resonance imaging in pediatric neurosurgery. J Neurosurg Pediatr. 2009; 4(5):467–474

[133] Nimsky C, Ganslandt O, Gralla J, Buchfelder M, Fahlbusch R. Intraoperative low-field magnetic resonance imaging in pediatric neurosurgery. Pediatr Neurosurg. 2003; 38(2):83–89

[134] Yousaf J, Avula S, Abernethy LJ, Mallucci CL. Importance of intraoperative magnetic resonance imaging for pediatric brain tumor surgery. Surg Neurol Int. 2012; 3 suppl 2:S65–S72

[135] Giese H, Hoffmann KT, Winkelmann A, Stockhammer F, Jallo GI, Thomale UW. Precision of navigated stereotactic probe implantation into the brainstem. J Neurosurg Pediatr. 2010; 5(4):350–359

[136] Winkler D, Lindner D, Richter A, Meixensberger J, Schober J. The value of intraoperative smear examination of stereotaxic brain specimens. Minim Invasive Neurosurg. 2006; 49(6):353–356

[137] Lobão CA, Nogueira J, Souto AA, Oliveira JA. Cerebral biopsy: comparison between frame-based stereotaxy and neuronavigation in an oncology center. Arq Neuropsiquiatr. 2009; 67 3B:876–881

[138] Woodworth GF, McGirt MJ, Samdani A, Garonzik I, Olivi A, Weingart JD. Frameless image-guided stereotactic brain biopsy procedure: diagnostic yield, surgical morbidity, and comparison with the frame-based technique. J Neurosurg. 2006; 104(2):233–237

[139] McGirt MJ, Woodworth GF, Coon AL, et al. Independent predictors of morbidity after image-guided stereotactic brain biopsy: a risk assessment of 270 cases. J Neurosurg. 2005; 102(5):897–901

[140] Winkler D, Trantakis C, Lindner D, Richter A, Schober J, Meixensberger J. Improving planning procedure in brain biopsy: coupling frame-based stereotaxy with navigational device STP 4.0. Minim Invasive Neurosurg. 2003; 46(1):37–40

[141] Cavalheiro S, Di Rocco C, Valenzuela S, et al. Craniopharyngiomas: intratumoral chemotherapy with interferon-alpha: a multicenter preliminary study with 60 cases. Neurosurg Focus. 2010; 28(4):E12

[142] Woodworth GF, McGirt MJ, Elfert P, Sciubba DM, Rigamonti D. Frameless stereotactic ventricular shunt placement for idiopathic intracranial hypertension. Stereotact Funct Neurosurg. 2005; 83(1):12–16

[143] Nimsky C, Buchfelder M. Neuronavigation in epilepsy surgery. Arq Neuropsiquiatr. 2003; 61 suppl 1:109–114

[144] Oertel J, Gaab MR, Runge U, Schroeder HW, Wagner W, Piek J. Neuronavigation and complication rate in epilepsy surgery. Neurosurg Rev. 2004; 27(3):214–217

[145] Polkey CE. Clinical outcome of epilepsy surgery. Curr Opin Neurol. 2004; 17(2):173–178

[146] Polkey CE. Resective surgery for hypothalamic hamartoma. Epileptic Disord. 2003; 5(4):281–286

[147] Stefan H, Nimsky C, Scheler G, et al. Periventricular nodular heterotopia: a challenge for epilepsy surgery. Seizure. 2007; 16(1):81–86

[148] Centeno RS, Yacubian EM, Sakamoto AC, Ferraz AF, Junior HC, Cavalheiro S. Pre-surgical evaluation and surgical treatment in children with extratemporal epilepsy. Childs Nerv Syst. 2006; 22(8):945–959

[149] Wurm G, Ringler H, Knogler F, Schnizer M. Evaluation of neuronavigation in lesional and non-lesional epilepsy surgery. Comput Aided Surg. 2003; 8(4):204–214

[150] Stone SS, Rutka JT. Utility of neuronavigation and neuromonitoring in epilepsy surgery. Neurosurg Focus. 2008; 25(3):E17

[151] Surbeck W, Bouthillier A, Weil AG, et al. The combination of subdural and depth electrodes for intracranial EEG investigation of suspected insular (perisylvian) epilepsy. Epilepsia. 2011; 52(3):458–466

[152] Van Gompel JJ, Meyer FB, Marsh WR, Lee KH, Worrell GA. Stereotactic electroencephalography with temporal grid and mesial temporal depth electrode coverage: does technique of depth electrode placement affect outcome? J Neurosurg. 2010; 113(1):32–38

[153] Benifla M, Sala F, Jr, Jane J, et al. Neurosurgical management of intractable rolandic epilepsy in children: role of resection in eloquent cortex. Clinical article. J Neurosurg Pediatr. 2009; 4(3):199–216

[154] Tovar-Spinoza ZS, Ochi A, Rutka JT, Go C, Otsubo H. The role of magnetoencephalography in epilepsy surgery. Neurosurg Focus. 2008; 25(3):E16

[155] Ochi A, Otsubo H. Magnetoencephalography-guided epilepsy surgery for children with intractable focal epilepsy: SickKids experience. Int J Psychophysiol. 2008; 68(2):104–110

[156] Park YS, Lee YH, Shim KW, et al. Insular epilepsy surgery under neuronavigation guidance using depth electrode. Childs Nerv Syst. 2009; 25(5):591–597

[157] von Lehe M, Wellmer J, Urbach H, Schramm J, Elger CE, Clusmann H. Epilepsy surgery for insular lesions. Rev Neurol (Paris). 2009; 165(10):755–761

[158] Chandra PS, Padma VM, Shailesh G, Chandreshekar B, Sarkar C, Tripathi M. Hemispherotomy for intractable epilepsy. Neurol India. 2008; 56(2):127–132

[159] Jea A, Vachhrajani S, Johnson KK, Rutka JT. Corpus callosotomy in children with intractable epilepsy using frameless stereotactic neuronavigation: 12-year experience at the Hospital for Sick Children in Toronto. Neurosurg Focus. 2008; 25(3):E7

[160] Modi H, Suh SW, Song HR, Yang JH. Accuracy of thoracic pedicle screw placement in scoliosis using the ideal pedicle entry point during the freehand technique. Int Orthop. 2009; 33(2):469–475

[161] Modi HN, Suh SW, Fernandez H, Yang JH, Song HR. Accuracy and safety of pedicle screw placement in neuromuscular scoliosis with free-hand technique. Eur Spine J. 2008; 17 (12):1686–1696

[162] Kosnik-Infinger L, Glazier SS, Frankel BM. Occipital condyle to cervical spine fixation in the pediatric population. J Neurosurg Pediatr. 2014;13(1):45–53

[163] Hott JS, Deshmukh VR, Klopfenstein JD, et al. Intraoperative Iso-C C-arm navigation in craniospinal surgery: the first 60 cases. Neurosurgery. 2004; 54(5):1131–1136, discussion 1136–1137

[164] Rajasekaran S, Kanna RM, Kamath V, Shetty AP. Computer navigation-guided excision of cervical osteoblastoma. Eur Spine J. 2010; 19(6):1046–1047

[165] Takahashi S, Morikawa S, Saruhashi Y, Matsusue Y, Kawakami M. Percutaneous transthoracic fenestration of an intramedullary neurenteric cyst in the thoracic spine with intraoperative magnetic resonance image navigation and thoracoscopy. J Neurosurg Spine. 2008; 9(5):488–492

Appendices

Appendix A.1 Peripheral nerve examination scoring tables

Score	BMRC nerve grading[1]		American nerve grading[3]	Modified highest classification[4]	LSUMC grading[2]		
	Motor	Sensory (autonomous)			Motor	Sensory	Whole nerve
0	No contraction	No sensation	No contraction	No recovery	None	None	None
1	Perceivable contraction proximal	Deep cutaneous pain	Perceivable contraction proximal	Recovery of deep pain + superficial pain	Trace contraction	Hyperparesthesias, deep pain recovery	Proximal M1–M2, sensation S0–S1
2	Perceivable contraction proximal and distal	Some cutaneous pain and tactile sensibility	Proximal muscles antigravity, distal muscles without perceivable contraction	Recovery of superficial pain and some touch sensibility + overresponse	Movement against gravity only	Sensory response sufficient for grip or slow protection; sensory stimuli mislocalized with overresponse	Proximal M3, sensation usually S3
3	All important muscle groups contract against resistance	S2, without dysesthesias + 2-point discrimination	Proximal muscles antigravity, distal muscles with perceivable contraction	Disappearance of overresponse, >15 mm s2pd >7 mm m2pd +7–15 mm s2pd 4–7 m2pd	Movement against mild resistance	Response to touch and pinprick; sensation mislocalized and some overresponse	Proximal M4; distal M3, Sensory usually S3
4	All synergistic and independent movements perceivable	Complete recovery	All important muscle groups contract against resistance	Complete recovery +2–6 mm s2pd 2–3 mm m2pd	Movement against moderate resistance	Response to touch and pinprick; response localize but sensation not normal, no overresponse	All proximal and some distal muscles M4. Sensory is S3 or better
5	Complete return of function	N/A	All synergistic and independent movements perceivable	N/A	Movement against maximal resistance	Sensation near normal to touch and pinprick	All muscles at least M4, sensory at least S4
6	N/A	N/A	Complete return of function	N/A	N/A	N/A	N/A

Abbreviations: m2pd, moving 2-point discrimination; s2pd, static 2-point discrimination.

Appendix A.2 Peripheral nerve examination pearls

Nerve	Motor distribution	Sensory distribution	How to distinguish from corresponding root pathology	Sign
Musculocutaneous (C5–7)	Biceps, coracobrachialis and brachialis	Radial forearm	C5 has deltoid weakness, C6 has sensory deficit in 1st 2 digits	Atrophy of biceps, brachialis, and coracobrachialis
Suprascapular (C5, 6)	Supra- and infraspinatus	Glenohumeral proprioception	C5 has biceps, deltoid, and cutaneous sensory	Infraspinatus atrophy, +/– deep shoulder pain
Axillary (C5, 6)	Deltoid + teres minor	Lateral upper arm	C5 has biceps and supraspinatus involved	Shoulder abduction <30 degrees
Dorsal scapular (C5)	Rhomboids	N/A	See above	Rhomboid atrophy, lateral movement of inferior scapula
Upper subscapular (C5, 6)	Subscapularis	N/A	See above	Weak internal rotation of humerus
Lower subscapular (C5–7)	Subscapularis, teres major	N/A	See above	Weak internal rotation of humerus
Long thoracic (C5–7)	Serratus anterior	N/A	See above	Winged scapula
Thoracodorsal (C6–8)	Latissimus dorsi	N/A	See above	Weak pull-up, asymmetric tone with cough *Good nerve transfer candidate
Median (C5–8, T1)	Forearm: flexors except FCU and lateral FDP Hand: LOAF muscles	First 3½ digits and thenar eminence	C6 has biceps and brachioradialis and supinator, no hand intrinsics	Thenar wasting Hand of benediction
AIN	Flexor pollicis longus, flexor profundus to 1st and 2nd digit	N/A	See above	Poor "OK sign"
Ulnar (C8, T1)	FCU, ulnar FDP, interossei, 3rd and 4th lumbricals, digiti minimi, adductor pollicis, FPB	Palmar ½ 4th and 5th digit	C8 all of 4th digit sensation, all hand intrinsics are weakened (including median nerve APB, OP)	Ulnar clawing
Radial (C5–8)	Finger, wrist, and arm extensors	Posterior cutaneous and dorsal hand	C7 has pectoralis, pronator, and median nerve flexion muscles	Wrist drop
PIN	Finger, wrist extensors	N/A	See above	Weak finger extension
Femoral (L2–4)	Knee extensors	Anterior thigh + saphenous	L3 also innervates leg adductors, knee jerk likely preserved	Weak leg extension, "knee buckling," saphenous symptoms rare
Obturator (L2–4)	Thigh adductors, internal rotators	Medial thigh	L3 would involve knee extensors	Hip eversion, adductor weakness +/– medial thigh numbness

Appendix A.2 (Continued)

Nerve	Motor distribution	Sensory distribution	How to distinguish from corresponding root pathology	Sign
Sciatic (L4–S3)	Hip flexors + tibial + peroneal	Posterior thigh, + tibial and peroneal	L4 has cutaneous distribution to anterior thigh, only dorsiflexion weakness	Foot drop, weak knee flexion, plantar flexion
Peroneal	Short biceps, peroneus longus, brevis and dorsiflexors/extensors	Lateral leg, dorsal foot	L5 has proximal sensory/motor distribution L5 effects ankle inversion	Foot drop Tinel's sign
Tibial (L4–S3)	Knee flexors—short biceps, foot and toe flexors	Medial leg, plantar foot	S1 has proximal sensory/motor distribution and peroneal innervations	Weak plantar flexion

Abbreviations: AIN, anterior interosseous nerve; APB, abductor pollicis brevis; FCU, flexor carpi ulnaris; FDP, flexor digitorum profundus; FPB, flexor pollicis brevis; LOAF, OP, opponens pollicis; PIN, posterior interosseus nerve.

*Most often associated with median/AIN, then radial, then ulnar,[5] overall 10 to 20% of the time associated with neural injury[6] and most common fracture around the elbow in children.[6]

Appendix A.3 Fracture Association

Fracture/dislocation	Fracture/injury type	Nerve injury	Mechanism/notes
Humerus	Proximal dislocation, humeral neck fracture[7]	Axillary, posterior cord and supra-scapular[8,9]	Humeral head forced down and posterior
	Humeral midshaft and distal one-third	Radial[9]	Most commonly injured peripheral nerve
	Supracondylar*	Ulnar	Flexion fracture
		Median/AIN[5,10,11]	Most commonly injured nerve with fracture type
		Radial nerve[10,11]	Posterior displaced fragment
Ulna	Monteggia's fracture	PIN[12]	PIN most commonly injured with anterior ulnar angulation and anterior radial head dislocation
	Midshaft	Radial[12]	Distal forearm fractures most common fracture type in pediatrics[15]
Radius	Galeazzi's fracture	Ulnar and AIN[14]	
	Distal physeal and metaphyseal fractures	Median and ulnar possible	Displaced fragments or compartment syndrome
Pelvis	Posterior ring	Sciatic	Near greater sciatic notch
	Anterior	Femoral	Rare (0.16%)[16]
Femur	Hip dislocation	Sciatic[17]	5% of posterior dislocations in children[17] Peroneal nerve component more easily injured[2,17]
	Femoral neck fracture	Sciatic	GSW and iatrogenic more common[18]
	Midshaft	Femoral (rare)[15]	Sciatic protected by adductor magnus
Fibula/knee	Dislocation	Peroneal	Most commonly injured nerve in the lower extremity
	Surgical neck fracture	Peroneal	
Tibia	Medial malleolus	Tibial	

Abbreviations: AIN, anterior interosseous nerve; GSW, gunshot wound; PIN, posterior interosseus nerve.
* Most often associated with median/AIN, then radial, then ulnar,[5] overall 10 to 20% of the time associated with neural injury[6] and most common fracture around the elbow in children.[6]

References

[1] Seddon HJ. Nerves Injuries Committee of the British Medical Research Council. In: Seddon HJ, ed. Peripheral nerve injuries. London: Her Majesty's Stationery Office, 1954. MRC Special Report Series, no. 282:10–11

[2] Kline DG, Hudson AR. Nerve injuries. Operative Results for Major Nerve Injuries, Entrapments and Tumors. Philadelphia, PA: W.B. Saunders Company; 1995

[3] Woodhall B, Beebe G, Eds. Peripheral Nerve Regeneration: A Follow Up Study of 3656 WWII Injuries. Washington, DC: VA Medical Monograph, US Government Printing Office; 1956

[4] Mackinnon SE, Dellon AL. Surgery of the Peripheral Nerve. New York, NY: Thieme Medical Publishers; 1988

[5] Dormans JP, Squillante R, Sharf H. Acute neurovascular complications with supracondylar humerus fractures in children. J Hand Surg Am. 1995; 20(1):1–4

[6] Hosalkar HS, Matzon JL, Chang B. Nerve palsies related to pediatric upper extremity fractures. Hand Clin. 2006; 22(1): 87–98

[7] Perlmutter GS, Apruzzese W. Axillary nerve injuries in contact sports: recommendations for treatment and rehabilitation. Sports Med. 1998; 26(5):351–361

[8] de Laat EA, Visser CP, Coene LN, Pahlplatz PV, Tavy DL. Nerve lesions in primary shoulder dislocations and humeral neck fractures. A prospective clinical and EMG study. J Bone Joint Surg Br. 1994; 76(3):381–383

[9] Pollock FH, Drake D, Bovill EG, Day L, Trafton PG. Treatment of radial neuropathy associated with fractures of the humerus. J Bone Joint Surg Am. 1981; 63(2):239–243

[10] McGraw JJ, Akbarnia BA, Hanel DP, Keppler L, Burdge RE. Neurological complications resulting from supracondylar fractures of the humerus in children. J Pediatr Orthop. 1986; 6(6):647–650

[11] Cramer KE, Green NE, Devito DP. Incidence of anterior interosseous nerve palsy in supracondylar humerus fractures in children. J Pediatr Orthop. 1993; 13(4):502–505

[12] Jessing P. Monteggia lesions and their complicating nerve damage. Acta Orthop Scand. 1975; 46(4):601–609

[13] Suganuma S, Tada K, Hayashi H, Segawa T, Tsuchiya H. Ulnar nerve palsy associated with closed midshaft forearm fractures. Orthopedics. 2012; 35(11):e1680–e1683

[14] Moore TM, Klein JP, Patzakis MJ, Harvey JP, Jr. Results of compression-plating of closed Galeazzi fractures. J Bone Joint Surg Am. 1985; 67(7):1015–1021

[15] Lyons RA, Delahunty AM, Kraus D, et al. Children's fractures: a population based study. Inj Prev. 1999; 5(2):129–132

[16] Noble J, Munro CA, Prasad VS, Midha R. Analysis of upper and lower extremity peripheral nerve injuries in a population of patients with multiple injuries. J Trauma. 1998; 45(1):116–122

[17] Cornwall R, Radomisli TE. Nerve injury in traumatic dislocation of the hip. Clin Orthop Relat Res. 2000(377):84–91

[18] Jiang D, Yu X, An H, Liang Y, Liang A. Hip and pelvic fractures and sciatic nerve injury. Chin J Traumatol. 2002; 5(6):333–337

Index

Note: Page numbers set **bold** or *italic* indicate headings or figures, respectively.

Index of Notation